*Cancer Surgery
for the General Surgeon*

Cancer Surgery for the General Surgeon

Editors

David P. Winchester, M.D.
Professor of Surgery
Northwestern University Medical School
Chicago, Illinois;
Chairman
Department of Surgery
Evanston Northwestern Healthcare
Evanston, Illinois

R. Scott Jones, M.D.
Professor and Chairman
Department of Surgery
University of Virginia
Charlottesville, Virginia

Gerald P. Murphy, M.D.
Director of Research
Pacific Northwest Cancer Foundation
Northwest Hospital
Seattle, Washington

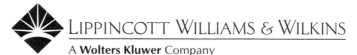

LIPPINCOTT WILLIAMS & WILKINS
A **Wolters Kluwer** Company
Philadelphia · Baltimore · New York · London
Buenos Aires · Hong Kong · Sydney · Tokyo

Manufacturing Manager: Kevin Watt
Production Manager: Robert Pancotti
Production Editor: Emily Harkavy
Cover Designer: Christine Jenny
Indexer: Kathrin Unger
Compositor: Circle Graphics
Printer: Maple Press

9 8 7 6 5 4 3 2 1

Library of Congress Cataloging-in-Publication Data

Cancer surgery for the general surgeon / editors, David P.
Winchester, R. Scott Jones, Gerald P. Murphy.
    p. cm.
    Includes bibliographical references and index.
    ISBN 0-397-58470-9 (alk. paper)
    1. Cancer—Surgery.   I. Winchester, David, 1937-   II. Jones, R.
Scott (Rayford Scott), 1936-   III. Murphy, Gerald Patrick.
    RD651 .C38 1998
    616.99′4059—dc21
                                 98-27799
                                   CIP

Contents

Contributing Authors

Nasser K. Altorki, M.D.
Professor of Cardiothoracic Surgery
Department of Cardiothoracic Surgery
The New York Hospital–Cornell Medical Center
525 East 68th Street
New York, New York 10021

Harry D. Bear, M.D., Ph.D.
Walter Lawrence, Jr., Distinguished Professor of
  Oncology
Professor and Chairman
Division of Surgical Oncology
Department of Surgery
Massey Cancer Center
Virginia Commonwealth University
1200 East Broad Street
Richmond, Virginia 23298

William E. Burak, Jr., M.D.
Assistant Professor
Department of Surgery
The Ohio State University
Arthur G. James Cancer Hospital and Research
  Institute
N914 Doan Hall
410 West 10th Avenue
Columbus, Ohio 43210

Bruce H. Campbell, M.D.
Associate Professor
Department of Otolaryngology
Medical College of Wisconsin
9200 West Wisconsin Avenue
Milwaukee, Wisconsin 53226-3522

Ara A. Chalian, M.D.
Assistant Professor
Director of Microvascular and Reconstructive
  Surgery
Department of Otorhinolaryngology: Head and
  Neck Surgery
University of Pennsylvania Health System
3400 Spruce Street
Philadelphia, Pennsylvania 19104

John M. Daly, M.D., F.A.C.S.
Lewis Atterbury Stimson Professor
Chairman, Department of Surgery
Surgeon-in-Chief
The New York Hospital–Cornell Medical Center
525 East 68th Street
New York, New York 10021

Wayne C. DeVos, M.D., Ph.D.
Assistant Professor of Surgery
Department of Surgery
Northwestern University Medical School
250 East Superior Street
Chicago, Illinois 60610

Jeffrey A. Drebin, M.D., Ph.D.
Assistant Professor of Surgery
Department of Surgery
Washington University School of Medicine
1 Barnes Hospital Plaza
St. Louis, Missouri 63110

Warren E. Enker, M.D.
Professor, Department of Surgery
Albert Einstein College of Medicine;
Vice Chairman and Chief, Colorectal Service
Beth Israel Medical Center
350 East 17th Street
New York, New York 10003

Thomas J. Fahey III, M.D.
Assistant Professor of Surgery
Chief, Section of Endocrine Surgery
Department of Surgery
The New York Hospital–Cornell Medical Center
525 East 68th Street
New York, New York 10021

William B. Farrar, M.D.
Associate Professor of Surgery
Department of Surgical Oncology
The Ohio State University
Arthur G. James Cancer Hospital and Research
  Institute
N924 Doan Hall
310 West 10th Avenue
Columbus, Ohio 43210

Yuman Fong, M.D.
Associate Attending Physician
Department of Surgery
Memorial Sloan-Kettering Cancer Center
1275 York Avenue
New York, New York 10021

Susan Galandiuk, M.D.
Associate Professor of Surgery
Department of Surgery
University of Louisville School of Medicine
550 South Jackson Street
Louisville, Kentucky 40292

Mark David Gendleman, M.D.
Assistant Clinical Professor
Department of Dermatology
Northwestern University Medical School
Chicago, Illinois 60611

Oreste D. Gentilini, M.D.
Department of Surgery
Istituto di Ricovero e Cura a Carattere
Scientifico
San Raffaele Hospital
Via Olgettina 60
Milano, 20132, Italy

Frederick L. Greene, M.D.
Clinical Professor of Surgery
Department of Surgery
University of North Carolina School of Medicine
Carolinas Medical Center
Charlotte, North Carolina 28232

Klaas Havenga, M.D., Ph.D.
Department of Surgery
Canisius-Wilhelmina Hospital
Weg Door Jonkerbos 100
6532 SZ Nijmegen
The Netherlands

Scott A. Hundahl, M.D., F.A.C.S.
Chief of Surgery
Department of Surgery
The Queen's Medical Center
1301 Punchbowl Street
Harkness 100
Honolulu, Hawaii 96813

Janardan D. Khandekar, M.D.
Professor of Medicine
Department of Medicine
Northwestern University;
Chairman, Department of Medicine
Evanston Northwestern Healthcare
2650 Ridge Avenue
Evanston, Illinois 60201

Robert J. Korst, M.D.
Clinical Assistant Surgeon
Department of Thoracic Services
Memorial Sloan-Kettering Cancer Center
1275 York Avenue
New York, New York 10021

Joseph Martz, M.D.
Resident
Department of Surgery
Beth Israel Medical Center
350 East 17th Street
New York, New York 10003

Jeffrey F. Moley, M.D.
Associate Professor
Department of Surgery
Washington University School of Medicine
660 South Euclid
St. Louis, Missouri 63110

Joseph P. Muldoon, M.D.
Assistant Professor
Department of Surgery
Northwestern University Medical School;
Chief, Colorectal Services
Evanston Northwestern Healthcare
2650 Ridge Avenue
Evanston, Illinois 60201

Jeffrey A. Norton, M.D.
Professor of Surgery
Department of Surgery
University of California, San Francisco;
Chief of Surgery
San Francisco Veterans Affairs Medical Center
4150 Clement Street
San Francisco, California 94121-1598

Edward E. Partridge, M.D.
Professor of Obstetrics and Gynecology
Department of Obstetrics and Gynecology
Division of Gynecologic Oncology
University of Alabama at Birmingham
618 South 20th Street
Birmingham, Alabama 35233-7333

John E. Phay, M.D.
Resident in General Surgery
Department of Surgery
Washington University School of Medicine
660 South Euclid
St. Louis, Missouri 63110

Peter W. T. Pisters, M.D.
Assistant Professor
Department of Surgical Oncology
University of Texas M.D. Anderson Cancer Center
1515 Holcombe Boulevard
Houston, Texas 77030

Raphael E. Pollock, M.D., Ph.D.
Head, Division of Surgery
Department of Surgical Oncology
University of Texas M.D. Anderson Cancer Center
1515 Holcombe Boulevard
Houston, Texas 77030

David S. Robinson, M.D.
Professor of Surgery
University of Missouri-Kansas City School of
  Medicine
308 Medical Plaza
4320 Wornall Road
Kansas City, Missouri 64111

Worthington G. Schenk III, M.D.
Associate Professor of Surgery
Department of Surgery
University of Virginia
Jefferson Park Avenue
Charlottesville, Virginia 22908

Nancy Schindler, M.D.
Resident in General Surgery
Northwestern University School of Medicine
250 East Superior Street
Chicago, Illinois 60201

Richard D. Schulick, M.D.
Chief Fellow, Surgical Oncology
Department of Surgery
Memorial Sloan-Kettering Cancer Center
1275 York Avenue
New York, New York 10021

Stephen F. Sener, M.D.
Professor of Surgery
Northwestern University Medical School;
Chief, Division of General Surgery
Evanston Northwestern Healthcare
2650 Ridge Avenue
Evanston, Illinois 60201

S. Eva Singletary, M.D.
Professor of Surgery
Chief, Surgical Breast Service
Department of Surgical Oncology
University of Texas M.D. Anderson Cancer Center
1515 Holcombe Boulevard
Houston, Texas 77030

Steven M. Strasberg, M.D., F.R.C.S., F.A.C.S.
Professor of Surgery
Department of Hepatobiliary Pancreatic Surgery
Barnes-Jewish Hospital
1 Barnes Hospital Plaza
St. Louis, Missouri 63110

Magesh Sundaram, M.D.
Assistant Professor of Surgery
Department of Surgery
University of Miami School of Medicine
1201 Northwest 16th Street
Miami, Florida 33125

Mark S. Talamonti, M.D.
Associate Professor
Department of General Surgery
Northwestern University Medical School
300 East Superior Street
Chicago, Illinois 60611-3010

Tianna Tsitsis, M.D.
Department of Internal Medicine
Evanston Northwestern Healthcare
2650 Ridge Avenue
Evanston, Illinois 60201

Thomas A. Victor, M.D., Ph.D.
Professor and Chairman, Department of
  Pathology
Northwestern University Medical School;
Chairman, Department of Pathology and
  Laboratory Medicine
Evanston Northwestern Healthcare
2650 Ridge Avenue
Evanston, Illinois 60201

Todd J. Waltrip, M.D.
Surgical Resident
Department of Surgery
University of Louisville School of Medicine
550 South Jackson Street
Louisville, Kentucky 40202

Randal S. Weber, M.D.
Gabriel Tucker Professor
Otorhinolaryngology: Head and Neck Surgery
University of Pennsylvania Health System
3400 Spruce Street
5th floor Ravdin Building
Philadelphia, Pennsylvania 19104

David J. Winchester, M.D.
Associate Professor of Surgery
Department of Surgery
Northwestern University Medical School;
Evanston Northwestern Healthcare
2650 Ridge Avenue
Evanston, Illinois 60201

Preface

The Society of Surgical Oncology promotes the continuing improved care of cancer patients by fostering research, education, and the dissemination of new knowledge. The Society accomplishes these objectives by sponsoring research fellowships, by sponsoring and setting the standards for clinical training programs for surgical oncology specialists, by sponsoring a journal for the dissemination of new knowledge, and by conducting an annual meeting that provides a forum for examination of new research and for extensive communication among scientists, surgical specialists, and surgeons devoted to the care of cancer patients. This textbook, *Cancer Surgery for the General Surgeon*, was developed in the spirit of the Society of Surgical Oncology to provide yet another instrument for enhancing cancer care by the dissemination of knowledge. Royalties of this book will go to the Society for Surgical Oncology to provide additional funds to support the mission of the Society and its important work.

This new book provides up-to-date practical and authoritative information on cancer surgery and cancer care for those general surgeons who are responsible for the management of patients with malignancies. The editors and authors of this volume obviously recognize the scientific biological basis for cancer care and the rate of important scientific discovery in this field. Nonetheless, they made a conscious choice for this book to concentrate on the cancer patient. The reader, therefore, will not find extensive discussions on the etiology and pathogenesis of cancer. The book is organized along a traditional organ system format and emphasizes those diseases traditionally treated by general surgeons. The authors, all of whom are recognized authorities in their fields, have responded with concise, easy-to-read, thoroughly up-to-date material about their topics.

By sponsoring this book, *Cancer Surgery for the General Surgeon*, the Society of Surgical Oncology recognizes an important issue in modern medical and surgical practice, particularly in surgical practice. That issue is the tension between generalism and specialism. Unquestionably, specialized centers and superspecialists will play ever-increasing roles in the provision of care and in the development of new knowledge. Without those specialists, new knowledge, improved treatments, and improved care would stagnate. It is also clear from recent publications that the outcomes and the morbidity and mortality for cancer operations, particularly cancer of the esophagus, cancer of the pancreas, and cancer of the colon, are better in the hands of those surgeons who have received special training in the field of cancer surgery or in the hands of those surgeons who do sufficient numbers of cancer surgery to maintain their expertise. However, it is also true that general surgeons will remain essential to provide the needed care to the increasing numbers of cancer victims in our nation. For the foreseeable future, general surgeons must be engaged in cancer care because of the sheer numbers of patients. Multidisciplinary cancer programs continue to flourish and to increase in effectiveness in small to mid-sized urban and community hospitals. Community general surgeons are becoming important resources in multidisciplinary cancer teams. In addition to supporting specialists and specialist centers, its leaders and our professional organizations, such as the Society of Surgical Oncology, should expend their energy and resources in making the general surgery workforce as effective as possible in fulfilling its role in providing the best care possible for our population.

This book is a visible commitment to that end. Drs. Winchester and Murphy deserve special recognition for their vision in developing this book, and they also deserve special recognition for the energy and effectiveness with which they pursued this timely production. It has been an educational and learning experience to have read this book. I sincerely believe that my colleagues in general surgery will share that opinion.

R. Scott Jones, M.D.

Introduction

The title of this book was thoughtfully chosen to reflect the continuing key role for the general surgeon in the evaluation and management of patients with cancer. The Society of Surgical Oncology, founded as the James Ewing Society in 1940, has evolved from a relatively small group of superspecialized oncologic general surgeons to a more diversified group of over 1,600 members. An analysis of the present membership profile redefines the field of surgical oncology. Our members now include the "traditional surgical oncologist," with 1 to 4 years of formal surgical oncology training after a general surgical residency, and the general surgeon who elected not to pursue formal postresidency surgical oncology training, but has self-selected into a general surgical practice with a majority interest in surgical oncology as evidenced by case mix, publications, oncologic teaching or research, involvement in American Cancer Society activities, involvement in the Commission on Cancer, American College of Surgeons, and a leadership role in hospital or community cancer activities. Other members include: general surgeons who have pursued additional training in basic science cancer research and those who have pursued fellowship training in colorectal surgery, breast cancer, or other specialized areas; and colleagues involved in various oncologic surgical subspecialties, including noncardiac thoracic, neurosurgery, gynecology, urology, and musculoskeletal areas. In addition, subspecialists in other disciplines, for example, surgical pathology, with a primary interest in cancer, have become members.

Thus, cancer patients are ably served by a large number of general surgeons and a much smaller number of surgical oncologists. The American Board of Surgery believes that cancer patients in this country will be best served by maintaining the integrity of general surgery, while recognizing that the maturing field of surgical oncology can enhance the oncologic knowledge base and skills of the general surgeon. The Board of Directors of the American Board of Surgery made this milestone decision in January 1998 by establishing an Advisory Council for Surgical Oncology. The issues to be considered by this newly conceived Advisory Council include but are not limited to: (a) training in oncologic surgery; (b) nominating consultants with surgical oncologic expertise to the qualifying examination and the recertification examination committees; and (c) establishing a relationship to other components of surgery and other specialties. The relationship between the American Board of Surgery and the Society of Surgical Oncology provides an opportunity for the general surgical and surgical oncology communities to work together in improving the care of the cancer patient. In the future, certification of the general surgeon by the American Board of Surgery will require a more rigorous and relevant oncology knowledge base.

All clinicians caring for cancer patients are coming under increased scrutiny by the public and payers of care for outcome. Complex procedures such as major liver resections, pancreatectomies, and extended resections for sarcoma may have outcomes related to the volume of cases performed. However, defining what the numbers should be is difficult, if not impossible, because of the variability of the primary disease, co-morbid conditions, the technical skill of the surgeon, and the quality of the ancillary services in the institution. Cancer care in these areas is evolving toward "superspecialists" who have made a career choice to do most or all of their work in a highly specific area. These individuals, located within the Society of Surgical Oncology, approved training programs and other large centers, and provide educational opportunities for the next generation of self-selecting superspecialists; but the general surgeon still must understand the fundamental principles associated with these complex diseases and procedures. The cancer practice profile of the general surgeon is not, and should not be, regulated or legislated. In the final analysis, a portion of the fellowship pledge of the American College of Surgeons defines the scope of one's practice: "I pledge myself to pursue the practice of surgery with scientific honesty and to place the welfare of my patients above all else; to advance constantly in knowledge; and to render willing help to my colleagues, regard their professional interest and seek their counsel when in doubt as to my own judgment."[1]

The Society of Surgical Oncology is proud to sponsor this book and to dedicate it to the enhanced knowledge of the general surgical community.

David P. Winchester
President, Society of Surgical Oncology, 1997–1998

---

[1] Stevenson GW. American College of Surgeons at 75. Chicago, American College of Surgeons, 1990:167.

Cancer Surgery
for the General Surgeon

CHAPTER 1

Cancer Susceptibility Genetics

John E. Phay and Jeffrey F. Moley

Malignant tumors are caused by alterations in normal cellular genes that result in transformation. Because some of these mutations can be inherited, there are a variety of syndromes that predispose individuals to develop certain types of cancer. In the beginning of this chapter, the nomenclature of these syndromes will be outlined, followed by a generalized approach to the patient with a possible inherited cancer syndrome. The remainder of the chapter will focus on the individual syndromes, grouped according to organ type.

Genetic mutations that are inherited from one's parents and are present in all cells of the body are **germ-line** or **constitutional** mutations. Non-germ-line mutations that are acquired during an individual's lifetime and cannot be passed on to one's children are **somatic** mutations. Radiation, chemicals, or other environmental factors are examples of carcinogens that cause these somatic mutations. When a tumor arises in an individual, it can be classified as either hereditary or sporadic. A **hereditary** case has as one of its genetic alterations, an inherited germ-line mutation. If the mutations are all somatic, then the tumor is classified as **sporadic**. The **index case**, or **proband**, is the individual who is first diagnosed as having the syndrome, even if earlier generations are later recognized as also having the syndrome. Rarely, a *de novo* case of a familial cancer arises when a spontaneous mutation occurs in a germ-line cell that has the capacity to be passed on to their offspring. The specific mutations responsible for hereditary and sporadic cancer often overlap. For example, familial adenomatous polyposis (FAP) is caused by a germ-line mutation in the adenomatous polyposis coli (APC) gene. More than 80% of sporadic colorectal cancers also have a somatic mutation of this same gene. Understanding inherited cancer genetics has provided insight into the mechanisms of all cancers.

Almost all inherited cancer syndromes are transmitted in an **autosomal dominant** manner to the next generation. Therefore, any individual who inherits one of these cancer susceptibility genes from either parent has a risk of developing the syndrome. Not all individuals will develop the disorder, because not all of these genes have complete penetrance. The **penetrance** of the gene is the likelihood that an individual will develop a phenotype from a specific genotype.

The penetrance can vary widely, ranging from close to 100%, such as for colon cancer in FAP, to below 50% for pheochromocytomas in neurofibromatosis. Penetrance can also vary considerably for different characteristics of the same syndrome. The factors determining penetrance remain largely unknown. A few exceptions to the autosomal dominant pattern of inheritance exist. Specifically, ataxia-telangiectasia (AT) and xeroderma pigmentosum are transmitted in an **autosomal recessive** manner. An individual must inherit a defective gene from each parent to develop these syndromes. Controversy surrounds the issue of whether a heterozygous individual has an increased risk for certain cancers.

Genes that lead to cancer are grouped into three categories: protooncogenes, tumor suppressor genes, or DNA mismatch repair genes. **Protooncogenes** are normal functioning genes found in all cells that become oncogenes when changed or amplified in a way that causes malignant transformation. **Oncogenes** produce an overexpressed or abnormally activated gene product. This protein typically has an important function in cellular proliferation or differentiation. Therefore, an abnormal *gain of function* of a protooncogene has occurred. Using a car as a metaphor of a cell, this activation has been compared to the accelerator being stuck in the depressed position. The RET protooncogene that is responsible for multiple endocrine neoplasia (MEN) 2A and 2B is an example of an inherited oncogene. Because these gene products must be functionally active, the mutations that cause them are usually restricted to a few sites in the gene.

Tumor suppressor genes normally produce proteins that regulate differentiation or programmed cell death, or inhibit cellular growth. During tumorigenesis these genes are altered, resulting in a *loss of function* of these gene products so that the cells are abnormally activated. In the car analogy, this would be similar to the loss of its brakes. Hereditary retinoblastoma is the prototypical familial cancer disorder caused by a tumor suppressor gene. Knudson's "two-hit" hypothesis is based on his observations of this disease. The "two-hit" hypothesis states that both copies of a tumor suppressor gene must be mutated or "hit" before a malignancy will develop. For familial cancer syndromes, one of these "hits" is inherited as a germ-

1

line mutation; therefore, these patients generally develop multifocal cancer at an earlier age. Most familial cancer syndromes are the result of a germ-line mutation in a tumor suppressor gene. Because these mutations make the gene product nonfunctional, mutations, deletions, or rearrangements may occur throughout the gene. This makes identification of a mutation in an individual or family more difficult.

The other class of genes that contributes to the development of cancer does so indirectly by improper maintenance of the cell's DNA. These genes encode proteins which act as caretakers of genome integrity. As every cell's DNA undergoes replication, there are a host of gene products that identify and correct mistakes made in the genetic code. When these gene products do not function properly, mutations are passed on and accumulate from cell to cell. When these mutations occur in protooncogenes and tumor suppressor genes, cells can undergo transformation to malignancy. Examples of such genes are MSH1 and MLH2, which are transmitted with germ-line mutations in hereditary nonpolyposis colorectal cancer (HNPCC) syndrome. These genes repair mismatches that occur in the cell's DNA. When they are not functioning, genome wide instability occurs, which results in mutations of other genes.

Familial cancer genes have been identified largely through the technique of positional cloning. **Positional cloning** locates genes through their position on a chromosome by linkage analysis, and not by their function or sequence. The genomes of individuals in a family with the syndrome are closely analyzed. The region of one of their chromosomes that is found to cosegregate with their phenotype is identified. This region is then gradually narrowed using a variety of techniques until the gene is located and verified by detecting mutations in the genes of affected individuals. Once the gene is identified, its function can be studied.

Another method which has been widely employed to identify tumor suppressor genes is through **loss of heterozygosity**. In order for a tumor suppressor gene to contribute to cancer, both copies of the gene must be altered. Typically, tumor cells lose large sections of chromosomes, which may be detectable in karyotypes (a gross visualization of all the chromosomes) as aneuploidy. Thus, one copy of the gene is deleted. The other copy is presumably mutated directly. When polymorphic markers are used to examine normal cellular DNA, there will often be heterozygosity due to the different alleles inherited from each parent. In a tumor cell, when a segment of a chromosome is lost, the tumor DNA will have loss of heterozygosity, or reduction to homozygosity, at that locus. Regions of chromosomes which have a high rate of loss of heterozygosity often contain a tumor suppressor gene.

BASIC PRINCIPLES WHEN EVALUATING A PATIENT WITH A SUSPECTED FAMILIAL CANCER SYNDROME

Several characteristics of familial cancer syndromes should be kept in mind when evaluating a patient with a possible inherited syndrome. Familial cancers tend to occur at an earlier

age than sporadic cases, because one of the mutations needed for neoplastic transformation is already present as a germ-line mutation. Several close relatives are usually affected by the cancer, especially different generations of a kindred. Inherited cancers often occur bilaterally in the same patient. Familial cancer syndromes are also not limited to a specific type of cancer, but can involve a variety of cancers. The Li-Fraumeni syndrome (LFS) can give rise to breast cancer, sarcomas, brain tumors, adrenocortical carcinomas, and others. If one finds any of these trends in a patient and their family, one should suspect a familial cancer syndrome.

A thorough family history should be taken on all patients with cancer. If an inherited cancer is suspected, then a family pedigree should be created (Fig. 1-1). Circles are drawn for all females and boxes for all males in rows by generation. All married couples are joined by a horizontal line. Their offspring are all connected to this line. Affected individuals are represented by a completely or partially filled circle or box often with the type of cancer and their age of diagnosis written next to them. All deceased individuals are represented by a diagonal slash through them. Once a pedigree is established, potential carriers of the gene can be identified and appropriate counseling and testing can be done.

The loss or addition of specific chromosomal material can provide important clues to the location of the gene responsible for a syndrome. A karyotype of the individual may be helpful in locating the defective gene. The initial clue that the APC gene resides on chromosome 5 was the karyotype of an institutionalized patient with polyposis, mental retardation, and congenital abnormalities, which revealed an interstitial deletion on the long arm of chromosome 5 (1).

GENETIC TESTING AND COUNSELING

Genetic testing should be considered when a patient presents with a suspected familial malignancy (Fig. 1-2). If a mutation is found, this patient will need close surveillance and possible prophylactic surgery. Testing and surveillance of the family and especially of the children of affected individuals should be recommended. In those found not to have inherited a mutation, the emotional stress and financial costs of surveillance can be eliminated. Conversely, a positive result will necessitate the need for lifelong testing and intervention; therefore, all outcomes must be thoroughly discussed beforehand.

The involvement of genetic counselors is an important complement to the nurses and surgeons who discuss therapeutic options with family members. In an evaluation of the use of the commercial APC gene test, over 30% of physicians misinterpreted the test results (2). Genetic counselors have an advanced degree in genetics, and are trained in the communication skills necessary for transmitting complicated information to family members. They are primarily involved in explaining test results and therapeutic options available in a nonbiased way. Patients consider them a valuable resource for obtaining information and understanding these complex issues. Proper pretesting counseling cannot be overemphasized.

Kindred 3

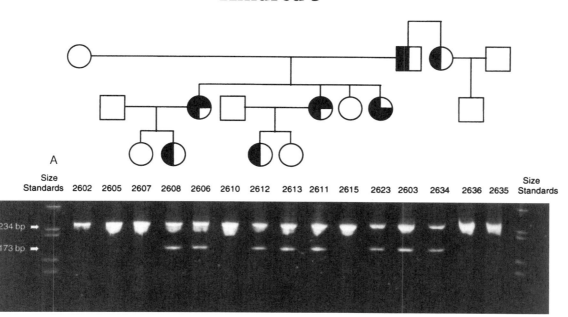

FIG. 1-1. **A:** Pedigree of kindred affected by MEN 2A. *Circles,* females; *squares,* males; *shaded left hemi-circle,* affected by medullary thyroid carcinoma; *shaded right upper quarter-circle,* hyperparathyroidism; *shaded right lower quarter-circle,* pheochromocytoma. **B:** Restriction digest patterns for the 15 family members shown in pedigree. The portion of the RET gene that is mutated in this family was amplified by polymerase chain reaction and then cut with a restriction enzyme which gives a different cleavage pattern for normal and mutant alleles. The normal allele contains one restriction site producing a fragment of 234 bp, whereas the mutant 234-bp fragment is cleaved into fragments of 173 and 61 bp (only the 173- and 234-bp fragments are resolved in the picture). bp, fragment size in base pairs; DNA size standard (1-Kb ladder). Two cleavage products (234-bp normal and 173-bp mutant) are resolved in the polyacrylamide gel shown. Seven individuals with clinical signs of MEN 2A (2608, 2606, 2612, 2611, 2623, 2603, 2634) demonstrate the mutant RET digestion pattern. One individual (2613) is a presymtomatic mutant RET gene carrier.The remaining seven individuals have inherited only the normal RET alleles. (From Chi DD, Toshima K, Donis-Keller H, Wells SA Jr. Predictive testing for multiple endocrine neoplasia type 2A (MEN 2A) based on the detection of mutations in the RET protooncogene. *Surgery* 1994; 116:128.)

SPECIFIC CANCER SYNDROMES

For all the cloned genes for familial cancer syndromes, see Table 1-1.

Patient or a relative with cancer

↓

Personal history of previous cancer
Family history of cancer
Multiple tumor types and/or associated abnormalities in the same patient or family members (see Table 1–1)
Multifocal or bilateral tumor
Early age at diagnosis

↓

Consider genetic testing (see Table 1–1) and referral to a genetic counselor or physician with genetic expertise (medical geneticist or surgical oncologist with genetic training)

FIG. 1-2. Algorithm for genetic testing for familial cancer.

Breast Cancer

Breast cancer is one of the most common cancers treated by the general surgeon. For over 100 years, it has been recognized that certain families have a very high incidence of breast and ovarian cancer. About 5% to 10% of breast cancers demonstrate an autosomal dominant inheritance pattern, accounting for 9,000 to 18,000 cases per year in the United States (3). For all inherited forms of breast cancer, family histories need to include the paternal as well as the maternal side, since defective genes can be passed on from either parent.

BRCA1 and BRCA2

The recent cloning of the BRCA1 and BRCA2 genes has provided a great deal of insight into these familial cancer syndromes, but has also raised difficult screening, treatment, and ethical issues. Hereditary early-onset breast cancer was initially linked to the long arm of chromosome 17 (17q 12-21) by King in 1990 (70). Four years later, after an intense international search, the BRCA1 gene was positionally cloned by Skolnick

TABLE 1–1. *Cloned genes of familial cancer syndromes*

Syndrome	Tumor	Associated features	Gene	Chromosome
Hereditary early-onset breast cancer (4,5)	Breast cancer	Ovarian cancer	BRCA1, BRCA2	17q21.1, 13q12-13
Li-Fraumeni syndrome (11)	Sarcoma, breast	Pediatric malignancies	p53, ? others	17p13
Cowden's disease (12)	Breast cancer	Facial lesions	PTEN[a]	10q23
Ataxia-telangiectasia	Leukemia, lymphoma, breast cancer	Cerebellar ataxia, oculocutaneous telanglectasias	ATM [a]	11q22-23
Familial adenomatous polyposis (17,18)	Colorectal cancer	Colonic polyposis, CHRPE, desmoids, osteomas, upper GI cancer	APC	5q21
Hereditary nonpolyposis colon cancer	Colorectal cancer	Endometrial and ovarian cancer	MLH1,MSH2, PMS1, PMS2, ? others	3p21, 2p16, 2q31, 7p22
MEN 1 (31)	Pancreatic islet cell	Parathyroid hyperplasia, pituitary adenoma	MENIN[a]	11q13
MEN 2A (33,34)	Medullary thyroid cancer	Pheochromocytoma, parathyroid hyperplasia	RET	10q11.2
MEN 2B	Medullary thyroid cancer	Pheochromocytoma, ganglioneuro-matosis, marfanoid habitus	RET	10q11.2
Familial medullary thyroid cancer	Medullary thyroid cancer		RET	10q11.2
Neurofibromatosis type I (43,44)	Neurofibrosarcomas	Neurofibromas, café-au-lait spots, Lisch nodules	NF1	17q11.2
Neurofibromatosis type II (45,46)	Neurofibrosarcomas	Neurofibromas, bilateral vestibular schwannomas	Merlin[a]	22q12
Familial atypical multiple-mole syndrome (50)	Melanoma	Atypical melanocytic nevi, pancreatic cancer	CDKN2[a] (p16), ? others	9p21
Familial retinoblastoma	Retinoblastoma	Development retardation, osteosarcomas	RB	13q14
Wilms' tumor syndromes	Wilms' tumor	WAGR, Denys-Drash syndrome	WT1[a]	11p13
Von Hippel-Lindau (55)	Hemangioblastoma, renal cancer	Multiple cysts, pheochromocytomas	VHL	3p25
Hereditary papillary renal carcinoma (61)	Papillary renal cancer		MET[a]	7q31-34
Peutz-Jeghers syndrome (71)	GI cancers	Hamartomas, mucocutaneous pigmentation	LKB1*	19p
Familial juvenile polyposis (72)	GI cancers	Hamartomas	SMAD4*	18q21

[a] Testing limited or not yet available.

(4) using the family pedigrees of the Mormon community. Just over 1 year later, a second hereditary early-onset breast cancer gene was identified on chromosome 13, BRCA2 (5). The highly publicized discovery of these genes has created great expectations from the general public and the medical community of being able to control these relatively prevalent diseases, but certain characteristics of these genes have made this difficult. BRCA1 is a large gene spanning about 100,000 nucleic acids, with over 250 different mutations reported, spread across the gene. About 100 different mutations have been reported for BRCA2, an even larger gene. This makes identifying a mutation, as well as determining the significance of a mutation, an arduous task. In order to detect a new mutation in an individual whose family has not been studied, the entire gene may need to be examined, not just a specific region of a gene. Different mutations in BRCA1 may have greatly varying risks of breast cancer associated with them (6). Finally, there is no functional assay of the BRCA gene products, which could provide the quickest method to screen for abnormalities. The normal functions of the genes are only beginning to be understood. There is evidence that the genes may act like a tumor suppressor gene or act as a caretaker of the genome.

For a physician and patient to make an informed decision regarding management of BRCA mutations, they need to know the lifetime risk of developing cancer. Current estimates have been based largely on genetic-linkage analysis of large families with multiple members with breast or ovarian cancer, or both. Assessment of risk based on these families may overestimate the risk for other families. Penetrance may depend on the specific BRCA mutation, other related genes, or environmental factors. Initial estimates reported that a BRCA1 mutation confers an 87% lifetime risk of developing breast cancer, as opposed to a 12% risk for the general public (6). The lifetime risk for carriers of BRCA2 mutations has been estimated to be 80%.

On the other hand, a recent study from the National Cancer Institute (NCI) of specific BRCA1 and BRCA2 mutations in the Ashkenazi Jewish population found the risk at age 70 to be only 56% (7). The difference between an 87% and a 56% risk may lead physicians and patients to make different decisions about prevention. Clearly, more broad based studies will need to be done to determine the actual risks for specific mutations. The Cooperative Breast Cancer Registry organized by the NCI will attempt to analyze 6,000 women with breast cancer over the next several years, which may provide better estimates of the risk of breast cancer in these patients.

Carriers of BRCA mutations are also at higher risk for other cancers, especially ovarian cancer. The estimates of the lifetime risk of ovarian cancer in a patient with a BRCA1 mutation have ranged from 16% to 84%, with a generally accepted rate of 40% to 60% (6). About 5% of all ovarian cancers are believed to arise from BRCA1 germ-line mutations. Compared with sporadic cases, patients with germ-line BRCA1 mutations who develop ovarian cancer appear to have a more favorable clinical outcome (8). For BRCA2 mutation carriers the risk of ovarian cancer is believed to be much lower than for BRCA1, closer to 15% to 20%. Prostate cancer appears to be more common in these kindreds, and a few studies have found colon cancer to be more prevalent. In contrast to BRCA1, men who are carriers for BRCA2 mutations appear to have a higher risk themselves of breast cancer, although not as high as women.

Mutations in the BRCA1 gene are generally believed to account for 45% of hereditary early-onset breast cancer and 5% of all breast cancers. These estimates again are based on large families with multiple members. A study based on all women (not only early-onset) with a family history of breast cancer found the rate of BRCA1 mutations to be only 16% for patients who had breast cancer with a positive family history (9). BRCA2 mutations are estimated to be responsible for 70% of the remaining cases of familial breast cancers. The accuracy of these numbers is important for counseling a family who has a negative genetic analysis for the BRCA genes.

Diagnosis and Screening

Currently there are two commercial laboratories which perform genetic analysis to detect mutations in the BRCA1 and BRCA2 genes (Myriad Genetics in Salt Lake City, Utah, and Oncormed, Inc. in Gaithersburg, Maryland). Unless a mutation is already known in a patient's family, a method which sequences the entire gene is preferable. These tests should only be used for patients at risk for having a mutation, and not as a screening test for the general population. Genetic counseling is essential before any test is administered, and should also be given with the test results. Because of the nature of these genes, genetic testing may identify a mutation of unknown significance, which the physician needs to be prepared to explain to the patient.

Treatment for carriers of BRCA 1 and 2 mutations has not been well defined. Prophylactic bilateral mastectomies may be a reasonable option for a high rate of penetrance. Unlike a total colectomy for colon cancer, the subsequent risk of cancer is not zero, due to the small amount of breast tissue invariably left behind. Therefore, if a patient's risk of developing cancer is not too dangerously high, other surveillance options should be considered. A decision analysis study based on a lifetime risk of breast cancer ranging from 40% to 85% found prophylactic bilateral mastectomies increased life expectancy 2.9 to 5.3 years for a 30-year-old woman, but only 0.2 to 0.5 years for a 60-year-old woman (10). Although the efficacy of prophylactic mastectomies has not been well established, this study assumed an 85% reduction in risk of breast cancer with surgical prophylaxis. From this decision analysis study, performing the surgery at a young age in gene carriers may be a reasonable option after appropriate genetic counseling. If mastectomies are performed, it is critical that the patient continues to have close follow-up of their remaining breast tissue.

While BRCA1 and BRCA2 comprise most of the inherited breast cancer cases, there are some other important syndromes which the clinician should consider when treating a patient with familial breast cancer.

Li-Fraumeni Syndrome

LFS is a rare autosomal dominant disease, also known as the SBLA—sarcoma, breast cancer, leukemia, and adrenocortical cancer—syndrome. It is characterized by an inherited predisposition to at least five childhood cancers—soft tissue sarcoma, osteosarcoma, leukemia, brain tumor, and adrenocortical carcinoma—and breast cancer. Other tumors have been reported in these patients, including germ cell tumors, neuroblastoma, malignant melanoma, Wilms' tumor, and carcinoma of the lung, prostate, and pancreas. Breast cancer is the most common cancer seen in LFS, and almost 90% of carriers develop it by age 50 in classic kindreds (3). Because the syndrome is rare, LFS accounts for less than 1% of all breast cancers. The penetrance for any invasive cancer is approximately 50% by age 30. Patients appear to have an increased sensitivity to radiation, since second primaries are prone to develop in the bed of an irradiated field.

Germ-line mutations in the TP53 tumor suppressor gene were identified in five LFS kindreds in 1990, and since then about 50% of LFS families have been found to have germ-line mutations in this gene (11). There are also a significant number of LFS kindreds who do not have a TP53 germ-line mutation, suggesting genetic heterogeneity. One possibility is that genes involved in regulation of TP53 may be mutated. Another study found germ-line TP53 mutations in a family without classic LFS characteristics, having a high rate of gastric cancer instead. Nonetheless, when a germ-line TP53 mutation is discovered in a kindred, genetic testing can identify carriers.

The TP53 gene is considered to be the most mutated gene in cancer. The protein product of the TP53 gene, p53, appears to function as a transcription factor. The product likely has a role in preventing DNA synthesis when damage has occurred to the cell's DNA. The types of germ-line mutations in LFS are similar to those TP53 mutations found in sporadic tumors, mostly occurring in exons 5 to 9.

Cowden's Disease

Cowden's disease (multiple hamartoma syndrome), named after the patient Rachel Cowden, is an autosomal dominant syndrome best characterized by cutaneous facial lesions, seen in 96% of patients. The spectrum of disease includes multiple facial trichilemmomas, oral papillomas, lingua plicata ("cobblestoning" of the tongue), acral keratoses, bilateral breast cancer, gastrointestinal (GI) hamartomas, and thyroid tumors. Lipomas, hemangiomas, macrocephaly, and brain tumors have also been reported. Breast cancer develops in 30% to 50% of patients by age 50. Linkage analysis located a region for a candidate gene on chromosome 10q23. Within this region, constitutional mutations in the gene PTEN (also known as MMAC1) have been found in affected individuals in four of five kindreds (12). The types of mutations found suggest the gene is a tumor suppressor gene. The protein appears to act as a tyrosine phosphotase. Since testing of this gene is not currently available, counseling should be based on family pedigrees and clinical judgment.

Ataxia-Telangiectasia

AT is an autosomal recessive disease in which homozygots for the mutation develop a varied phenotype including progressive cerebellar ataxia, oculocutaneous telangiectasias, progeric skin changes, immune dysfunction, and increased cancer susceptibility. The hallmark of AT is the cerebellar ataxia, often seen at a very young age. Most individuals are unable to walk by age 10. They are extremely sensitive to ionizing radiation. Cells from individuals display characteristics suggesting that the AT gene plays a role in DNA repair. The putative gene for AT (termed ATM) has been cloned and is located on the long arm of chromosome 11. ATM appears to be required for the transcription of TP53 in response to radiation damage. Most of the mutations in the gene lead to a truncation of the protein; therefore, a protein truncation assay may be useful for detection in the future. At the time of this writing, genetic testing is done only at the research level.

Homozygous carriers are prone to a variety of cancers, particularly leukemia and lymphoma, but also breast cancer, as well as pancreatic, stomach, bladder, and ovarian cancer. Heterozygous carriers also are reported to have an increased risk of breast cancer, as much as a five to eightfold increase over the normal population, and an earlier incidence of cancer. Since about 1% of the population are heterozygous carriers of AT, these individuals may account for up to 7% of all breast cancer (13). A recent study of 401 women with early onset breast cancer found only 0.5% of them to be AT carriers, suggesting that the gene may not be involved in as large a number of cases as originally believed (14).

Colorectal Cancer

There are about 150,000 new cases of colorectal cancer diagnosed annually in the United States, making this a disease frequently encountered by the general surgeon. Familial cancers may account for as many as 15% of these cases (15). Although there are several rare hereditary syndromes associated with colorectal cancer, most known hereditary colorectal cancer can be divided into two main categories: familial adenomatous polyposis (FAP) and hereditary nonpolyposis cancer (HNPCC) syndrome. Historically, FAP has received the greatest amount of attention, since it is characterized by an obvious phenotype, florid colonic polyposis, and its inherited nature was appreciated by 1900. During the explosion of molecular genetics, the research community has used this disease as a paradigm for familial cancer, leading to the identification of the responsible gene, APC. More recently, HNPCC, lacking a striking precancerous phenotype, has gained recognition as the more prevalent form.

Although 5% of colorectal cancer has been ascribed to defined inherited syndromes, another 10% of colorectal cancer appears to have a hereditary component. The genes or factors responsible for these cases are unknown. One explanation is that certain mutations in cancer related genes, which initially appear harmless, actually make the region more likely to be mutated. The inherited mutation does not alter the function of the gene but makes further mutations more common during DNA replication. Volgelstein (16) reported one such mutation in the APC gene in Ashkenazi Jews, which doubled an individual's risk for colorectal cancer.

Familial Polyposis Syndromes

FAP is an inherited autosomal dominant disease caused by mutations in the tumor suppressor gene, APC. The penetrance is extremely high with greater than 90% of affected individuals developing colorectal cancer if not treated. Carriers typically develop adenomatous polyps that progress to carpet the large intestine during the second or third decades of life. The polyps are histologically indistinguishable from sporadic polyps, and individually these polyps do not have a greater propensity to undergo malignant transformation than sporadic polyps. Because of the enormous number of polyps (typically hundreds to thousands) and the early age at which the polyps develop, the risk that one of these will undergo further genetic changes to progress to malignancy is close to 100%. The median age of cancer diagnosis for untreated individuals is 39 years, almost 30 years earlier than the median age for sporadic colorectal cancer. Affected individuals are also prone to develop duodenal, gastric, and ileal polyps, and are at risk for developing duodenal, stomach, periampullary, thyroid, and other cancers.

After cytogenetic analysis of a patient with congenital abnormalities and intestinal polyposis suggested that the gene was on the long arm of chromosome 5 (5q), the APC gene was positionally cloned in 1991 (17,18). The gene encodes a 300-kd protein expressed in a variety of cell types, but its normal function is not clearly known. The protein contains a domain that binds microtubules and beta-catenin, suggesting it may function in cell adhesion and/or signaling. A mouse model has been developed in which the mice carry a germ-line mutation in the mouse homologue of the APC gene and develop multiple intestinal neoplasia (MIN).

Germ-line mutations have been found in many FAP kindreds. Somatic mutations in the APC gene also occur in over 80% of sporadic cases of colorectal cancer as well as sporadic adenomas. These mutations have been found in early adenomas, suggesting these mutations are one of the early genetic events in the development of colonic malignancy.

The complex relationship between genotype and phenotype is just becoming clear (19). Different locations of a mutation within the gene can produce different phenotypes. Congenital hypertrophy of the retinal pigment epithelium (CHRPE), which was once thought to be a signature of the disease, is associated with mutations between codons 463 and 1387. There are several phenotypic variations of FAP that were once thought to be distinct syndromes, but are probably a family of disorders related to the APC gene. Gardner syndrome, associated with mutations in codons 1403 to 1578, is characterized by desmoid tumors (especially of the abdominal wall and mesentery), osteomas of the mandible or skull, and sebaceous cysts. Hereditary flat adenoma syndrome is another variant of FAP, characterized by ordinary adenomas as well as flat adenomas. Turcot's syndrome is associated with malignant central nervous system tumors, GI polyposis, and colorectal cancer.

At the genetic level, it is unclear why some patients have a relatively sparse number of polyps, 100 to 200, whereas others have more than 5,000. Genes that modify or regulate the APC gene have been postulated to cause this discrepancy. Two MIN mice can have a significant variation in the number of GI polyps, even though they posses identical mutations in the mouse APC homologue gene. Apparently, this variation of polyp number is due to a gene on a different chromosome, MOM1 (modifier of MIN), which affects the mouse APC homologue.

Screening and Diagnosis

Because of the high penetrance and the short time course in which tumors develop, close surveillance is essential. For children of an affected individual, the colon should be examined via flexible sigmoidoscopy beginning in their preteenage years. After a baseline procedure, sigmoidoscopy should be done annually.

Currently there are at least ten centers in North America which perform linkage analysis for the APC gene. In addition to the at-risk individual, testing requires other affected and unaffected individuals within the kindred. A few laboratories offer direct analysis of the gene. Over 95% of the mutations result in a truncated protein product. This allows a more rapid protein truncation test to be effective in detecting many mutations. At this time only a few places offer this test, including Mount Sinai Hospital in Toronto and Washington University School of Medicine in St. Louis.

Genetic testing may eliminate some of the emotional stress and financial cost of surveillance, if the patient is found not to have inherited a mutation. Two to three sigmoidoscopies should still be done to guard against a false-negative result. Genetic testing is also appropriate when a patient presents with a large number of intestinal polyps, with or without the presence of colorectal cancer. If a mutation in the APC gene is found, they will require not only management of colorectal neoplasia, but lifelong surveillance of the upper GI tract for a second malignancy, and genetic counseling of family members.

Surgical Management

The primary treatment for FAP is surgical. Surgery should be done when florid polyposis is detected, usually in the late teen years or early twenties. Unlike breast and ovarian cancer, prophylactic surgery can completely eliminate the risk of colorectal cancer if a total proctocolectomy is performed. Generally, if the patient is relatively young, there are two procedures to remove the colon: either a total proctocolectomy with an ileoanal anastomosis or a colectomy with an ileorectal anastomosis. By leaving rectal mucosa after an ileorectal anastomosis, there is still a significant risk for developing rectal cancer. Close surveillance of this mucosa is necessary. Iwama (20) found the risk for rectal carcinoma after ileorectal anastomosis to be 24% at 15 years for 322 patients who underwent rectum-preserving surgery. Two factors were found to correlate with an increased risk of rectal cancer: length of the rectal stump greater than 7 cm and a high rectal polyp density. Ambroze (21) reported the rates to be 13% at 25 years from St. Marks Hospital, 12% at 20 years from the Cleveland Clinic, and 20% at 20 years from the Mayo Clinic. Generally, rectal screening should be done every 6 months and possibly more frequently, especially after the age of 45.

Total proctocolectomy with ileoanal anastomosis also has disadvantages: sphincter dysfunction, greater morbidity including loss of sexual function in men, and more technically challenging surgery. Because many FAP patients are asymptomatic at the time of surgery, these patients may not tolerate the functional problems of an ileal-pouch as well as patients who undergo this surgery for ulcerative colitis. Multiple factors should be considered when deciding the appropriate surgical procedure including extent of rectal disease, location of any cancer, sphincter function, extracolonic disease, surgeon experience, and patient follow-up.

After the colorectal cancer risk, the greatest risk of mortality is from upper GI cancer, primarily periampullary, duodenal, and stomach tumors. Jejunal and ileal cancers are rare. Upper endoscopic surveillance is strongly recommended for these individuals. Generally, duodenal polyposis progresses slowly, but the natural history of this entity is not well understood (22). Lynch (23) suggests an upper endoscopy every 3 years for screening. Polypectomy, if possible, is thought to be adequate treatment for most polyps, followed by annual screening. Currently, prophylactic resection is not recommended.

Desmoids appear as a phenotypic characteristic in 10% to 20% of FAP patients. Although not malignant, they can be locally aggressive and a significant cause of mortality. Desmoids often arise in surgical scars or in the small bowel mesentery after abdominal surgery. Diffuse fibrosis may lead to ureteral, vascular, or GI obstruction. Further surgical resection may not be possible, and after initial success, desmoids often recur. Rodriguez-Bigas (24) found only nine of 21 patients who underwent surgery for desmoids were potentially cured, and seven of these nine had a recurrence at a median of 61 months postoperatively. Overall, only two of 21 were thought to have a long-term cure. Desmoids may also prevent an ileorectal anastomosis from being converted to a restorative proctectomy. Radiation, suldinac, and tamoxifen have been used to treat desmoids with varying success.

Hereditary Nonpolyposis Colorectal Cancer Syndrome

HNPCC, also known as Lynch syndromes I and II, is an autosomal dominant disease caused by one of at least four DNA mismatch repair genes. HNPCC accounts for about 5% of all colorectal cancers. When Lynch initially described this syndrome, he divided kindreds into those having only colorectal cancer (Lynch syndrome I) and those who also had extracolonic cancers (Lynch syndrome II), which is the more common form. The penetrance of the disease has not been well defined, but it is likely high. As in sporadic and FAP colorectal cancer cases, these patients still develop cancer through the progression of adenomatous polyps to frank malignancy, but they lack the diffuse colonic polyposis seen in FAP. The incidence of polyps is believed to be equal to that seen in individuals who develop sporadic colorectal cancer. Once a polyp develops there appears to be an increased rate of tumor progression. Unlike sporadic tumors, about 10% of HNPCC patients develop a colorectal cancer within 5 years after colonoscopy or colon resection, with the median age of cancer development being 44 years (25).

HNPCC was initially defined based on its clinical manifestations, which are termed the Amsterdam criteria. These criteria consist of the following: (a) a family with at least three relatives having proven colorectal cancer, and one individual being a primary relative of the other two, (b) at least two generations being affected, and (c) one individual being diagnosed before age 50. There are several other clinical characteristics of these cancers. The lesions have a right-sided colon predominance (70% proximal to the splenic flexure). There is an excess of synchronous and metachronous colorectal cancers. Anecdotal reports suggest that these patients do better, stage for stage, than their sporadic counterparts. Extracolonic malignancies are also seen, especially endometrial and ovarian cancer. Other associated cancers include small bowel, stomach, larynx, pancreas, urologic tract, bladder, and possibly breast cancer.

The process that led to the discovery of the responsible genes is interesting, aided both by linkage analysis in affected families and by microbiologists studying mutations in bacteria and yeast. Tumor DNA of affected patients were found to have widespread instability in short repeat sequences, termed microsatellite instability, detected as extra bands on PCR amplified short repetitive segments of DNA. Similar DNA instability is seen in bacteria and yeast which have induced mutations in their DNA mismatch repair genes. This led scientists to locate germ-line mutations in the human versions of the same genes, MSH2, MLH1, PMS1, and PMS2, in families with hereditary colorectal cancer. Currently MSH2 and MLH1 are estimated to account for two-thirds of HNPCC, and PMS1 and PMS2 cause less than 5% of cases. When the normal corresponding allele to one of these mismatch repair genes is mutated, the cell cannot repair mistakes made by DNA polymerase during DNA replication, leading to genome wide mutations. The mutation rate in tumors of these patients has been shown to be two to three times higher than in normal cells (19). Consequently, mutations in protooncogenes and tumor suppressor genes occur much more frequently, leading to cancer.

Microsatellite instability is seen in 10% to 15% of sporadic tumors. These sporadic tumors also occur predominately in the proximal colon (25). Some, but not all, have somatic mutations in the genes that cause HNPCC. There is an inverse relationship between microsatellite instability and aneuploidy, suggesting that one of these two forms of instability is found in all colorectal cancer (26).

Screening and Treatment

Currently, genetic testing for MSH2 and MLH1 is only done at a few centers, largely within research protocols. For individuals known to carry a germ-line mutation or strongly suspected to have one, Lynch (25) suggests screening with colonoscopy beginning between the ages of 20 to 25 years. This procedure should be repeated every two years until age 30, at which point it should be done annually. Women carriers should undergo endometrial aspiration curettage annually beginning at age 30. Surveillance for ovarian cancer is limited, but transvaginal ultrasound and CA-125 should be considered.

Treatment for HNPCC kindreds has not been well defined. Without accurate knowledge of the penetrance for the different mutations, guidelines cannot be made. If a germ-line mutation is found in an individual, then prophylactic surgery could be considered. The same general principles of treatment exist as for FAP, but a colectomy with an ileorectal anastomosis may be a more reasonable alternative since these tumors have a proximal predilection. Alternatively, nonoperative management with screening colonoscopy every 1 to 2 years in known gene carriers is a reasonable option. At this point there have been no significant clinical trials examining the various treatment options. Prophylactic total abdominal hysterectomy and bilateral salpingo oophorectomy could be considered for women who have completed their families. Carriers need to be forewarned that removal of both ovaries, even if they appear histologically normal, does not completely eliminate the risk of ovarian cancer.

Muir-Torre Syndrome

Muir-Torre syndrome (MTS) is a rare autosomal dominant disorder, characterized by the presence of at least one sebaceous gland tumor and a visceral cancer. The sebaceous gland tumors often appear as yellow facial papules and are considered a hallmark of this syndrome. The most common internal malignancy is colorectal cancer, but other tumors occur, especially genitourinary. There are several clinical similarities with HNPCC, which led Lynch to describe it as a variation of HNPCC. Both are characterized by an inherited susceptibility to colorectal cancer at an early age. Both have a tendency to form proximal colon cancers, and patients tend to have better survival than for sporadic cancers. Recently, genetic similarities have strengthened this association. Microsatellite instability is found in the sebaceous tumors and other malignancies in about half of the affected individuals (27). Germ-line mutations have been found in both the MSH2 and MLH1 genes in different kindreds (28).

Peutz-Jeghers Syndrome

Peutz-Jeghers syndrome (PJS) is a rare autosomal dominant disease, characterized by GI polyposis and mucocutaneous pigmentations. The pigmentations are melanin deposits which can occur on and around the lips, oral mucosa, hands, feet, perianal region, and umbilical area, usually appearing in childhood. Those on the skin may fade, but generally not those of the mucous membranes. The GI polyps are hamartomas with a prominent smooth muscle component derived from the muscularis mucosa. These polyps are distinctly different from those seen in FAP and HNPCC. Their malignant potential is uncertain, but it is likely that carcinomas arise from coexisting adenomatous polyps. Hamartomas can be found anywhere along the GI tract, but are more frequent in the small bowel and are usually multiple. Obstruction, intussusception, and bleeding are the most common manifestations.

Malignancies of the GI tract occur with increased frequency, including pancreatic cancer. The relative risk of death from a GI cancer was estimated by Spigelman (29) to be 13 times higher than for a matched population. There appears also to be an increased risk of extra GI malignancies. Although it is generally believed that the rate of GI malignancy is low (2% to 3%) (30), Spigelman followed a series of 72 patients and found the mortality from any cancer by age 57 was 50%. Iwama reported a prevalence of 17% of GI tumors among the 420 cases of PJS in the Japanese literature.

Recently, the LKB1 gene has been linked to PJS (71), but genetic testing is not yet available. These patients should have a baseline upper endoscopy and colonoscopy around age 20 with frequent surveillance thereafter. Some have advocated a subtotal colectomy if the polyps are too numerous to follow.

Familial Juvenile Polyposis

Familial juvenile polyposis (FJP) is another rare autosomal dominant disease characterized by hamartomatous polyposis. The polyps, usually numbering 50 to 200, primarily occur in the colon and rectum, but can be found in the stomach and duodenum. A typical juvenile polyp consists of stromal elements overlaid with normal epithelium, and is found as a solitary lesion in children with no known malignant potential. In FJP, the polyps may be "atypical," containing epithelial dysplasia, or "mixed," containing regions that resemble an adenoma. Individuals usually present with diarrhea during childhood or rectal bleeding during the second decade. Associated congenital abnormalities include cerebral and pulmonary arteriovenous malformations, cardiac anomalies, polydactyly, malrotation, and cranial malformations.

The lifetime risk for developing colorectal cancer is estimated to be 50%, usually at an early age. This has led to the recommendation for prophylactic colon resection during the second decade. The procedure is usually a subtotal colectomy with ileorectal anastomosis, since the predilection for these polyps is in the right colon. Some surgeons have noted a rapid rate of recurrence in the retained rectum. For this reason some advocate a restorative proctocolectomy with ileoanal anastomosis. Periodic surveillance of the ileal pouch needs to be done, because polyps may arise in the ileal pouch. Recently, Howe (72) identified germ-line mutations in the SMAD4 gene that are associated with FJP.

Endocrine Cancers

The MEN syndromes are a group of familial endocrinopathies which include MEN 1, MEN 2A, and MEN 2B. Five years ago, the RET protooncogene was found to be the predisposition gene for MEN 2A, MEN 2B, and familial, non-MEN medullary thyroid cancer (FMTC). This made possible the institution of presymptomatic genetic testing for at-risk members of affected kindreds, and led the way to early, preventative treatment of gene carriers. The predisposition gene for MEN 1 was cloned and characterized very recently (31), and presymptomatic genetic screening is being developed. These recent discoveries and their influence upon clinical management reflect the rapid changes in clinical medicine which are occurring as a result of advances in basic science research. Now it is possible to recommend an operation based on the results of a genetic test. Surgeons must exercise particular diligence and attention to detail when performing preventative operations and when recommending treatment and follow-up of patients and their relatives.

Multiple Endocrine Neoplasia Type 1

In MEN 1, patients develop tumors of the parathyroid glands, the pancreatic islet cells and the pituitary gland. Lipomas, carcinoids, and benign tumors of the thyroid and adrenal cortex may also develop. Hyperparathyroidism occurs in virtually all patients with MEN 1. Clinical evidence of pituitary and pancreatic islet cell tumors develop in 25% to 50% of patients, respectively. Wilcox and associates, in an autopsy study of patients with MEN 1, found neoplasia of the parathyroid glands, the pituitary gland, and the pancreatic islets even though patients did not manifest clinical evidence of hyperfunction from each of these tissues. The diagnosis of MEN 1 is confirmed by the presence of at least three of these four criteria: primary hyperparathyroidism, pancreatic islet cell tumor [Zollinger-Ellison syndrome, insulinoma, vasoactive intestinal polypeptide-secreting tumor (VIPoma)], a pituitary tumor, or a positive family history. The gene responsible for MEN 1 is the tumor suppressor gene, MENIN, located on chromosome 11q13.31 Routine presymptomatic diagnostic testing is not widely available at the present time, but will be in the near future. Relatives of patients with MEN 1 should be screened for this disorder starting in their early teens. Because hyperparathyroidism is almost always the first detectable abnormality in patients with MEN 1, serum calcium measurements should be performed yearly on asymptomatic kindred members at risk for the disease. If the history or physical examination suggests pituitary or pancreatic tumors, an appropriate diagnostic evaluation, including biochemical testing and radiological imaging studies, should be initiated. Few patients present with renal stones or bone disease. Patients with MEN 1 have generalized (four-gland) parathyroid enlargement. Occasionally there is a marked discrepancy in the size of the parathyroid glands, but patients should be treated as if they have four gland disease. Surgery is the appropriate treatment of choice for these patients. Three and one-half gland parathyroidectomy is the procedure of choice of many surgeons. However, there are reported rates of persistent or recurrent hypercalcemia of up to 50% and of hypoparathyroidism of up to 25%. Therefore, we perform total parathyroidectomy with autotransplantation of parathyroid tissue to the forearm. This achieves an immediate cure rate of over 90% with an incidence of hypoparathyroidism of less than 5%. Approximately 50% of patients having total parathyroidectomy and autotransplantation will develop graft dependent hyperparathyroidism, but this can be effectively managed by resecting a portion of the autografted tissue (32).

Pituitary tumors occur in 40% of patients with MEN 1. The most common type of tumor is a benign prolactin-producing adenoma, although a few patients have tumors which produce growth hormone or adrenal corticotrophic hormone (ACTH). Patients present with headache, diplopia, and symptoms referable to hormone overproduction. Prolactinomas cause amenorrhea-galactorrhea in females and impotence in men. Hypopituitarism may also be present. Patients with growth hormone-producing tumors present with symptoms of acromegaly, and patients with ACTH-producing tumors present with Cushing's disease. Effective inhibition of prolactin production can be achieved by administration of bromocriptine, an ergot derivative with dopaminergic activity. Use of this drug may also reduce tumor bulk, and obviate the need for surgical intervention, although trans-sphenoidal hypophysectomy may be necessary in patients who fail bromocriptine treatment, and in patients with growth hormone producing tumors. Patients with MEN 1 who do not have known pituitary disease should be screened by monitoring serum prolactin and growth hormone levels.

Pancreatic islet cell tumors occur in 60% of patients with MEN 1. Though these tumors often secrete more than one type of polypeptide hormone they rarely produce a mixed clinical picture. Several distinct clinical syndromes have been described. The most common islet cell tumor in patients with MEN 1 is a gastrinoma, which produces the clinical picture of the Zollinger-Ellison syndrome. VIPomas, insulinomas, glucagonomas, and somatostatinomas are also encountered. As opposed to the management of sporadic islet cell tumors, the management of pancreatic tumors in patients with the MEN 1 syndrome is complicated by the fact that the pancreas is usually diffusely involved with islet cell hyperplasia and multifocal tumors. Islet cell tumors (particularly gastrinomas) may also be found in the proximal duodenum and peripancreatic areas (gastrinoma triangle), and the tumors are virtually always malignant. Therefore, the treatment of these tumors must be focused on two goals: relief of symptoms related to excessive hormone production, and cure or palliation of the malignant process. Patients with islet cell tumors almost always suffer from the systemic effects of overproduction of a specific hormone rather than a space occupying mass. Prior to surgical exploration for an islet cell tumor the patient should be evaluated for the presence of an adrenal tumor by measuring urinary excretion rates of glucocorticoids, mineralocorticoids, and sex hormones.

Follow-up of Patients With Known MEN 1

Patients with known MEN 1 and their children should be closely followed for development of new abnormalities and recrudescence of endocrinopathies already treated. This should include yearly determinations of plasma calcium, glucose, gastrin, fasting insulin, VIP, prolactin, growth hormone, and beta-human gonadotropin hormone. In addition, a detailed history and physical examination should be directed toward detecting abnormalities in the parathyroid, pituitary or pancreatic islet cell systems. Because the gene responsible for MEN 1 has been identified, routine genetic testing will soon allow identification of MEN 1 gene carriers in affected families, and this will obviate the need to continue following individuals found not to have inherited the mutation.

Multiple Endocrine Neoplasia Type 2

Multiple endocrine neoplasia type 2A is an autosomal dominant inherited syndrome with almost complete penetrance by age 40. Medullary cancer of the thyroid (MTC) develops in all carriers of the gene, while pheochromocytoma develops in approximately 50% and hyperplasia of the parathyroid glands in approximately 25%. MEN 2B is a variant of MEN 2A, in which patients develop MTC and pheochromocytomas, as well as megacolon, ganglioneuromatosis, and a characteristic physical appearance, with hypergnathism of the mid-face, marfanoid body habitus, and multiple mucosal neuromas. They do not develop hyperparathyroidism (Fig. 1-3). Familial, non-MEN MTC (FMTC) is caused by mutations in the same gene that causes MEN 2A and 2B. In FMTC, patients

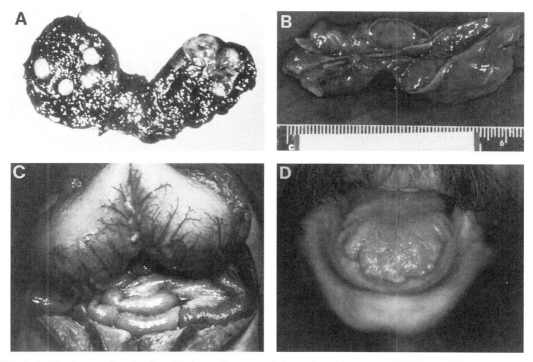

FIG. 1-3. Features of patients with hereditary medullary thyroid cancer (MTC). **A:** Bisected thyroid gland from a patient with MEN 2A showing multicentric, bilateral foci of MTC. **B:** Adrenalectomy specimen from patient with MEN 2B demonstrating pheochromocytoma. **C:** Megacolon in patient with MEN 2B. **D:** Midface and tongue of patient with MEN 2B showing characteristic tongue notching secondary to plexiform neuromas. (Reprinted with permission from Moley JF. Medullary thyroid cancer. In: Clark O, Duh Q, eds. *Textbook of endocrine surgery.* Philadelphia: WB Saunders, 1997:109.)

develop MTC only. In all of these disorders, MTC develops on a background of C-cell hyperplasia, and pheochromocytomas arise in the setting of hyperplastic adrenal chromaffin cells. Pheochromocytomas can occur sporadically or as part of other genetic syndromes, especially neurofibromatosis type 1 (NF1) and von Hippel–Landau (VHL) disease. Most pheochromocytomas in patients with MEN 2A and MEN 2B are not invasive and have a low metastatic potential. Similarly, MTC shows a spectrum of histologic and clinical malignancy that ranges from C-cell hyperplasia to generally minimally aggressive disease in patients with FMTC, intermediate grade behavior in patients with MEN 2A, and very aggressive growth in patients with MEN 2B. Predicting the clinical behavior of these tumors based on the histologic appearance alone is frequently difficult.

Diagnosis and Screening

Because the MEN 2 disorders are inherited in an autosomal dominant fashion, first degree relatives and children of patients with the disorder have a 50% chance of inheriting the gene for the disease. Mutations in the RET protooncogene were identified in the constitutional DNA of MEN 2A and FMTC patients by two groups (33,34). RET encodes a transmembrane tyrosine kinase receptor, whose ligands are glial cell line–derived neurotrophic factor (GDNF) and neurturin.

The mutations found in MEN 2A, 2B and FMTC cause constitutive activation (tyrosine phosphorylation) of the RET protein, which presumably drives tumorigenesis through mechanisms that are currently being elucidated. These mutations are gain-of function mutations as compared to loss-of function mutations, which are found in the disease genes responsible for VHL, neurofibromatosis type 1, and MEN 1. Activating mutations of RET, which have been described in MEN 2A and FMTC, affect exon 10 (codons 609, 611, 618, or 620), exon 11b (codons 630 or 634), exon 13 (codon 768), or exon 14 (codon 804). Patients with MEN 2B usually have a mutation in codon 918 (35). Testing for the presence of a RET gene mutation is done by polymerase chain-based methods which involve restriction digestion, band migration on acrylamide gels, or direct sequencing. The clinician requesting the test need only obtain the patient's blood after informed consent and send it to an appropriate lab. It is strongly recommended that genetic counselors speak to patients before genetic testing is done. Genetic testing is available at a number of institutions, including Washington University School of Medicine in St. Louis, Missouri.

Biochemical Testing. C-cells and MTC cells make calcitonin, which can be measured in the blood, and has been invaluable in screening patients for recurrent or residual disease after treatment for MTC. We have found the sequential infusion of calcium gluconate and pentagastrin to be a very potent calcitonin secretagogue, and to provide more reliable results than basal or unstimulated calcitonin levels. Blood samples are collected before and at 1, 2, 3, and 5 minutes following injection, and calcitonin levels are measured by radioimmunoassay (36).

Surgical Management of MTC

Since MTC in patients with MEN 2A and MEN 2B is virtually always present in both thyroid lobes, the preferred treatment is total thyroidectomy with resection of lymph nodes in the central region of the neck. Central node dissection entails removal of all nodes and fatty tissue between the carotid sheaths from the level of the hyoid to the innominate artery. We generally also perform parathyroidectomy with autotransplantation of parathyroid tissue into the forearm (MEN 2A) or sternocleidomastoid (MEN 2B, FMTC, sporadic disease).

Patients who are at risk for development of MTC because they are in known MEN 2A, MEN 2B, or FMTC kindreds should undergo genetic testing for the presence of a mutation in the RET protooncogene, and stimulated calcitonin testing. If an individual is found to have a mutation (in families with a known mutation, the mutation will of course be the same in all affected family members) they should undergo screening for a pheochromocytoma, and if there is no evidence of pheochromocytoma, thyroidectomy should be performed. At our institution, over the last 5 years, we have studied 235 kindred members at direct risk for inheriting MEN 2A, FMTC or MEN 2B (37,38). We have performed over 60 "preventative" thyroidectomies in patients found to be RET gene mutation carriers. Over half of the patients were under 15 years of age. The operative treatment was total thyroidectomy, regional lymph node dissection, and autotransplantation of the parathyroid to the forearm (MEN 2A patients) or sternocleidomastoid muscle (MEN 2B patients). In all except two patients (5 years old and 13 years old), a C-cell disorder was identified in the resected specimen. Three patients were found to have lymph node metastases (two 10-year-old patients with MEN 2A and one 6-year-old patient with MEN 2B), and in one patient (the 6-year-old MEN 2B patient), the immediate postoperative stimulated calcitonin level was elevated. This series and others indicate that genetic testing allows earlier intervention in these patients which will result in more long-term cures. In addition, family members who are found not to have inherited a mutation are spared the inconvenience and discomfort of further testing.

Pheochromocytomas in MEN 2

Most patients with MEN 2A and MEN 2B who develop pheochromocytomas do so subsequent to development of MTC. Only about 10% of patients present with symptoms of pheochromocytomas prior to the detection of MTC. Screening for pheochromocytomas should be done at the same time as screening for MTC in these patients. This procedure should consist of measurement of 24 hour urinary excretion rates of catecholamines, VMA, and metanephrine. If urinary values are positive, C.T. or M.R.I. evaluation of the adrenals is obtained. It is critical to identify pheochromocytomas in these patients prior to performing other surgeries, since the mortality rate in patients undergoing operations who have an undetected pheochromocytoma is high.

Parathyroid Carcinoma

A hereditary predisposition to parathyroid hyperplasia with hyperparathyroidism is seen in MEN type 1, MEN type 2A, and non-MEN familial hyperparathyroidism. Parathyroid carcinomas, while rare, have been described in 25% of families affected by non-MEN familial hyperparathyroidism. These patients may also have fibroosseous tumors of the mandible or maxilla, and Wilms' tumor. The gene for this disorder, HRPT2, has been mapped to the long arm of chromosome 1 (39).

Sarcoma

Sarcomas have been identified in several familial cancer syndromes. Li-Fraumeni syndrome (LFS) (previously described in the Breast Cancer section) was initially described linking childhood rhabdomyosarcomas with other childhood cancers. A large variety of sarcomas have been reported within LFS kindreds including both soft tissue sarcomas and osteosarcomas. TP53 mutations are the germ-line mutation responsible for many cases of LFS. These mutations also are extremely common in sporadic sarcomas and are associated with a more aggressive histologic grade (40).

Retinoblastoma

Familial retinoblastoma is characterized primarily by bilateral retinoblastomas in infants and young children but also by an increased risk of sarcomas in affected individuals, especially in irradiated beds. The syndrome is an autosomal dominant inherited disorder with 90% penetrance. The retinoblastoma gene, RB, is located on chromosome 13q14. Most familial cases have no prior family history, indicating that they are de novo cases. Early screening includes ophthalmological examinations every 3 month to age 2, then every 4 months to age 4, and then every 6 months to age 10, which can reduce mortality by 55%. Treatment includes cryocoagulation, photocoagulation, radiation, or enucleation for advanced cases.

Neurofibromatosis

Neurofibromatoses are a group of inherited neurocutaneous syndromes which confer a much greater risk for developing neurofibrosarcomas. These syndromes primarily affect neural crest derived tissues and have a wide clinical heterogeneity. Predisposition genes for two distinct forms have been cloned: neurofibromatosis type I and neurofibromatosis type II. Neurofibromatosis type 1 (NF1), also called "von Recklinghausen disease," is a common autosomal dominant disorder, affecting more than 80,000 people in the United States. The three hallmarks of the disease are multiple neurofibromas, café au lait spots, and Lisch nodules (benign iris hamartomas). Neurofibromas are benign tumors composed of Schwann cells, fibroblasts, and endothelial cells, and can occur anywhere nerves are found. Surgical excision may be required for pain, functional impairment, or cosmetic reasons. Complete surgical resection is often needed because of the aggressive nature of the tumors. Neurofibromas can also occur along the GI tract, resulting in bleeding, obstruction, or intussusception. Although greater than 90% of NF1 patients demonstrate each of the three characteristic features, the number of lesions can be extremely variable. Other characteristics of NF1 include learning disabilities, macrocephaly, scoliosis, short stature, seizures, pseudoarthrosis, and malignancies (41). NF1 tends to be a progressive disease, with many of these features appearing in childhood.

Neurofibromatosis type 1 patients have a much greater likelihood to develop neurofibrosarcomas, and are also at risk for pheochromocytomas, CNS tumors, and leukemias. The increased risk for developing a neurofibrosarcoma is estimated to be 10,000 to 100,000 times greater than for the normal population (42). This results in 3% to 6% of all patients with NF1 developing neurofibrosarcomas. These tumors are believed to arise from neurofibromas, especially the plexiform type. Neurofibrosarcomas can be aggressive and invasive. An enlarging mass, localized pain, or neuropathy should be considered a neurofibrosarcoma until proven otherwise. After a tissue diagnosis is made, complete surgical removal should be performed as early as possible. These tumors are generally resistant to radiation and chemotherapy.

The gene responsible for NF1 was positionally cloned in 1990 to the long arm of chromosome 17 at q11.2 and is termed the NF1 gene (43,44). The gene is extremely large, spanning more than 350 kb of DNA with at least 59 exons. Within one of its introns are three other genes that are read in the opposite orientation. The gene product, neurofibromin, has a GTPase-activating protein (GAP) domain, which has been shown to down regulate the protooncogene p21-ras. This suggests a role of NF1 as a tumor suppressor gene. Further support is demonstrated by the fact that neurofibrosarcomas have a somatic mutation in the other allele of NF1, and no protein product is found in these tumors. Occasionally this locus is deleted in other sporadic tumors, especially colon cancer. Presently there are fifteen to twenty centers which provide genetic testing for the NF1 gene. Many offer only linkage analysis, but most offer prenatal diagnosis.

Neurofibromatosis type 2 (NF2) is a much more rare disorder, characterized by the defining feature of bilateral vestibular schwannomas (previously referred to as acoustic neuromas). The syndrome shares similarities with NF1, namely skin neurofibromas and café au lait spots. The syndrome also is characterized by cataracts and other CNS tumors, including gliomas, meningiomas, schwannomas, and neurofibromas.

NF2 is inherited in an autosomal dominant manner with a high degree of penetrance. In 1993 the gene, called "Merlin"

or "Schwannomin," was cloned and localized to chromosome 22 q11.1–13.1 (45,46). Its predicted protein product has sequence similarity to the exrin family of proteins which play a role in attaching the cell cytoskeleton to the cell membrane. Studies of neurofibrosarcomas and meningiomas have found somatic mutations in this gene, suggesting that it is a tumor suppressor gene. Currently, very few places test for the gene. Massachusetts General Hospital and Athena Diagnostic in Worchester, Massachusetts are two places that perform this service. An important study to follow carriers is gadolinium-enhanced magnetic resonance imaging to detect CNS and spinal tumors.

Melanoma

The incidence of cutaneous malignant melanoma has been rising faster than any other cancer. Approximately 10% of melanoma cases are familial, often associated with multiple atypical moles. These moles have been suggested as precursor lesions for melanoma. In 1820, Norris probably described the first family with familial atypical multiple-mole melanoma syndrome (FAMMM). The syndrome has been called several names, including "dysplastic nevus syndrome," "B-K mole syndrome," and "large atypical nevus syndrome." Because these syndromes have not been defined uniformly either clinically or histopathologically, controversy has surrounded their description, inheritance, and predisposition towards melanoma. The number and size of the moles can vary considerably, as well as their associated risk of developing melanoma. The NIH Consensus Conference defined FAMMM as having the following characteristics: (a) the occurrence of malignant melanoma in one or more first- or second-degree relatives, (b) a large number of melanocytic nevi, usually more that 50, some of which are atypical and variable in size, and (c) melanocytic nevi that have certain histopathologic features, which are an asymmetric architectural disorder, subepidermal fibroplasia, and lentiginous melanocytic hyperplasia with spindle or epithelial melanocyte nests (47). The lesions predominantly occur on the trunk, but are also found on the buttocks, scalp, and lower extremities. Previously, the syndrome was believed to have an autosomal dominant inheritance, but a Genetics Analysis Workshop Study Group focusing on melanoma concluded this was not the case (48). They also found that the most difficult issue in the analysis of this syndrome was the definition of affected individuals. The increased risk for developing melanoma in the presence of FAMMM is significant, but has not been well established. The relative risk based on nine studies of patients with atypical moles ranged from 1.6 to 70, but most studies found the range to be from 5 to 11 when multiple atypical moles were present (49).

The diverse clinical and histopathologic definitions of FAMMM have also made cloning the genes by linkage analysis difficult. Initial studies pointed to a gene on the short arm of chromosome 1. Four independent studies since have shown no linkage to this area. Overwhelming evidence based on linkage, cytogenetic studies, and LOH, has implicated the region

9p21 as having at least one tumor suppressor gene related to melanoma. Approximately half of all kindreds have germ-line mutations in this area. Germ-line mutations in 13 of 18 kindreds were found in a cell cycle gene, CDKN2, also called p16 (50). CDNK2 encodes a 16-kd protein (p16INK4), which inhibits cyclin-dependent kinase 4 (CDK4). Normally, CDK4 combines with cyclin and phosphorylates the retinoblastoma (Rb) protein. This releases Rb-bound transcription factors necessary for the transition from the G1 to the S phase in the cell cycle. When p16INK4 binds to CDK4, Rb does not become phosphorylated, thus keeping the cell in G1. Knocking out CDKN2 removes a brake on the cell cycle leading to uncontrolled cell growth. Another candidate for a 9p tumor suppressor gene is p15 INK4B, which is located close to the CDKN2 gene and has structural and functional homology. Abnormalities in 9p have been found in a high number of dysplastic nevi as well as melanomas, suggesting it plays an early role in tumor development. The penetrance of melanomas in three 9p kindreds was calculated to be 53% by age 80 (51). Gene carriers that developed melanoma were found to have more sun exposure than those that did not develop melanoma suggesting environmental and other genetic factors may be involved.

Screening

Presently, testing for CDKN2 is not available at a commercial level. There are several measures that should be taken for members of FAMMM kindreds and others with a strong family history of malignant melanoma (49). These patients should have physical examinations yearly, which should include a total cutaneous exam where they are completely undressed. In a prospective study of patients with atypical moles, the only melanomas found greater that 0.76-mm-thick were those in patients who did not have routine skin examinations (52). Screening should begin around puberty. A recent study found the median age for melanoma diagnosis was 34 for 19 9p kindreds. For patients who have a large number of moles, baseline photographs may be helpful. Patients should examine their own skin regularly. Suspicious lesions should undergo biopsy. Regular ophthalmologic examinations should also be a part of their care, since there is an increased risk of ocular nevi and ocular melanoma. Sun exposure should be avoided. Other malignancies have been related to mutations in the CDKN2 gene, especially pancreatic cancer (53,54).

Kidney Cancer

The kidney is host to several forms of hereditary cancer including three types of renal carcinoma—those associated with VHL, hereditary clear cell renal carcinoma (HCRC) (also called "hereditary renal carcinoma"), and hereditary papillary renal carcinoma (HPRC)—as well as Wilms' tumor—an embryonic malignancy arising from immature kidney remnants in children. Estimates are that up to 4% of adult renal carcinomas are familial. Histologically, the most common type of renal carcinoma is clear cell, while the pap-

illary variant represents a small subset (5% to 15%). VHL patients develop exclusively clear cell renal carcinoma.

The first clues to a gene responsible for renal carcinoma came from a kindred with multifocal clear cell carcinoma who had a translocation from the short arm of chromosome 3 (3p) to chromosome 8. Translocations of 3p have been shown to be a common trait of these kindreds. Loss of heterozygosity (LOH) of 3p has been found in 90% of all sporadic renal carcinomas, but not in papillary renal carcinomas, strongly suggesting the presence of a tumor suppressor gene for nonpapillary cancer in this area. The VHL gene was subsequently localized on 3p25-p26, cloned (55), and found to be mutated frequently (more than 50%) in sporadic clear cell renal carcinomas (56). No mutations in the VHL gene have been found in papillary renal cell carcinomas. Despite frequent 3p deletions in other types of cancers, VHL mutations have not been found in other sporadic tumors, including pheochromocytomas, lung, ovarian, colon, or bladder cancers.

Von Hippel–Lindau Disease

VHL is an autosomal dominant inherited familial cancer syndrome in which benign and malignant tumors develop in a variety of organs. Organs involved include the kidneys, brain, spine, eyes, adrenal glands, pancreas, inner ear, and epididymis. The penetrance of the VHL gene is about 90% by age 65, with the mean age at diagnosis being 26 years. Maher (57) found the frequency of the different tumors to be 59% for retinal hemangioblastomas, 59% for cerebellar hemangioblastomas, 28% for renal cell carcinomas, 13% for spinal hemangioblastomas, and 7% for pheochromocytomas. The median age for diagnosis of retinal hemangioblastomas (25.4 years) and of cerebellar hemangioblastomas (29 years) was significantly less than that for renal cell carcinomas (44 years). Multiple, bilateral renal cysts are also common, with up to 75% of VHL patients developing cysts, tumors, or both. Pancreatic and epididymal cysts can also occur and are usually asymptomatic. The number of renal cysts can be greater than 1,000, with up to 600 clear cell carcinomas. Tumors can even be found growing inside renal cysts. The cancers have been found to metastasize in up to 40% of untreated patients. The life span of VHL patients seems to be shortened, with renal cell carcinoma and cerebellar hemangioblastomas being the most common cause of death.

The function of the VHL protein appears to be the regulation of the transcription of DNA to mRNA by RNA polymerase II. Normally, the VHL product binds to two subunits (elongin B and C), which prevents them from binding elongin A. The conglomerate of elongin A, B, and C activates RNA polymerase II. By mutating VHL, transcription proceeds without one of its controls. VHL has also been proposed to regulate vascularization by altering the stability of vascular endothelial growth factor (VEGF).

There is extensive clinical variation of the disease, and several investigations have examined the correlation between genotype and phenotype. Crossey (58) found that greater than

80% of kindreds with pheochromocytomas had missense mutations, compared to 25% of families without pheochromocytomas. Mutations causing a truncation of the protein were much more common in kindreds without pheochromocytomas than those with them. Other studies have found a specific mutation to be correlated with a phenotype having pheochromocytomas, but not renal cell carcinomas. This discovery has led to classifying VHL into different types based on phenotypes. In type I, pheochromocytomas do not occur. In type 2A, pheochromocytomas are present, but renal cell carcinomas do not occur, while in type 2B, both pheochromocytomas and renal cell carcinomas occur. This classification may prove to be helpful in presymptomatic counseling and screening.

Screening and Management

The management of VHL patients requires a multidisciplinary approach. Direct testing of the gene as well as prenatal testing is possible in a handful of centers. This enables physicians to tailor presymptomatic screening. Renal cysts should be regarded as potentially malignant, particularly any solid or rapidly growing areas, since their epithelial lining can undergo malignant transformation. Because renal cell carcinomas in VHL are usually bilateral and multiple, nephron-sparing surgery is the treatment of choice to preserve as much renal function as possible (59). The rate of recurrence is 40% to 50%, necessitating close follow-up. Renal transplantation has also been used successfully for extensive disease. Retinal hemangioblastoma frequently are symptomatic and are usually controlled with laser treatment. Therefore, regular examinations by an ophthalmologist can lower the risk of blindness. Spinal and cerebellar hemagioblastomas should be removed so that functional damage does not occur. Pheochromocytomas should be removed when discovered.

Hereditary Clear Cell Renal Carcinoma

HCRC is characterized by the early onset of clear cell carcinomas that are often bilateral or multifocal. This disorder is fairly rare and not well understood. A common characteristic of these kindreds is a translocation of part of chromosome 3p, which is more proximal than the VHL gene. As opposed to VHL, HCRC does not have a predilection for the development of other tumors, suggesting that another gene besides VHL is responsible.

Hereditary Papillary Renal Carcinoma

HPRC was only recognized as a distinct form of familial renal carcinoma in 1994. HPRC is characterized by the development of multiple, bilateral papillary renal cell carcinomas. Based on an investigation of 10 kindreds, the median age of survival is 52 years (60). The carcinomas were often detected incidentally in asymptomatic patients or during screening of asymptomatic patients. None of the kindreds have VHL or other 3p mutations, suggesting the role of a distinct gene. Recently, the MET protooncogene on chromosome 7q31-34 was found to be the predisposition gene (61). The MET protooncogene encodes a transmembrane tyrosine kinase receptor which is activated by hepatocyte growth factor and induces cellular proliferation, motility, and invasiveness. This receptor has been found to be overexpressed in a variety of cancers (62,63). The gene is similar to the RET protooncogene, and its mutations are homologous to those seen in RET, suggesting that they cause constitutive activation of the protein. The RET and MET genes are the only known protooncogenes to cause a human inherited cancer syndrome by gain-of-function mutations, as compared to other syndromes which are caused by loss-of-function mutations in tumor suppressor genes.

Wilms' tumor

Wilms' tumor, or nephroblastoma, is the most common intraabdominal solid tumor in children. The peak incidence occurs at age 3 to 4 years. Bilateral tumors occur in 5% to 10% of cases, with the peak incidence of these cases occurring between age 2 and 3. Most tumors are sporadic, with one percent being inherited. There are three distinct syndromes which have a genetic predisposition to Wilms' tumor: WAGR Syndrome (**W**ilms' tumor, **A**nirida [a congenital abnormality of the iris], **G**enitourinary malformations, and mental **R**etardation), Denys-Drash dsyndrome (DDS) and Beckwith-Wiedemann syndrome (BWS), as well as a familial form that lacks any other associated conditions. The first gene linked to Wilms' tumor was discovered through the investigations of the WAGR syndrome. Within this syndrome there is a greater than 30% chance of developing a Wilms' tumor. Karyotypic analysis of patients with WAGR found deletions in chromosome 11q13. This deletion has been found to encompass several genes, including PAX6, which causes aniridia, and WT1, which is a Wilms' tumor suppressor gene. While loss of only one allele of the PAX6, gene causes aniridia, both alleles of WT1 must be mutated in order for a Wilms' tumor to develop. The product of WT1 contains four "zinc finger" domains, indicating a possible role as a transcription factor. The genes which WT1 may help regulate are not known. The tissue distribution of WT1 expression is limited, unlike some other tumor suppressor genes, such as p53 and Rb, which are found throughout the body. Renal expression is limited to blastemal cells, renal vesicles, and glomerular epithelium, and peaks at birth only to fall rapidly with age. WT1 expression is also found in mesothelial cells, Sertoli cells of the testis, and granulosa cells of the ovary. WT1 mutations are found only in 10% of sporadic cases of Wilms' tumors implying that other genes are involved. Another gene has already been named WT2 and lies in the 11p15 area.

DDS is characterized by Wilms' tumors, mesangial sclerosis leading to progressive renal failure, and ambiguous genitalia. The severity of the genital anomalies is highly variable, and there can be phenotypic overlap with WAGR. Germ-line point mutations in the WT1 gene can be found in most DDS patients (64).

BWS is characterized by overgrowth, congenital malformations (especially omphalocele), and a predisposition to embryonic malignancies, the most common of which is Wilms' tumor. The overgrowth can involve half the body in the form of hemihyperplasia, or it can be regional, such as of an extremity or certain organs like the tongue, kidneys, pancreas, adrenal cortex, and liver. Patients with hemihyperplasia appear to have a greater risk for malignancy (12.5%). Besides Wilms' tumors, other cancers include hepatoblastoma, neuroblastoma, rhabdomyosarcoma, and adrenocortical carcinoma. BWS is usually sporadic, but when inherited it follows an autosomal dominant pattern with variable penetrance. The genetic locus for BWS has been narrowed to chromosome 11p15, with a subset of these patients having chromosomal duplication. Presently it is unclear whether the gene causing BWS is WT2. BWS is a genetically heterogeneous disorder, probably affected by imprinting from different methylation patterns from the paternal and maternal allele (65).

Finally, Wilms' tumor can be familial without any of the associated syndromes. Little is known about the genetics of this disorder except that it is heterogeneic. WT1 as well as 11p15 have been excluded as possible candidate loci.

Screening and Management

The best method for surveillance for patients with a predisposition to Wilms' tumor is with abdominal ultrasound. Generally, it is agreed that the examinations should occur every 3 months until age 5 to 7 (66). A baseline abdominal CT should be performed in those patients at risk for other malignancies. Genetic testing is only available at a few centers and is done largely on a research basis, but it can be helpful in identifying a high-risk individual. In the presence of aniridia, genetic evaluation can distinguish whether only the PAX6 gene has a mutation, or if the WT1 gene is also deleted. The treatment of Wilms' tumor consists of resection for local control and chemotherapy for most patients, and radiation therapy for advanced disease. Generally, Wilms' tumors have a cure rate greater than 80%.

Pancreatic Cancer

Because of the fairly high incidence of pancreatic cancer and its extremely high mortality rate, discovering genes that predispose to pancreatic cancer could provide a significant improvement in health care. Genetic factors are thought to play a role in 3% to 5% of all pancreatic cancers (67). There are several inherited syndromes that have pancreatic cancer as a component of their disorder, including hereditary pancreatitis, FAMMM, HNPCC, and possibly AT. Endocrine pancreatic tumors are seen in MEN type 1 (reviewed earlier), but this section will focus on pancreatic adenocarcinomas. There have also been reports of familial pancreatic cancer which is not related to any other syndrome.

Inherited pancreatitis usually affects individuals at an early age (frequently in childhood) with recurrent episodes of pancreatitis. Affected patients often develop the sequelae of chronic pancreatitis, namely diabetes, pancreatic insufficiency, and pseudocysts, and can also develop portal and splenic vein thrombosis. The syndrome is transmitted in an autosomal dominant fashion by an unknown gene. The prevalence of pancreatic cancer was found to be 20% in 21 kindreds (68). This is a higher rate of pancreatic cancer than found in individuals with pancreatitis for other reasons. The longer period of time for which the patients with the inherited form of pancreatitis are exposed to this insult may account for this difference. Presently, it is unknown whether the increased risk of pancreatic cancer is due to a genetic susceptibility or if it is due to the pancreatitis itself.

FAMMM (previously described) has been known to have a higher incidence of other cancers besides malignant melanoma. This syndrome has been linked to the gene CDKN2 on chromosome 9p. Some of those families with increased risk of pancreatic cancer have germ-line mutations in this gene (54). Studies have shown that kindreds with mutations in this gene which affect the function of its protein, p16, have a greater risk of pancreatic cancer by a factor of 13 to 22 than those kindreds with mutations that do not affect the gene product function (53). In sporadic pancreatic tumors this genetic region was found to be lost in 85% of the cases, suggesting that this gene plays an important role in all pancreatic cancers (69).

CONCLUSIONS

Inherited cancer syndromes have provided tremendous insight into the genetics of cancer. This understanding has translated into elucidating the mechanisms of sporadic cancer as well as improved treatment for those with familial cancer. A new paradigm in surgery has emerged: the recommendation that an operation be performed based on the results of a genetic test. Surgeons must now face a number of related, and sometimes unfamiliar, issues related to genetic testing: ethics, confidentiality, liability, and insurance coverage. It is an exciting and challenging time for clinicians involved in care of these patients. The field of inherited cancer susceptibility is growing so rapidly that it is impossible for a book to provide the most current information. New predisposition genes are constantly being isolated; therefore, enlisting the input of a genetic counselor can help keep one abreast of the changing field. Overall, genetic testing with appropriate genetic counseling adds considerable strength to the surgeon's armamentarium in their treatment of cancer.

REFERENCES

1. Herrera L, Kakati S, Gibas L, Pietrzak E, Sandberg AA. Gardner syndrome in a man with an interstitial deletion of 5q. *Am J Med Genet* 1986;25:473.
2. Giardiello FM, Brensinger JD, Petersen GM, et al. The use and interpretation of commercial APC gene testing for familial adenomatous polyposis. *N Engl J Med* 1997;336:823.
3. Radford DM, Zehnbauer BA. Inherited breast cancer [Review]. *Surg Clin North Am* 1996;76:205.

4. Miki Y, Swensen J, Shattuck-Eidens D, et al. A strong candidate for the breast and ovarian cancer susceptibility gene BRCA1. *Science* 1994; 266:66.

5. Wooster R, Bignell G, Lancaster J, et al. Identification of the breast cancer susceptibility gene BRCA2. *Nature* 1995;378:789. [For erratum, see *Nature* 1996;379:749.]

6. Easton DF, Ford D, Bishop DT. Breast and ovarian cancer incidence in BRCA1-mutation carriers. Breast Cancer Linkage Consortium. *Am J Hum Genet* 1995;56:265.

7. Struewing JP, Hartge P, Wacholder S, et al. The risk of cancer associated with specific mutations of BRCA1 and BRCA2 among Ashkenazi Jews. *N Engl J Med* 1997;336:1401.

8. Rubin SC, Benjamin I, Behbakht K, et al. Clinical and pathological features of ovarian cancer in women with germ-line mutations of BRCA1. *N Engl J Med* 1996;335:1413.

9. Couch FJ, DeShano ML, Blackwood MA, et al. BRCA1 mutations in women attending clinics that evaluate the risk of breast cancer. *N Engl J Med* 1997;336:1409.

10. Schrag D, Kuntz KM, Garber JE, Weeks JC. Decision analysis—effects of prophylactic mastectomy and oophorectomy on life expectancy among women with BRCA1 or BRCA2 mutations. *N Engl J Med* 1997;336:1465. [For erratum, see *N Engl J Med* 1997;337:434.]

11. Frebourg T, Barbier N, Yan YX, et al. Germ-line p53 mutations in 15 families with Li-Fraumeni syndrome. *Am J Hum Genet* 1995;56:608.

12. Liaw D, Marsh DJ, Li J, et al. Germline mutations of the PTEN gene in Cowden disease, an inherited breast and thyroid cancer syndrome. *Nat Genet* 1997;16:64.

13. Athma P, Rappaport R, Swift M. Molecular genotyping shows that ataxia-telangiectasia heterozygotes are predisposed to breast cancer. *Cancer Genet Cytogenet* 1996;92:130.

14. FitzGerald MG, Bean JM, Hegde SR, et al. Heterozygous ATM mutations do not contribute to early onset of breast cancer. *Nat Genet* 1997;15:307.

15. Houlston RS, Collins A, Slack J, Morton NE. Dominant genes for colorectal cancer are not rare. *Ann Hum Genet* 1992;56:99.

16. Laken SJ, Petersen GM, Gruber SB, et al. Familial colorectal cancer in Ashkenazim due to a hypermutable tract in APC. *Nat Genet* 1997;17:79.

17. Kinzler KW, Nilbert MC, Su LK, et al. Identification of FAP locus genes from chromosome 5q21. *Science* 1991;253:661.

18. Groden J, Thliveris A, Samowitz W, et al. Identification and characterization of the familial adenomatous polyposis coli gene. *Cell* 1991; 66:589.

19. Kinzler KW, Vogelstein B. Lessons from hereditary colorectal cancer [Review]. *Cell* 1996;87:159.

20. Iwama T, Mishima Y. Factors affecting the risk of rectal cancer following rectum-preserving surgery in patients with familial adenomatous polyposis. *Dis Colon Rectum* 1994;37:1024.

21. Ambroze WL Jr, Orangio GR, Lucas G. Surgical options for familial adenomatous polyposis [Review]. *Semin Surg Oncol* 1995;11:423.

22. Debinski HS, Spigelman AD, Hatfield A, Williams CB, Phillips RK. Upper intestinal surveillance in familial adenomatous polyposis. *Eur J Cancer* 1995;31A:1149.

23. Lynch HT, Smyrk T, Watson P, et al. Hereditary colorectal cancer [Review]. *Semin Oncol* 1991;18:337.

24. Rodriguez-Bigas MA, Mahoney MC, Karakousis CP, Petrelli NJ. Desmoid tumors in patients with familial adenomatous polyposis. *Cancer* 1994;74:1270.

25. Lynch HT, Smyrk T, Lynch J, Fitzgibbons R Jr, Lanspa S, McGinn T. Update on the differential diagnosis, surveillance and management of hereditary non-polyposis colorectal cancer [Review]. *Eur J Cancer* 1995;31A:1039.

26. Lengauer C, Kinzler KW, Vogelstein B. Genetic instability in colorectal cancers. *Nature* 1997;386:623.

27. Honchel R, Halling KC, Schaid DJ, Pittelkow M, Thibodeau SN. Microsatellite instability in Muir-Torre syndrome. *Cancer Res* 1994;54: 1159.

28. Bapat B, Xia L, Madlensky L, et al. The genetic basis of Muir-Torre syndrome includes the hMLH1 locus [Letter]. *Am J Hum Genet* 1996;59: 736.

29. Spigelman AD, Murday V, Phillips RK. Cancer and the Peutz-Jeghers syndrome. *Gut* 1989;30:1588.

30. Reid JD. Intestinal carcinoma in the Peutz-Jeghers syndrome. *JAMA* 1974;229:833.

31. Chandrasekharappa SC, Guru SC, Manickam P, et al. Positional cloning of the gene for multiple endocrine neoplasia type 1. *Science* 1997; 276:404.

32. Wells SA Jr, Farndon JR, Dale JK, Leight GS, Dilley WG. Long-term evaluation of patients with primary parathyroid hyperplasia managed by total parathyroidectomy and heterotopic autotransplantation. *Ann Surg* 1980;192:451.

33. Mulligan LM, Kwok JB, Healy CS, et al. Germ-line mutations of the RET protooncogene in multiple endocrine neoplasia type 2A. *Nature* 1993;363:458.

34. Donis-Keller H, Dou S, Chi D, et al. Mutations in the RET proto-oncogene are associated with MEN 2A and FMTC. *Hum Mol Genet* 1993;2:851.

35. Goodfellow PJ, Wells SA Jr. RET gene and its implications for cancer [Review]. *J Natl Cancer Inst* 1995;87:1515.

36. Wells SA Jr, Baylin SB, Linehan WM, Farrel RE, Cox EB, Cooper CW. Provocative agents and the diagnosis of medullary carcinoma of the thyroid gland. *Ann Surg* 1978;188:139.

37. Wells SA Jr, Chi DD, Toshima K, et al. Predictive DNA testing and prophylactic thyroidectomy in patients at risk for multiple endocrine neoplasia type 2A. *Ann Surg* 1994;220:237.

38. Wells SA Jr, Moley JF, DeBenedetti MK, Skinner MA. Prophylactic thyroidectomy in patients with MEN 2A and familial medullary thyroid carcinoma. Presented at the Sixth International Workshop on Multiple Endocrine Neoplasia and Von Hippel–Lindau Disease, Leeuwenhorst Congress Center, Noordwijkerhout, The Netherlands, 1997.

39. Szabo J, Heath B, Hill VM, et al. Hereditary hyperparathyroidism-jaw tumor syndrome: the endocrine tumor gene HRPT2 maps to chromosome 1q21-q31. *Am J Hum Genet* 1995;56:944.

40. Kawai A, Noguchi M, Beppu Y, et al. Nuclear immunoreaction of p53 protein in soft tissue sarcomas. A possible prognostic factor. *Cancer* 1994;73:2499.

41. Goldberg Y, Dibbern K, Klein J, Riccardi VM, Graham JM Jr. Neurofibromatosis type 1—an update and review for the primary pediatrician [Review]. *Clin Pediatr* 1996;35:545.

42. Riccardi VM, Powell PP. Neurofibrosarcoma as a complication of von Recklinghausen neurofibromatosis [Review]. *Neurofibromatosis* 1989;2:152.

43. Wallace MR, Marchuk DA, Andersen LB, et al. Type 1 neurofibromatosis gene: identification of a large transcript disrupted in three NF1 patients. *Science* 1990;249:181. [For erratum, see *Science* 1990;250: 1749.]

44. Cawthon RM, Weiss R, Xu GF, et al. A major segment of the neurofibromatosis type 1 gene: cDNA sequence, genomic structure, and point mutations. *Cell* 1990;62:193. [For erratum, see *Cell* 1990;62: after p. 608.]

45. Rouleau GA, Merel P, Lutchman M, et al. Alteration in a new gene encoding a putative membrane-organizing protein causes neurofibromatosis type 2. *Nature* 1993;363:515.

46. Trofatter JA, MacCollin MM, Rutter JL, et al. A novel moesin-, ezrin-, radixin-like gene is a candidate for the neurofibromatosis 2 tumor suppressor. *Cell* 1993;75:826.

47. Anonymous. NIH Consensus conference. Diagnosis and treatment of early melanoma [Review]. *JAMA* 1992;268:1314.

48. Risch N, Sherman S. Genetic Analysis Workshop 7: summary of the melanoma workshop. *Cytogenet Cell Genet* 1992;59:148.

49. Slade J, Marghoob AA, Salopek TG, Rigel DS, Kopf AW, Bart RS. Atypical mole syndrome: risk factor for cutaneous malignant melanoma and implications for management [Review]. *J Am Acad Dermatol* 1995;32:479.

50. Hussussian CJ, Struewing JP, Goldstein AM, et al. Germline p16 mutations in familial melanoma. *Nat Genet* 1994;8:15.

51. Cannon-Albright LA, Kamb A, Skolnick M. A review of inherited predisposition to melanoma [Review]. *Semin Oncol* 1996;23:667.

52. Tucker MA, Fraser MC, Goldstein AM, Elder DE, Guerry D IV, Organic SM. Risk of melanoma and other cancers in melanoma-prone families. *J Invest Dermatol* 1993;100:350S.

53. Goldstein AM, Fraser MC, Struewing JP, et al. Increased risk of pancreatic cancer in melanoma-prone kindreds with p16INK4 mutations. *N Engl J Med* 1995;333:970.

54. Whelan AJ, Bartsch D, Goodfellow PJ. Brief report: a familial syndrome of pancreatic cancer and melanoma with a mutation in the CDKN2 tumor-suppressor gene. *N Engl J Med* 1995;333:975.

55. Latif F, Tory K, Gnarra J, et al. Identification of the von Hippel–Lindau disease tumor suppressor gene. *Science* 1993;260:1317.
56. Gnarra JR, Tory K, Weng Y, et al. Mutations of the VHL tumour suppressor gene in renal carcinoma. *Nat Genet* 1994;7:85.
57. Maher ER, Yates JR, Harries R, et al. Clinical features and natural history of von Hippel–Lindau disease. *Q J Med* 1990;77:1151.
58. Crossey PA, Richards FM, Foster K, et al. Identification of intragenic mutations in the von Hippel–Lindau disease tumour suppressor gene and correlation with disease phenotype. *Hum Mol Genet* 1994;3: 1303.
59. Steinbach F, Novick AC, Zincke H, et al. Treatment of renal cell carcinoma in von Hippel–Lindau disease: a multicenter study. *J Urol* 1995;153:1812.
60. Zbar B, Glenn G, Lubensky I, et al. Hereditary papillary renal cell carcinoma: clinical studies in 10 families [Review]. *J Urol* 1995;153:907.
61. Schmidt L, Duh FM, Chen F, et al. Germline and somatic mutations in the tyrosine kinase domain of the MET proto-oncogene in papillary renal carcinomas. *Nat Genet* 1997;16:68.
62. Di Renzo MF, Olivero M, Katsaros D, et al. Overexpression of the Met/HGF receptor in ovarian cancer. *Int J Cancer* 1994;58:658.
63. Ferracini R, Di Renzo MF, Scotlandi K, et al. The Met/HGF receptor is over-expressed in human osteosarcomas and is activated by either a paracrine or an autocrine circuit. *Oncogene* 1995;10:739.
64. Coppes MJ, Huff V, Pelletier J. Denys-Drash syndrome: relating a clinical disorder to genetic alterations in the tumor suppressor gene WT1. *J Pediatr* 1993;123:673.
65. Weksberg R, Squire JA. Molecular biology of Beckwith-Wiedemann syndrome [Review]. *Med Pediatr Oncol* 1996;27:462.
66. Clericuzio CL, Johnson C. Screening for Wilms' tumor in high-risk individuals [Review]. *Hematol Oncol Clin North Am* 1995;9:1253.
67. Lynch HT, Smyrk T, Kern SE, et al. Familial pancreatic cancer: a review [Review]. *Semin Oncol* 1996;23:251.
68. Kattwinkel J, Lapey A, Di Sant'Agnese PA, Edwards WA. Hereditary pancreatitis: three new kindreds and a critical review of the literature. *Pediatrics* 1973;51:55.
69. Caldas C, Hahn SA, da Costa LT, et al. Frequent somatic mutations and homozygous deletions of the p16 (MTS1) gene in pancreatic adeno-carcinoma. *Nat Genet* 1994;8:27. [For erratum, see *Nat Genet* 1994;8:410.]
70. Hall JM, Lee MK, Newman B, et al. Linkage of early-onset familial breast cancer to chromosome 17q21. *Science* 1990; 250:1684.
71. Hemminki A, Markie D, Tomlinson E, et al. A serine/threonine kinase gene defective in Peutz-Jeghers syndrome. *Nature* 1998: 391:184.
72. Howe JR, Roth S, Ringold JC, et al. Mutations in the SMAD4/DPC4 gene in juvenile polyposis [comment in: *Science* 1998: 280:1036]. *Science* 1998; 280:1086.

CHAPTER 2

New Approaches in the Preoperative Staging for Gastrointestinal and Abdominal Malignancies

Frederick L. Greene

The approach to effective cancer management by the general surgeon must be based on complete staging of gastrointestinal (GI) and abdominal malignancy preoperatively. This information will not only assist in making appropriate decisions for surgical management but, more importantly, will direct the surgeon and other members of the cancer management team to alternative methods of treatment that might improve quality of life and potential outcome for the patient. Since the mid-1980s, a worldwide agreement to use the TNM system has assured that a common language is spoken among all of those who care for cancer patients (1). Proper surgical management is based on using clinical information derived from taking appropriate histories, by performing adequate examinations, and through the use of appropriate imaging studies. The extent of local and regional disease as well as the possibility of diffuse metastases may be assessed by using appropriate preoperative modalities, and information from these studies must be in place before surgical decision making is finalized.

Identification of tumors involving the abdominal cavity is readily assessed using conventional contrast radiographic techniques, computerized tomography (CT), magnetic resonance imaging (MRI), and percutaneous ultrasound (US). The use of these modalities has traditionally given information that is valuable to the operative surgeon. A recent enhancement of CT, such as spiral CT, has enabled an increased sensitivity in assessing for abdominal and thoracic malignancy. In some centers, positron emission tomography (PET) scanning has proven to be particularly enlightening in the identification of small hepatic metastases (2). Because of economic and logistical necessities, however, PET scanning is today only rarely used, but it may become a more common imaging technique in the future assessment of cancer.

The most exciting concepts in preoperative staging are those relating to intraoperative ultrasound (IOU) and endoluminal ultrasound (EUS), as well as the use of laparoscopy for preoperative abdominal assessment in the management of a variety of tumors. These techniques used either alone or in combination have a high sensitivity and selectivity for cancers of the GI tract and hepatobiliary anatomy.

ENDOSCOPIC ULTRASOUND

Endoscopic US may be effectively used to stage esophagogastric (3), pancreatic (4), and colorectal (5) tumors. Since staging is based on depth of tumor penetration in the GI tract, EUS is an ideal tool for preoperative assessment and may be much more sensitive than traditional CT or percutaneous US imaging. By placing the US transducer inside the GI tract, interference and artifacts caused by bone and soft tissue in the chest and abdominal wall from pulmonary and intestinal gas are largely eliminated (6). EUS uses higher frequencies than percutaneous US. These frequencies are usually in the range of 7.5 to 20 MHz. EUS is based on instrumentation that is a combination of both an endoscope and an US probe. This technology uses rotating transducers with variable frequencies. A 360-degree rotation is produced, which gives a circumferential evaluation of the GI tract. Evaluation of images produced by EUS may be initially difficult and should be evaluated as a team by the surgeon and his or her GI endoscopic colleague. It is important for the surgeon to understand endoscopic US images as currently necessitated in evaluation using percutaneous US techniques. The involvement of the sonographer from the Department of Diagnostic Radiology may be important in the interpretation of the images obtained during EUS.

Using EUS at 7.5 to 12 MHz frequency, the wall of the GI tract can be imaged as a five-layered structure of alternating bright (hyperechoic) and dark (hypoechoic) bands (Fig. 2-1). The first two inner layers correspond to the superficial and deep mucosae; the third layer to the submucosa; the fourth to the muscularis propria; and the fifth to the serosa or adventitia. Using EUS to stage GI cancers, especially those of the esophagus and gastric wall, frequencies of 7.5 to 12 MHz have been employed. Preoperative assessment of tumors of the foregut may be enhanced using EUS and give an indication of depth of tumor penetration as well as nodal involvement in these

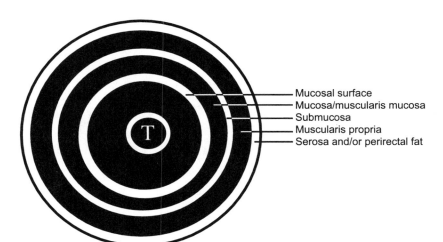

FIG. 2-1. Five-layer anatomic model for interpretation of endorectal ultrasonographic scans. Three echogenic *(white lines)* and two echo-poor, or hypoechoic *(dark lines)*, are visualized.

tumors. The greatest strength of EUS lies in its ability to image the wall of the GI tract in greater detail than any other current method (7). The diagnosis of esophageal or gastric cancer is based on upper GI endoscopy and biopsy. EUS is limited in its ability to distinguish between neoplastic tissue and inflammation or fibrosis. EUS may become beneficial in detecting minute submucosal cancer, such as seen in Barrett's esophagus (8). The technology of EUS must be improved before routine dysplastic lesions are identified. EUS cannot be used to definitively differentiate benign from malignant ulcers. Routine GI endoscopy and biopsy must be performed for diagnostic evaluation in such a patient. In the evaluation of esophageal cancer, EUS is highly accurate in determining depth of primary cancer invasion or the T-stage. Combined results in the staging of esophageal cancer in 739 patients from 14 centers showed an overall accuracy of 85% (9). In staging regional nodal disease, overall accuracy was 79%. The most difficult stage of esophageal tumor to identify by EUS was T2 cancer. EUS has been valuable in differentiating early stage (T1 to T2) from later stage (T3 to T4) tumors. Currently, EUS may not be totally reliable in differentiating benign lymph nodes frm malignant nodes. The size of the imaged lymph node may be an unreliable criterion of malignancy. Malignant nodes tend to be rounded, sharply defined and hypoechoic compared with benign nodes that tend to be elongated, or hazy in outline and more echogenic. Catalano et al. (10) studied preoperative endosonographic features thought to characterize lymph node metastases in 100 patients with esophageal carcinoma. The likelihood of N1 disease was 86% when lymph nodes were imaged. When no lymph nodes were noted on EUS, the likelihood of N0 disease was 79%. In this study, N1 disease could be predicted with 100% accuracy when a hypoechoic echo pattern, sharply demarcated borders, rounded contour, and size greater than 10 mm. were noted. More recently, the opportunity to perform fine-needle aspiration (FNA) using EUS has increased preoperative assessment and diagnosis of involved lymph nodes (11) (Table 2-1). Obviously, EUS is limited when esophageal stenosis is present and the endoscope cannot be passed in this area. Esophageal dilatation before EUS results in more complete examination but adds risk to diagnostic tests and is probably contraindicated. Preoperative staging of gastric cancer, using EUS, has shown that the layers of the stomach are more easily imaged than those of the esophagus. Use of this modality in gastric cancer, however, has been slightly less accurate than when utilized for patients with esophageal cancer. Review of the literature concerning the use

TABLE 2-1. *Endoscopic ultrasound–guided fine-needle aspiration results*

Type of lesion	Patients (n)	Mean lesion size (cm)	Mean no. of passes attempted (range)	Diagnostic accuracy[a]
Mediastinal mass/LN	43	2.1 × 1.8	3.2 (1–8)	41/43, 95%
Pancreatic masses	121	3.4 × 3.3	3.4 (2–9)	103/121, 85%
Submucosal lesions	27	2.8 × 2.7	3.8 (2–8)	22/27, 81%
Perirectal masses	4	3.5 × 4.0	5.3 (2–10)	4/4, 100%
Intraabdominal LN Celiac (n = 7) Peripancreatic (n = 4) Periportal (n = 2)	13	2.9 × 2.8	3.0 (1–5)	11/13, 85%

[a] Diagnostic accuracy is calculated by comparing the EUS-guided FNA cytology results to the final diagnosis based on surgery findings or long-term clinical follow-up.
LN, lymph node.

of EUS for gastric cancer shows a 78% accuracy for the T-stage and a 73% accuracy for assessing nodal status (12). In view of the significant increase in number of cases of adenocarcinoma of the distal esophagus and gastric cardia, EUS may play a greater role in preoperative staging of these lesions. The future use of EUS-guided FNA in preoperative assessment may be especially important when tumors of the distal esophagus and proximal stomach are evaluated. A recent report by Gress et al. (13) of 208 consecutive patients referred for suspected GI or mediastinal masses showed that overall diagnostic accuracy was 87% with a sensitivity of 89% and a specificity of 100%. EUS FNA provided an adequate specimen in 90% of patients. These authors observed immediate complications in four of 208 (2%) patients. These complications consisted of bleeding and pancreatitis in two patients each. The use of EUS-directed aspiration cytology will play an even greater role in the future as this technology becomes more easily performed. The ability to access lymph nodes and masses adjacent to the GI tract will aid in the preoperative assessment and will be important in selecting those patients who may benefit from preoperative radiation or chemotherapy.

There is a significant amount of data which indicates that EUS with or without aspiration cytology is the most accurate means for preoperative T- and N-staging of tumors of the esophagus, stomach, pancreas, and rectum (Figs. 2-2 to 2-4) One important issue is whether EUS-guided FNA could lead to the seeding of tumor cells and the inadvertent spread of malignancy. Percutaneous biopsies using CT have resulted in track seeding although the incidence is low (14). Since EUS-FNA is performed with 22-gauge or smaller needles, the likelihood of seeding is low and no reports of this complication are available to date. Because the portion of the GI tract that is penetrated is usually removed as part of the operative specimen, the issue of seeding may be moot. Long-term follow-up studies are indeed needed to assess whether seeding is an actual or theoretical risk.

Endosonography is technically demanding and the interpretation of EUS images may be difficult. The surgeon and gastroenterologist should institute this technology together in order to more fully assess the patient preoperatively and to identify those patients with GI malignancy whose tumors may not benefit by initial resection. The interpretation of EUS must also be improved by relating all studies to eventual pathologic staging of the specimens. An experienced cytopathologist must also be involved in order to make FNA assessment more meaningful. EUS-guided FNA should only be performed if the results of the biopsy will materially change the patient management. A patient who should undergo surgical resection regardless of the FNA results should certainly not have this procedure performed. The technique may help in assessing patients with mediastinal adenopathy who may not benefit by operative intervention if periesophageal masses show positive tumor. It remains controversial as to whether FNA of mediastinal adenopathy is routinely indicated in the staging of esophageal carcinoma. FNA is indicated when enlarged celiac nodes are identified in patients with squamous cell carcinoma of the esophagus. In these patients, palliation with radiation and chemotherapy may be more productive than surgical resection. In pancreatic cancer, EUS with FNA may help to stage this disease and to rule out patients with advanced local regional disease who are not candidates for curative resection (Table 2-1). EUS-guided FNA has been used for aspiration of pleural or ascitic fluid in the diagnosis of malignant effusions and ascites. Further studies are needed which will confirm the sensitivity and safety of EUS-guided FNA.

Endoscopic US is gaining a large role in the preoperative staging of rectal cancer. Since sphincter-saving procedures are becoming more common, complete preoperative assessment is mandatory to select patients who may avoid a permanent colostomy. Conventional modalities, such as CT and MRI, are accurate for assessing advanced rectal cancer, especially when adjacent organs are invaded. These modalities, however, are unable to distinguish reliably the extent of rectal wall invasion of an early cancer. Similarly, CT is suboptimal in determining lymph node metastasis, and overall ac-

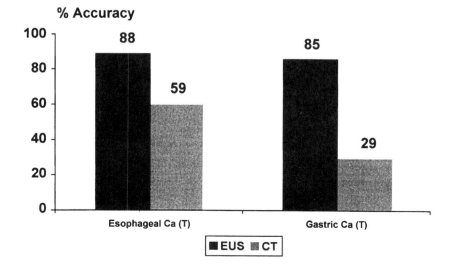

FIG. 2-2. Composite results showing accuracy of staging for depth of invasion (T) for esophageal and gastric cancer, comparing results of EUS and CT in the same patient.

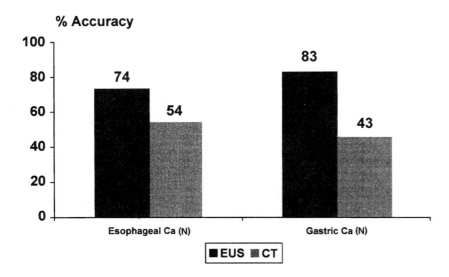

FIG. 2-3. Composite results showing accuracy of staging for regional lymph node metastases *(N)* for esophageal and gastric cancer, comparing results of EUS and CT in the same patient.

curacies of 40% to 45% are reported. Endorectal ultrasonography has proven to be accurate in assessing tumor depth and lymph node involvement (15). As noted in the proximal GI tract, a five-layer structure is identified in the rectum. An ultrasonographic Stage T-1 is a malignant lesion confined to the mucosa and submucosa (Table 2-2). A T2N0 lesion is confined to the rectal wall with invasion but not through the muscularis propria. A T3N0 lesion denotes invasion into the perirectal fat, whereas a T4N0 lesion indicates a lesion invading an adjacent organ such as the prostate, vagina, or bladder. The major advantage of endorectal sonography over other imaging modalities is the ability to determine the depth of bowel wall invasion by the rectal neoplasm. Overall, an 88% accuracy for depth of invasion may be achieved, whereas 4% of patients may be understaged and 8% are overstaged (16). Endorectal US may be effectively used to assess large villous tumors of the rectum. This technique reliably determines whether a villous tumor harbors any areas of invasive malignancy.

Endorectal ultrasonography is proven to be a reliable predictor of lymph node status in patients with rectal cancer (17). The technique demonstrates 82% accuracy, a 70% sensitivity, and an 87% specificity in determining lymph node status (18). Generally, normal lymph nodes and "reactive" nodes are not visualized on ultrasonographic scan. The presence of a hypoechoic lesion in the perirectal region is indicative of a metastatic lymph node. Unfortunately, endorectal sonography cannot differentiate islands of tumor outside of the wall from involved nodes. Lymph node size is of little value in differentiating true positives from reactive nodes.

A number of studies have been performed comparing the efficacy of endorectal sonography, CT scanning, and digital examination in the preoperative staging of rectal cancer (19). Several studies have shown the superiority of endorectal ultrasonography. As the technology of this imaging modality increases, it is anticipated that overall accuracy, especially when compared with traditional imaging studies, will improve. As was true with the esophagus, stenosis preventing

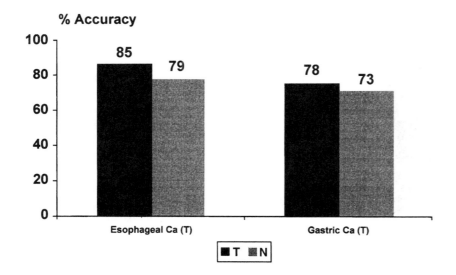

FIG. 2-4. The accuracy of EUS for esophageal and gastric staging for T and N stages where EUS findings were compared with surgical pathology.

TABLE 2–2. *Correlation of AJCC pathologic stage with EUS findings*

Stage	EUS (abnormal)
T1 (mucosa/submucosa)	First three layers
T2 (muscularis propria)	Fourth layer
T3 (through adventitia/serosa)	Fifth layer
T4 (adjacent organ)	Adjacent organ

the advancement of the probe through the rectal lumen is a limitation of the procedure. Lesions of the upper rectum are less easily examined than distal or mid-rectal lesions. As is true with EUS of the upper GI tract, endorectal US has a steep learning curve and requires pathologic confirmation of US findings to help the learning process. In addition to its role in preoperative staging of rectal cancer, endorectal ultrasonography will play an increasing role in the follow-up of patients undergoing resection of rectal cancer.

RADIOLABELED MONOCLONAL ANTIBODY IMAGING

The aim of preoperative assessment is to identify by any means possible the likelihood of distant metastases, especially in solid organs or the retroperitoneum. Although conventional imaging techniques are important in this goal, using information about the biology of a tumor will enhance the opportunity of identifying early and potentially resectable distant foci of disease.

Radioimmunoscintigraphy (RIT) involves the injection of radioactively labeled antibody raised against tumor or tumor byproduct followed by external imaging with a nuclear gamma camera to localize primary and metastatic deposits in patients with carcinoma. This modality has been used to assess a variety of neoplasms but may be quite useful in the assessment of staging of colorectal cancers. Current trials have confirmed the relative safety of intravenous administration of murine monoclonal antibodies to patients (20). Clinical utility of this relatively newer technique in the management of patients with colon and rectal cancer has been supported. From the initial studies in the late 1940s (21), it has become clear that a variety of isotopes may be injected which selectively bind to tumor protein. Radiolabeled antibodies to fibrin or fibrinogen may also be used. A particular pitfall noted in using fibrin is that this substance is known to be present in tumors as a result of the inflammatory process which accompanies tumor invasion. Using fibrin as a marker may thus reduce the specificity and decrease the effective staging using this modality. Since the discovery of carcinoembryonic antigen (CEA) in 1964, a variety of markers have been used that selectively bond to CEA (22). The presence of CEA in primary and metastatic tumors is of paramount importance for successful tumor visualization. More recently, monoclonal antibodies have been labeled with I-123 instead of I-131 (23). The administration of larger scanning doses is possible with I-123, permitting imaging at 6 to 12 h after administration. Delaloye et al. (24) re-

ported 23 of 24 primary tumors or local recurrences of colorectal cancers that were detected with anti-CEA monoclonal antibody. The short half-life of the I-123 system does not permit protracted and delayed imaging of suspected lesions. Recently, the use of indium-111 has been found to enhance the results with isotopic staging (25). The current work with anti-TAG-72 monoclonal antibody B72.3 has been shown to further enhance the benefit of this technique. In a pilot study of 15 patients with metastases from colorectal cancers, 18 of 20 lesions, including lymph node metastases, 1.5 cm or less were imaged (20). The smallest lymph node detected measured 1.3 cm, and the identification was confirmed by CT scan performed 6 months later. These studies show that only 25% of liver metastases were seen as areas of increased concentration of radiolabeled antibody. Monoclonal antibody B72.3 is a murine IgG that was prepared using a membrane-enriched extract of human breast carcinoma metastasis to the liver (26). This antibody recognizes a mucin-like substance known as tumor-associated glycoprotein (TAG-72). TAG-72 is expressed in several epithelial-derived malignancies, including 85% of colonic adenocarcinomas, 70% of breast carcinomas, 95% of ovarian carcinomas and 50% of non–small cell lung carcinomas as well as the majority of pancreatic, gastric, and esophageal cancers (27). Combining the measurement of serum TAG-72 with CEA increased the percentage of patients diagnosed with advanced GI cancer from 63% to 80% (28). Preliminary clinical trials conducted with B72.3 labeled with I-131 showed positive tumor localization in 8 of 12 patients with peritoneal carcinomatosis following intraperitoneal injection of the labeled antibody (27). Excellent correlation between positive scans and surgical findings was provided in seven patients. Significant improvement in tumor detection was achieved when In-111, instead of I-131, was used to label monoclonal antibody B72.3. A total of 127 patients with colorectal cancer received approximately 5 mCi of In-111 site-specific labeled B72.3 (CYT-103, Cytogen Corporation, Princeton, NJ, U.S.A.) preoperatively at doses of 0.2, 1, 2, or 20 mg. Antibody images were positive in 74% of patients and 73% of tumors. This preliminary trial indicated that In-111 CYT-103 is a safe and promising RIT agent for preoperative staging of patients with colorectal carcinoma (29). In another series of 116 patients with colorectal carcinoma, In-111 CYT-103 immunoscintigraphy yielded true-positive results in 70% of patients and true-negative results in 90% of patients (30). In-111 CYT-103 imaging was superior to CT in detecting local pelvic recurrences (83.3% versus 63.6%). These results indicate a definite use for RIT in the preoperative work-up of patients with primary colorectal carcinomas.

Immunoscintigraphy with Indium-labeled monoclonal antibodies offers the advantage of detecting lesions at multiple sites simultaneously. It could thus be used as the primary diagnostic modality once the diagnosis of primary colorectal carcinoma is established to document the singularity of this lesion as well as the absence of extraabdominal metastases. In a primary setting, antibody scans showing extensive local and regional spread show that benefits may be derived from preoperative and intraoperative radiotherapy. Monoclonal antibody scans demonstrating synchronous colon lesions argue for extended hemicolectomy or subtotal colectomy. Preoperative identification of hepatic metastases by monoclonal antibody scan would alter the operative approach to include a more extensive workup to determine the extent and resectability of these hepatic deposits.

LAPAROSCOPY AND PREOPERATIVE STAGING

The general surgeon plays an important role in the management of abdominal malignancy and uses endoscopic methods in many clinical strategies. These include diagnosis, surveillance, surgical management, and patient follow-up. Each of these phases depends on physical examination and laboratory tests, as well as direct or indirect visualization of both the entire GI tract and abdominal cavity. It is imperative that the surgeon managing abdominal malignancy appreciate the mechanical and interpretive issues as well as the outcomes realized through endoscopic means.

Benefits of Laparoscopy Versus Imaging Studies

Cost of imaging studies and diagnostic procedures varies from institution to institution and may not be easily determined because of the problems in equating "charges" and "costs" relating to patient management. The additional difficult issue is to determine the appropriate procedure as a function of its outcome in relating to the overall management of the cancer patient. Outcome management has been defined as "technology of patient experience designed to help patients." Payors and providers make rational medical care–related choices based on better insight into the effect of these choices on the patient's life (31). An additional issue is to clarify both the functional state and overall well-being of the patient over a period of time as these relate to any medical or surgical intervention. With this unique population, the type of malignancy, nutritional and metabolic derangements, stage of disease, as well as psychological and functional issues affect the patients' outcomes.

Traditional preoperative evaluation of cancer patients depended primarily on indirect methods represented by radiological imaging studies that depended heavily on interpretive skills of the individual radiologist. Although recent CT and MRI improved the ability to clinically stage and localize disease preoperatively, interpretation still plays a major role in the usefulness of these techniques. In addition, there is a tendency to perform multiple imaging studies in order to achieve an "additive" effect and to arrive at the best possible estimate of disease location and bulk prior to determining treatment options. Several studies now support the idea that the addition of laparoscopy increases both the sensitivity and specificity of disease recognition when compared to these conventional imaging studies. In addition, the overall "accuracy" is higher when laparoscopy is used for assessment of abdominal malignancy (32).

Evaluation of Esophageal Carcinoma

Esophageal carcinoma is a good example of the importance of a multimodality approach, not only for diagnosis but also for treatment. Endoluminal endoscopy is important in order to visualize the tumor and to obtain adequate tissue for diagnosis. With the unique ability of esophageal cancer to manifest "skip" areas, endoscopy is also important for staging and evaluation prior to surgical intervention. Once the diagnosis is made, however, assessment of regional metastatic disease is completed with CT, MRI, percutaneous US, or radionuclide scanning techniques. These additional modalities rely on indirect interpretation. Laparoscopy becomes important because it allows direct visualization and biopsy within the abdominal cavity in order to evaluate metastatic disease and satisfy requirements for complete pathological staging.

The following characteristics of esophageal cancer are associated with an improved likelihood of survival: (a) the tumor is less than 5 cm in length, (b) no tumor extends beyond the esophageal wall, and (c) lymph nodes are free of disease. DeMeester et al. (33) found that in patients with one or more of the predictors of outcome, only metastasis to lymph nodes and tumor penetration of the esophageal wall had a significant independent influence.

Many patients who present with dysphagia are incurable or unresectable at the time of diagnosis. Studies have shown that laparoscopy is more sensitive than conventional imaging studies in the evaluation of the patient with advanced esophageal carcinoma. Dagnini et al. (34) found that in their study of 369 patients with cancer of the esophagus, preoperative evaluation detected metastatic disease in 88 patients. The sensitivity was 88% with a specificity close to 100%. They concluded that laparoscopy is more reliable than CT scan and US.

Molloy et al. (35) described the use of laparoscopy in the evaluation of the patient with cancer of the gastric cardia and esophagus. The patients all had untreated, biopsy-proven carcinoma of the esophagus or gastric cardia. All patients were evaluated with US, contrast-enhanced CT, and laparoscopy. Rigid bronchoscopy was carried out in all patients with upper and middle third lesions of the esophagus. Laparoscopy was performed separately under general anesthesia, using a 30-degree endoscope. Thirty-eight percent had local or metastatic disease detected on laparoscopy. Three of 244 patients had isolated liver metastases not seen on laparoscopy. The patients identified as having no hepatic, omental, or peritoneal metastases underwent esophagastrectomy.

The evaluation of esophageal carcinoma with laparoscopy is an important modality to avoid the unnecessary laparotomy in the patient with distant metastatic disease. If the patient is not resectable, effective palliative treatment may be performed. This includes laser ablation, dilatation of malignant strictures, introduction of after-loading catheters for high-dose-rate brachytherapy (HDRB) or placement of stents using endoscopic techniques. It is important for the surgeon-endoscopist to be aware of all the possible intervention modalities which determine resectability in the patient with esophageal carcinoma (Fig. 2-5).

Gastric Carcinoma

In the last five to six decades, the incidence of primary gastric carcinoma has fallen significantly in the United States, but remains a significant tumor in the Far East and in Central and South America. Resection continues to be the primary modality in the management of gastric carcinoma even in cases of palliative management.

Endoscopic evaluation of the stomach is generally performed along with esophagoscopy and should include visualization of the duodenum and ampullary area. The stomach must be empty of food for total visualization of the gastric wall. Gastroscopic inspection is more difficult than esophagoscopy since blind areas are present in the stomach. The anatomy requires an experienced endoscopist to evaluate the greater and lesser curvatures and gastroesophageal junction. When taking a biopsy of an ulcerated lesion, it is important to take adequate tissue which should include the inner rim of the ulcer crater. The central ulceration should be avoided because it may contain only necrotic tissue which is not adequate for cancer diagnosis. The localization of each biopsy specimen should be well documented since this plays a significant role in planning sur-

gical intervention. Endoluminal endoscopy and biopsy, while effectively diagnosing and localizing gastric cancer, does not contribute greatly to overall staging of these tumors.

Laparoscopy may be important in the evaluation of visceral and nodal metastases prior to planned gastric resection. Kriplani and Kapur (36) reported laparoscopic examination in 40 patients with gastric carcinoma who had imaging studies that suggested resectability. Using laparoscopic approaches, distant metastases were found in five patients (12.5%), whereas locally advanced disease indicating uresectability was noted in 11 patients (27.5%). A total of 16 patients (40%) avoided unnecessary laparotomy for unresectable disease. The overall diagnostic accuracy of laparoscopic evaluation was 92% and proved quite beneficial in overall surgical planning. Small peritoneal implants and liver metastases may be visualized that were not evident on CT or US studies. Possik et al. (37) evaluated 360 patients laparoscopically with a diagnosis of gastric carcinoma. Evidence of tumor penetration, nodal involvement, and liver metastasis was reported. Laparoscopy was compared to liver scintigraphy, US, and alkaline phosphatase levels as indicators of liver involvement. The sensitivity was 87% for laparoscopy and 78.7% and 78.6% for scintigraphy and US, respectively. Alkaline phosphatase was the least sensitive indicator. Although gastric resection may be excellent palliation for advanced gastric neoplasia, the dismal 5-year overall survival of

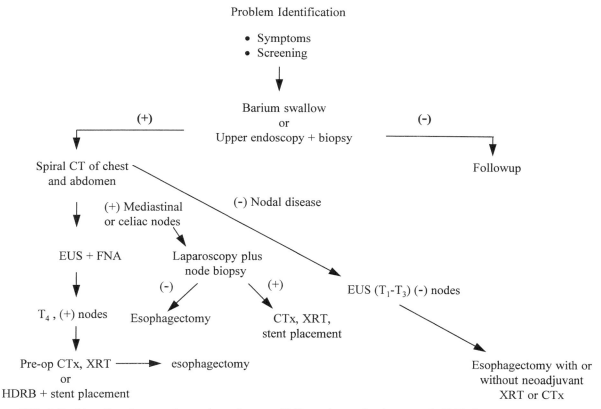

FIG. 2-5. Algorithm for esophageal carcinoma. *EUS,* endoscopic ultrasound; *FNA,* fine-needle aspiration; *CT,* computerized tomography; *XTR,* external beam radiation therapy; *CTx,* chemotherapy; *HDRB,* high-dose rate brachytherapy.

10% to 15% indicates that most patients have unrecognized disease in the peritoneal cavity at the time of gastric resection.

The addition of peritoneal lavage at the time of laparoscopy may aid in the identification of intraperitoneal free cancer cells (IFCC) which may help to identify a subset of patients at risk for recurrence following gastric resection (38). The rate of detection of IFCC in published reports ranges from 14% to 47% at the time of laparotomy for gastric cancer (39). IFCC were detected in 41% of patients during staging laparoscopy (38). The presence of ascites increases the likelihood of obtaining IFCC during laparoscopic evaluation. Positive cytology, however, may occur in the absence of ascites but is frequently associated with gastric serosal invasion. Laparoscopy with peritoneal cytology might be used as a predictor of extent of surgical treatment in gastric cancer patients. Unresectable tumors had higher positivity of IFCC than those who underwent palliation or curative gastrectomy (38). The use of laparoscopy will help identify those patients who will not benefit from surgical intervention. Unfortunately, no effective systemic multimodal therapy is currently available for these patients.

Lymphoma

In the past, laparotomy was a common method used in the staging of lymphoma. Glatstein et al. (40) found that the pathologic stage was upgraded 30% with specific techniques, such as liver biopsies, splenectomy, node dissection, and general inspection of the peritoneal cavity. Currently, operative staging is recommended only if imaging studies are suggestive of intraabdominal disease and documentation of these findings would lead to a change in overall management.

The role of laparoscopy became more popular for lymphoma staging in the mid-1980s and now all components of operative staging (liver and nodal biopsy, splenectomy, oophoropexy) can be accomplished laparoscopically (41). Laparoscopy has been used not only for initial evaluation but also as a second-look modality to evaluate the effects of therapy on intraabdominal disease and to confirm recurrence. The use of CT and US to evaluate abdominal Hodgkin's disease has been complimented by laparoscopy. Hepatic involvement is an especially challenging problem since most metastatic deposits may be too small to be visualized with CT or nuclear scanning. False negative studies were found in 20% and false positives may be as high as 15% to 20% with CT or US when subsequent laparoscopy is used (42).

The important consideration in measuring the outcome of patients with Hodgkin's disease is to realize that those who are appropriately staged may be more appropriately treated using radiation or chemotherapeutic approaches singularly or in combination. Proper endoscopic staging may now replace traditional celiotomy as a method to further promote these improvements in patient outcome.

Pancreatic Carcinomas

Accurate staging for pancreatic carcinoma is mandatory so that appropriate patient selection for pancreatic resection with curative intent can be accomplished (Fig. 2-6). Palliative approaches, such as stent placement via endoscopic retrograde cholangioscopy, percutaneous biliary decompression, and laparoscopic gastrojejunal and biliary bypass have reinforced the need to identify unresectable disease in order to avoid unnecessary laparotomy. Staging procedures are especially challenging in the patient with pancreatic carcinoma because of the retroperitoneal location of the pancreas. Although radiologic modalities have improved, allowing for more accurate diagnosis of metastatic disease, the accuracy of staging, even using combinations of modalities, may not be optimal. Failure to detect occult metastatic cancer can result in early tumor recurrence, whereas identification can change the intervention toward palliative aspects of therapy. Laparoscopic US will assume a greater role in the evaluation of pancreatic and periampullary tumors. John et al. (43) found in a prospective study that occult disease was present in 35% of their patient population and laparoscopic US confirmed unresectable tumor in 59%. Additional staging information occurred in 53% of their population, which led to a change in resectability in 25%. Bemelman et al. (44) used laparoscopy and laparoscopic US to evaluate the resectability of patients diagnosed by percutaneous US and endoscopic retrograde cholangiopancreatography with stage I pancreatic head carcinoma. Seventy of 73 patients were subsequently evaluated by laparoscopy with ultrasonography. Sixteen of 21 patients were diagnosed with distant metastasis. Laparotomy was avoided in 19% with a positive predictive value of 93%.

Laparoscopic Ultrasonography

Precise staging of malignant disease is mandatory to allow for adequate and effective treatment planning. The use of conventional imaging studies, such as CT and transcutaneous US, will generally only identify lesions that are 1 cm or larger in diameter. These modalities are also limited in the identification of infiltrating tumor into adjacent structures. Laparoscopy has allowed complete evaluation of the abdominal cavity with two- and three-dimensional imaging of the anatomy. It has also facilitated identification of lesions not seen with CT or transcutaneous US. In addition, the ability to perform laparoscopic biopsy within the abdominal cavity has allowed for appropriate staging and the avoidance of unnecessary laparotomy. The drawback of laparoscopy is the lack of tactile sensation and the inability to evaluate structures below the surface of solid organs or within the retroperitoneal space.

The benefit of laparoscopic US is to overcome the limitations of routine laparoscopy in the staging of patients with abdominal malignancy. The ability to more accurately guide needle biopsy or cryotherapy of hepatic metastasis is realized with laparoscopic ultrasonography (Fig. 2-7). Hünerbein et al. (45) found that laparoscopy provided additional information in 40% of patients, whereas laparoscopic ultrasonography enhanced the identification of metastases, causing a change of stage in one-third of their patients with upper GI tract tumors. These authors concluded that the combination

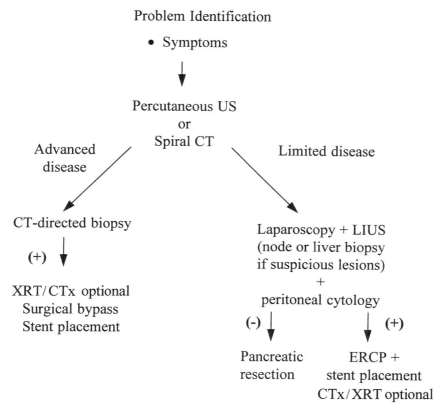

FIG. 2-6. Algorithm for pancreatic carcinoma. *US,* ultrasound; *CT,* computerized tomography; *LIUS,* laparoscopic intraoperative ultrasound; *ERCP,* endoscopic retrograde cholangiopancreatography; *XTR,* external beam radiation therapy; *CTx,* chemotherapy.

of diagnostic laparoscopy and intraabdominal US aided in the upstaging and downstaging of their patients. Surgery was abandoned in 16 patients and downstaging occurred in seven patients who then subsequently underwent surgical resection.

The ability to visualize suspected neoplastic tissue makes laparoscopy a more accurate procedure than CT-guided biopsy.

An evaluation of the dimension of the specimen and avoidance of injuring surrounding structures are benefits of laparoscopy and concomitant US. These techniques allow for avoidance of necrotic tumor, more accurate retrieval of biopsy specimens and more selective localization of parenchymal metastases. The addition of laparoscopic US in evaluating lymph nodes and the

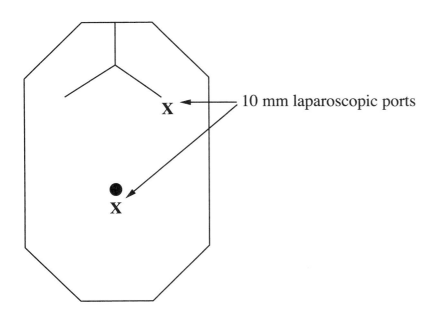

FIG. 2-7. Port position for laparoscopic ultrasound examination.

retroperitoneum, which is not well visualized by laparoscopy alone, has allowed significant advances in the diagnosis and staging of abdominal malignancies (46,47).

Second-Look Procedures

The role of laparoscopy in performing "second-look" evaluation of the abdominal cavity is not well defined. The eventual benefit of endoscopic evaluation will be in conjunction with CT, US, and tumor markers to help identify patients who might benefit from further surgical and nonsurgical interventions. The limitation of laparoscopy in this area is the inability to identify anatomic landmarks or residual tumor in the presence of adhesions from previous operations. Gynecologic oncologists traditionally have used second-look laparoscopy for evaluation of ovarian carcinomas. Marti Vincente et al. (48) found that 48% of their studies revealed residual tumor. This identified a subset of patients who might benefit from reoperation and debulking procedures. A negative laparoscopic examination on its own, however, cannot definitely place the patient in a disease-free category, and certain patients may benefit from a formal celiotomy. This is an important point for the surgeon-laparoscopist to keep in mind.

The use of a laparoscopic "second-look" in patients with colorectal carcinoma is debatable. CEA levels have traditionally helped to identify patients with disease recurrence. The addition of laparoscopic US may help to identify recurrence in this patient population in a more accurate fashion and to enhance information gained from tumor markers. In addition, using tagged monoclonal antibodies along with laparoscopic probes to identify uptake of these substances may facilitate the identification of occult abdominal disease in the near future.

Outcome assessment comparing laparoscopy, laparoscopic US, and radiologic and ultrasonic imaging techniques will be required to continually evaluate the various modalities used in tumor staging. Recently, PET scanning using 18F-fluorodeoxy glucose (18 FDG) has been applied to the detection of metastatic deposits in the liver. Vitola et al. (2) report 24 patients who were studied with the FDG PET scan along with either concomitant conventional CT, CT portography, or both to assess the possibility of detecting hepatic metastases from colorectal cancer. Fifty-five suspicious intrahepatic lesions were identified. Eventual biopsy confirmed 39 malignant lesions and 16 benign deposits in this group. Of significance is that FDG PET imaging had a higher accuracy rate (93%) than the other two modalities (76%) in the detection of hepatic metastases. PET scanning altered surgical plans in six (25%) of the 24 patients studied. Although laparoscopy was not used in this study, the obvious next step is to include a "laparoscopic arm" in the subsequent assessments.

Contraindications and Complications

The major contraindication to laparoscopy occurs when the information obtained from the study will not enhance the diagnosis or change the patient's need to undergo abdominal exploration. Other contraindications include problems of trocar insertion (adhesion or sepsis) or difficulty in the establishment of a safe pneumoperitoneum (bowel distension due to ileus or mechanical obstruction). Patients undergoing general anesthesia who have advanced cardiac and pulmonary disease may also have difficulties with arrhythmia and reduced cardiac output secondary to establishing a carbon dioxide pneumoperitoneum (49). Local and regional anesthetic techniques have been advocated for the performance of diagnostic laparoscopy, and, in the cooperative patient, these may be quite appropriate. In the performance of complete abdominal staging, most patients will tolerate a more complete examination when general anesthesia is used. There are no studies, however, comparing local versus general anesthetic techniques in the overall diagnostic outcome of laparoscopic management.

The surgeon performing procedures for cancer must carefully evaluate his or her patients to insure that those undergoing minimal access staging will derive benefit. The potential hazard of any procedure must be carefully realized in any risk-benefit equation. In addition, as the cost of procedures and the additive effect of diagnostic studies becomes more important in the era of managed care, the surgeon must continue to take the lead in deciding whether laparoscopic studies should be performed. Thus far, the greatest benefit of abdominal staging procedures, with respect to cost, may be that the expense of unnecessary celiotomy and resection in the face of advanced disease may be reduced.

Tumor Implantation

Tumor implantation in trocar sites following laparoscopy was first noted in the gynecologic literature but has been seen as a consequence of seeding from gastric, pancreatic, biliary tract, and colon carcinomas as well as lymphoma (50). Serosal involvement with tumor or positive peritoneal cytology may be significant factors in the promotion of trocar site metastases. Evaluation of anecdotal reports of abdominal wall implantation as well as recent studies involving animal models (51) suggest that the effect of the pneumoperitoneum and manipulation of intraabdominal organs may play a primary role in trocar site metastases (52). It is anticipated that implantation in the abdominal wall may become more prevalent as laparoscopic staging of abdominal malignancy becomes more popular. Placement of specimens into appropriate plastic bags or other receptacles prior to extraction from the peritoneal cavity will hopefully reduce the occurrence of metastatic implantation of trocar sites and counter incisions which are created for organ removal. Outcome studies will be extremely important to further evaluate the importance of trocar site metastases. Individual surgeons have a prime responsibility in recording such episodes in their own patient populations.

REFERENCES

1. Hutter RP. At last—a worldwide agreement on the staging of cancer. *Arch Surg* 1987;122:1235.

2. Vitola JV, Delbecke D, Sandler MP, et al. Positron emission tomography to stage suspected metastatic colorectal cancer to the liver. *Am J Surg* 1996;171:21.
3. Zuccaro G., Sivak M, Rice T. Endoscopic ultrasound and the staging of esophageal and gastric cancer. *Gastrointest Endosc Clin North Am* 1992;2:625.
4. Tio T. Endosonography in diagnosing and staging of pancreatic and ampullary cancer. *Gastrointest Endosc Clin North Am* 1992;2:673.
5. Boyce GA. Colorectal cancer staging. *Gastrointest Endosc Clin North Am* 1992;2:729.
6. Kimmey M, Martin R. Fundamentals of endosonography. *Gastrointest Endosc Clin North Am* 1992;2:557.
7. Massari M, Cioffi U, DeSimone M, et al. Endoscopic ultrasonography for preoperative staging of esophageal carcinoma. *Surg Laparosc Endosc* 1997;7:162.
8. Srivastava A, Vanagunas A, Kamel P, Cooper R. Endoscopic ultrasound in the evaluation of Barrett's esophagus. *Gastrointest Endosc* 1991;37:244.
9. Lightdale CJ. Endoscopic ultrasonography in the diagnosis, staging, and follow-up of esophageal and gastric cancer. *Endoscopy* 1992;24 [Suppl 1]:297.
10. Catano MF, Sivak MV, Rice T, et al. Endosconographic features predictive of lymph node metastases. *Gastrointest Endosc* 1994;40:442.
11. Stotland BR, Kochman ML. Diagnostic and therapeutic endosonography: endoscopic ultrasound-guided fine-needle aspiration in clinical practice. *Gastrointest Endosc* 1997;45:329.
12. Rosch T. Classen M. *Gastroenterologic endosonography.* Stuttgart: Thieme, 1992.
13. Gress F, Hawes R, Savides T, Ikenberry S, Lehman G. Endoscopic ultrasound-guided fine-needle aspiration biopsy using linear array and radial scanning endosonography. *Gastrointest Endosc* 1997;45:243.
14. Chaboneau WJ, Reading CC, Welch TJ. CT and sonographically guided needle biopsy: current techniques and new innovations. *Am J Roentgenol* 1990;154:1.
15. Wong W, Orrom W, Jensen L. Preoperative staging of rectal cancer with endorectal ultrasonography. *Perspect Colon Rectal Surg* 1990;3:315.
16. Zainea GG, Lee F, McLeary RD, et al. Transrectal ultrasonography in the evaluation of rectal and extrarectal disease. *Surg Gynecol Obstet* 1989;169:153.
17. Hildebrandt U, Klein T, Feifel G, et al. Endosonography of pararectal lymph nodes: *in vitro* and *vivo* evaluation. *Dis Colon Rectum* 1990;33:863.
18. Beynon J, Mortensen N, Foy D, et al. Preoperative assessment of mesorectal lymph node involvement in rectal cancer. *Br J Surg* 1989;76:276.
19. Rifkin MD, Ehrlich SM, Marks G. Staging of rectal carcinoma: prospective comparison of endorectal US and CT. *Radiology* 1989;170:319.
20. Nabi HA, Doerr RJ. Radiololabeled monoclonal antibody imaging of colorectal cancer: current status and future perspectives. *Am J Surg* 1992;163:448.
21. Pressman D. The development and use of radiolabeled antitumor antibodies. *Cancer Res* 1980;40:2960.
22. Goldenberg DM, DeLand F, Kim E, et al. Use of radiolabeled antibodies to carcinoembryonic antigen for the detection and localization of diverse cancers by external photoscanning. *N Engl J Med* 1978;298:1384.
23. Epenetos AA, Mather S, Granowska M, et al. Targeting of iodine-123 labeled tumor associated monoclonal antibodies to ovarian, breast, and gastrointestinal tumors. *Lancet* 1982;2:999.
24. Delaloye B, Bischof-Delaloye A, Buchegger F, et al. Detection of colorectal carcinoma by emission-computerized tomography after injection of I-123 labeled Fab or F(ab')2 fragments from monoclonal anticarcinoembryonic antigen antibodies. *J Clin Invest* 1986;77:301.
25. Kuhn JA, Corbisiero RM, Buras R, et al. Intraoperative gamma detection probe with presurgical antibody imaging in colon cancer. *Arch Surg* 1991;126:1398.
26. Colcher D, Horan-Hand P, Nuti M, Schlom J. A spectrum of monoclonal antibodies reactive with human mammary tumor cells. *Proc Natl Acad Sci USA* 1981;78:3199.
27. Carrasquillo JA, Sugarbaker P, Colcher D, et al. Radioimmunoscintigraphy of colon cancer with iodine-131 labeled B72.3 monoclonal antibody. *J Nucl Med* 1988;29:1022.
28. Guadagni F, Roselli M, Amato T, et al. Complementarity between serum tumor-associated glycoprotein–72 and CEA levels in the longitudinal evaluation of patients with adenocarcinomas of the GI tract. *Proc Am Assoc Cancer Res* 1990;31:165.
29. Maguire RT, Schmelter RF, Pascucci V, Conklin JJ. Immunoscintigraphy of colorectal adenocarcinoma; results with site-specific radiolabeled B72.3. *Antibody Immunocong Radiopharm* 1989;2:257.
30. Doerr RJ, Abdel-Nabi H, Krag D, Mitchell E. Radiolabeled antibody imaging in the management of colorectal cancer: results of a multicenter clinical study. *Ann Surg* 1991;214:118.
31. Ellwood P. Shattuck lecture. Outcome management: a technology of patient experiences. *N Engl J Med* 1988;318:1549.
32. Watt I, Stewart I, Anderson D, et al. Laparoscopy ultrasound and computed tomography in cancer of the oesophagus and gastric cardia: a prospective comparison for detecting intra-abdominal metastases. *Br J Surg* 1989;76:1036.
33. DeMeester TR, Zaninotto G, Johansson KE. Selective therapeutic approach to cancer of the lower esophagus and cardia. *J Thorac Cardiovasc Surg* 1988;95:42.
34. Dagnini G, Caldironi M, Marin G, et al. Laparoscopy in abdominal staging of esophageal carcinoma. *Gastrointest Endosc* 1986;32:400.
35. Molloy RG, McCourtney JS, Anderson JR. Laparoscopy in the management of patients with cancer of the gastric cardia and oesophagus. *Br J Surg* 1994;82:352.
36. Kriplani AK, Kapur BM. Laparoscopy for pre-operative staging and assessment of operability in gastric carcinoma. *Gastrointest Endosc* 1991;37:441.
37. Possik RA, Franco EL, Pires DR, et al. Sensitivity, specificity and predictive value of laparoscopy for the staging of gastric cancer for the detection of liver metastases. *Cancer* 1986;58:1.
38. Ribeiro U, Gama-Rodrigues J, Bitelman B, et al. Value of peritoneal lavage cytology during laparoscopic staging of patients with gastric carcinoma. *Surg Laparosc Endosc* 1998;8:132.
39. Juhl H, Stritzel M, Wroblewski A. Immunocytological detection of micrometastatic cells: comparative evaluation of findings in the peritoneal cavity and the bone marrow of gastric, colorectal and pancreatic cancer patients. *Int J Cancer* 1994;57:330.
40. Glatstein E, Guernsey JM, Rosenberg SA, et al. The value of laparotomy and splenectomy in the staging of Hodgkin's disease. *Cancer* 1969;24:709.
41. Greene FL, Cooler AW. Laparoscopic evaluation of lymphomas. *Semin Laparosc Surg* 1994;1:13.
42. Moormeier JA, Williams SF, Golomb HM. The staging of Hodgkin's disease. *Hematol Oncol Clin North Am* 1989;3:237.
43. John TG, Greig JD, Carter DC, et al. Carcinoma of the pancreatic head and periampullary region. Tumor staging with laparoscopy and laparoscopic ultrasonography. *Ann Surg* 1995;221:156.
44. Bemelman WA, deWit LT, Van Delden OM, et al. Diagnostic laparoscopy combined with laparoscopicc ultrasonography in staging of cancer of the pancreatic head region. *Br J Surg* 1995;82:820–824.
45. Hünerbein M, Rau B, Schlag PM. Laparoscopy and laparoscopic ultrasound for staging of upper gastrointestinal tumors. *Eur J Surg Oncol* 1995;21:50.
46. Stein HJ, Kraemer S, Feussner H, Fink U, Siewert J. Clinical value of diagnostic laparoscopy with laparoscopic ultrasound in patients with cancer of the esophagus or cardia. *J Gastrointest Surg* 1997;1:167.
47. Tandan VR, Asch M, Margolis M, Page A, Gallinger S. Laparoscopic vs. open intraoperative ultrasound examination of the liver: A controlled study. *J Gastrointest Surg* 1997;1:146.
48. Marti Vincente A, Sainz S, Soriano G, et al. Utilidad de la laparoscopica como metado de *second-look* en las neoplasias de ovario. *Rev Esp Enform Apar Dig* 1990;77:275.
49. Dorsay DA, Greene FL, Baysinger CL. Hemodynamic changes during laparoscopic cholecystectomy monitored with transesophageal echocardiography (TEE). *Surg Endosc* 1995;9:128.
50. Nduka CC, Monson JRT, Menzies N, et al. Abdominal wall metastases following laparoscopy. *Br J Surg* 1994;81:648.
51. Alendorf JD, Bessler M, Kayton ML. Tumor growth after laparotomy or laparoscopy. *Surg Endosc* 1995;9:49.
52. Treat MR, Bessler M, Whelan RL Mechanisms to reduce incidence of tumor implantation during minimal access procdures for colon cancer. *Semin Laparosc Surg* 1995;2:176.

CHAPTER 3

Nutrition and the Cancer Patient

Oreste D. Gentilini, Thomas J. Fahey III, and John M. Daly

Malnutrition is commonly associated with cancer. In fact, more than 50% of patients with cancer present with weight loss at the time of diagnosis (1). The tumor syndrome characterized by involuntary weight loss, anorexia, abnormal metabolism, and tissue wasting is termed "cachexia," a word derived from the Greek words *kakos* and *hexis,* which mean bad condition.

Many cancer-related conditions are responsible for the development of cachexia, but in general it is possible to divide them into two main causes: reduced nutrient intake (including malabsorptive syndromes) and metabolic imbalance.

Reduced nutrient intake can be the result of anorexia, learned food aversions, and alterations in taste, leading to poor food intake. Tumors of the lower gastrointestinal (GI) tract may produce obstruction, whereas oropharyngeal and esophageal cancers can cause odynophagia or dysphagia, all of which can lead to decreased food intake. Malabsorption may be the result of exocrine insufficiency (i.e., secondary to carcinoma of the pancreas) or due to bacterial overgrowth associated with a blind loop syndrome.

Cancer treatment strategies may further impact on the nutritional status of patients with cancer. Antineoplastic therapies may produce toxicity that further interferes with nutrient intake or absorption, as well as increase metabolic demands. Surgery can be complicated by prolonged ileus, infection, or postresection syndromes. Chemotherapy is often associated with nausea, vomiting, anorexia, altered taste, mucositis, stomatitis, and diarrhea. Similar complications can be seen with radiation therapy, depending on the site, dose, and volume of tissue irradiated (Table 3-1).

In normal subjects, the physiological response to diminished food intake is a decrease in the resting energy expenditure (REE). REE consists of all the energy-requiring processes of vegetative function and accounts for 75% of total energy expenditure in normal people. In theory, all of the conditions mentioned above should induce adaptive changes found in the setting of semistarvation, particularly a reduction in REE. On the contrary, tumor-bearing hosts react without decreasing REE and exhibit altered carbohydrate, fat, and protein metabolism (2). Glucose production and utilization are enhanced, insulin-resistance often occurs,

and there is equal mobilization of fat and skeletal proteins without sparing of the muscle protein. This energetic and metabolic impairment of tumor-bearing hosts contributes to protein breakdown and tissue wasting, and to some extent is analagous to the metabolic responses characteristic of stress and sepsis (Table 3-2).

ETIOLOGY OF CANCER CACHEXIA

Although much has been learned over the past decade, at present, the mechanisms underlying cancer cachexia remain incompletely defined. Experimental studies have suggested that cachexia is caused by circulating factors either produced by the tumor itself or by the host in response to the tumor. These host-derived factors may be abnormal products or normal factors synthetized by the host in attempt to control the tumor. This latter model of normal host factors causing cancer cachexia when produced or released inappropriately suggests a paradigm for understanding the similarities between cancer cachexia and the weight loss seen in chronic infections or acute illness. Current concepts have shifted their focus from tumor-derived factors produced autonomously to host-derived factors that are produced in response to the presence of malignant cells.

Experimental evidence in animal models has suggested that a number of cytokines contribute to cancer cachexia, including tumor necrosis factor (TNF), interleukin-1 (IL-1), interleukin-6 (IL-6), and gamma-interferon (γ-IFN).

TNF is a pluripotent cytokine, produced mainly by macrophages, that has been shown to reproduce many aspects of cancer cachexia when administered to animals chronically, including decreases in body weight, food intake, and negative nitrogen balance. Antibodies against TNF reversed all of these derangements in tumor-bearing animals (3). The administration of low doses of TNF over several days induced tolerance in animals with a protective effect from cancer cachexia, while an increase in the dose administered produced cachexia in previously tolerant animals (4). However, serum levels of TNF do not correlate with clinical findings of cachexia in either humans or animals with tumor (5). It is hypothesized that the lack of

TABLE 3–1. *Factors contributing to reduced food intake or absorption in cancer cachexia*

Reduced food intake
  Anorexia
  Nausea and vomiting
  Altered taste and smell
Local effects of tumor
  Odynophagia and dysphagia
  Early satiety
  Intestinal or gastric outlet obstruction
  Malabsorption
Effects of cancer treatment
  Surgery
    Altered mastication and swallowing
    Postgastrectomy syndromes
    Pancreatic insufficiency
    Anastomotic stricture
  Chemotherapy
    Nausea and vomiting
    Altered taste and smell
    Stomatitis and mucositis
    Diarrhea
  Radiation therapy
    Anorexia, nausea, and vomiting
    Altered taste and smell
    Xerostomia and mucositis
    Gastrointestinal mucosal damage
    Late strictures
  Psychosocial
    Depression and grief
    Anxiety
    Learned food aversion

correlation between circulating TNF levels and cachexia may be due to a cyclical secretion of TNF, or due to paracrine effects that do not require measurable levels in the blood. The mechanisms by which TNF causes cachexia are multiple and are not completely understood. TNF induces alterations in both carbohydrate and fat metabolism. Additionally, it may produce central effects on the satiety center in the hypothalamus (6) or more peripheral effects by reducing gastric emptying (7).

IL-1 is a proinflammatory cytokine produced by a variety of cell types that is a critical mediator of septic shock, infections, and injury. It has been shown to be more powerful than TNF in inducing anorexia. The relationship between IL-1 and cancer cachexia has been confirmed in animal studies. Administration of antibodies against IL-1 in animal models reversed the development of cachexia (3). As with TNF, it is difficult to correlate IL-1 plasma levels and cachexia. IL-1 also exerts effects on the central nervous system, perhaps inducing corticotropin-releasing factor (CRF) production by the hypothalamus. IL-1 may also produce its effects through the prostaglandin pathway. In fact, pretreatment of animals with ibuprofen prior to IL-1 infusion have been demonstrated to block the anorexic effect of IL-1. Similar results have been achieved by reducing prostaglandin production, using a diet high in ω-3 fatty acids (8).

IL-6 is a multifunctional cytokine, expressed by a variety of cells under complex regulatory mechanisms, that may act both as a proinflammatory mediator and a marker of injury. IL-6 has been found in the serum of tumor-bearing mice (9),

TABLE 3–2. *Metabolism imbalance in the tumor-bearing host and differences between starvation and cancer cachexia*

	Starvation	Cancer cachexia
Metabolic rate		
REE	Decreased	Normal/increased
Respiratory quotient	Decreased	Unchanged
O_2 consumption, CO_2 production	Decreased	Unchanged
Nitrogen balance	Negative	Negative
Protein metabolism		
Whole body protein turnover	Decreased	Unchanged
Urinary nitrogen excretion	Decreased	Unchanged
Skeletal muscle anabolism	Decreased	Decreased
Skeletal muscle catabolism	Decreased	Increased
Glucose metabolism		
Whole body glucose turnover	Decreased	Increased
Hepatic gluconeogenesis	Increased	Increased
Glucose tolerance	Decreased	Decreased
Insulin sensitivity	Decreased	Decreased
Blood glucose	Decreased	Unchanged
Serum insulin	Decreased	Unchanged
Blood lactate	Unchanged	Increased
Cori cycle activity	—	Increased
Fat metabolism		
Lipolysis	Increased	Increased
Lipoprotein lipase activity	Unchanged	Decreased
Serum triglycerides	—	Increased

and it has been reported that increased IL-6 serum levels correlate with tumor burden and poorer survival in animals (10). Further evidence for IL-6 involvement in the development of cancer cachexia arises from the observation that resection of the tumor induced a decrease in IL-6 concentration in mice, with subsequent weight gain. Moreover, treatment with a monoclonal antibody against IL-6 was able to reverse cachexia in mice (11).

γ-IFN has also been noted to be a potential mediator of cancer cachexia. Administration of γ-IFN to non–tumor-bearing animals simulates the effects of cachexia, while passive immunization against γ-IFN is able to reverse these alterations in a rat model (12).

Recently, a circulating factor has been isolated from the tumor cell line MAC16 that may contribute to the development of the cachectic state. This factor has been purified and found to be a proteoglycan that induces catabolism of skeletal muscle. This substance was also found in the urine of cachectic cancer patients but was absent in normal subjects, patients with weight loss due to trauma, and cancer patients with little or no weight loss. Though further investigation is warranted, it appears that this circulating factor also contributes to cancer cachexia (13).

CONSEQUENCES OF MALNUTRITION IN THE CANCER PATIENT

The association between cancer malnutrition and poor outcome has been known for many years (14,15). Moreover, malnourished patients are at high risk for increased morbidity and mortality after surgery. Poor wound healing, an increased wound infection rate, prolonged postoperative ileus, and longer hospital stay have all been linked to compromised nutritional status associated with cancer (16). Furthermore, there is evidence that nutritional depletion causes impairment of both cellular and humoral immune function, making patients more susceptible to infectious complications (17,18).

It has been shown in both human and animal studies that nutritional repletion can reverse anergy and ameliorate cell-mediated immunity. Bone marrow transplant recipients who received prophylactic total parenteral nutrition (TPN) before and during marrow transplantation had longer survival and disease-free survival than those who were not nutritionally supported (19). A subsequent trial demonstrated equal effectiveness by using enteral formulas (20). However, nutritional support has been shown to reduce morbidity and mortality after surgery only in severely malnourished cancer patients (16).

In order to detect specific nutrient deficits and to identify severely malnourished patients who are at high risk for increased morbidity and mortality during treatment, a nutritional evaluation of the cancer patient should be performed at the time of the diagnosis. Patients who may benefit from nutritional support can then receive the appropriate intervention.

TABLE 3–3. *Assessing degrees of malnutrition*

	Normal	Mild/moderate	Severe
Weight loss	0%	<9%	≥10%
Albumin (g/dl)	3.5–5.0	3.0–3.4	<3.0
Transferrin (mg/dl)	200–400	100–200	<100

NUTRITIONAL ASSESSMENT

Nutritional status can be assessed by employing clinical and laboratory parameters to determine whether a given patient is either well nourished or presents with a mild, moderate, or severe degree of malnutrition (Table 3-3). Sophisticated tests, like evaluation of total body potassium, total body nitrogen or creatinine-height index, are largely reserved for research settings.

Clinical Parameters

A complete history and a thorough physical examination by an experienced physician still represents the simplest and most reliable method for determining an individual's nutritional status, and it is usually enough to define the presence of severe depletion.

A recent (within 3 months) loss of 10% or more of the usual body weight is indicative of significant malnutrition and of increased risk of morbidity and mortality. Patients should also be asked about recent dietary changes, onset of anorexia, food aversions, or altered taste and bowel habits. The patient should be questioned regarding the presence of GI symptoms such as nausea, early satiety, vomiting, abdominal pain, and diarrhea. Previous gastric or intestinal resections and underlying chronic diseases may affect both food intake and absorption. Physical examination can reveal changes in skin (dry and atrophic), hair (brittle, easy pluckability), and nails (ridged and spooned) or evidence of muscle wasting.

Depletion in the tumor-bearing host usually stems from a combination of marasmus (reduced intake of both protein and calories) and kwashiorkor (protein deficiency with an adequate calorie intake). Patients affected mostly by marasmus may present with decreased subcutaneous fat, as suggested by redundant skin folds, and diminished lean muscle mass, while those suffering in most part from kwashiorkor may also have anasarca, ascites or hepatomegaly.

Anthropometrics

Anthropometric measurements are useful in estimating body fat and lean muscle composition based on patient's body weight, height, skinfold thickness, and upper arm circumference. Values are compared to standard, age- and sex-matched population controls. However, unless a patient is significantly malnourished, anthropometrics may be helpful only after serial evaluations to monitor change.

The triceps skinfold (TSF) thickness is an indirect measure of body fat, and is determined with calipers placed at a point between the acromial process and the olecranon of the non-dominant arm. The arm should be relaxed and hanging freely at the patient's side or folded across the chest. A lengthwise fold of skin is pinched 1 cm above the midline, pulled away from the underlying muscle, and measured at a depth equal to the thickness of the fold.

Mid-arm muscle circumference (MMC) is an indirect assessment of lean muscle and is calculated from the arm circumference with an adjustment for the subcutaneous fat as measured by the TSF [MMC = arm circumference (cm) − (0.134 × TSF (mm)]. The arm circumference is assessed by placing a tape midway between the acromial process and the olecranon of the nondominant arm without constricting the skin.

Skin testing for delayed cutaneous hypersensitivity (DCH) is not a sensitive indicator of mild or moderate depletion, nor is it a specific test for nutritional depletion and therefore it is not recommended as a routine method of clinical assessment.

Laboratory Tests

The degree of visceral protein depletion can be estimated by determining serum levels of albumin, transferrin (TFN), pre-albumin, and retinol-binding protein (RBP). The concentration of these proteins reflects the patient's nutritional status but can also be affected by changes in salt and water balance. For instance, the serum albumin (Alb) concentration usually decreases early after starting a patient on TPN as a result of hydration. The normal concentration of Alb ranges between 3.5 and 5.0 g/dL. Levels below 3 g/dL are associated with higher morbidity and mortality and represent a marker of severe depletion. Further, in determining the nutritional status and in monitoring the effects of nutritional support one has to consider the half-life of the marker proteins—20 and 8 days for albumin and TFN, respectively, and 2 and 0.5 days for prealbumin and RBP. Hence, albumin and TFN are related more to overall nutritional status, whereas prealbumin and RBP can be modified by recent dietary changes. Significant increases in TFN concentration occur after 7 to 10 days of effective nutritional support, while Alb levels may take up to 4 weeks to recover.

In an attempt to find a single method to quantify the extent of malnutrition and to correlate it with the risk of postoperative complications, the prognostic nutritional index (PNI) has been proposed. This is a scoring system based on the TSF, serum albumin (Alb), TFN levels, and DCH and can be calculated as follows:

$$PNI (\%) = 158 - 16.6 \times (Alb) - 0.78 \times (TSF) - 0.20 \times (TFN) - 5.8 \times (DHC)$$

where albumin is in g/dL, TSF is in mm, TFN is in mg/dl, and DHC is scored as 0 = negative, 1 = less than 5 mm reactivity, and 2 = more than 5 mm activity.

In a large retrospective study, surgical patients with a PNI less than 30% had a 12% complication rate and 2% mortality, whereas patients with a PNI more than 60% had an 81% morbidity and 59% mortality (21). Though the PNI is a useful predictive measure of morbidity and mortality as related to nutritional status, it is not widely applied, probably because it includes assessment of DCH.

PREOPERATIVE NUTRITIONAL SUPPORT

Once the need for nutritional support is established, the surgeon has to answer three questions: (a) For how long do I have to feed the patient? (b) Which route and regimen are preferable for this patient? (c) What are the patient's nutritional requirements?

Length of Preoperative Nutritional Support

Patients with severe malnutrition should receive at least 7 days of nutritional support during their workup and preparation for a major elective procedure. Severely malnourished patients should also receive postoperative nutritional support until oral intake is adequate. Of course, the urgency of an operation determines the length of time available to correct existing nutritional deficits before the operation.

Choice of Nutritional Route and Regimen

As a general rule, nutritional support should be provided via the enteral route whenever possible. Enteral feeding has fewer complications and is easier to administer, less expensive, and more physiological than TPN. In fact, enteral feeding prevents some of the alterations related to the lack of use of the GI tract during parenteral feeding, such as villous atrophy with subsequent loss of the gut barrier and the possible development of bacterial translocation. Therefore, a patient should be put on TPN only when enteral feeding is contraindicated. Current indications for TPN in cancer patients are listed Table 3-4.

The safest and most effective route for delivering hypertonic TPN solutions in adults has been the use of infraclavicular, percutaneous subclavian catheters. Tunnelling of the catheters subcutaneously and use of the Seldinger method of placement may reduce catheter related infections.

Parenteral nutrition is usually started by administering approximately 750 mL of the hypertonic solution over 24 h using an infusion pump. Once the initial flow rate is tolerated, the rate can be increased up to the target rate (usually around 2,000 mL over 24 h) over a course of 2 to 3 days. Within 2 to

TABLE 3-4. *Current indications for TPN in cancer patients*

Malabsorption or severe, intractable diarrhea
Mechanical intestinal obstruction
High-output intestinal fistula (>600 cc/day)
Short bowel syndrome

3 days most adults are able to tolerate their total caloric and protein requirements intravenously.

The best way to provide short-term enteral feeding is a nasoenteric tube. Small-bore (8 to 10 French) flexible tubes of polyurethane and silicone elastomer have reduced major patient discomfort caused by larger-bore tubes. The smallest bore that allows the formula to flow without clogging should be used for greater patient acceptance. Gastric feeding is performed by placing a soft tube (usually ~90 cm) with its tip in the stomach and is generally well tolerated because of the distensibility and the dilutional function of the stomach, as well as pyloric regulation of emptying into the duodenum. However, gastric feeding has a higher risk of aspiration than jejunal feeding. Thus, patients with severe gastroesophageal reflux, absent gag reflex, or altered mental status are not candidates for gastric feeding. For such patients, nutritional therapy should be provided via a nasojejunal tube (109 cm-long with weighted tip) after the correct position of the catheter tip has been documented by x-ray.

If preoperative nutritional support is indicated for more than 4 to 6 weeks, as in patients undergoing multimodality treatment, a gastrostomy or a jejunostomy should be considered. The gastrostomy tube may be placed with a percutaneous endoscopic technique, a laparoscopic technique, or a minor surgical procedure under local, regional, or general anesthesia. The percutaneous endoscopic gastrostomy (PEG) has become quite popular as a cost-effective and less morbid method for permanent gastric intubation.

Jejunostomy tubes are indicated in patients at high risk for aspiration and patients with cancers involving the stomach, pylorus, or duodenum. Jejunostomy tubes can be placed at the time of laparotomy or as a separate procedure by using a standard Witzel technique and tacking the bowel to the anterior abdominal wall. Alternatively, a laparoscopic approach can be employed.

The enteral solutions used should be nutritionally adequate, well tolerated, easy to prepare, and economical. Four types of enteral formulas are available: blenderized formulas, nutritionally complete commercial formulas, chemically defined liquid diets, and modular formulas.

Blenderized tube feedings may be composed of any food that can be blenderized. The caloric concentration varies from 0.6 to 1.3 kcal/mL. These formulas are the less expensive but require a long time for preparation and a large-bore tube (at least 14 French) for infusion due to viscosity.

Nutritionally complete commercial formulas are the regimen of choice because of the relatively low cost, easy preparation, and adequacy of nutrients. These are polymeric formulas with intact proteins. Most are isotonic with a caloric density of 1 kcal/mL but are also available as high-calorie, high-nitrogen, hyperosmolar formulas that provide 1.5 to 2 kcal/mL. Continous pump infusion is recommended for delivery into the stomach or jejunum to avoid GI complications associated with overly rapid feedings.

Chemically defined formulas contain hydrolyzed proteins and crystalline amino acids and are more promptly absorbed.

Elemental diets are indicated in patients with special requirements as a consequence of deficits in absorption, e.g., patients with severe radiation enteritis, or intestinal fistulae.

Modular formulas consist of core modules of protein or carbohydrate or fats. Modules of vitamins or minerals are also available. This type of enteral nutrition can be used as supplements in combination with other enteral formulas or combined in different ways to meet special requirements.

Except for blenderized formulas, all enteral feeding should be delivered by continous gravity or pump infusion. We recommend initiating feedings 24 h after tube placement with an isotonic solution at 20 to 30 mL/h. The rate of infusion can be increased by 20 to 30 mL every 12 to 24 h as tolerated by the patient, up to the nutritional goal rate. Tube feedings can then be gradually cycled, ultimately providing the required volume at a more rapid rate for 12 to 16 h overnight. This kind of regimen is usually well tolerated, improves quality of life, and allows for better compliance by the patient.

Daily Requirements

Whatever route or regimen has been selected, the daily requirements for calories, proteins, fluids, electrolytes, vitamins, and trace elements should be satisfied. An accurate measurement of the REE is obtained by indirect calorimetry that determines gas exchanges in a thermoneutral environment. However, the high costs of this method prohibit their routine use outside of a research setting. Caloric requirements can also be calculated based on sex, age, weight, and height by using the Harris-Benedict formula. The basal energy expenditure is then adjusted by a correction factor related to the level of activity and the clinical conditions of the patient (Table 3-5).

Practically, daily caloric requirements can be met by providing 1000 kcal above the patient's basal energy expenditure or by giving 150% of the calculated or measured REE. Nonprotein calories are supplied as a combination of carbohydrates and fat usually in a percentage of 70% for carbohydrates and 30% for lipids. The maximal rate of glucose oxi-

TABLE 3–5. *Harris-Benedict equation and correction factors for determination of energy requirements*

Condition or level of activity	Correction factor
Confined to bed	1.2
Ambulatory	1.3
Elective surgery	1.2
Fever	1.0 + 0.13 per °C
Peritonitis	1.2–1.5
Soft tissue trauma	1.2–1.4
Major sepsis	1.4–1.8
Starvation	0.7

Basal energy expenditure (BEE) for women (kcal/day): BEE = 655 + [9.6 × weight (kg)] + [1.7 × height (cm)] − [4.7 × age (years)].

Basal energy expenditure (BEE) for men: BEE = 66 + [13.7 × weight (kg)] + [5.0 × height (cm)] − [6.8 × age (years)]

Resting energy expenditure (REE) = BEE × correction factor.

dation in the adult is 7 g/kg/day. Patients with high caloric requirements or severe glucose intolerance should be given calories in excess of this calculated rate as lipid.

The average protein requirement in normal subjects is 0.8 g/kg/day for maintenance and is 1.2 to 1.5 g/kg/day for anabolism. Hospitalized cancer patients have increased requirements and should be provided with 1.5 to 2.0 g/kg/day. Dietary nitrogen should be supplied with a calorie-to-nitrogen ratio ranging from 125 to 150 calories per gram of nitrogen (1 g of nitrogen = 6.25 g of protein). A 24-h urine collection for urinary urea nitrogen can be performed to calculate nitrogen balance for a more precise estimate of protein delivery.

In addition to calories and protein, electrolytes, vitamins, and trace elements are required nutrients. Daily requirements of electrolytes are as follows: sodium, 60 to 120 mEq; potassium, 60 to 100 mEq; chloride, 60 to 120 mEq; magnesium 8 to 10 mEq; calcium, 200 to 400 mg; phosphorus, 300 to 400 mg. Ongoing urinary and GI losses of fluid and electrolytes must be considered and specific electrolyte, vitamin, or mineral deficiences identified and corrected. Required daily vitamins and minerals are included in most enteral formulas or can be provided as multivitamin and trace element preparations. Vitamin and trace element formulas are commercially available to provide daily parenteral requirements.

COMPLICATIONS OF NUTRITIONAL SUPPLEMENTATION

Both enteral nutrition and TPN are associated with potential complications, though the enteral route is considered safer because complications associated with enteral feeding are usually less severe than those seen with TPN.

Enteral nutrition can be affected by GI, mechanical, metabolic, and infectious complications. GI complications include nausea, vomiting, cramping, bloating, and diarrhea and are frequently related to hyperosmolarity or the infusion rate of the formula (Table 3-6). Mechanical complications can be produced by tube malfunction or displacement, and most frequently are related to clogging of the feeding tube (Table 3-7). Metabolic abnormalities include hyperglycemia, and electrolyte or fluid imbalances (Table 3-8). Aspiration pneumonia, bacterial overgrowth within the feeding tube, and, occasionally, abdominal wall cellulitis can also occur.

Complications during TPN may be infectious, mechanical, or metabolic. A central venous line must be considered as a possible source of infection whenever an unexplained fever occurs in a patient receiving TPN. If this is suspected, the central line should be changed over a sterile guide wire and the tip of the catheter cultured. If a line infection is confirmed, the central line must be removed and a new catheter should

TABLE 3–6. *Gastrointestinal complications associated with enteral feeding*

Complication	Diagnosis	Therapy	Prevention
Offensive smell	Smell, nausea, vomiting	Add flavorings	Use polymeric formulas
Gastric retention	Nausea, vomiting, gastric residual > 100 ml after a bolus, or >115% volume/h	Dilute formula	Dilute formula and then gradually increase the concentration
Overly rapid infusion	Nausea, vomiting	Decrease rate, advance 25 ml/h every 12 to 24 h	Start feeding at 20–30 ml/h, advance 20–30 ml/h every 12–24 h
Lactose intolerance	Diarrhea, nausea, vomiting; review history; lactose tolerance test	Switch to non–lactose-based formula	Use formulas with low lactose content
Excessive fat in diet	Nausea, vomiting; review history	Switch to low-fat diet	Provide <30–40% of calories as fat
Fat malabsorption	Steatorrhea; review history; 72-h fecal fat assessment	Pancreatic enzyme supplements	Use low-fat formulas
Hyperosmolar solution	Diarrhea, increased stool water content; formula osmolality > 300 mOsm	Dilute to isotonicity, stop for 12 h, resume at slow rate, use Kaopectate, Lomotil	Use isotonic solutions, start at slow rate and increase at 12–24-h increments
Cold feelings	Diarrhea; tubing cold to touch	Discontinue feedings until formula is warm	Start recently refrigerated formulas at slow rate
Protein malnutrition	Diarrhea; albumin < 3g/dl	Dilute solution to isotonicity, use antidiarrheal	Start feeding at 20–30 ml/h, advance 20–30 ml/h every 12–24 h
Diarrhea	Diarrhea	Decrease flow rate or discontinue if severe and persistent	Use parenteral feeding
Dehydration	Orthostatic hypotension, dry mucous membranes, constipation	Supplemental fluids	Monitor intake and output
Impaction	Rectal examination	Digital disimpaction	Monitor intake and output
Bowel obstruction	Nausea, vomiting, bloating, constipation, obstipation; obstructive series	Surgery	—

Adapted from Callans LS, Daly JM. Nutritional support in the cancer patient. In: *Manual of oncologic therapeutics.* 3rd ed. Philadelphia: JB Lippincott, 1995:409.

TABLE 3–7. *Mechanical complications associated with enteral feeding*

Complication	Diagnosis	Therapy	Prevention
Nasopharyngeal discomfort	Mouth breathing, sore throat, hoarseness	Sugarless gum, gargling with warm water and mouth-wash, anesthetic lozenges	Use soft small-bore tubes
Nasal erosions	Erosions of nasal ala	Tape tube without pressure on nasal ala	Use soft small-bore tubes, proper taping
Abscess of nasal septum	Pain, fever, chills	Remove tube, drainage, antibiotics	Use soft small-bore tubes
Acute sinusitis	Pain, nasal congestion, fever, malodorous breath	Remove tube, hot compresses, analgesic	Use soft small-bore tubes
Acute otitis media	Severe throbbing ear pain, fever, chill, dizziness	Change tube to other nostril, antibiotics	—
Rupture of esophageal varices	Hematemesis, melena, radiographic studies	Remove tube	Use soft small-bore tubes
Esophagitis	Heartburn, substernal and epigastric burning pain	Remove tube	Keep head of bed at 45° angle
Esophageal ulceration	Dysphagia, odynophagia, radiologic studies, esophagoscopy	Remove tube	Use of small-bore tube; consider a jejunostomy tube or PEG
Tracheoesophageal fistula	Fistula present	Symptomatic	Use of small-bore tube; use gastric or jejunostomy tube
Knotting tube	Unable to remove tube	Cut tube and allow to pass per rectum, use McGill forceps to bring tube out mouth to cut tube	—

Adapted from Callans LS, Daly JM. Nutritional support in the cancer patient. In: *Manual of oncologic therapeutics.* 3rd ed. Philadelphia: JB Lippincott, 1995:409.

be inserted at a distant site. Usually, bacteria responsible for catheter infections are gram-positive skin commensals, suggesting that careful catheter placement and meticulous care during maintenance are required to reduce the incidence of infections. Single lumen catheters are associated with lower infection rates than multilumen catheters, and thus are more suitable for patients requiring TPN.

Mechanical complications of TPN administration include pneumothorax, hydrothorax, or hemothorax and are possible consequences of erroneous catheter placement (Table 3-9). Metabolic complications (Table 3-10) can be avoided by carefully assessing daily requirements and by closely monitoring the glucose, electrolyte, and fluid balance of the patient.

TABLE 3–8. *Metabolic complications associated with enteral feeding*

Complication	Causes	Therapy	Prevention
Hypokalemia	Diarrhea, severe malnutrition, insulin administration	K+ supplements	Check electrolytes
Hypophosphatemia	Insulin administration, severe malnutrition	Phosphate supplements	Check electrolytes
Hyponatremia	Overhydratation	Water restriction	Check electrolytes
Hyperphosphatemia	Renal insufficiency	Switch to low-phosphate feeding	Check electrolytes
Hypomagnesemia	Decreased carrier protein, inadequate delivery	Magnesium supplements	Check electrolytes
Elevated transaminases	Activation of hepatic enzymes, excess caloric load	Reduce carbohydrates	Check liver function tests
Vitamin K deficiency	Inadequate delivery	Vitamin K replacement	Check liver function tests
Essential fatty acid deficiency	Low linoleic acid	Parenteral fat; 5 ml safflower daily	Give balanced formula, including lipids

Adapted from Callans LS, Daly JM. Nutritional support in the cancer patient. In: *Manual of oncologic therapeutics.* 3rd ed. Philadelphia: JB Lippincott, 1995:409.

TABLE 3-9. *Mechanical complications associated with total parenteral nutrition*

Complication	Diagnosis	Therapy	Prevention
Pneumothorax following central line placement	Dyspnea, chest pain, chest x-ray	Tube thoracostomy, observation	Avoid placement in subclavian vein in emergency situation; use Trendelenburg position
Hemothorax, hydrothorax	Dyspnea, chest pain, chest x-ray	Tube thoracostomy, remove catheter, serial CXR, possible thoracotomy	Avoid placement in subclavian vein in emergency situation; use Trendelenburg position
Venous thrombosis	Inability to cannulate	Remove catheter, heparin therapy	Use silicon catheters, add heparin
Air embolism	Dyspnea, cyanosis, hypotension, tachycardia, precordial murmur	Trendelenburg, left lateral decubitus positions	Trendelenburg position, Valsalva maneuver; tape connections
Catheter embolism	Sheared catheter	Fluoroscopic retrieval	Never withdraw catheter through needle
Arrhythmias	Catheter tip in atrium	Withdraw catheter to SVC	—
Subclavian artery injury	Pulsatile red blood	Remove needle, apply pressure, chest x-ray	Trendelenburg position with roll between scapulae
Catheter tip misplacement	Chest film	Redirect with a guidewire	Direct bevel of needle caudally

RQ, respiratory quotient; *SVC*, superior vena cava; *TPN* total parenteral nutrition.
Adapted from Callans LS, Daly JM. Nutritional support in the cancer patient. In: *Manual of oncologic therapeutics*. 3rd ed. Philadelphia: JB Lippincott, 1995:412.

TABLE 3-10. *Metabolic complications associated with total parenteral nutrition*

Complication	Diagnosis	Therapy	Prevention
Hyperglycemic, hyperosmolar non-ketotic coma	Dehydration with osmotic diuresis, disorientation, lethargy, stupor, convulsions, coma; glucose > 1,000 mg/dl; Osm > 350 MOsm/l	Discontinue TPN, administer 5% dextrose half-normal saline at 250 ml/h; insulin 10–20 units/h, bicarbonate; monitor glucose, potassium, pH	—
Hypoglycemia	Headache, sweating, thirst, convulsions, disorientation, paresthesias	D_{50} intravenously as a bolus push	Taper TPN by one half for 12 h; then 12 h of D_{50} at 100 ml/h
CO$_2$ retention	Ventilator dependence, high RQ	Reduce glucose load	Provide 30–40% calories as lipid
Azotemia	Dehydration, elevated blood urea nitrogen	Reduce protein load	Monitor fluid balance
Hyperammonemia	Lethargy, malaise, coma, seizures	Discontinue amino acid infusions, infuse arginine	Avoid casein or fibrin hydrolysate
Essential fatty acid deficiency	Xerosis, hepatomegaly, impaired healing, bone changes	Fat administration	Provide 25–50 mg/kg/day of essential fatty acids
Hypophosphatemia	Lethargy, anorexia, weakness, arrythmias	Supplemental phosphate	Treat causative factors: alkalosis, gram-negative sepsis, vomiting, malabsorption, provide 20 mEq/1,000 kcal
Abnormal liver function tests	Fatty infiltrate	Evaluate for other causes	Provide balanced TPN solutions
Hypomagnesemia	Weakness, nausea, vomiting, tremors, depression, hyporeflexia	Infuse 10% MgSO$_4$	Supply magnesium in dose of 0.35–0.45 mEq/day; monitor serum levels
Hypermagnesemia	Drowsiness, nausea, vomiting, coma, arrhythmia	Dialysis, infuse calcium gluconate	Monitor serum levels

Adapted from Callans LS, Daly JM. Nutritional support in the cancer patient. In: *Manual of oncologic therapeutics*. 3rd ed. Philadelphia: JB Lippincott, 1995:412.

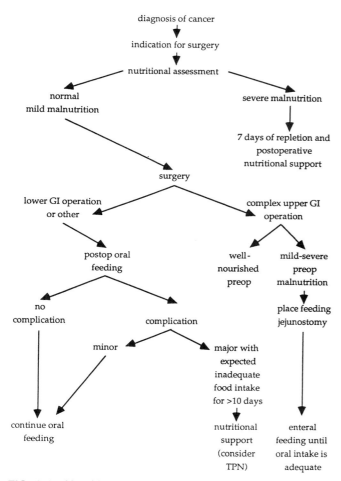

FIG. 3-1. Algorithm defining indications for nutritional support in patients undergoing surgery alone. *GI*, gastrointestinal; *TPN*, total parenteral nutrition.

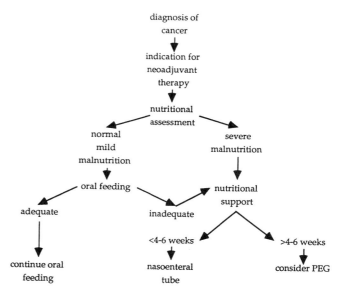

FIG. 3-2. Algorithm defining indications for nutritional support in cancer patients undergoing neoadjuvant treatment. *PEG*, percutaneous endoscopic gastrostomy.

POSTOPERATIVE NUTRITIONAL SUPPORT

The American Society of Parenteral and Enteral Nutrition has recommended that postoperative nutritional support should be provided for patients who are severely malnourished before surgery; well nourished before surgery, but have complications that result in more than 10 days of inadequate food intake; or well nourished before surgery, but expected to have inadequate intake for more than 10 days because of the nature of their surgery (22).

Patients undergoing complex upper-GI procedures such as esophagogastrectomy, total gastrectomy, and pancreaticoduodenectomy who have experienced moderate to severe weight loss preoperatively should have a feeding jejunostomy placed for postoperative nutritional support.

In patients who are candidates for postoperative nutrition, TPN is indicated when enteral nutrition cannot be accomplished by jejunostomy. Use of TPN is also suggested in patients who develop a major postoperative complication that does not allow resumption of adequate enteral or oral feeding (Fig. 3-1).

MULTIMODALITY TREATMENT

Current concepts on cancer therapy are frequently based on multimodality treatment with patients undergoing surgery plus radio- and chemotherapy given pre- or postoperatively. It is well known that these therapies, especially when provided in an aggressive fashion, may induce damages to both the immune system and to the GI tract, sometimes resulting in a decrease in food intake and in a subsequent worsening of the nutritional status.

A metaanalysis by Detsky et al. (23), evaluating the effectiveness of perioperative intravenous nutrition in the cancer patient, concluded that the routine use of this approach was not justified. However, data from a randomized controlled study by Daly et al. (24) showed an increase in hospital admissions for patients given oral feeding alone versus patients who received supplemental enteral feeding. Additionally, there was a 61% cross-over rate to the tube feeding regimen because of the onset of diarrhea, dehydration, inanition, or other complications during radiation or chemotherapy (24).

The correct management of patients undergoing multimodality treatment is still controversial. As a general recommendation, patients who have a feeding jejunostomy should be supplemented during radiation or chemotherapy, particularly if food intake is not adequate, so that the development of cachexia may be prevented (Figs. 3-2 and 3-3).

SPECIALIZED FORMULAS

When immune dysfunction is caused by malnutrition only, nutritional repletion is usually able to reverse anergy. In cancer patients immune system impairment is multifactorial and may be a consequence of the tumor itself, cancer cachexia, reduced

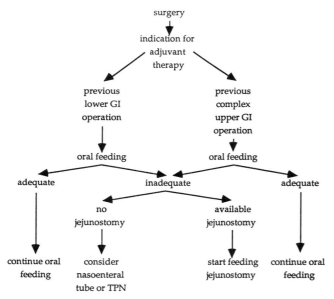

FIG. 3-3. Algorithm defining indications for nutritional support in patients undergoing adjuvant therapy. *GI*, gastrointestinal; *TPN*, total parenteral nutrition.

food intake, or the effect of multimodality treatment. Therefore, it is not surprising that, in tumor-bearing patients, nutritional support frequently fails to restore normal immune competence. Whether particular amino acid deficiencies contribute to this problem has been widely studied and is addressed below.

Arginine

Arginine (Arg) is an amino acid classically considered as nonessential since it can be synthetized *in vivo* via the urea cycle. However, it becomes essential under particularly stressful conditions, such as trauma or sepsis, when its requirements increase dramatically. For this reason Arg has come to be regarded as a semiessential amino acid. Arg has been demonstrated to have many important activities not dependent on being a simple source of nitrogen. Two pathways have been identified as potential effectors of the immunomodulatory actions *in vivo*, although to date the real mechanisms of the pharmacologic activity of Arg remain unclear. First, the arginase pathway, in which Arg is converted to ornithine with the production of urea, generates polyamine synthesis by the action of the enzyme ornithine decarboxylase. A second more recently described pathway of Arg metabolism leads to the generation of nitric oxide through the action of the nitric oxide synthase (NOS).

Arg has been recognized to possess metabolic, immunostimulatory, and antitumor properties. In both animals and humans, there has been evidence that Arg has anabolic effects by reducing urinary nitrogen losses, increasing nitrogen retention and wound healing. Also, Arg has secretagogue properties, inducing the production of growth hormone and prolactin by the pituitary gland and of insulin and glucagon by the pancreas. The relationship between anabolic and secretagogue effect of Arg is not yet well established, but some authors have suggested that an intact hypothalamopituitary axis is essential for Arg to mediate its effect (25).

The immunostimulatory properties of Arg are potentially very useful in cancer patients. It seems that Arg exerts beneficial actions over a variety of different cell populations, including ameliorating lymphocyte, neutrophil, and macrophage function. Animal studies have demonstrated that Arg supplementation produces thymotrophic activity, increases the total number of thymic lymphocytes, as well as their responsiveness to mitogens, and enhances cellular immunity as suggested by the increase in skin allograft rejection and the improvement in delayed hypersensitivity response and survival in burned rats (26,27). In human trials, Arg increased CD4 expression and lymphocyte blastogenesis in both healthy volunteers (28) and patients undergoing major cancer surgery (29). Ornithine (Orn) shares the same thymotropic activities as Arg either by the same mechanism or because Arg increases Orn availability.

Arg also appears to play a key role in polymorphonuclear neutrophil (PMN) function. A direct transport system of L-Arg into PMNs has been identified. PMNs express NOS, and Arg supplementation has been demonstrated to increase bacterial phagocytosis in healthy volunteers (30) and to regulate PMN chemotaxis *in vitro* (31). Recently, a randomized controlled trial was reported in which patients received pre- and postoperatively either standard or enriched enteral diets. In this trial patients who were given Arg-enriched diets had an earlier recovery in PMN phagocytosis and respiratory burst after surgery than patients fed a standard diet (32).

The antitumor activity of Arg seems to be related to improvement in cellular immune function, particularly for macrophages and natural killer (NK) cells. Animal studies have demonstrated that Arg increases cell lysis of tumor targets by macrophages and NK cells (33). Whether Arg is capable of reducing infectious complications in surgical patients remains controversial. In our experience with two different randomized controlled studies, a significant reduction in infectious wound complications was seen in the group fed postoperatively with an enriched formula as compared to the standard enteral formula group (11 versus 37%, $p = 0.02$; and 10 versus 43%, $p < 0.05$) (34,24). Although other authors have not observed a significant reduction in the number of postoperative complications, they have reported a significant decrease in the severity of postoperative infections and shorter hospital stays for patients who received Arg-supplemented diets (35).

RNA and ω-3 Polyunsaturated Fatty Acids

Formulas used for clinical trials are enriched not only with Arg but also with other nutrients that are thought to have pharmacologic properties and immunomodulatory activity, such as RNA and ω-3 polyunsaturated fatty acids (ω-3 PUFA). RNA has been shown to be essential for the continued maturation of T cells in animal models. Absence of RNA from the diet results in depressed cell-mediated immune function, decreased survival after **Staphylococcus aureus** injection, and diminished rejection of allograft (36). Administration of RNA significantly improved host immune responsiveness and host survival to a septic change with **Candida albicans** (37).

The ω-3 PUFA influence the production of prostanoids from the dienoic to the trienoic variety, the latter of which are much less immunosuppressive (38). A major biologic effect of dietary PUFA is the change in cell membrane composition and receptor enzyme functions. Diets high in ω-3 PUFA decrease prostaglandin E_2 (PGE_2) synthesis and suppress TNF production after stimulation. Both animal and human studies evaluating mononuclear cells, Kupffer's cells, and peritoneal macrophages demonstrate suppression of IL-1β secretion after increasing ω-3 PUFA in the diet (39).

Glutamine

Glutamine, a nonessential amino acid, is the most abundant amino acid in the circulation and in the free intracellular amino acid pool. It is supposed to have both immunomodulatory activity and structural function for the gut wall. Research in our laboratory has shown that macrophage superoxide, nitric oxide production, **Candida killing**, and tumor cytotoxicity are enhanced with increasing glutamine concentration *in vitro*. In rats, glutamine-supplemented TPN has been found to improve peritoneal and macrophage function (40).

Other experimental results have proven that glutamine is important for manteinance of integrity of gut structure. In fact, in animal studies glutamine supplementation increased mucosal disaccaridase activity, protected liver from fatty infiltration, improved glucose absorption, and decreased bacterial translocation (41). Most enteral feeding formulas contain a significant amount of glutamine, but parenteral glutamine supplementation remains limited because glutamine is relatively unstable in TPN solutions, and thus it is usually not included in commercially available formulas.

Though there is some evidence that nutritional formulas that possess immunomodulatory properties can improve the clinical outcome of patients following surgery by improving immune response capability and gut function, further studies are required to clarify whether these enriched enteral formulas are cost effective in providing optimal nutritional support for cancer patients.

CONCLUSIONS

Malignancy is frequently associated with nutritional compromise due to tumor effects that result in decreased nutrient intake, metabolic abnormalities, or both. Malnutrition in cancer patients can lead to decreased ability to tolerate medical or surgical therapy. A thorough history and physical examination represents the most effective method to define the nutritional status of cancer patients, though additional useful information can be obtained by determining serum levels of albumin and TFN. Anthropometric measurements, skin testing, RBP, prealbumin levels, and PNI are not recommended for routine clinical assessment but may be of interest in selected cases.

Available data suggest that preoperative nutritional support is only beneficial for patients with severe malnutrition. Postoperative nutritional supplementation should be given via an enteric route whenever possible. Placement of a feeding jejunostomy at the time of laparotomy in any patient who is undergoing a complicated abdominal tumor resection is advocated, even if there is evidence of only mild or moderate malnutrition on their nutritional assessment. Future studies should be aimed at elucidating what enteric formulation provides optimal nutritional supplementation in cachectic cancer patients.

REFERENCES

1. De Wys WD, Begg D, Lavin PT. Prognostic effect of weight loss prior to chemotherapy in cancer patients. *Am J Med* 1980;69:491.
2. Knox LS, Crosby LO, Feurer ID, et al. Energy expenditure in malnourished cancer patients. *Ann Surg* 1983;197:152.
3. Gelin J, Moldawer LL, Lonroth C, Sherry B, Chizzonite R, Lundholm K. Role of endogenous tumor necrosis factor alpha and inteleukin 1 for experimental tumor growth and the development of cancer cachexia. *Cancer Res* 1991;51:415.
4. Tracey KJ, Wei H, Manogue KR, et al. Cachectin/tumor necrosis factor induces cahcexia, anemia and inlammation. *J Exp Med* 1988;167:1211.
5. Socher SH, Martinez D, Craig JB, Kuitn JG, Oliff A. Tumor necrosis factor not detectable in patients with clinical cancer cachexia. *J Natl Cancer Inst* 1988;80:595.
6. Tracey KJ, Morgello S, Koplin BK, et al. Metabolic effect of cachectin/tumor necrosis factor are modified by the site of production. *J Clin Invest* 1990;86:2014.
7. Patton JS, Peters PM, McCabe J, et al. Development of partial tolerance to the gastrointestinal effects of high doses of recombinant tumor necrosis factor–alpha in rodents. *J Clin Invest* 1987;80:1587.
8. Hellerstein MK, Meydani SN, Meydani M, Wu K, Dinarello CA. Inteleukin 1–induced anorexia in the rat. Influence of prostaglandins. *J Clin Invest* 1989;84:228.
9. McIntosh K, Jablons DM, Mule JJ, et al. *In vivo* induction of IL-6 by administration of endogenous cytokines and detection of de novo serum levels of IL-6 in tumor-bearing mice. *J Immunol* 1989;143:162.
10. Jablons DM, McIntosh JK, Mule JJ, Nordan RP, Rudikoff S, Lotze MT. Induction of interferon-beta₂/interleukin-6 by cytokine administration and detection of circulating interleukin-6 in the tumor-bearing state. *Ann NY Acad Sci* 1989;557:157.
11. Strassmann G, Fong M, Kennedy JS, Jacob CO. Evidence for the involvement of interleukin-6 in experimental cancer cachexia. *J Clin Invest* 1992;89:1681.
12. Langstein HN, Doherty GM, Frakler DL, Buresh CK, Norton JA. The roles of gamma-interferon and tumor necrosis factor alpha in an experimental model of cancer cachexia. *Cancer Res* 1992;51:2302.
13. Todorov P, Cariuk P, McDevitt T, Coles B, Fearon K, Tisdale M. Characterization of a cancer cachectic factor. *Nature* 1996;379:739.
14. Warren S. The immediate cause of death in cancer. *Am J Med Sci* 1932;184:610.
15. Nixon DW, Heymsfield SB, Cohen AE. Protein-calorie malnutrition in hospitalized cancer patients. *Am J Med* 1980;68:683.
16. Meguid M, Mughal MM, Debonis D, et al. Influence of nutritional status on the resumption of adequate food intake in patients recovering from colorectal operations. *Surg Clin North Am* 1986;66:1167.
17. Harvey KB, Bath A, Blackburn GL. Nutritional assessment and patient outcome during oncological therapy. *Cancer* 1979;43[Suppl]:2065.
18. Daly JM, Dudrick SJ, Copeland EM. Intravenous hyperalimentation: effect on delayed cutaneous hypersensitivity in cancer patients. *Ann Surg* 1980;192:587.

19. Weisdorf SA, Lysne J, Wind D, et al. Positive effect of prophylactic total parenteral nutrition on long-term outcome of bone marrow transplantation. *Transplantation* 1987;43:833.
20. Szeluga DJ, Stuart RK, Brookmyer R, et al. Nutritional support of bone marrow transplant recipients: a prospective, randomized clinical trial comparing total parenteral nutrition to an enteral feeding programme. *Cancer Res* 1987;47:3309.
21. Buzby GP, Mullen JL, Mathews DL, et al. Prognostic nutritional index in gastrointestinal surgery. *Am J Surg* 1980;139:160.
22. American Society of Parenteral and Enteral Nutrition Board of Directors. Guidelines for use of total parenteral nutrition in the hospitalized adult patient. *JPEN J Parenter Enteral Nutr* 1986;10:441.
23. Detsky AS, Baker JP, O'Rourke K, et al. Perioperative parenteral nutrition: a meta-analysis. *Ann Int Med* 1987;107:195.
24. Daly JM, Weintraub FN, Shou J, Rosato EF, Lucia M. Enteral nutrition during multimodality therapy in upper gastrointestinal cancer patients. *Ann Surg* 1995;221:327.
25. Barbul A, Rettura G, Levenson SM, Seifter E. Wound healing and thymotropic effects of arginine: a pituitary mechanism of action. *Am J Clin Nutr* 1983;37:786.
26. Barbul A, Wasserkrug HL, Sisto DA et al. Thymic and immunostimulatory actions of arginine. *JPEN J Parenter Enteral Nutr* 1980;4:446.
27. Barbul A, Wasserkrug HL, Seifter E, et al. Immunostimulatory effects of arginine in normal and injured rats. *J Surg Res* 1980;29:228.
28. Barbul A, Rettura G, Wasserkrug HL, et al. Arginine stimulates lymphocyte immune responses in healthy volunteers. *Surgery* 1981;90:244.
29. Daly JM, Reynolds J, Thom A, et al. Immune and metabolic effect of arginine in the surgical patient. *Ann Surg* 1988;208:512.
30. Moffat FL, Han T, Li ZM, et al. Supplemental L-arginine augments bacterial phagocytosis in human polymorphonuclear leukocytes. *J Cell Physiol* 1996;168:26.
31. Belenky SN, Robbins RA, Rennard SI, Gossman GL, Nelson KJ, Rubinstein I. Inhibitors of nitric oxide synthase attenuate human neutrophil chemotaxis *in vitro. J Lab Clin Med* 1993;122:388.
32. Braga M, Gianotti L, Cestari A, et al. Gut function and immune and inflammatory responses in patients perioperatively fed with supplemented enteral formulas. *Arch Surg* 1996;131:1257.
33. Tachibana K, Mukai K, Hiraoka I, et al. Evaluation of the effect of arginine enriched amino acid solution on tumor growth. *JPEN J Parenter Enteral Nutr* 1985;9:428.
34. Daly JM, Lieberman MD, Goldfine J, et al. Enteral nutrition with supplemental arginine, RNA and omega-3 fatty acids in patients after operation: immunologic, metabolic and clinical outcome. *Surgery* 1992;112:56
35. Gianotti L, Braga M, Vignali A, et al. Effect of route of delivery and formulation of postoperative nutritional support in patients undergoing major operations for malignant neoplasms. *Arch Surg* 1997;132:1222.
36. Rudolph RF, Kulkami AD, Schandle VB, et al. Involment in dietary nucleotides in T-lymphocyte function. *Adv Exp Med* 1984;165:175.
37. Kulkarni AD, Fanslow WC, Drath DB, et al. Influence of dietary nucleotide restriction on bacterial sepsis and phagocytic cell function in mice. *Arch Surg* 1986;121:169.
38. Kinsella J, Lokesh B, Broughton S, et al. Dietary polyunsaturated fatty acids and eicosanoids: potential effect on the modulation of inflammatory and immune cells: an overview. *Nutrition* 1990;6:24.
39. Mean C, Martin J. Fatty acids and immunity. *Adv Lipid Res* 1993;16:127.
40. Shou J, Lappin J, Minnard E, et al. Total parenteral nutrition, bacterial translocation and host immune function. *Am J Surg* 1994;167:145.
41. Zhang W, Franlel WL, Singh A, et al. Improvement of structure and function in orthotopic small bowel transplantation in the rat by glutamine. *Transplantation* 1993;56:512.

CHAPTER 4

Cost-Effective Preoperative and Postoperative Treatment Testing in a Managed Care Environment

Janardan D. Khandekar

Ours is a society of styles and fads. At present, "cost-effective analysis," "efficacy studies," and "managed care" are very much in vogue. These buzz words represent a real, new discipline in medicine that involves assessment of relative utility and costs of different diagnostic and therapeutic measures. This discipline, known as "outcome analysis," is often labeled as a third revolution in medicine, preceded by the discovery of antibiotics and the era of biotechnology as the first and second revolutions, respectively.

The worldwide interest in escalating health care costs stems from two realities confronting health policy decision-makers: the availability of health-related interventions considerably exceeds the societal ability to afford them; and current practice patterns are inadequate to guide choices between interventions that are likely to yield the most benefit for the population (1). An individual physician often faces a schizophrenic choice between providing the best care for a patient under his/her care, and the societal needs of controlling health care costs. Although these are not new developments, the rapid progress in medicine in recent years has reached to a point where technology evaluation has become almost mandatory.

In this chapter, I shall examine the utility of various diagnostic tests conducted in the pre- and postoperative settings for common solid tumors with the principal emphasis on breast and colon cancers. Prior to examining the usefulness of various tests in this setting, it will be useful to examine the following: (a) a brief review of current status of managed care (2,3); (b) principles of analysis of cost-effectiveness (CE) (1); and (c) decision analysis which underpins the evaluation of diagnostic tests.

MANAGED CARE

The United States is not alone in its concern about rapidly rising health care costs. These concerns are shared by almost every industrialized nation, including Canada, Great Britain,

and Germany (4). These industrialized nations who have national health care have tried to address this issue through rationing of care. The United States has tried to apply the principles of market forces for this dilemma (2). The economic data for containing health care costs are compelling (1,5,6). Between 1965 to 1995, the share of the U.S. gross domestic product devoted to health care grew from 5% to 15%, and over $1 trillion were spent in 1995 on health care. It is expected that by the year 2000, $1.5 trillion will be spent on health care. Health care costs grew at twice the cost of inflation. For Medicare, the case for cost containment is even more compelling. This program accounts for approximately 11% of the federal budget, and grew at a 17% annualized rate.

Managed care has evolved as a market force to contain the health care costs (2). In 1994, 51 million individuals were enrolled in health maintenance organizations (HMOs). It is estimated that an equal number, if not more, are enrolled in preferred provider organizations (PPOs), which also follow many of the policies of the HMOs. Managed care has thus become a big business, and many of the large managed care companies are traded on Wall Street (7). Almost two-thirds of all Americans working for medium-sized and large firms are enrolled in the managed care plans. Further, there is increasing pressure to shift the Medicare population from a fee-for-service system to managed care.

The HMOs, as a prepaid group practice, had a humble beginning in Tacoma, Washington in 1910. This was followed by Kaiser plans around the country, but HMO enrollment was modest. However, in late 1973, Congress passed legislation to provide federal funding for the expansion of HMOs (6). Excessive congressional regulations on HMOs precluded their expansion, and it was only in the early 1980s that Corporate America moved aggressively to shift its workforce from indemnity insurance to one or another variant of managed care (8). The impact of managed care on costs began to occur only in the 1990s when the health care costs began to decelerate, primarily as the result of surplus capacity of hospitals and the weakening of the labor movement. There was also a decrease in physician resistance to the HMOs as a result of the burgeoning number of physicians. The HMOs were able to meet the twin demands of a slowing of premiums for health care costs, while making a substantial profit for the officers of the corporation, and the stockholders. At present, HMOs and PPOs decide the kinds of treatments available to the patients as well as the site of service. As a result of the growing power of these organizations, physicians and hospitals have been relegated to a secondary role in the care of patients.

Simultaneous with these developments, there has been a marked shift in the managed care companies themselves. They are in an era of consolidation. Many provider-owned HMOs and PPOs are being acquired by large managed care companies (7).

Moreover, there is a continuing debate about the future of managed care. Some have questioned whether the slower growth of expenditures is a onetime phenomena or is a continuing process (3,6). Those who argue that managed care will continue to provide cost containment point out that development of clinical guidelines will be a major factor in reducing or eliminating costly procedures as a key feature. However, there continues to be some evidence, at least in the Medicare population, that the healthier patients enroll, while the sicker ones leave the organizations (9). Although no one has a crystal ball to see the future of managed care, recently Malik M. Hasan (10), Chief Executive Officer of Foundation Health Systems was quoted as saying, "The managed health care system is here, and it is not going to go away . . . the war is coming, which will make what has happened until now look practically like a picnic." It therefore behooves every practicing physician to be acquainted with managed care and the CE that these companies demand.

PRINCIPLES OF COST-EFFECTIVE ANALYSIS

Cost-effective analysis is basically a method that compares cost and years of life gained for a given intervention (1). The commonly used terms are as follows: *CE analysis* is the incremental cost of obtaining a unit of health effect (such as dollars per year of life expectancy) from a given health intervention. When compared to an alternative, ideally the new intervention should be more effective and less costly than the alternative. *Cost-benefit analysis* is a tool that estimates net societal benefit of a program or intervention, less the increased cost with benefits and costs measured in dollars.

The results of the analysis such as that conducted for screening for breast cancer, for bypass surgery, for coronary artery disease, or dialysis in renal failure are usually summarized as *cost-effective ratios,* i.e., the cost of achieving one unit of health outcome such as one year of life gain (1,11). This kind of analysis helps decision-makers in different fields such as HMOs and state and federal governments make judgments about intervention. However, there are many caveats to the problem of measuring CE.

In determining cost analysis, the economic assessment is based on the following: (a) prospective analysis of costs and benefits of intervention; (b) determination of the source of data (for example, there is a considerable difference between cost versus charges, because each economic entity has a markup to the cost, this should be properly evaluated); (c) determination of the components of costs (see below); and (d) the type of study (was it prospective or retrospective?).

The principal aim for health services is to maximize the years of healthy life gained for its population in return for a given level of investment. However, predicting return on investments, particularly in medicine, is difficult. The economic model to evaluate the costs of goods and services are not applicable to health care. The benefits side of the intervention are often uncertain and time frames not very precise. Thus, these benefits cannot be listed at quarterly intervals as is customary on Wall Street, as the returns have long horizons. For example, the lowering of cholesterol will not produce returns in terms of decreased cardiovascular events for many years. On the other side of the coin, the "costs" are also different. The customary economic models do not include time required for intervention (time taken off from work for various tests) or undesirable side effects that may occur as a result of the interventions. As a result of the uncertainty of measuring these cost-to-benefit ratios, there has been a high degree of variability in the reports. For example, mammography, which reduces breast cancer mortality, has been variously estimated to cost from $3,000 to $80,000 per year of life saved. As a result of these discrepancies, the U.S. Public Health Service appointed a group of 13 nongovernment scientists and scholars with expertise in cost-effective analysis, and charged them with the task of assessing the current state of science in the field and provide specific recommendations for conducting such analysis. The panel has streamlined the process of calculating costs and benefits (1).

COMPONENTS OF COST

Various components of cost include the following:

1. Monetary
   A. The use of health care resources
   B. Indirect costs
      (1) Changes in the use of nonhealth care resources
      (2) Changes in the employment status, i.e., lost time to the employer
      (3) Changes in the use of time of caregiver
2. Human cost (obtained from patients)
   A. Pain and suffering
   B. Role disruption
   C. Social isolation

Determining total cost as a result of illnesses and intervention requires a thorough analysis of each of the factors mentioned above. It is therefore important that the sources that have been used to generate this data be identified to accurately estimate the costs and benefits (outcome) incurred as a result of therapy.

OUTCOME ANALYSIS

Outcome analysis, which is defined as a product of treatment, has evolved to address the issues of alternative treatments. In recent years, there has been an increasing emphasis on secondary endpoints such as ability to tolerate treatment and impact of treatment on the functional status and overall quality of life. The methodological challenges posed for the assessments of these secondary endpoints are considerable. These outcomes can be divided into two categories: (a) *disease outcome*—which measures principally disease-free survival in surgical oncology, but also measures response rate and duration of responses in medical oncology; and (b) *patient outcome*—which translates the effects of treatment on the patient in terms of quality of life and survival. However, quality of life is subjective, and in part definitional. It is measured differently by different individuals and is currently the subject of intensive studies.

The standard that is often used as cost-benefit procedure is $50,000 per year for quality adjusted extension of survival. For example, surgery for the left anterior descending artery results in a $4,000 to $8,000 of adjusted life survival per year. Screening for alpha-fetoprotein in the prenatal diagnosis costs $5,000 to $10,000 per year for 1 year of life extended. Control of diastolic blood pressure between 90 to 95 mm Hg costs between $30,000 and $40,000 per year of life extended. Heart transplant costs about $125,000 per year of life saved (1,11). These figures give some perspectives on how cost analysis can provide guidance for obtaining diagnostic tests or carrying interventions.

As observed by Eisenberg (12), "the application of economics to medical practice does not necessarily mean that less should or can be spent; rather the use of resources might be more efficient." However, more efficient use of resources require an understanding of decision analysis, i.e., principles that govern utilities of various diagnostic tests and interventions.

PRINCIPLES OF DECISION ANALYSIS

In interpreting the various diagnostic tests, *truth* is an important variable. For example, in a study of hepatic lesions with CT scans, if only pathologically confirmed cases were accepted as accurate, while all other unconfirmed cases considered false-negative, the CT was accurate only 31% of the time. On the other hand, if all unconfirmed cases were considered as correct by CT, then 87% of the cases were diagnosed correctly (13). It is therefore important to understand the concepts used in analyzing various diagnostic tests.

Physicians early in their career have a passion for acquiring facts. Facts, critical as they are, have no clinical value unless they are applied in solving clinical problems. The rapid introduction of technology in the medical practice has created further uncertainty about tests that one should choose in di-

agnosing and following patients. About 20 years ago, Fineberg and Hiatt (14) called for technology assessment, including development of guidelines in medical practices. The *decision matrix* is one such method of evaluating sensitivity, specificity, and predictive values of tests; the knowledge of which is essential in the practice of medicine.

DECISION MATRIX

This is the term most commonly applied to the simple decision of whether disease is present, D^+, or absent, D^-, when a test is abnormal (i.e., positive, T^+) or normal (i.e., negative, T^-) (15,16). When these two binary results are plotted on a two by two table, four possible combinations form the following ratios, as shown below:
True-positive (tP) ratio

$$\frac{a}{a + b}$$

represents the proportion of positive tests in all patients who have the disease. The TP ratio then expresses the sensitivity of the test.

False-positive (FP) ratio is the proportion of positive tests in all patients who do not have the disease, or

$$\frac{c}{c + d}$$

True-negative (TN) ratio is the proportion of negative tests in all patients who do not have the disease, or

$$\frac{c}{c + d}$$

This expresses specificity of the examination.
False-negative (FN) ratio is the proportion of negative tests in all patients with the disease, or

$$\frac{b}{a + b}$$

The *sensitivity,* which is defined as the likelihood of a positive test in a population with the disease, can be calculated as:

$$\frac{\text{diseased persons with positive test}}{\text{all diseased subjects tested}} \times 100$$

Simply stated, the sensitivity of a test is determined by the false-negative rate. The sensitivity of a test under consideration is usually determined by evaluating its efficacy against a known standard. Depending on the sensitivity of that standard, the sensitivity can be spuriously high or low. For example, the sensitivity of a bone scan is usually evaluated in relation to x-rays, a technique which is not very sensitive. Therefore, the sensitivity of bone scans is very high, in the vicinity of about 99%. On the other hand, in a study from Roswell Park, the false-negative rate of bone scans was 4.5%. This will give a lower sensitivity of the test.

The other term often used is the *specificity,* which is the likelihood of a negative test in the population without the disease. It is determined by the false-positive rate. Specificity is as follows:

$$\frac{\text{nondiseased persons negative to test}}{\text{all nondiseasd subjects tested}} \times 100$$

In order to determine specificity of the test, one must have adequate controls. For example, the relative increase in uptake of the bone scanning agents is noted in disease processes that produce a regional increase in blood flow, new bone formation, increased surface area of exchange, and/or as a result of increase in local extraction efficiency. This gives false-positivity to a bone scan. The instance of false-positive rate for bone scans in various series ranges from 3% to 64%. This depends on the criteria used in reading the bone scans. Implications of this variability are discussed later.

When sensitivity and specificity of a test are determined, it is important to know what its *predictive value* will be (17). That is, what is the likelihood that a subject yielding a positive test actually has the disease? Conversely, what is the likelihood that a subject with a negative test does not have the disease? This likelihood is related to the actual prevalence of the disease in the total population. More simply stated, predictive value for positive tests may be defined as a percentage of time that positive tests will detect the diseased individual. The *predictive value of a positive test* may be calculated as follows:

$$PV = \frac{\text{number of diseased subjects (or proportion) with positive test}}{\text{total number (or proportion) of subjects with positive test}} \times 100$$

The predictive value of a negative test is a percentage of time that a negative test will detect a nondiseased person. The *predictive value of a negative test* may be calculated as follows:

$$PV = \frac{\text{number (or proportion) of non-diseased persons with positive tests}}{\text{total number (or proportion) of persons with negative test}} \times 100$$

Thus, if the prevalence of the target disease in the population is high, and the sensitivity and specificity are high, then the predictive value for positive tests is also high. On the other hand, if the prevalence of the disease is low, and the sensitivity and specificity are also low, then the predictive value of a positive test is low.

Other biases also effect the interpretation of the various diagnostic tests (15). These include the following:

1. Lead-time bias: As shown in Fig. 4-1, for a patient who develops symptoms at a particular point in life, and who will die at a subsequent point, the aim of the screening test is to detect the disease before symptoms fully develop, and intervene

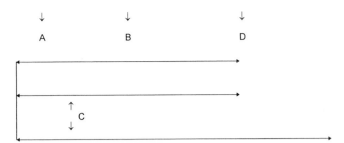

FIG. 4-1. Lead-time bias. In this example, let us say the natural history of disease is survival from point A to D, while B represents the point at which disease is diagnosed by conventional tests. If a new test diagnoses a condition at point C (i.e., earlier) but survival is still at point D, the test has made no impact on survival (lead-time bias); on the other hand, if diagnosing a condition at point C leads to extension of survival up to point E, the mortality rate will be reduced.

promptly, thereby prolong the patient's life. However, in the phenomena of lead-time bias, as shown in the figure, the test does indeed detect the disease early in the course of the evolution of the disease, but has no impact on overall survival. In other words, although the patient seems to be "under care" for a longer period of time and thus gives the appearance of improved survival, actually there was no impact on the mortality. Therefore, unless a particular screening test has been shown to decrease mortality, as has been the case for mammography, a screening diagnostic test cannot be routinely recommended.

2. Length bias: The biological behavior of cancer can be either aggressive or indolent. Cancers detected in the asymptomatic phase could be slow growing, and therefore detected at the time of screening, while more aggressive cancers occur in between the screening tests, giving an illusion that screening has led to detection of cancer with favorable outcome.

In this example, let us say the natural history if disease is survival from point A to D, while B represents the point at which disease is diagnosed by conventional tests. If a new test diagnoses a condition at point C (i.e., earlier) but survival is still at point D, the test has made no impact on survival (lead-time bias); on the other hand, if diagnosing a condition at point C leads to extension of survival up to point E, the mortality rate will be reduced.

EVALUATION OF VARIOUS TESTS USED IN COLON AND BREAST CANCERS

Various imaging techniques and tumor markers may be used in the diagnosis, prognosis, and recurrence of cancer. The American Society of Clinical Oncology (ASCO) established an expert panel to evaluate the use of tumor markers in breast and colon cancers (18,19). The panel modified the scale developed by the Canadian Task Force on Periodic Health Examination to evaluate the various tests (20) (Table 4-1). A similar process for developing guidelines was followed by another ASCO panel evaluating breast cancer surveillance guidelines (19). These guidelines were developed on the

TABLE 4–1. *Modified Canadian criteria for evaluating diagnostic test evidence*

Level of evidence	Type of evidence for recommendation
Level 1 (highest level)	Meta-analysis or large high-powered concurrently controlled studies with a primary objective to evaluate the utility of a given test
Level 2	Prospective clinical trials designed to test given hypothesis
Level 3	Large size retrospective trials
Level 4	Similar to level 3, but even less reliable; comparative and correlative descriptive and case study can be included
Level 5	Case reports and clinical examples

Data from refs. 19 and 20.

basis of criteria established by the Canadian task force on periodic health examination (20).

BREAST CANCER

Preoperative Evaluation of Breast Cancers

In the year 1998, approximately 180,300 new cases of breast cancer will be diagnosed in the United States (21). With more widespread use of mammography, breast cancer is being increasingly detected at an earlier stage of the disease. The work-up of a breast cancer patient depends on the clinical stage of the disease as well as the patient's symptoms. A complete history and physical examination is essential in order to establish the clinical stage of the patient. Apart from mammography (which is being discussed elsewhere), magnetic resonance imaging (MRI) to identify the presence of mammographically undetectable single or multifocal carcinoma is under evaluation. Although the preliminary reports indicate that MRI may be able to detect additional foci of disease in 20% to 35% of patients, further perspective studies are needed to establish its clinical role in the routine practice (22).

Patients undergoing surgical therapy for breast cancer should receive the laboratory tests needed for any patient undergoing general anesthesia. Thus, the patients should have a blood count, chemistry profile, urine analysis, electrocardiogram, and a chest x-ray (22,23) (Table 4-2). Patients with ductal carcinoma *in situ* do not require any further screening tests for metastatic disease.

Role of Bone Scans

Twenty years ago, bone scans were routinely recommended in the preoperative evaluation of breast cancer patients (16,24,25). Subsequent studies showed that positivity of bone scans in asymptomatic stage I and II breast cancer is between 4% and 5% (16,25). The false-positive rate of bone scan is around 10% to 15%. Therefore, the predictive value for positive test is only about 20%. In other words, if a patient with a stage I or II breast cancer had a positive bone scan, four out of five such scans will be false-positive. On the other hand, in patients with stage III disease, bony metastases are identified by scanning in 20% to 25% of asymptomatic patients, making this a worthwhile screening procedure in this group

of women. However, if the patient is symptomatic with pain, bone scans should be obtained.

It has been suggested that baseline scans may be useful in interpretation of later diagnostic scans (24). As pointed out earlier, in stage I and II breast cancers, the predictive value for positive tests is low, and therefore patients exhibiting positive tests will have to needlessly undergo a series of further diagnostic tests to confirm or refute the presence of metastasis. It therefore makes equal sense to submit a patient for similar diagnostic procedures when the scan is performed in response to the patient's symptoms later in the course of their disease. It has also been suggested that a positive bone scan may serve as a predictive test for future recurrence of the disease. Other studies have suggested that in those who have questionable abnormality on bone scan at the time of diagnosis, the conversion rate (i.e., development of disease) occurred in 26% of the patients. This rate was similar to a 29% recurrence rate among other patients who had no evidence of disease on imaging studies at the time of initial surgery, refuting arguments about the value of baseline scans.

Role of Screening Liver Scans

When the sensitivity and the specificity of old radionucleotide liver scans was evaluated, only 2 out of 529 patients had a positive liver scan consistent with metastasis in absence of abnormalities of the liver enzymes. Although CT scans have replaced radionucleotide scans, false-positive scans are common, and therefore liver imaging should be reserved for

TABLE 4–2. *Preoperative tests in breast cancer*

CBC
Chemistry
EKG
Mammograms (if not previously obtained)
Chest x-ray
Bone scan[a]
Liver CT[b]
Brain CT[c]

[a] Only in stage III patients and patients with symptoms.
[b] Only in patients with abnormal liver function tests and/or with symptoms.
[c] Only in patients with neurological symptoms.

patients with an abnormal liver chemistry or symptoms and signs suggestive of hepatic metastasis (22).

Radionucleotide and CT Brain Scans

Many studies have shown that in early breast cancer patients who are neurologically asymptomatic, negative radionucleotide and CT brain scans are almost never positive (22). Therefore, routine scanning is not indicated. Similarly, internal mammary lympho-scintigraphy has been advocated by some but the sensitivity and specificity of tests is not available.

Serum Tumor Markers

Hayes et al. (26) defined the marker which represents qualitative or quantitative alteration or deviation from normal of a molecule, substance, or process that can be detected by some type of assay. This includes measurement of a gene, RNA, or a product such as protein carbohydrate and lipid, and a process such as vascular density (26):

1. *Carcinoembryonic antigen (CEA):* This is a serum glycoprotein with the molecular weight of 180 kd, and it is one of at least 19 related molecules that are members of the immunoglobulin genes superfamily. CEA functions as an intracellular adhesion molecule, and although first detected in colorectal carcinomas, has also shown to be overexpressed by breast and other cancers. CEA is elevated in over 60% of patients with advanced breast cancer, and its level may correlate with the tumor burden. However, because of its low sensitivity in early-stage disease, CEA is not recommended in the screening or diagnosis of breast cancer.

2. *CA-15-3:* This measures the serum level of a mucin-like membrane glycoprotein which is shed from tumor cells into the blood stream. Recently, the Food and Drug Administration approved the Truquant assay which uses a monoclonal antibody, CA-27-29, to measure CA-15-3-like antigen. CA-15-3 has been evaluated in early-stage breast cancer, and in stage I only 9% of the women had an elevated CA-15-3. The incidence of positivity increased to 19% in women with stage II disease, while it increased to 38% and 75% in patients with stage III and IV disease, respectively. On the basis of lack of clear data on the utility of measuring CA-15-3, the ASCO panel has concluded that, at present, there is no role of CA-15-3 measurement in early-stage breast cancer.

Once the tissue is obtained for the diagnosis of breast cancer, various additional tests and markers are evaluated on the specimen, such as receptor status, DNA flow cytometry, p53 measurements, HER-2/neu. The utility of these markers in the decision-making process for the treatment of breast cancer is discussed elsewhere in chapter 22.

Follow-up After Primary Treatment

Following the primary treatment of breast cancer, follow-up of patients is directed at screening for new primary or local or regional recurrence, as well as diagnosis of metastatic breast cancers. Patients with a history of breast cancer are at a high risk for developing recurrence in the contralateral breast. Further, patients subjected to lumpectomy and radiation can also develop ipsilateral recurrence. Lastly, patients undergoing mastectomy can develop local recurrence. Patients with breast cancer also have a high risk for developing ovarian and colon cancer, and this risk is particularly high (16% to 44% for ovarian cancer) in women with a family history suggesting inheritance of BRCA1 or BRCA2 genes (27).

Recommended Breast Cancer Follow-up Schedule

There have been only two prospective trials to evaluate the impact of a multitude of tests on the overall survival and quality of life in breast cancer patients (28,29). However, about 20 years ago, Winchester et al. (30) reviewed patterns of recurrence and methods of detection in 87 patients with recurrent breast cancer. In only three asymptomatic patients was recurrence documented by "routine" chest x-rays or by abnormalities in the liver enzymes or liver scan. Subsequent to this study, a large number of retrospective studies have analyzed the values of various diagnostic tests in the follow-up of breast cancer patients.

Two Italian trials have prospectively studied the effects of intensive follow-up program on outcome in breast cancer patients. Rosselli Del Turco et al. (29) followed 1,243 patients with physical examination every 3 months for 2 years, and then every 6 months for the next 3 years. All patients also had a yearly mammogram. The intensively followed patients also had chest x-rays and bone scan every 6 months. Although in the intensively followed patients, there was lower relapse-free survival, 5-year overall mortality was not different in the two groups (18.6% versus 19.5%). The GIVIO investigators added liver echography in the arm which was being followed with intensive testing. At a median follow-up of 71 months, overall mortality rate was 20% in the intensive group, versus 18% in the control group.

These studies (31) have asked and tried to answer some of the following questions: (a) Can our present technology diagnose early recurrences in breast cancer, and, if so, are these tests cost-effective? (b) Is the early detection of recurrences simply indicative of lead-time bias or leads to better therapy and thus improved survival? (c) Are there any other diagnostic tests that can detect asymptomatic recurrent disease, the treatment of which will lead to improved quality of life?

Recently, ASCO developed guidelines for follow-up of breast cancer patients based on their exhaustive literature review. The issues raised in the ASCO guidelines have been reviewed earlier (19).

History and Physical Examination

Following the studies of Winchester et al. (30), Tomin and Donegan (32) reviewed the records of 230 women with recurrent breast cancer, and reported that in only 47 patients recurrence was local. Aggressive therapy of local recurrence led to a 50% 5-year survival, but it could be argued that these patients may have a biologically inert disease. Literature indicates that only 12% to 22.3% of the recurrences occur in truly asymptomatic women. In the prospective intergroup for cancer care evaluation (GIVIO) trial, in the intensely investigated group 31% of the recurrences were detected in asymptomatic patients, as compared to 21% of the recurrences in the control group (28,29).

Some authorities have even questioned the value of even routine physical evaluations (33). In one study, recurrences were found five times more often during spontaneous visits than during routine visits (an example of lead-time bias). These authors suggest that negative physical examinations may give a false assurance to a patient, leading to even further delay in the diagnosis of recurrence. The ASCO guidelines recommend that a careful history be performed every 3 to 6 months for the first 3 years after primary therapy, and then every 6 to 12 months for the next 2 years (19). The only study which has tried to determine the frequency with which patients should be followed is that of Scanlon et al. (23). They observed that 43% of the recurrences were detected within 3 months of the last examination, and therefore suggested that patients be examined every 3 months for the first 3 years after the primary therapy of breast cancer (23). During the visit, patients should undergo a complete history and physical examination, as about 15% of the recurrences are detected by physical examination. It is important to evaluate breast(s), local and regional lymph nodes, as well as symptoms or signs for systemic disease.

In conclusion, a vast majority of the recurrences are detected by history and physical examination (30). It is unclear at this time whether detection during these visits has any impact on overall survival. Since the costs of such services is between $100 and 200 per anum per patient and allows one to evaluate other parameters such as the effects of primary therapy, and the physical and psychosocial status of the patient, as well as detection of ipsilateral or contralateral breast cancer, it is recommended that patients should return at 3- to 6-month intervals for the first 5 years (19,31,34).

Patient Education About Breast Self-Examination and Symptoms of Recurrence

There is a general expert consensus that all women should be instructed in the detection of abnormalities in the breasts (22,35). This is particularly relevant in women with a history of breast cancer, as they are at a higher risk for developing contralateral breast cancer. In women who have undergone mastectomy with reconstruction or who have undergone breast conservation with radiation, there are intrinsic changes in the configuration of the breast, and the patient should be carefully instructed to recognize them so that during the follow-up they can identify any changes that may occur. There have been no studies that have addressed the effect of breast self-examination on the stage of the cancer at presentation or on the survival after a second primary breast cancer is detected by a woman.

Since the majority of recurrences occur between scheduled visits, it would be prudent to educate women about the symptoms of recurrence. The most common symptomatic site for recurrence of breast cancer is the skeleton, and therefore bone pain may indicate such a recurrence. Breast cancer can also recur locally, regionally, in the lungs, liver, or brain. Although intuitively one would consider that such an educational exercise will be of value in detecting a recurrence, there have been no studies to document its usefulness in clinical practice.

Mammography

Patients with breast cancer are at a higher risk of developing contralateral breast cancer. Therefore, all women undergoing unilateral mastectomy should undergo a contralateral mammography on a yearly basis for detecting evidence of a new primary tumor. Women who have been treated with conservative techniques can develop local recurrences, which does not preclude a potential long-term cure. The ASCO panel recommends that first posttreatment mammography be performed 6 months after the completion of radiotherapy, and then annually, unless there are specific indications for more frequent surveillance.

The mammography surveillance should include a two-view mammogram performed in a nationally licensed institution. In the GIVIO trial from Italy, which randomized patients between intensive follow-up versus routine observation, the incidence of contralateral breast cancer detected was 11.4% in the intensive group, versus 6.6% in the routine follow-up group only. There is also evidence that routine screening mammograms can increase the proportion of second breast cancer diagnosed as *in situ* or in stage I disease from 58% to 74%. There is no evidence at this time whether such an increase in the percentage of early-stage breast cancers will lead to an improved overall survival. However, it would be reasonable to expect that such would be the case.

Pelvic Examination

Women with breast cancer are at an increased risk for developing ovarian cancer. Additionally, women who are on tamoxifen have about a 1% risk of developing endometrial cancer at 5 years. Periodic pelvic examination, which includes Pap test and bimanual rectal/vaginal examination is therefore indicated. The Pap smear is also helpful in detecting cervical cancer. There continues to be controversy in the literature about the routine annual endometrial biopsy or transvaginal ultrasound in detecting endometrial cancer in women receiving tamoxifen, and at present such tests are not routinely indicated in asymptomatic women (22).

Blood Counts and Chemistry

An abnormal blood count is rarely seen as a first indicator of recurrent breast cancer. In one study, in only eight of 430 patients, elevated erythrocyte sedimentation rate, gammaglutamyl transferase, and alkaline phosphatase values denoted recurrence. Bone marrow involvement may be reflected by an abnormal blood count or peripheral smear. This is a rare clinical scenario, and therefore routine blood tests may not be of any value. Lastly, patients who are receiving alkylating chemotherapy can develop leukemia, but the risk is small. At the present time, the ASCO panel recommends that routine blood tests should not be performed in the follow-up of breast cancer patients (19).

An abnormal chemical value as a first evidence of recurrent breast cancer is seen in approximately 1% to 12% of the patients. The combined sensitivity and specificity of the tests for elevated alkaline phosphatase and gammaglutamyl transferase, recurrence was 55% and 91%, respectively. In a large retrospective review, alkaline phosphatase was found to be elevated in about a third of the patients with bone metastasis, but less than 2% of the tests performed routinely over a 2-year period were abnormal (36). In the GIVIO study, alkaline phosphatase and gammaglutamyl transpeptidase were prospectively followed, and there was no evidence that survival was altered with the addition of the tests in the intensive surveillance group (28,29).

Chest X-Rays

Several investigators have reported on the value of yearly chest x-rays in patients with breast cancer (37). Only 0.2% to 0.4% of the x-rays are abnormal in asymptomatic patients. In only 2.7% of the patients, first recurrence was detected by chest x-ray. However, pulmonary recurrences can cause significant morbidity and impair quality of life because of pleural effusion or lymphangitic spread of the tumor (34). The ASCO panel recommends that routine chest x-rays are of unproven value, but this author concurs with Loprinzi that a yearly chest x-ray may be prudent, at least in the first 3 years after primary therapy, to detect pulmonary metastasis (19,34). Earlier treatment, although unlikely to have any significant impact on survival, may allow improved quality of life.

Bone Scan

In 1979, on the basis of decision analysis, it was proposed that since there is no evidence that early detection and intervention for metastatic breast cancer will alter the natural history of the patient, bone scan should be performed only in symptomatic patients (16). Since then, several studies (38–40), including the National Surgical Adjuvant Breast and Bowel Program (NSABP) B-09 trial, confirmed this finding (38). In that study, 1,989 patients were followed. Of 779 patients who developed treatment failure, about 20% had their recurrences to bone. However, in only 52 (0.6%) of the patients, a screening scan was useful in detecting asymptomatic patient. In the prospective GIVIO trial, bone metastases were detected in 8% of the patients in the group receiving bone scans every 6 months, as compared to 8.9% in the routinely

followed patients in whom the scans were obtained only when they became symptomatic. More importantly, the 5-year mortality rate was not different in the two groups (28,29). It is a general consensus at this time that routine bone scans are not indicated in the follow-up of breast cancer patients (19,31,34,35).

Other Imaging Techniques

Earlier studies conducted with technetium-99m for colloid and hepatic ultrasound detected asymptomatic liver metastasis in only 0.1% to 0.2% of the patients (40). Computed tomography (CT) and MRI scans have more sensitivity and specificity than ultrasound, but studies that have been conducted indicate that these tests should be reserved for patients with abnormal physical examination, or with elevated liver function tests. Schapira and Urban (40) conducted a prospective trial that included liver echography, and found no survival benefit when compared to the group who had only minimal surveillance. At present, there have been no prospective or retrospective studies that have addressed the utility of CT in follow-up of breast cancer patients.

Tumor Markers, Including CA-15-3 and CEA

As pointed out earlier, CA-15-3 is a serum cancer antigen whose level is elevated in patients with advanced disease. The level of CA-15-3 is highest in patients with liver or bone metastasis. The ASCO panel evaluated 12 studies that have reported on the value of CA-15-3 in detecting asymptomatic recurrent breast cancer (18). Out of these 12 studies, only seven could be properly analyzed. Among 1,672 patients followed in these trials, 352 developed recurrence. About two-thirds of these recurrences were detected by elevated CA-15-3 before other parameters revealed recurrence, with a mean lead-time from marker elevation to clinical diagnosis of 5 to 7 months (41). A more recent study with B-27-29 antibody showed the mean lead-time for detection with antibody at 53 months over all methods. However, the sensitivity of the test was only 57% to 79%. As this marker is not exquisitely sensitive to detecting early recurrence, and as there is no curative therapy for macrometastatic breast cancer, this probably represents lead-time bias. Both of the ASCO panels strongly recommend that this marker should not be routinely used in the follow-up of breast cancer patients (18,19). Further, these panels observed that CEA was an even less reliable marker than the CA-15-3. On the basis of a large number of studies, at this time, routine CEA measurement is not recommended. The above recommendations are summarized in Table 4-3 (19,31,34,42).

Implications for Health Care Costs

As discussed earlier, in today's managed care environment, cost containment is a major issue. Developing standards of care with critical pathways for various illnesses has evolved as a necessary tool to maintain adequate quality of care while

TABLE 4–3. *Summary of recommendations for follow-up of asymptomatic breast cancer patients[a,b]*

Procedure	Low-risk	High-risk
History and physical examination	Every 3 months × 2 years, then every 6 months × 3 years, then yearly	Every 3 months × 2 years, then every 6 months × 3 years, then yearly
Complete blood count and chemistry	Every 6 months × 2 years, then yearly[c]	Every 3 months × 2 years, then every 6 months × 3 years, then yearly[c]
Markers: CEA, CA-15-3	—	—
Mammogram	Yearly	Yearly
Chest x-ray	Yearly[c]	Yearly[c]
Scans (bone, liver)	—	—

Patients with DCIS should be seen every 6 months for 5 years and then yearly. Annual mammogram is recommended. ASCO, American Society of Clinical Oncology; DCIS, ductal carcinoma *in situ*.

[a] Low-risk: patients who have negative nodes and/or positive receptors; High-risk: patients who have positive nodes and/or have received chemotherapy.

[b] Modified from: Khandekar JD. Recommendations on follow-up of breast cancer patients following primary therapy. *Semin Surg Oncol* 1996;12;346–351.

[c] ASCO Guidelines do not recommend blood tests and chest x-ray.

keeping a lid on the health care costs (43). The Society of Surgical Oncology has recently issued practice guidelines (35). A comprehensive cost-effective analysis for the tests in breast cancer have not been conducted. In the only prospective trial conducted by GIVIO investigators, no such analysis was available (28,29). Moreover, this trial was conducted in Italy where the health care delivery system is quite different from that in the United States. Schapira claims a saving of about $636 million in 1990 costs and about $1 billion in the year 2000 when a minimal follow-up approach, as proposed here, is employed (42). However, as discussed in the section on cost-effective analysis, much more work needs to be undertaken to reach a firm conclusion on the cost-benefit ratio of various tests.

COLON CARCINOMA

Adenocarcinoma of the large bowel effects about one person in 20 in the United States, with more than 155,000 new cases diagnosed each year. Once the diagnosis of colorectal carcinoma is made, the preoperative work-up should be undertaken. Much of the evaluation is similar for colon and rectal cancer, but some additional work-up is indicated for rectal cancers.

Preoperative Evaluation

A history and physical evaluation is important. During history taking, particular emphasis should be on family history of colorectal cancer, polyps, and other cancers. On physical evaluation, check for hepatomegaly, ascites, and lymphadenopathy. In women, pelvic pathology and breast cancer should be ruled out during examination. A rectal examination should be a part of the initial evaluation in all patients.

Laboratory Tests

A routine blood count and chemistry, including liver function tests, should be performed. Patients exhibiting abnormal liver function tests should be further evaluated with CT scan and other tests, as necessary (see the following).

Value of CEA

CEA is produced by normal cells, but its level is elevated in many adenocarcinomas, including colon, rectum, breast, and lung. CEA is cleared by liver. Many benign conditions such as alcoholic cirrhosis, acute inflammatory bowel disease, emphysema, bronchitis, or history of smoking can cause elevation of CEA (18,44). Several studies have evaluated preoperative CEA as a prognostic factor. Unfortunately, at this time there is no literature proving that preoperative CEA testing has impact on survival, quality of life, and CE. Nevertheless, there are studies that indicate that preoperative CEA can serve as a prognostic marker. The NSABP conducted a study on 945 patients, and observed that the preoperative CEA of more than 2.5 ng/mL indicated an increased risk of recurrence by 1.62-fold in Dukes B patients. Further, if a preoperative CEA value was more than 10 ng/mL, the risk was increased by 3.25-fold. It was also reported that time for recurrence was shorter if the CEA was more than 5 ng/mil. Since 35% of the Dukes D patients will have a CEA value of less than 5 ng/mL and 25% to 45% of Dukes B and C patients have a CEA value of more than 5 ng/mL, a preoperative CEA value is of no value in staging. The ASCO panel presently recommends that CEA can be ordered preoperatively if a surgeon thinks that it will assist in staging and surgical treatment planning (18). The Society of Surgical Oncology Practice Guidelines recommends that no CEA be obtained (34).

Imaging Studies

A full colonoscopy and double contrast barium enema to evaluate the entire colon is indicated. In addition, a preoperative chest radiograph is appropriate.

Abdominal CT or Liver Ultrasound

The role of conventional CT scan and conventional MRI in staging colon cancer has been extensively studied (45). In general, these techniques have a low staging accuracy, and this is related to the fact that neither method can assess the depth of tumor infiltration within the bowel wall and have difficulty in diagnosing malignant adenopathy. The mean overall accuracy of staging of primary colon tumors by these techniques is approximately 70%. The sensitivity for detecting malignant lymphadenopathy is only about 45%. However, in patients with abnormal liver function tests or in those whose history or physical findings suggest metastasis, CT and MRI are very useful in detecting metastatic spread to liver, adrenals, lung, etc.

The usefulness of preoperative CT is higher in patients with rectal cancer. A CT or MRI scan will give a better indication to surgeons as to whether the patient should receive preoperative radiation therapy. The technique also allows the surgeon to evaluate whether the patient can undergo a sphincter-saving procedure, and is certainly used by radiation oncologists for their port placement. Any adenopathy in the perirectal area can be considered malignant, as benign adenopathy is not seen in this area. Therefore, in patients with rectal cancer, CT scan or MRI is of benefit.

In patients with rectal carcinoma, a comparative trial of CT and MRI was undertaken. The overall accuracy of CT staging was 80%, while with MRI it was only 59%. The detection of lymph node metastasis was also more accurate with CT at 65% versus 39% with MRI. The reason is that high sensitivity is at 40% for CT as compared with MRI at only 13%. These individuals can be further evaluated with transrectal ultrasound or MRI with endorectal coils. The transrectal ultrasound evaluation is performed at a lower cost, is less time consuming, and can guide a surgeon in deciding choice of operative intervention.

The prognosis of colorectal carcinomas is dependent on many factors, including tumor size, node involvement, and grade of the tumor. Many tumor biological features such as blood group antigens, presence or absence of growth factors, and flow cytometry are being evaluated to assess prognosis of these patients. This aspect is beyond the scope of the present chapter.

Postoperative Follow-up of Colon Cancer Patients

The goals of the follow-up strategy include the following: to detect a new primary or colorectal neoplasia and to detect recurrent cancer; to treat postoperative complications that may occur as a result of therapy; to detect other cancers; to provide psychosocial support to the patient (46–49). Intuitively, one feels that metastasis diagnosed at an earlier stage, preferably at an asymptomatic phase, will be more treatable than a recurrence discovered later in the phase of the disease. This assumption is based on the belief that metastasis behaves like a primary disease and can be appropriately treated by local therapy. Many descriptive studies of postoperative screening for colorectal cancer metastasis have looked at tests such as CT scans, CEA, and other markers such as CA-19-19 (18). However, there has been no prospective randomized study, as is available in breast cancer, to address the question as to whether intensive surveillance leads to an improved survival and is cost-effective.

There have been publications suggesting that aggressive therapy of local recurrent disease leads to an improved survival. This probably represents a lead-time bias. The average percent of the total colorectal cancer population who benefited by postoperative screening and rendered disease-free through second-look surgery is 0.7% (0.2% to 1.7%).

Bruinvels et al. (46) conducted a metaanalysis on 3,283 patients published in seven reports. In each of these studies, the two groups had a different follow-up intensity. The metaanalysis showed that there was no difference in the 5-year survival between the two groups, although there was a trend toward improved survival when CEA is used as a part of follow-up protocol. However, none of the studies were prospective randomized trials. Based on the studies, the following schema is proposed for follow-up of colon cancer patients. The patients should be followed with history and physical evaluation every 3 months for the first 2 years, then every 6 months for the next 3 years. The patients should be particularly probed for change in bowel habits or symptoms suggesting recurrent disease. Colonoscopy is indicated every year for 3 years, and then every 2 or 3 years if no adenomas have been found. Women with colorectal carcinoma should undergo breast examination, mammography, and pelvic examination, as deemed appropriate.

Role of CEA

CEA has a high sensitivity (94%) and specificity (96%) with an accuracy of 94% in the detection of liver metastasis. CEA can detect a recurrent disease 1 to 30 months before detection by any other means, but the issue of quality adjusted survival remains unclear. The ASCO panel as well as DeVita's textbook on oncology recommend that despite uncertainty, CEA should be monitored at 2- to 3-month intervals for up to 2 years after curative resection of colorectal cancer. The ASCO panel recommends that a patient with stage II or III disease, and who can undergo hepatic resection if recurrence develops, should be followed with postoperative serum CEA testing every 2–3 months. An elevated CEA level should be confirmed by retesting, and the patient evaluated further for metastatic disease. However, no adjuvant therapy should be given based on elevated CEA alone. This recommendation was based on the observation that resection of isolated metastasis, particularly in the liver, increases survival compared with unresected patients or those given chemotherapy alone. In the study from the Mayo Clinic, there was a significant increase in survival for patients who had liver metastasis detected because of elevated serum CEA levels, as compared to those whose liver lesions were detected by an abnormal physical examination, symptoms, or liver function tests. In the study of Bruinvels et al. (46) discussed above, there was a 9% increase in survival for patients who had close monitoring. In the group who had undergone the intensive follow-up, more asymptomatic recurrences were detected (45%) versus 8% in the group who had a routine follow-up. Recurrences were 20% more likely to be resected with curative intent in patients

TABLE 4–4. *Summary of recommendations for follow-up of asymptomatic colon cancer patients*

Procedure	Low-risk[a]	High-risk[b]
History and physical examinations	Every 6 months × 5 years, then yearly	Every 3 months × 2 years, then every 6 months × 3 years, then yearly
CEA[c]	Every 6 months × 5 years[c]	Every 3 months × 5 years
Colonoscopy	Yearly × 2–3 years, and then every 3–5 years	Yearly × 2–3 years, and then every 3–5 years
Chemistry, scans	—	—

[a] Low-risk: Dukes A ($T_1 N_0 M_0$) survival >90%; B_1 ($T_2 N_0 M_0$) survival 85%; B_2 ($T_3 N_0 M_0$) survival 70–85%. Some studies indicate that B_2 tumors with aneuploidy on flow cytometry and with deletion of DCC gene on 18q are poor risk.
[b] High-risk: B_3 ($T_4 N_0 M_0$); C_1–C_3 (any $T_1 N_{1-3} M_0$) survival 30–60%.
[c] ASCO guidelines state patients who are suitable candidates for hepatic resection if need arises should have CEA measured.

with intensive follow-up, but the survival advantage was only significant when clinical follow-up included routine CEA testing.

Kievit et al. (44) used a CE model to study the usefulness of CEA monitoring after definitive surgery. They concluded that the net benefit of improved quality adjusted survival was between 0 and 13 days in the group followed with CEA. The CE ranged from $34,688 per year of life saved to $200,333 per year of life saved. A randomized controlled trial of postoperative CEA monitoring showed that a serial testing provided a 5-month lead-time compared to the control group, but there was no improved survival.

Radiologic Techniques

Many authorities recommend a yearly chest x-ray in the follow-up. The value of this in colon cancer has not been proven. It is generally believed that CT scans of the liver become abnormal only in the presence of abnormal liver function tests. Although no formal trial has been undertaken, the general consensus is not to undertake routine CT scans in the postoperative patient.

Another consideration in the postoperative follow-up of rectal cancer pertains to colostomy that may have to be undertaken in patients undergoing AP resection. In these individuals, colostomy management, irrigation techniques, and prevention of skin irritation is important and will necessitate consultations with an enterostomal therapist. Women who have undergone surgical castration or pelvic irradiation can develop menopausal problems requiring psychosocial and other intervention (50).

Radioimmunoguided Surgery

CEA can provide an effective target for radiolabeled antibodies. Technetium-99m labeled anti-CEA monoclonal antibody as well as indium-111 oncoscint (antibodies against TAG-72) labeled antibody against colon cancer have been used to detect recurrences. Although there are studies indicating the usefulness of these techniques, it has not been

demonstrated by prospective studies. Table 4-4 shows the postoperative follow-up of colon cancer patients.

Nelson (47) recently calculated the total cost of performing various tests, including once a year CT scan, CEA, blood counts, x-ray, and colonoscopy in the postoperative management of colon cancer patients. Although these are crude estimates, he estimates that the cost will over $1 billion for the follow-up studies (47). There is an ongoing study in Denmark in which patients are being followed either more intensively at 6 months intervals, versus at 5-year intervals. Once the results of this study will be available one can make a better recommendation on the postoperative follow-up of colorectal cancer patients.

In conclusion, the U.S. health care system is undergoing a paradigm shift whereby there is increasing emphasis on prevention and early detection, as well as focusing on improving quality of life of patients. It is abundantly clear that market forces are beginning to govern the health care delivery system. The economic principles that govern all trades are playing an increasing role in the health care market. As physicians, while advocating and fighting for what is best for our patients, we need to be cognizant of economic realities and change our behavior accordingly. Outcome analysis will certainly help us towards this goal. The development of guidelines, which have been criticized by some as a "cookbook" approach to medicine, will also help physicians against medicolegal cases. In our litigenous society, the guidelines can serve to protect physicians against frivolous lawsuits, while improving quality and overall survival of patients in a cost-effective manner.

ACKNOWLEDGMENT

I thank Karen Rector for her skillful secretarial assistance.

REFERENCES

1. Gold MR, Russell LB, Siegel JE, Weinstein MC, eds. *Cost-effectiveness in health and medicine.* New York: Oxford University Press, 1996.
2. Kongstvedt PR. *The managed health care handbook*, 3rd ed. Gaithersburg, MD: Aspen Publishers, 1996.

3. Kassirer JP. Is managed care here to stay? [Editorial]. *N Engl J Med* 1997;336:1013.

4. Gesensway D. Trouble in Canadian health care: money woes plague a popular system. *ACP Observer* 1997;17:1.

5. Angell M. Fixing Medicare [Editorial]. *N Engl J Med* 1997;337:192.

6. Ginzberg E, Ostow M. Managed care—a look back and a look ahead. *N Engl J Med* 1997;336:1018.

7. Kertesz L. Managed change. *Modern Healthcare* 1997;27:58.

8. Rosenberg H. HMO fever—Wall Street may be making a faulty prognosis. *Barron's* 1985 Jan 28:13.

9. Morgan RO, Virnig BA, DeVito CA, Persily NA. The Medicare-HMO revolving door—the healthy go in and the sick go out. *N Engl J Med* 1997;337:169.

10. Iglehart JK. Listening in on the Duke University Private Sector Conference. *N Engl J Med* 1997;336:1827.

11. Lee TH. Cost effectiveness of tissue plasminogen activator [Editorial]. *N Engl J Med* 1995;332:1443.

12. Eisenberg JM. Clinical economics. A guide to the economic analysis of clinical practice [Review]. *JAMA* 1989;260:2879.

13. Levitt RG, Sagel SS, Stanley RJ, Jost RG. Accuracy of computer tomography of the liver and the biliary tract. *Radiology* 1977;124:123.

14. Fineberg HV, Hiatt HH. Evaluation of medical practices. The case for technology assessment. *N Engl J Med* 1979;301:1086.

15. McNeil BJ, Keller E, Adelstein SJ. Primer on certain elements of medical decision making. *N Engl J Med* 1975;293:211.

16. Khandekar JD. Role of routine bone scans in operable breast cancer: an opposing viewpoint. *Cancer Treat Rep* 1979;63:1241.

17. Vecchio TJ. Predictive value of a single diagnostic test in unselected populations. *N Engl J Med* 1966;274:1171.

18. Clinical practice guidelines for the use of tumor markers in breast and colorectal cancer. *J Clin Oncol* 1996;14:2843.

19. Recommended breast cancer surveillance guidelines. *J Clin Oncol* 1997;15:2149.

20. The periodic health examination. The Canadian task force on the Periodic Health Examination. *Can Med Assoc J* 1979;121:1193.

21. Landis SL, Murray T, Bolden S, Wingo PA. Cancer statistics, 1998. *CA Cancer J Clin* 1998;48:6.

22. Harris JR, Morrow M, Norton L. Malignant tumors of the breast. In: DeVita VT, Helman S, Rosenberg SA, eds. *Cancer: principles and practice of oncology. Vol. 2.* 5th ed. Philadelphia: Lippincott–Raven Publishers, 1997:1557.

23. Scanlon EF, Oviedo MA, Cunningham MP, et al. Preoperative and follow-up procedures on patients with breast cancer. *Cancer* 1980;46 [Suppl 4]:977.

24. Gerber FH, Goodreau JJ, Kirchner PT, Fouty WJ. Efficacy of preoperative and postoperative bone scanning in the management of breast carcinoma. *N Engl J Med* 1977;297:300.

25. Burkett FE, Scanlon EF, Garces RM, Khandekar JD. The value of bone scans in the management of patients with carcinoma of the breast. *Surg Gynecol Obstet* 1979;149:523.

26. Hayes DF, Bast RC, Desch CE, et al. Tumor marker utility grading system: a framework to evaluate clinical utility of tumor markers [Review]. *J Natl Cancer Inst* 1996;88:1456.

27. Burke W, Daly M, Garber J, et al. Recommendations for follow-up care of individuals with an inherited predisposition to cancer. II. BRCA1 and BRCA2 [Review]. *JAMA* 1997;277:997.

28. Impact of follow-up testing on survival and health-related quality of life in breast-cancer patients. A multicenter randomized controlled trial. The GIVIO Investigators. *JAMA* 1994;271:1587.

29. Rosselli Del Turco M, Palli D, Cariddi A, et al. Intensive diagnostic follow-up after treatment of primary breast cancer. A randomized trial. *JAMA* 1994;271:1593.

30. Winchester DP, Sener SF, Khandekar JD, et al. Symptomatology as an indicator of recurrent or metastatic breast cancer. *Cancer* 1979;43:956.

31. Khandekar JD. Recommendations on follow-up of breast cancer patients following primary therapy [Review]. *Semin Surg Oncol* 1996;12:346.

32. Tomin R, Donegan WL. Screening for recurrent breast cancer—its effectiveness and prognostic value. *J Clin Oncol* 1987;5:62.

33. Dewar JA, Kerr GR. Value of routine follow-up of women treated for early carcinoma of the breast. *BMJ* 1985;291:1464.

34. Loprinzi CL. It is now the age to define the appropriate follow-up of primary breast cancer patients [Editorial]. *J Clin Oncol* 1994;12:881.

35. Morrow M, Bland KI, Foster R. Breast cancer surgical practice guidelines. Society of Surgical Oncology Practice Guidelines: breast cancer. *Oncology* 1997;11:877.

36. Crivellari D, Price KN, Hagen M, et al. Routine tests during follow-up of patients after primary treatment of operable breast cancer. *Ann Oncol* 1995;6:769.

37. Vestergaard A, Herrstedt J, Thomsen HS, et al. The value of yearly chest x-ray in patients with stage I breast cancer. *Eur J Cancer Clin Oncol* 1989;25:687.

38. Wickerham L, Fisher B, Cronin W. The efficacy of bone scanning in the follow-up of patients with operable breast cancer. *Breast Cancer Res Treat* 1984;4:303.

39. Pandya KJ, McFadden ET, Kalish LA, et al. A retrospective study of earliest indicators of recurrence in patients on Eastern Cooperative Oncology Group adjuvant chemotherapy trials for breast cancer. A preliminary report. *Cancer* 1985;55:202.

40. Schapira DV, Urban N. A minimalist policy for breast cancer surveillance. *JAMA* 1991;265:380.

41. Chan DW, Beveridge RA, Muss H, et al. Use of Truquant BR radioimmunoassay for early detection of breast cancer recurrence in patients with stage II and stage III disease. *J Clin Oncol* 1997;15:2322.

42. Schapira DV. Breast cancer surveillance—a cost-effective strategy. *Breast Cancer Res Treat* 1993;25:107.

43. Kattlove H, Liberati A, Keeler E, Brook RH. Benefits and costs of screening and treatment for early breast cancer. Development of a basic benefit package. *JAMA* 1995;273:142.

44. Kievit J, van de Velde CJ. Utility and cost of carcinoembryonic antigen monitoring in colon cancer follow-up evaluation. A Markov analysis. *Cancer* 1990;65:2580.

45. Thoeni RF. Colorectal cancer. Radiologic staging [Review]. *Radiol Clin North Am* 1997;35:457.

46. Bruinvels DJ, Stiggelbout AM, Kievet J, et al. Follow-up of patients with colorectal cancer. A meta-analysis. *Ann Surg* 1994;219:174.

47. Nelson RL. Postoperative evaluation of patients with colorectal cancer. *Semin Oncol* 1995;22:488.

48. Makela JT, Laitinen SO, Kairalouma MI. Five year follow-up of radical surgery for colorectal cancer. Results of a prospective randomized trial. *Arch Surg* 1995;130:1062.

49. DeCosse JJ, Cennerazzo WJ. Quality-of-life management of patients with colorectal cancer. *CA Cancer J Clin* 1997;47:198.

50. Cohen AM, Minsky BD, Schilsky RL. Cancer of the gastrointestinal tract. In: DeVita VT, Helman S, Rosenberg SA, eds. *Cancer: principles and practice of oncology. Vol. 1.* 5th ed. Philadelphia: Lippincott–Raven Publishers, 1997:1140.

CHAPTER 5

Vascular Access

Worthington G. Schenk III

Surgically installed permanent or semi-permanent vascular access devices are useful for chemotherapy, transfusion, pain control, supplemental fluid and nutrition administration, plasma and cell pheresis, hemodialysis, and parenteral medications. Each indication has preferred devices, and each device has its own nuances for installation and maintenance. This chapter discusses the available devices, the choice of device for specific cancer treatment scenarios, techniques for surgical installation, and hints for enhancing patient safety and satisfaction. The list of available vascular access products changes continuously, and those mentioned here are but examples, not an inclusive compendium. The conscientious surgeon must continuously evaluate new devices for safety, cost, and patient benefit before incorporating them into his daily practice.

IMPLANTABLE VASCULAR ACCESS DEVICES

Subcutaneous Port

The totally implanted vascular access port (Portacath, Bard-Port, and others) consists of a subcutaneous reservoir with a puncture diaphragm, permanently attached to an intravascular catheter. The reservoir or port is implanted subcutaneously in an accessible area, typically in the infraclavicular fossa, and the attached catheter is passed into a central venous location. The device is used to establish venous access by puncturing the diaphragm transcutaneously with a special noncoring needle using sterile technique. The device is valuable in patients with limited or exhausted intravenous sites, and is used typically in those with an established rhythm of chemotherapy treatments (Fig. 5-1). The principal **advantage** of the buried port is that it is a completely implanted device; it permits ordinary bathing or showering, it is less visible cosmetically, and tends to be lower maintenance between uses. It requires only intermittent flushing with heparinized saline, typically once a month, which for most patients already on a monthly visit schedule, makes it virtually maintenance-free. The principal **disadvantage** is that a needle stick is still required for use. A double-lumen device is also available, with a double-lumen catheter con-

nected to a port with two separate reservoirs (Fig. 5-2). This modification permits simultaneous administration of chemically incompatible solutions, although it should be recommended with discretion, since its installation has somewhat higher morbidity. Subcutaneous ports are popular with patients and generally well-tolerated. Ports may be used for blood sampling as well as fluid and drug administration. A well-functioning port has a virtually indefinite lifetime, certainly several years. The diaphragm is good for as many as two thousand punctures, depending upon needle size and adherence to proper techniques.

External Central Venous Catheters

Central venous catheters can be tunneled or non-tunneled, cuffed or un-cuffed, single or multi-lumen. Most surgically installed permanent catheters in oncology patients are dual-lumen, cuffed, and tunneled (Hickman, Leonard, and others). The typical design includes nonreactive, non-thrombogenic silicone rubber material, a cuff of Dacron felt to promote tissue adherence, permanently attached luer-lock hubs, and a simple straight catheter tip design which is cut to proper length at the time of insertion (Fig. 5-3). Catheters are also available with a second silver-impregnated cuff (VitaCuff). The antimicrobial effect of the silver-impregnated cuff has been shown to retard tunnel colonization in studies done using bedside insertion of nontunneled catheters in hospitalized patients; (1) the magnitude of the benefit when extrapolated to outpatient use of surgically-installed catheters is probably less, although the theory is sound: the local antibacterial effect of silver ions near the catheter exit site dissipates after several weeks, at which time tissue ingrowth into the felt cuff is established, forming a dense mechanical barrier to bacterial migration in the tunnel. The **advantage** of an external catheter is that no needle stick is required for use. This is appreciated by patients particularly when used frequently or continuously, such as for daily parenteral nutritional supplementation. The catheter generally has lower resistance/higher flow rate, which may be helpful if frequent transfusions are likely. The external catheter may be pre-

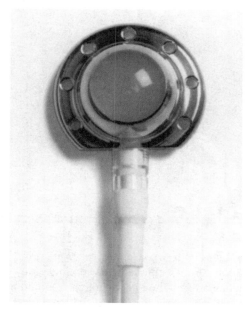

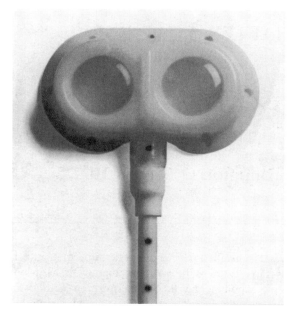

FIG. 5-1. Subcutaneous port. The reservoir base is constructed of either titanium or plastic. The membrane can be punctured approximately 2,000 times. The intravascular tubing may be permanently attached or, as shown here, user-attachable. (Courtesy of Bard Access Systems, Inc., with permission.)

FIG. 5-2. A double-lumen subcutaneous port. The device is intended to permit simultaneous infusion of chemically incompatible medications. Caution must be exercised during subsequent use to avoid accidental puncture of the same port with two needles. (Courtesy of Bard Access Systems, Inc., with permission.)

ferred over a buried port in cases of severe obesity, where placing a port which is both secure and easily palpable may be problematic—this issue is discussed further below under Surgical Techniques. The transcutaneous exposed nature of the catheter is also its **disadvantage**—it is more visually ob-

vious, possibly more prone to infection (2), and requires regular dressing care. Patients require better training in sterile technique, are usually constrained from bathing, swimming, and showering, and frequently require training or home-health assistance in catheter flushing. These catheters are

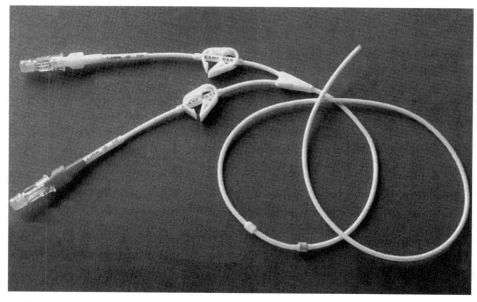

FIG. 5-3. The Hickman catheter. Illustrated is the double-lumen 10-French catheter with both the polyester felt (tissue ingrowth) and silver impregnated (antibacterial) cuffs. This style catheter must be tunneled first from the desired exit site, then cut to the appropriate length, then inserted into the vessel. (Courtesy of Bard Access Systems, Inc, with permission.)

flushed with heparinized saline more frequently than ports; once a week or every two weeks are common protocols, although some centers use a daily flush routine. Caps can be contaminated or lost; catheters can be damaged from repeated clamping, or even transected during dressing changes. Even in the best educated and motivated patients, catheters are occasionally dislodged or accidentally removed, a risk not shared with totally implanted ports.

Valve-end Catheters

Groshong catheters are manufactured with a bi-directional valve incorporated into the tip (Fig. 5-4). The most commonly used catheter is a double-lumen 9.5 French (F) variety, although single-lumen and pediatric size variations are available. The alleged advantage of the valve-end catheter is reduced rate of clot formation within the lumen and reduced risk of air embolism by prevention of unintentional blood ingress, and fluid/air egress, by the valve. The catheter is manufactured with a closed tip without an end-hole, which also improves the ease of radiographic identification of the tip location. Instead of an end-hole, the catheter has an elongated lateral slit which behaves as a low-resistance two-way valve (Fig. 5-5). A very small pressure gradient opens the valve in either direction, but without a gradient, the valve mechanically prevents blood backwash, or even diffusion of clotting factors, into the lumen of the catheter. This feature is designed to make the catheter lower maintenance, to decrease the frequency of catheter flushing, and to reduce or eliminate the need for heparin in the flush. While this could be important in a patient with heparin-induced thrombocytopenia (HIT) Syndrome, many

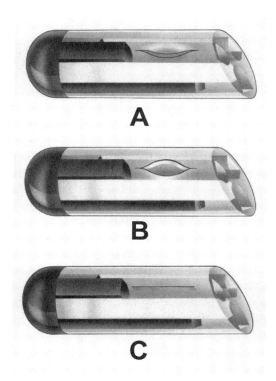

FIG. 5-5. The Groshong valve. **A:** With slight negative pressure applied to the lumen, the valve opens inward for blood sampling. **B:** With slight positive pressure, the valve opens outward, permitting fluid infusion into the patient. **C:** With neutral pressure, the valve remains closed, reducing the incidence of thrombus formation within the lumen. (Courtesy of Bard Access Systems, Inc, with permission.)

practitioners find this advantage largely hypothetical (3), and use the same flush and care protocol as with open-end catheters. One prospective study in the pediatric population, comparing valve-end to open end catheters, found no advantage to valve-end catheters with respect to thrombotic complications or ease of care (4). Air embolism risk is decreased, but not entirely eliminated, with the Groshong catheter (5). The greatest **advantage** of this style catheter may well be that it is slightly simpler to install and somewhat easier to place the tip in precisely the desired location, as described below in Surgical Techniques. One minor **disadvantage** is that the closed-end design makes the device more difficult to replace or change with an angiographic guide wire, although it is possible, with persistence, to manipulate a .025 in. guide wire through the lumen and out the lateral slit valve. The valve is also considered to be a source of potential trouble for infusion of cellular or viscous solutions; if frequent transfusions, plasma, platelets, or nutritional supplements are to be infused, an open-end catheter might be preferred.

Temporary Catheters

For short or intermediate term intravenous access (1-4 weeks), a Peripherally-Inserted Central Catheter (PICC) is

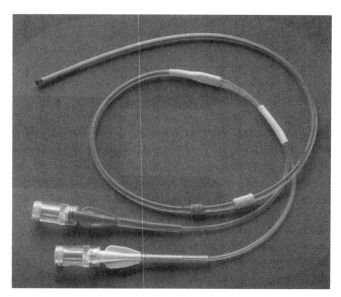

FIG. 5-4. The Groshong catheter. The luer-lock hubs are attached following insertion. This catheter design permits insertion of the catheter first, followed by subcutaneous tunneling, with the hubs attached last. (Courtesy of Bard Access Systems, Inc, with permission.)

frequently employed. This device is a long small bore catheter which, as its name implies, is inserted into a central venous location from an entry site in a peripheral vein. If an adequate size visible upper extremity superficial vein were available, use of the device could probably be precluded by ordinary peripheral intravenous catheters and a home health agency, so PICC lines are often placed under ultrasound or fluoroscopic guidance by radiologists, or by cut-down by surgeons, in the cephalic, basilic, or brachial vein, in the upper arm (Fig. 5-6). The main **advantage** of the PICC line is its ease and safety of insertion. Most of the mechanical risks of conventional central access, such as pneumothorax, hemothorax, arterial puncture, and thoracic duct injury, can be avoided completely. Its **disadvantages** include cost, and a small but significant incidence of thrombotic complications (6) which can confound subsequent access efforts. Whenever intermittent home intravenous care service can be provided using conventional intravenous catheters, this strategy will be less costly than PICC management. For patients with a predictable recurrent need for parenteral access, it is well to remember that after a second PICC line has been used, the cost of placement of a more permanent access device has probably been exceeded.

Prior to the development of permanent central venous catheters, simple percutaneous polyethylene catheters were inserted for chemotherapy or parenteral nutrition, usually

into the subclavian vein, and there was limited success with leaving these temporary catheters in place for many months. The contemporary tunneled and cuffed silastic or silicone permanent catheter is more durable and infection-resistant, but also more costly and complex to insert. A compromise device for patients requiring parenteral access for one to three months is the Hohn catheter, a cuffed but nontunneled smaller (typically 5 or 7 F) catheter which can be inserted using the Seldinger technique and a standard infraclavicular subclavian approach (Fig. 5-7). The catheter is small enough to be carried into a central venous location with a vascular guidewire only, without the added complexity and risk of the tearaway sheath needed for larger devices. For intermediate-term parenteral access, the Hohn catheter is a good alternative to the PICC, and generally better tolerated by patients because of its more conveniently located exit site. Whether there are fewer infectious complications with the cuffed Hohn catheter than with an uncuffed PICC has not been prospectively studied.

Pheresis and Hemodialysis Catheters

Cell pheresis for the collection of peripheral stem cells requires a two-way circuit carrying about 75 ml/min in each direction, a flow rate which cannot consistently be maintained with a conventional Hickman or similar catheter. For a limited number of treatments over two to three weeks, a simple percutaneous 11-French double-lumen polyurethane catheter (Sorensen, Mahurkar, and others) is adequate, although for more durable access, a 13.5-French Silastic tunneled and cuffed catheter, as shown in Fig. 5-8, may be useful (7). Hemodialysis, while not a cancer therapy per se, may also be employed in oncology patients. Hemodialysis requires approximately 300 ml/min in each of two lumens. Either of the two catheters described for pheresis is acceptable; the Perm-Cath is also available for semipermanent access for hemodialysis, a dual lumen 18-French Silastic catheter. The **advantage** of the dual lumen central venous catheter for hemodialysis is its immediate availability for use, compared to an arteriovenous fistula or graft, which typically requires four to six weeks before use. The most significant **disadvantage** of central catheters for hemodialysis is the incidence of venous stenosis, which can preclude ipsilateral permanent arteriovenous access 30% to 40% of the time.(8, 9)

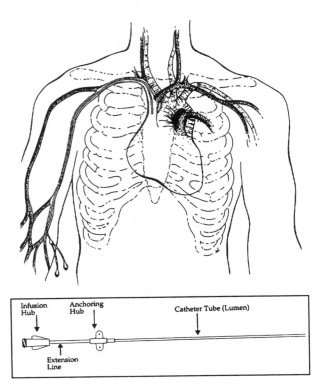

FIG. 5-6. The PICC (peripherally inserted central catheter). The device is inserted into a more peripheral vein (cephalic, basilic, or brachial), and threaded into a central venous position. It is intended for temporary use, but may be kept for several weeks.

Infusion Hub
Anchoring Hub
Catheter Tube (Lumen)
Extension Line

CHOICE OF VASCULAR ACCESS DEVICE

The initial consideration of any device for vascular access should include contemplation of both the desired purpose and the anticipated user. If a home health agency is to be involved, the familiarity and preference of the specific agency for a specific device may be quite important.

For example, if the patient has a blood-borne disease such as hepatitis or human immunodeficiency virus (HIV), which represents a hazard to health care workers, is it better to avoid

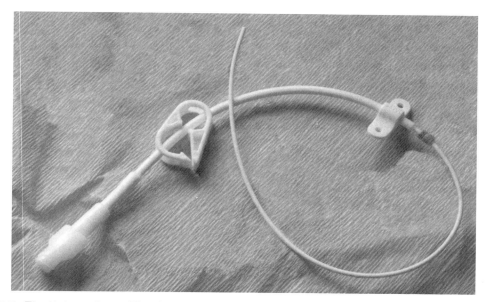

FIG. 5-7. The Hohn catheter. The device is intended for medium-term cannulation of a central vein. It is designed to be placed in the subclavian vein, but with a simplified untunneled technique. The single silver-impregnated cuff is placed under the skin at the insertion site; the catheter is not truly tunneled. The device is available in both single lumen and double lumen types. (Courtesy of Bard Access Systems, Inc, with permission.)

exposure to the organism (blood), or exposure to the vector (needles). Some home health agencies have a policy prohibiting the use of ports in such patients, to minimize exposure of their staff to needles, which are not necessary for external catheters. Other agencies prefer to limit potential blood exposure, largely from capping and uncapping external ports, by recommending implanted reservoir devices rather than external catheters. The optimum outcome in this situation requires that the ultimate user be identified so the choice can be resolved in advance.

For patients with an established rhythm of intermittent chemotherapy and exhausted superficial venous sites, installation of a subcutaneous port/catheter system is generally favored. Although the device itself is somewhat more costly than an external catheter, it requires less intensive maintenance, such that the port becomes more cost-effective after about two months' use (2). The devices are well tolerated by patients and are successfully used for the entire duration of intended therapy over 95% of the time (10).

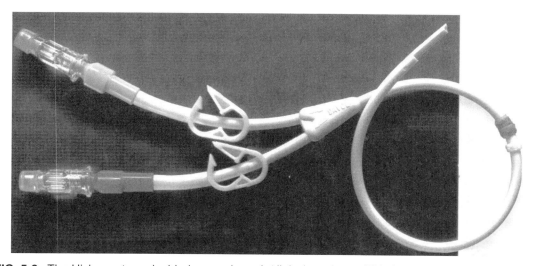

FIG. 5-8. The Hickman-type double-lumen pheresis/dialysis catheter. This larger 13.5-French catheter is designed to permit 300 ml/min in each of two lumens. Aspiration from the patient is through the shorter port, to reduce recirculation. Several overall lengths (40 to 60 cm) are available. (Courtesy of Bard Access Systems, Inc., with permission.)

An external catheter is a better choice for patients requiring more continuous use and more intensive therapy. For example, for intensive chemotherapy and bone marrow transplantation, it can be anticipated that the patient will require supplemental fluid administration, red cell and platelet transfusions and probably nutritional support and pain controls in addition to administration of parenteral medication, and frequently all at the same time. For such a patient, an external triple lumen large bore (12.5 F) Hickman or similar catheter is a more practical choice. For patients with less intensive needs, but who still require long-term daily therapy, such as for pain control or nutritional supplementation, an external catheter which does not require continuous transcutaneous needle access may still be preferred over a buried port. When the need for such support is anticipated for a shorter time, one to three months, a PICC or Hohn catheter may be adequate. If cell pheresis or dialysis is needed, a specialized larger bore double lumen catheter is needed, as described above. Finally, when a patient needs change, it is always possible to exchange one device for another, frequently by rewiring the new device in the same site with a modified Seldinger technique.

SURGICAL TECHNIQUES

There are a number of specific tasks which are common to the installation of many vascular access devices. These ubiquitous tasks include: selection of vascular approach, initial access of the desired vessel, using the Seldinger technique to access the central circulation, and tunneling or installing the desired device. These individual steps will be described separately, with emphasis on any modifications which are device-specific.

Selection of Approach

The classic approach for permanent or semi-permanent central venous catheters and ports is the infraclavicular approach to the subclavian vein. The three reasons for this preference are: constant relationship to surface landmarks, lower infection rate (for untunneled catheters) than the internal jugular (IJ) approach, and a more convenient and comfortable exit site or port site in the infraclavicular region. The approach has several disadvantages: it has a higher incidence of pneumothorax than the IJ approach, its risk of thrombosis or chronic venous obstruction is higher, and it occasionally results in catheter fracture and embolization. This latter problem, while unusual, is a direct consequence of the classic subclavian venipuncture technique. This approach specifically targets, for puncture and subsequent catheter insertion, the region of the subclavian vein over the first rib, behind the clavicular head, and anterior to the scalenus anterior, because it is in this small window that the location of the vein is predictable and constant with respect to surface landmarks. Unfortunately, this approach also tethers the foreign body precisely at the point where it is most likely to cause repeated trauma to the vein with motion of the arm, shoulder, or neck, which makes this zone particularly prone to puncture-related subclavian venous stenosis or occlusion. As illustrated in Fig. 5-9, this phenomenon of repeated flexing at a fixed spot can also result in a fatigue frac-

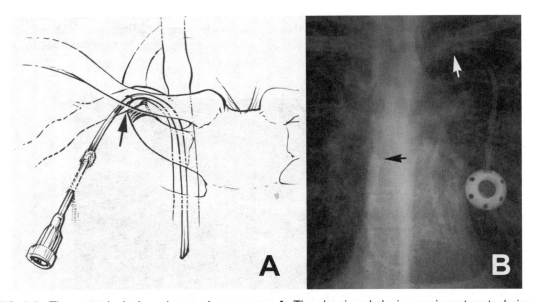

FIG. 5-9. The costoclavicular scissors phenomenon. **A:** The classic subclavian venipuncture technique tethers the catheter at its point of entry into the subclavian vein, where both the catheter and vein are subsequently prone to repeated trauma. The clavicle and first rib, like the blades of scissors, slide across each other with motion of the neck, arm, shoulder, and chest. Catheter-related stenosis of the subclavian vein usually occurs at this point. **B:** A stress fracture of a chronically implanted intravascular catheter virtually always occurs at the same point, and for the same reason. Illustrated is a subcutaneous port with the tubing fracture where it crosses the first rib *(white arrow)* and embolization of the distal fragment into the right heart *(black arrow)*. (Reprinted with permission from Schenk WG. Pitfalls in ambulatory vascular access surgery. In: Schirmer BD, Rattner D, eds. *Ambulatory surgery.* Philadelphia: WB Saunders, 1988.)

ture of the catheter. The phenomenon can be ameliorated by modifying the approach to actually puncture the axillary vein peripheral to where it becomes the subclavian vein, permitting the catheter to be in a mobile intraluminal position as it crosses the danger zone over the first rib.

This more peripheral approach frequently results in a more gentle curve from the subclavian vein to the innominate vein, particularly from the right side, which can make subsequent steps easier and safer (see below). A more peripheral approach to the axillary vein is relatively blind with respect to surface landmarks, however, and generally requires imaging assistance, as described in the next section. The alternative approach is an IJ approach, which has a substantially lower incidence of significant thrombosis or stenosis (9), has a greatly reduced risk of pneumothorax, has no bony impingements of concern, and, particularly from the right side, offers an essentially straight line course to the desired ultimate device insertion target in the superior vena cava (SVC) or right atrium (RA). The IJ approach introduces additional issues regarding tunneling the device to a convenient location, and also has less constant landmarks than the classic subclavian approach, which makes imaging, such as with ultrasound, beneficial for this approach. Indeed, if one uses ultrasound in the armamentarium for central access, it is useful to survey the potential targets with duplex ultrasound prior to committing to an approach.

In patients who have exhausted the conventional approaches, increasing desperation can foster increasingly creative vascular approaches, including catheters placed in the intercostal, azygous (11), femoral, iliac (12), even hepatic (13) veins. For individuals with complete obstruction of the SVC or both brachiocephalic veins from tumor, thrombosis, or fibrosis, the most practical option at this time is direct translumbar puncture of the inferior vena cava (IVC) for introduction of a catheter into the RA from below. The translumbar approach appears to have fewer thrombotic and infectious complications than catheter entry into either the femoral or saphenous vein (14).

Initial Vascular Access

The most commonly employed approach is the Seldinger technique wherein the desired vessel is punctured, a spring steel guide wire is passed through the needle, and subsequent manipulations follow the guide wire. One of the fundamental principles of the Seldinger technique is that the initial access is done with a needle only large enough to pass the wire regardless of the size of the device eventually to be installed, typically an 18 gauge thin-wall needle to pass a .035 or .038 in. wire. Puncture of either the subclavian or IJ can be accomplished with reference to surface landmarks only, with success rates of about 90% and 85%, respectively. Intraoperative imaging techniques can improve on the success and safety of this stage of the procedure, and the best advantage will be enjoyed by employing ultrasound not only to identify the course of the target, but also to puncture it under real-time observation (15, 16). An example of the use of intraoperative ultrasound to puncture the IJ is shown in Fig. 5-10. Using

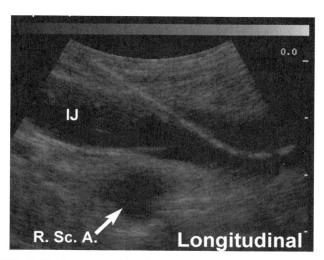

FIG. 5-10. Intraoperative ultrasound B-mode imaging. Illustrated is a right parasagittal image of the neck. The longitudinal image of the right internal jugular vein *(IJ)* is demonstrated and valve leaflets are visualized. The parallel common carotid artery is not seen because it is out of the plane of the image. The right subclavian artery *(R.Sc.A)* is seen as a transverse image, crossing deep to the jugular vein. The puncture has been completed and the intravascular position of the guidewire is illustrated.

real-time ultrasound assistance, the risk of arterial puncture is reduced by a factor of five, and there is similarly a five-fold decrease in the time required to establish successful access, compared to attempts using external landmarks alone (17). This advantage is particularly useful for the IJ approach, where there is more variability in the relationship between the vein and the accompanying carotid artery. In clinical ultrasound surveys, the vein lies in the expected location anterolateral to the common carotid artery only 45% to 70% of the time (18, 19). Furthermore, this relationship frequently is dependent upon the position of the patient (20), and even upon cardiac cycle (Fig. 5-11). The risk of mechanical complication at this stage is a direct function of the number of passes taken with the needle to enter the vein: one pass—4.3%, two passes—10.9%, three or more—24% (21). First pass success is greatly enhanced with real-time ultrasound (17).

The advantages of intraoperative ultrasound represent another reason for the general surgeon to establish proficiency in ultrasound imaging. While some education and practice are necessary, this proficiency is certainly attainable by the properly motivated operator. Other than requiring a certain amount of expertise, the only disadvantage to intraoperative ultrasound is cost. Amortization of the instrument and disposable supplies can add $100 to $150 to the procedure, but this cost is offset by reduced operating time, reduction in duplicate insertion kits and guide wires from unsuccessful attempts (15), and enhanced patient safety. The technology is not foolproof, however. The most common error directly attributed to ultrasound is the Skew Plane phenomenon (Fig. 5-12). The slice width of the ultrasound image can be as thin as 1mm, or approximately the width of the needle. While intentionally scoring the needle

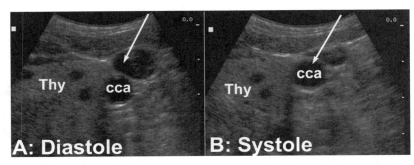

FIG. 5-11. The systolic fling phenomenon. The relationship between the internal jugular vein *(white arrow)* and common carotid artery *(cca)* can vary dramatically with the phase of cardiac cycle. **A:** In diastole, the vein appears to be a good target for puncture without threat to the adjacent artery. **B:** During each systole, the artery displaces laterally and effaces the vein lumen from behind. Note the relative change in position of the artery with respect to the adjacent thyroid *(Thy)*. Without real-time imaging to demonstrate this phenomenon, the vein could be punctured perfectly, and the artery could impale itself on the needle tip with the next systole, resulting in either inadvertent arterial cannulation, or hematoma formation. (Reprinted with permission from Schenk WG. Pitfalls in ambulatory vascular access surgery. In: Schirmer BD, Rattner D, eds. *Ambulatory surgery.* Philadelphia: WB Saunders, 1988.)

near the tip with a scalpel blade enhances imaging of the needle, it is still quite easy for the needle plane to be slightly skew with respect to the plane of the image, so that the shaft of the needle passes partly through the image, and the operator can be misled into mistaking the end of the needle image for the actual tip of the needle. As shown in the illustration, the tip of the needle can then invisibly threaten adjacent structures.

The lost art of the venous cutdown should perhaps not be completely forgotten as an option for this phase. For an im-

planted port, where an incision for the port pocket must be made anyway, a cutdown on the cephalic vein in the deltopectoral groove is an acceptable option, with the port pocket developed overlying the pectoral fascia through the same incision. A cutdown may also be used for exposure and access for a PICC line, using the deep brachial or superficial basilic or cephalic vein in the upper arm. A cutdown might be considered in the presence of a coagulopathy when one wishes to avoid the possibility of uncontrolled internal bleed-

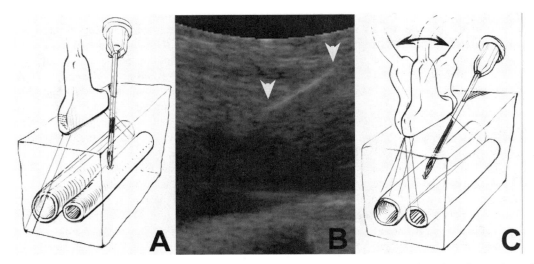

FIG. 5-12. The skew-plane phenomenon. **A:** During real-time ultrasound imaging, the plane of needle insertion can easily be slightly skew with respect to the plane of the ultrasound image. In this circumstance, the shaft of the needle will pass through, and out of, the plane of the image, permitting it to invisibly threaten adjacent structures. **B:** The ultrasound image represents the skew-plane phenomenon illustrated in A. Only a portion of the shaft of the needle appears in the image *(white arrows)*. The tip of the needle is not seen in the image, and can threaten adjacent structures. **C:** The plane of needle insertion must remain within the plane of the ultrasound transducer image. With experience, the operator learns to recognize the characteristic ultrasound signature of the machined needle tip. (Reprinted with permission from Schenk WG. Pitfalls in ambulatory vascular access surgery. In: Schirmer BD, Rattner D, eds. *Ambulatory surgery.* Philadelphia: WB Saunders, 1988.)

ing from a percutaneous approach, and it is an option if one wishes to reduce radiation exposure as much as possible, such as during the first trimester of pregnancy, since a cutdown permits direct passage of the catheter through the vein, largely avoiding the fluoroscopy necessary for the Seldinger technique. Radiation exposure can also be avoided by using a modified EKG technique for catheter positioning (22).

Access to the Central Venous Circulation

Once the desired vessel has been cannulated, the next phase involves passage from this entry site to the desired target in the central venous circulation. With a cutdown, this involves threading the installed catheter directly, but with the more common Seldinger technique, this step involves passing first a flexible spring steel guide wire. Passage of the wire into the central circulation is then corroborated by fluoroscopy, or manipulated into the right heart under fluoroscopic observation. For subclavian or IJ entry sites, I recommend passing the guide wire through the right atrium and well down the IVC.

If the wire tip is left in the right atrium (or worse, in the right ventricle), there is a greater danger of subsequently passed devices causing internal trauma. After passage of the wire, the original needle is removed and replaced by a vascular dilator, or graduated series of dilators, passed over the wire. The dilator passage is potentially hazardous, particularly because of the common but erroneous assumption that a properly located guide wire prevents an errant dilator. Because the wire is more flexible and has a lower resistance to bending than most dilators, the relatively stiff dilator can fail to negotiate a turn, despite the properly located wire, as illustrated in Fig. 5-13. This hazard is greatest from a right subclavian approach and least from the right IJ approach. It is also greater as the discrepancy between stiffness of wire and dilator, respectively, increases; if the largest dilator to be inserted is 10 F, the risk of an errant dilator is quite small. If the tract must be dilated to 18 F, the risk is substantially increased, and I prefer to dilate progressively (10,12,14,16 F, etc.) with liberal use of fluoroscopy whenever a curve must be negotiated. This risk is also reduced by progressing slowly, and checking that the

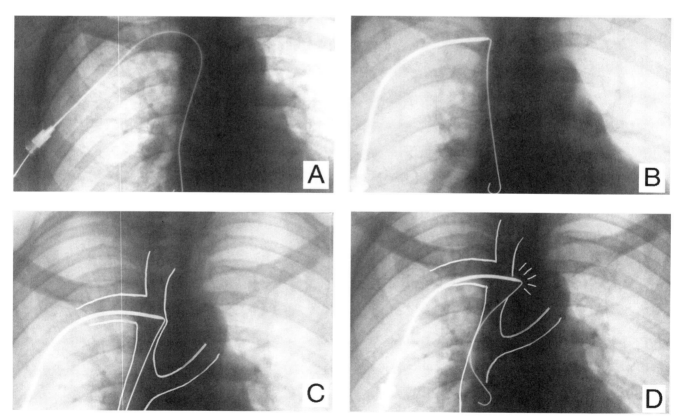

FIG. 5-13. The errant-dilator phenomenon. A guidewire that passes from puncture site to the right atrium does not guarantee that a dilator passed over the wire will do the same. **A:** The guidewire negotiates a fairly tight radius curve at the junction of the right subclavian and brachiocephalic veins. **B:** Whether a dilator passed over the wire will negotiate the same curve depends on the relative bending resistance or stiffness of the dilator with respect to the wire. If the dilator has a greater bending resistance, the wire bends, not the dilator. Bending resistance increases with increasing diameter of the dilator. **C:** Once the wire has been bent, the wire trails, rather than leads, the dilator. **D:** Serious vascular injury can result. (Reprinted with permission from Schenk WG. Pitfalls in ambulatory vascular access surgery. In: Schirmer BD, Rattner D, eds. *Ambulatory surgery.* Philadelphia: WB Saunders, 1988.)

wire moves freely in and out of the dilator after each centimeter or so of insertion—if the wire binds, it is being acutely angled against the dilator tip by impingement against the intimal surface, and any further insertion could damage the vessel wall. It is also well to remember that the vessel itself is not being dilated with these devices—it is the soft tissue tract and the hole into the vessel which is being dilated. Therefore, except to carry a tear-away sheath well into the vessel, it is usually not necessary to pass a dilator its entire length into the right heart—a few centimeters is frequently all that is needed. If a dilator or catheter simply will not follow the guide wire safely, because of either too tight a turn or a tortuous S-curve, it may be possible to exchange the wire for a stiffer one (Fig. 5-14). Once the more flexible wire has been successfully manipulated down the IVC, a flexible exchange catheter can be passed over the wire into the IVC, then the wire upgraded to a stiffer one, such as the Amplatz Super Stiff. With the stiffer wire in place, the larger dilator and/or catheter can then safely negotiate the course. If this technique is utilized, it is wise to insert the ultimate catheter or other device well longer than desired because any tortuosity which has been straightened by a stiffer wire is likely to recoil, leaving the more flexible device considerably shorter than expected. In this situation it is generally easy to incrementally withdraw the catheter to the desired position—and frequently impossible to insert it any farther if it is too short.

Installing the Device

With a guide wire in the central venous circulation and the tract suitably dilated, simple untunneled catheters can then be just advanced through the tract over the wire. A more involved carrier is not needed for catheters which are relatively small bore, tapered, and/or relatively stiff. However, a very floppy Silastic catheter with a full bore untapered end, particularly if greater than 12 F, will usually require the additional step of placing a relatively stiff plastic sheath over the wire first, through which the desired device can be passed. A relatively common problem at this phase is flattening or kinking of the introducer sheath once the carrier dilator is removed, preventing passage of the catheter through the sheath. The common response to this dilemma is replacement with a larger sheath, which unfortunately will be more kink-prone than the sheath with the smaller diameter. If the kink is ex-

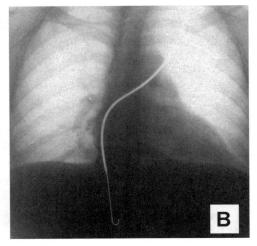
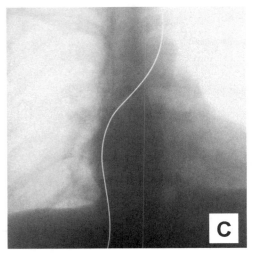
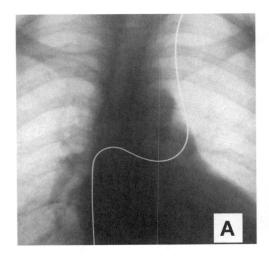

FIG. 5-14. The S-curve phenomenon. **A:** Shown from a left internal jugular approach, the guidewire follows an S-curve route to the right heart. The phenomenon is exaggerated by aortic ectasia and uncoiling. The wire is shown in the preferred location well down the IVC. A relatively stiff dilator or catheter advanced over this wire would preferentially perforate the left brachiocephalic vein rather than follow the S-curve to the right heart. **B:** A small flexible dilator or exchange catheter is passed over the wire first. The flexible catheter more safely negotiates the S-curve. **C:** A stiffer guidewire is then exchanged through the catheter, under fluoroscopic observation, to straighten the S-curve. A stiffer dilator or introducer can then be safely advanced to the right heart from the left internal jugular approach. (Reprinted with permission from Schenk WG. Pitfalls in ambulatory vascular access surgery. In: Schirmer BD, Rattner D, eds. *Ambulatory surgery*. Philadelphia: WB Saunders, 1988.)

travascular, usually from angulation beneath the clavicle, a more successful strategy is to dilate the tract with a larger **dilator**, such as up to 12-French for a 10-French sheath, then return to the smallest sheath which will pass the desired catheter. If the angulation of the sheath occurs intravascularly, most commonly at the junction of right subclavian and innominate veins, trying to overcome this with a larger dilator is both unsuccessful and hazardous. It might be possible to use a stiffer (not larger) sheath, but a safer strategy is to place the end of the sheath as close as possible to the junction under fluoroscopy, without kinking it, and pass the trouble spot with the softer catheter on its own. The kinked sheath phenomenon can also be avoided by making the initial subclavian venipuncture with a skin entry site further away from the clavicle, or by puncturing the axillary vein more peripherally under ultrasound imaging. Alternatively, the problem can be avoided altogether by using a jugular approach.

Tunneled devices are not all installed using the same sequence: Straight bore central catheters (Hickman and others) have one or more large luer-lock hubs attached to the external end, thus the catheter must be brought through the tunnel first, then the internal end of the catheter cut to the proper length, then inserted through the sheath. Valve-end (Groshong) catheters cannot have the internal end cut without defeating the valve, so these are inserted first, then tunneled, then attachable hubs are connected to the external end of the catheter. This feature probably makes the Groshong catheter easier and more reliable with respect to precise placement location, since the tip placement is accomplished first, and subsequent manipulations are keyed to that position. This type of catheter probably also has a more secure exit site, since the skin puncture for catheter exit never has to be larger than the buried cuff. Pheresis or dialysis catheters have specialized features on both ends, and neither end can be cut, although more than one length is available. For these catheters, it is best to mark the desired catheter tip location, then measure the approximate course length on the patient, using the catheter as a template, so that a properly located exit site can be selected. I find it best to mark the tip target under fluoroscopy, and plan for any imbedded cuff to be located midway between vascular entry site and skin exit site, to allow maximum last-minute position adjustability. Implanted ports come either with permanently attached or user-attached catheters. Pre-attached tubing must obviously be cut to length before insertion. User-attachable catheters can at least hypothetically be inserted to the desired length first, then tunneled, then cut and attached to the port. However, I find it difficult to accomplish this without inadvertently withdrawing the catheter shorter than the desired length. I find it more reliable to secure the tubing to the port prior to suturing the port into the pocket, then tunnel the tubing if necessary, cut the tubing based on a fluoroscopically selected target, then insert the tubing last.

The precise location of the desired target for a catheter tip depends upon its type and intended use. A PICC line or Hohn catheter for six weeks of antibiotic administration will function fine at the innominate-caval junction, although catheters coming from the left side may have a tendency to flip into the azygous vein orifice and may do better if left well past this zone (see Fig. 5–18 below). For administration of potentially sclerotic agents (hypertonic nutrients and most cytotoxic agents), it is better not to leave the tip close to the tricuspid valve—a location at, or just above, the atrial-caval junction is desired. Pheresis or dialysis catheters, which must sustain higher flow rates simultaneously in each of two channels, are the most unforgiving of minor imperfections in tip position and orientation. The offset-port catheters are designed to aspirate from the shorter shoulder port and return blood via the tip orifice of the longer lumen. If too short, with the red shoulder in the SVC, the catheter may aspirate against the intimal surface of the SVC and obstruct—too long, and the blue tip will be intermittently occluded by the diaphragmatic surface of the right atrium. In addition, the asymmetric design of the catheter frequently results in better function depending upon which side of the atrial-caval junction the catheter tends to lie—the red port should face the opposite way (Fig. 5-15).

Finally, positioning of the intravascular device can be confounded by anatomic shifting of location. Nicknamed the Tectonic Shift phenomenon (23), and more prevalent with subcutaneous ports than other devices, this problem is caused by motion of the soft tissues to which the device is anchored, with subsequent occult withdrawal of part of the attached intravascular tubing (Fig. 5-16). The most consistent risk factor for this phenomenon is obesity, where there is a greater degree of relative motion of the superficial tissues with changes in position. This is a bigger problem with ports, not only because the reservoir is larger and more effected by gravity, but also because the reservoir must be positioned reasonably close beneath the dermis, where soft tissues are more mobile, or needle access of the port could be difficult or impossible. The problem can be avoided by consistent suture attachment of the port to the pectoral fascia, but in obese patients, this could result in a functionally unusable device. Another strategy is to place the port as close as possible to the entry site of the tubing—immediately beneath the clavicle for a classic infraclavicular subclavian approach—to minimize the impact of any tectonic shift. The phenomenon can still occur if any part of the catheter, not only the port, is tethered to mobile tissues, and this also applies to tunneled external catheters: in an obese patient, if the entry site incision is too small, the catheter can become tethered to the dermis and, with subsequent shifting because of changes in patient position, become partially withdrawn out of the vein. The entry site incision, through which the initial access and Seldinger exchange are conducted, should be large enough to permit displacement of the subsequently tunneled catheter entirely within a plane well beneath the mobile dermis. Simply leaving the catheter a little too long will not always avoid this problem: repeated shifting of any tethered point toward and away from the point of intravascular entry can eventually deliver an enlarging loop of catheter into the subcutaneous plane. In patients at high risk for Tectonic Shift, placing the buried reservoir or external catheter exit site in the midline

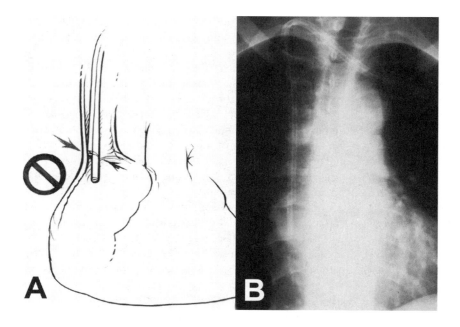

FIG. 5-15. The red-port reversal phenomenon. **A:** This problem is characteristic of high-low catheters with offset internal ports. Aspiration from the patient is through the shorter port. If this port lies up against an internal wall, aspiration from the patient will be interrupted. **B:** If the catheter tends to lie along either internal surface, the shorter port should face in the opposite direction. (Reprinted with permission from Schenk WG. Pitfalls in ambulatory vascular access surgery. In: Schirmer BD, Rattner D, eds. *Ambulatory surgery.* Philadelphia: WB Saunders, 1988.)

over the manubrium can be very helpful. In this location, not only is the subcutaneous plane thinner, but also less mobile with respect to the underlying pectoral fascia. A port in this location is rigidly secured, easily palpated, supported by the underlying sternum, and more comfortable and convenient

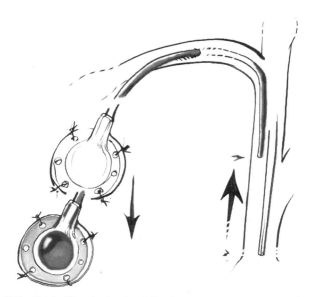

FIG. 5-16. The tectonic shift phenomenon. If the subcutaneous port is attached to mobile tissue, the attached catheter, and thus the internal end, migrates outward with the patient in an upright posture. A device that appears perfectly placed in a supine position in the operating room may prove substantially too short on the upright chest film. The phenomenon is aggravated by obesity. (Reprinted with permission from Schenk WG. Pitfalls in ambulatory vascular access surgery. In: Schirmer BD, Rattner D, eds. *Ambulatory surgery.* Philadelphia: WB Saunders, 1988.)

for many patients. If a midline position is anticipated, the right IJ vascular approach is the most practical, with the tubing tunneled beneath the platysma (Fig. 5-17).

COMPLICATIONS: PREVENTION, RECOGNITION, TREATMENT

Early Mechanical Complications

In a series of 821 central catheters for chemotherapy at M. D. Anderson, the overall mechanical complication rate was 10.5%. These included pneumothorax, arterial puncture, hematoma, and catheter malposition. The risk of a mechanical complication was found to increase with the number of needle passes taken, as described above, and decrease with operator experience (21). Several authors have described the value of intraoperative ultrasound imaging to improve first-pass success and decrease mechanical complications (15, 16, 17). This is corroborated by my own personal experience of 500 surgically installed central venous devices with a single carotid artery puncture/hematoma as the only mechanical complication. In the absence of unrecognized anatomic anomaly, catheter malposition should be largely avoidable with liberal use of intraoperative fluoroscopy. This should be augmented with the post-op upright chest x-ray, which will pick up a small pneumothorax, or a catheter left inadvertently too short, too long, or lodged in a side branch, and the problem can be promptly corrected. From the left side, an SVC catheter can pass quite easily into the orifice of the azygous vein (Fig. 5-18). Such a malposition can result in suboptimal function and, rarely, more serious complications such as broncho-venous fistula (24), so it should probably not be left uncorrected. The position-specific nuances of dialysis or pheresis catheters have been discussed above, as has the problem of late shift in position of subcutaneous ports.

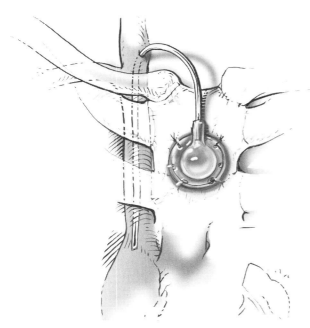

FIG. 5-17. The midline position for a subcutaneous infusion port. The port is sutured to the pectoral fascia over the manubrium, and the catheter enters the right internal jugular vein. This is an effective solution to the problem of tectonic shift because the pectoral fascia is quite immobile in this area. The overlying soft tissues are relatively thin, even in obesity, facilitating palpation and access of the port. (Reprinted with permission from Schenk WG. Pitfalls in ambulatory vascular access surgery. In: Schirmer BD, Rattner D, eds. *Ambulatory surgery.* Philadelphia: WB Saunders, 1988.)

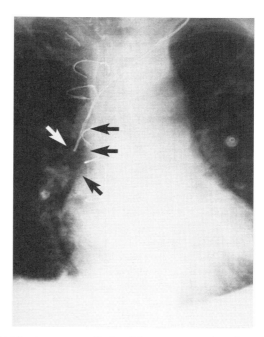

FIG. 5-18. Azygous catheter. The postoperative chest film of a catheter that would not aspirate. On the film, the catheter tip *(white arrow)* appears to extend beyond the lateral border of the superior vena cava *(black arrows).* The catheter is wedged in the azygous vein.

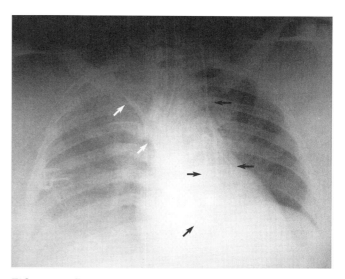

FIG. 5-19. Persistent left superior vena cava. A catheter placed from a left internal jugular approach *(black arrows)* functions properly for pulmonary artery pressure monitoring, but never crosses the midline. The catheter descends through a persistent left superior vena cava, through the coronary sinus into the right heart. Coincidental note is made of a temporary dialysis catheter *(white arrows),* which reaches the right heart from a right subclavian approach. Therefore, by inference, the patient must have a normal right superior vena cava as well. If an alternate route to the right heart is available, it is preferable to avoid leaving the catheter across the coronary sinus.

Anatomic Abnormalities

The most common anatomic problem is acquired central venous stenosis or occlusion from prior vascular access procedures or attempts. In patients with multiple prior bilateral procedures, and especially if a history is elicited of intraoperative difficulties, a pre-op central venogram can be invaluable. Similarly, if intraoperative difficulties are encountered, an intraoperative contrast injection under fluoroscopy can facilitate passage of the device, or demonstrate its futility prior to potentially dangerous persistence. The most commonly encountered congenital anomaly is Persistent Left Superior Vena Cava, although this has only about a 3% incidence. If encountered, the anomoly may or may not also have a normal right SVC, and if present, there may or may not be a communicating left innominate vein. The key anatomic feature of this developmental anomaly is the entry of the left SVC into the coronary sinus, and from there into the right atrium (Fig. 5-19). Since thrombosis of the coronary sinus can have fatal results in this situation (25), it is better not to leave a catheter through the left SVC and coronary sinus. When there is only a unilateral left SVC, a variant occurring in about 1.5% of the population (26), successful long-term cannulation of the RA across the coronary sinus has been reported SVC (27).

Thrombosis

Clot formation within the catheter lumen is prevented by routine flushing with saline, usually containing some concentration of heparin, although specific protocols vary. There is some success with further prevention of luminal thrombosis in the oncology population with concomitant administration of low-dose oral anticoagulation (coumadin, 1 mg/day) (28). If luminal obstruction occurs, it can almost always be restored with thrombolysis with a small volume of saline containing 50,000 u of urokinase instilled into the lumen (29). If older more mature thrombus cannot be dislodged with a power flush, thrombolysis, or an angiographic guide wire, replacement of the device may be necessary.

Catheter-related venous thrombosis is a different problem. Intravascular thrombosis of central veins occurs 6% of the time with peripherally inserted catheters (6), 30% with subclavian insertion (8), 10% with IJ insertion (9). However, the lesion is infrequently associated with any long-term disability, and rarely with serious embolization (30). In this regard, it should be distinguished from effort-related or spontaneous upper extremity venous thrombosis, which have a much higher incidence of chronic symptomatic sequelae (31), and from lower extremity thrombosis, which has a significant risk of both chronic post-phlebitic syndrome and pulmonary embolization. Clinical judgment is needed in the aggressiveness with which catheter-related venous thrombosis is treated, taking into account the severity of presenting symptoms and how desperately the device is needed. In one extreme, asymptomatic thrombosis, due to a catheter which is no longer needed, can be treated just with removal of the device, perhaps augmented with a short period of prophylactic oral Coumadin. On the other end of the spectrum, symptomatic venous hypertension in a patient with sepsis and pancytopenia who desperately needs vascular access should be treated with leaving the device and systemic thrombolysis, followed by therapeutic, then prophylactic anticoagulation (32). In one report from the University of Nebraska, where the incidence of thrombosis was as high as 12% depending upon the device, success with thrombolytic therapy was 70% (33). Since there were no long-term sequelae with or without thrombolytic success, it seems hard to justify a more aggressive approach. Although difficult to quantitate the long-term benefit, preservation of future access options may be one justification for treatment to a demonstrated clot-free end-point.

Infection

Catheter-related infection episodes are quite common, especially among immunosuppressed and/or leukopenic patients, although the majority can be treated with preservation of the intravascular device. The type of infection determines the most appropriate treatment: localized exit site infection should be distinguished from bacteremia, and both are treated differently from a tunnel infection with purulent drainage, presumably involving the buried cuff, expressed from the exit site. The incidence of bacteremia is probably lower with totally implanted ports than with external catheters (2). Localized cellulitis at a catheter exit site can be treated with antibiotics until clinical resolution. In a reported series from University of Maryland, in 690 patients with external catheters undergoing intensive chemotherapy, the incidence of documented bacteremia was 57.5%, although the majority were treated successfully with appropriate antibiotics without catheter removal (34). The success rate with this strategy in most series is about 60%. Generally accepted indications to remove the device for infection treatment include: documented failure to clear bacteremia within 48 hours of initiation of appropriate antibiotic therapy, purulent tunnel infection, and Candida fungemia in the absence of an alternate anatomic source.

CONCLUSIONS

The use of permanently implanted vascular access devices enhances efficacy of cancer treatment, effectiveness of palliation, and patient comfort. The surgical techniques involved with their installation are quite basic, but attention to details avoids complications. Selection of the best device, familiarity with the nuances of different available products, and liberal use of intraoperative imaging improve success, safety, and patient satisfaction. The majority of devices will remain complication-free for the duration of treatment.

ACKNOWLEDGMENT

Hickman, Hohn, Groshong, Leonard, and BardPort are trademarks of C. R. Bard, Inc. (Salt Lake City, Utah). VitaCuff is a trademark of Vitaphore Corporation (Los Angeles, California). Portacath is a trademark of Pharmacia Deltec Inc. (St. Paul, Minnesota). Mahurkar and PermCath are trademarks of Quinton Instrument Company (Bothell, Washington). Silastic is a trademark of Dow Corning, Inc. (Midland, Michigan). Dacron is a trademark of E.I. duPont de Nemours and Co., Inc. (Wilmington, Delaware). Sorensen is a trademark of Sorensen Research Corporation (Salt Lake City, Utah). Amplatz Super Stiff is a trademark of Boston Scientific Corp. (Boston, Massachusetts).

REFERENCES

1. Smith HO, DeVictoria CL, Garfinkel D, et al. A prospective randomized comparison of an attached silver-impregnated cuff to prevent central venous catheter-associated infection. *Gynecol Oncol* 1995;58:92–100.
2. Greene FL, Moore W, Strickland G, McFarland J. Comparison of a totally implantable access device for chemotherapy (Port-A-Cath) and long-term percutaneous catheterization (Broviac). *South Med J* 1988;81:580–583.
3. Mayo DJ, Horne MK, Summers BL, Pearson DC, Helsabeck CB. The effect of heparin flush on patency of the Groshong catheter: a pilot study. *Oncol Nurs Forum* 1996;23:1401–1405.
4. Warner BW, Haygood MM, Davies SL, Hennies GA. A randomized, prospective trial of standard Hickman compared with Groshong central venous catheters in pediatric oncology patients. *J Am Coll Surg* 1996;183:140–144.

5. Waggoner SE. Venous air embolism through a Groshong catheter. *Gynecol Oncol* 1993;48:394–396.

6. Salem RR, Ward BA, Ravikmar TS. A new peripherally implanted subcutaneous permanent central venous access device for patients requiring chemotherapy. *J Clin Oncol* 1993;11:2181–2185.

7. Hahn U, Goldschmidt H, Salwender H, Haas R, Hunstein W. Large bore central venous catheters for the collection of peripheral blood stem cells. *J Clin Apheresis* 1995;10:12–16.

8. Vanherweghem JL, Yassine T, Goldman M, et al. Subclavian vein thrombosis: a frequent complication of subclavian vein cannulation for hemodialysis. *Clin Nephrol* 1986;26:235–238.

9. Schillinger F, Schillinger D, Montagnac R, Milcent T. Post catheterisation vein stenosis in haemodialysis: comparative angiographic study of 50 subclavian and 50 internal jugular accesses. *Nephrol Dial Transplant* 1991;6:722–724.

10. Pettengell R, Davies AJ, Harvey VJ. Experiance with an implantable venous access system for chemotherapy. *N Z Med J* 1991;104:284–285.

11. Pokorny WJ, McGill CW, Harberg FJ. Use of the azygous vein for central venous catheter insertion. *Surgery* 1985;97:362.

12. Mathur MN, Storey DW, White GH, Ramsey-Steward G. Percutaneous insertion of long-term venous access catheters via the external iliac vein. *Aust N Z J Surg* 1993;63:858–863.

13. Azizkhan RG, Taylor LA, Jaques PF, et al. Percutaneous translumbar and transhepatic inferior vena caval catheters for prolonged vascular access in children. *J Pediatr Surg* 1992;27:165–169.

14. Lund GB, Lieberman RP, Haire WD, et al. Translumbar inferior vena cava catheters for long-term venous access. *Radiology* 1990;174:31–35.

15. Downie AC, Reidy JF, Adam AN. Tunneled central venous catheter insertion via the internal jugular vein using a dedicated portable ultrasound device. *Br J Radiol* 1996;69:178–181.

16. Randolph AG, Cook DJ, Gonzales CA, Pribble CG. Ultrasound guidance for placement of central venous catheters: a meta-analysis of the literature. *Crit Care Med* 1996;24:2053–2058.

17. Denys BG, Uretsky BF, Reddy PS. Ultrasound assisted cannulation of the internal jugular vein. A prospective comparison to the landmark-guided technique. *Circulation* 1993;87:1557–1562.

18. Dickson CS, Roth SM, Russell JM, et al. Placement of internal jugular vein central venous catheters: anatomic ultrasound assessment and literature review. *Surg Rounds* 1996;19:102–107.

19. Troianos CA, Kuwik RJ, Pasqual JR, Lim AJ, Odasso DP. Internal jugular vein and carotid artery anatomic relationship as determined by ultrasonography. *Anesthesiology* 1996;85:43–48.

20. Sulek CA, Gravenstein N, Blackshear RH, Weiss L. Head rotation during internal jugular cannulation and the risk of carotid artery puncture. *Anesth Analg* 1996;82:125–128.

21. Mansfield PF, Hohn DC, Fornage BD, et al. Complications and Failures of subclavian vein catheterization. *N Engl J Med* 1994;331:1735–1738.

22. Madan M, Shah MV, Alexander DJ, et al. Right atrial electrocardiography: a technique for the placement of central venous catheters for chemotherapy or intravenous nutrition. *Br J Surg* 1994;81:1604–1605.

23. Schenk WG. Pitfalls in ambulatory vascular access surgery. In: Schirmer BD, Rattner D, eds. *Ambulatory surgery*. Philadelphia: WB Saunders, 1998.

24. Beauregard JF, Matsumoto AH, Paul MG, Holt RW. Venobronchial fistula: a complication associated with central venous catheterization for chemotherapy. *Cathet Cardiovasc Diagn* 1990;19:49–52.

25. Gerlis LM, Gibbs JL, Williams GL, Thomas GD. Coronary sinus atresia and persistent left superior vena cava. A report of two cases, one associated with atypical coronary artery thrombosis. *Br Heart J* 1984;52:648–653.

26. Pugliese P, Murzi B, Aliboni M, Eufrate S. Absent right superior vena cava and persistent left superior vena cava. Clinical and surgical considerations. *J Cardiovasc Surg* 1984;25:134–137.

27. Ronnevik PK, Abrahamsen AM, Tollefsen I. Transvenous pacemaker implantation via a unilateral left superior vena cava. *Pacing Clin Electrophysiol* 1982;5:808–813.

28. Lokich JJ, Bothe A, Benotti P, Moore C. Complications and management of implanted venous access catheters. *J Clin Oncol* 1985;3:710–717.

29. Hurtubise MR, Bottino JC, Lawson M, McCredie KB. Restoring patency of occluded central venous catheters. *Arch Surg* 1980;115:212–213.

30. Black MD, French J, Rasuli P, Bouchard AC. Upper extremity deep venous thrombosis: underdiagnosed and potentially lethal. *Chest* 1993; 103:1887–1890.

31. Lambert D, Drew R. Aetiology influences late morbidity following axillary-subclavian vein thrombosis. *Br J Surg* 1988;75:391.

32. Druy EM, Trout HH, Giordino JM, Hix WR. Lytic therapy in the treatment of axillary and subclavian vein thrombosis. *J Vasc Surg* 1985;2: 821–827.

33. Haire WD, Lieberman RP, Edney J, et al. Hickman catheter-induced thoracic vein thrombosis. Frequency and long-term sequelae in patients receiving high-dose chemotherapy and marrow transplantation. *Cancer* 1990;66:900–908.

34. Newman KA, Reed WP, Schimpff SC, Bustamante CI, Wade JC. Hickman catheters in association with intensive cancer chemotherapy. *Support Care Cancer* 1993;1:92–97.

CHAPTER 6

Operative Complications in Pelvic Surgery

Warren E. Enker, Klaas Havenga, and Joseph Martz

The traditional complications of surgery for rectal cancer have been reviewed elsewhere (1) (Tables 6-1 to 6-3). The profusion of complications which are associated with mobilization of the rectum are testimony to the lack of understanding that prevails regarding the planes of pelvic anatomy. Sharp dissection under direct vision along the areolar pelvic tissue planes drastically reduces the complications which most surgeons associate with conventional pelvic surgery. The goal of this article is to outline the complications which may be associated with circumferential or total mesorectal excision (CME or TME) for rectal cancer, as a guide to dissecting within the pelvis.

COMPLICATIONS

Principles of TME

The majority of patients with rectal cancer present with regional disease, i.e., either full thickness penetration of the rectal wall, $T_3N_0M_0$, or the involvement of regional mesorectal lymph nodes, $T_{any}N_{1-2}M_0$. Operations for rectal cancer should achieve the following: (a) cure, i.e., the prevention of systemic spread; (b) local control, i.e., the avoidance of pelvic recurrence; (c) sphincter preservation, i.e., the restoration of continuity and preservation of anorectal function; and (d) the preservation of sexual and urinary functions, i.e., preserving the integrity of the pelvic autonomic nervous system (2).

Conventional surgery, as commonly practiced worldwide (i.e., blunt or blind dissection within the pelvis) without knowledge of or regard for specific planes of dissection, has failed to achieve these goals. Blunt or manual dissection often encounters areas of resistance at the level of the rectosacral ligament creating the following problems. The surgeon is forced to choose between inadequate planes and/or operative complications. Blunt pelvic dissection is notorious for major hemorrhage. Because of the fear of avulsing the presacral veins, surgeons usually elect to deviate forward, often violating the mesorectum, leaving cancer-containing fat attached to the pelvic side wall. This mishap generally results in a 30%

worldwide rate of local, pelvic recurrence. The same surgeon often finds that it is difficult to mobilize the rectum beyond the rectosacral ligament. As a result, blunt dissection has been associated with common use of abdominoperineal excision of the rectum. An inadequate mesorectal resection is associated with a 60% to 65% incidence of systemic metastases in stages $T_3N_0M_0$ and $T_{any}N_{1-2}M_0$, plus high rates of impotence and of sexual and urinary dysfunction resulting from the blind cutting of the pelvic autonomic nerves (3).

Pathophysiology of Pelvic Recurrence

In 1986, Quirke and associates documented that local recurrence is attributable to involved circumferential margins and incomplete resection of the mesorectum during conventional resections which were deemed curative by experienced operating surgeons (4). Portions of mesorectal fat containing involved lymph nodes remain attached to the pelvic sidewall. This persistent disease is manifest clinically as recurrent disease, on average, 18 months later. The results of Quirke have been reproduced by other investigators (5,6). With uninvolved circumferential margins, i.e., lateral margins, local recurrence rates average 10% or less. After curative resections, when the lateral margins are unsuspectedly involved, the local failure rates are as high as 85% to 90% (5). The primary goal of surgery is the complete excision of all potential regional mesorectal disease, enveloped within an intact visceral layer of the pelvic fascia, with negative lateral or circumferential margins (2).

Selected series have now confirmed a marked decline in abdominoperineal resections which may be reserved for patients with cancers of the distal rectum situated 0 to 5 cm from the anal verge, i.e., distal to the tip of the coccyx and in direct proximity to the levator ani muscles (7). Marked declines in the rates of local recurrence, from 30%, to 5% to 8%, are reported in patients with stages $T_3N_0M_0$ or $T_{any}N_{1-2}M_0$, the so-called high-risk stages which would qualify patients for combined radiation and chemotherapy in the NIH Consensus (2). Patients with classical Dukes B and C stages have rates of distant metastases as low as 25% as opposed to a reported in-

TABLE 6–1. *Operative mortality*

Reference	Year	Percentage mortality	Operation
Hedberg (1)	1963	7–9%	
Localio (1)	1978	1.7%	Anterior resection
		2.3%	Abdominoperineal resection
Rosen (1)	1982	1.7%	Abdominoperineal resection
Enker (2)	1995	0.8%	Anterior resection and abdominoperineal resection
Enker (16)	1997	2.0%	Abdominoperineal resection

Factors associated with operative mortality: ***Patient-related***—coronary artery disease (comorbidity or complications), sepsis (i.e., anastomotic leakage), age, obesity, diabetes, hypertension, chronic obstructive pulmonary disease; ***tumor-related***—obstruction, bleeding, perforation, adjacent organ invasion.

cidence of 60% to 65%. Cure rates in these stages approach 75%. Autonomic nerve preservation (ANP) has preserved sexual and urinary functions in men and women. Together the technical advances which are responsible for these changes are known as either TME, or TME with ANP.

These dramatic improvements are all attributable to a fundamental change in operative technique. The technical distinction between TME and conventional surgery has to do with the techniques of total rectal mobilization. In contrast to conventional or blunt dissection, TME uses sharp dissection under direct vision, following a defined plane between the visceral and the parietal layers of the pelvic fascia (Fig. 6-1). The visceral fascia envelopes the rectum and the mesorectum. The parietal fascia covers the musculoskeletal and vascular boundaries of the sidewalls, including the pelvic autonomic nerves and plexuses.

The techniques of sharp dissection are not new, being routinely applied in the head and neck, in thoracic surgical oncology, and in upper GI surgery. However, the use of sharp technique in the pelvis is new to most surgeons; the pelvis being previously considered an anatomical black box in which operating is associated with the fear of bleeding, causing impotence, etc.

It should come as no surprise that sharp dissection under direct vision would become the appropriate operative tech-

TABLE 6–2. *Intraoperative complications*

Bleeding
    Pelvic presacral veins
    Internal iliac vessels
    Splenic injury
    Anastomotic hemorrhage
Adjacent organ injury
    Ureter
    Bladder
    Vagina
    Prostate urethra

TABLE 6–3. *Postoperative complications*

Abdominal
    Anastomotic leakage
    Ileus
    Sepsis
    Hemorrhage
    Fistulae
    Intestinal obstruction
Systemic
    Pulmonary embolism
    Myocardial infarction
    Renal failure
Infections
    Wound abscess
    Pelvic or intraabdominal abscess
    Consequences of inadequate preparation due to obstruction or perforation
    Peritonitis
Other
    Urinary retention and neurogenic bladder
    Stoma management and placement
    Perineal wound infection
    Persistent perineal sinus
    Sexual dysfunction

nique for rectal cancer, once the anatomic planes of the pelvis were appreciated.

Practicing surgeons, who have not been previously trained in the art of sharp dissection within the pelvis, need to adopt new methods of dissection if the advantages of TME are to

THE VISCERAL COMPARTMENT OF THE RECTUM AND THE MESORECTUM

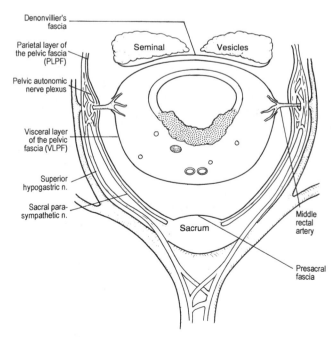

FIG. 6-1. The visceral compartment of the rectum and mesorectum, with the visceral and parietal fascial layers. In some areas, these layers are known by their special names, i.e., presacral fascia.

be available to all patients. In addition to the advantages of survival and lower rates of local recurrence, sharp dissection is associated with sphincter preservation, with ANP, and with reduced blood loss, which in theory has been associated with immunosuppression and the risk of cancer progression. The learning curve can be shortened by utilizing many of the available educational tools ranging from publications and videos to preceptorship and workshops.

Principles of Operative Technique

This operation is performed using sharp dissection throughout. As such, a reminder of the principles guiding operative technique is warranted. These principles include: traction and countertraction at the site of dissection, exposure including good lighting, a working knowledge of the planes of dissection, and then proceeding with the dissection itself. Good lighting is imperative, and a headlight or an overhead light which diffuses the column of projected light across the operative field are both helpful in different hands.

Proper Position of the Patient

The patient undergoes operation in the Trendelenburg lithotomy position. We utilize the Lloyd-Davies stirrups which provide support for the calves in a neutral or universal position. These stirrups allow for the use of additional padding, the use of sequential compression devices, and the avoidance of pressure along the tibial tuberosity, i.e., the location of the peroneal nerves. The latter minimizes the incidence of peroneal nerve palsy, i.e., foot drop. The sacrum rests on a double folded silastic pad minimizing the impact of long periods of pressure on the lumbar spine.

Modifying the Abdominal Incision

Most surgeons operate upon rectal cancer through a midline incision which usually ends at the transverse suprapubic skin fold. The focus of this article is the avoidance of complications. To do so requires that the entire operation be conducted under direct vision. When a midline laparotomy incision is retracted with many self-retaining retractors, i.e. the Balfour retractor, the lower end of the incision actually rides upward, further obscuring the pelvis. The first step in achieving visibility of the entire pelvis is the completion of the midline incision to the symphysis pubis. This often requires a skin incision down to the lowest edge of the mons pubis or to the suspensory ligament of the penis.

Modifying the Use of Self-Retaining Retractors

Lateral retraction to open the most common abdominal incision obscures visibility within the pelvis. A retractor system that spreads the abdominal incision in both a lateral and a downward direction opens the pelvis to a complete view, allowing one to proceed with sharp dissection under direct vision. I find that the bar system retractors (i.e., the Thompson retractor system) perform better in this respect than the circle or elliptical ring retractors (i.e., the Bookwalter system) and better duplicate the exposure that would be achieved by human effort. Under optimal conditions, the elliptical retractors may be modified by placing the lower edge of the ring well distal to the symphysis pubis. Often, however, this is not possible, particularly in the stocky male patient. The elliptical ring retractors are also associated with a small, however real, incidence of femoral nerve compression which may occur because of the depth of the retractor blades. The body wall retractor blades of the Thompson system are shallow and less likely to contact the pelvic sidewalls. Between the choice of abdominal incision and the utilization of appropriate retraction, the pelvis is fully exposed for sharp dissection.

The use of appropriate self-retaining retraction makes possible the same type of operation with the same or less manpower in the operating room. This is an important consideration in today's economic climate.

Surgeon's Tray: Special Instruments for TME

Because of the depth of the pelvis, and the need to dissect sharply from the sacral promontory to the anal hiatus in the levator ani, the standard operating tray is not appropriately equipped for executing the resection of rectal cancer in accordance with the principles of TME. Long instruments and special hand-held retractors are needed for the surgeon to accomplish the type of resection which is advocated. Among the needed instruments are items which are common to the cardiac or thoracic setup, including long (12-inch) DeBakey Forceps, 11- to 12-inch scissors, an insulated extension for the electrocautery tip, a Cooley suction tip, St. Marks retractors (deep and superficial), Sarot clamps, and a variety of right angle bowel clamps, including the DeBakey, Potts-Block, and Deddish designs.

Dissection of the pelvis begins at the level of the sacral promontory. To either side, the hypogastric nerves are identified and sharply dissected away from the mesorectum (Fig. 6-2). These nerves are dissected from the aortic bifurcation to the pelvic autonomic nerve plexus (PANP).

Sharp dissection continues downward or caudad between the visceral and parietal planes of the pelvic fascia (Fig. 6-1). At the level of the sacral curvature, the rectosacral ligament is encountered, and is sharply divided, exposing the lower half of the true pelvis to view (Fig. 6-3).

Dissection continues circumferentially around the mesorectum and medial to the parasympathetic nerves. These nerves are identified as they exit the sacral foramina and course toward the PANP. Alternatively, the PANP, which is located anterolaterally at the level of the seminal vesicles or the cervix, is identified first, and the dissection continues in a retrograde fashion. The lateral ligaments are really the attachments of the PANP to the mesorectum, through which course the pelvic autonomic nerves to the pelvis (Fig. 6-4). The connections binding the mesorectum to the PANP are dissected meticulously, and divided medial to the PANP.

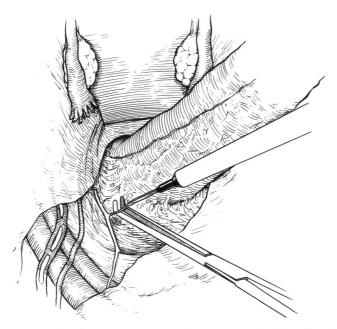

FIG. 6-2. Dissection of the left hypogastric nerves just distal to the aortic bifurcation. Branches to the rectum are serially divided. The plane between the VLPF and the PLPF is now apparent.

After complete dissection bilaterally, the mesorectum is completely mobilized and the pelvic autonomic nerves and plexuses remain intact (Fig. 6-5). Overlying the posterior portion of the mesorectum is the visceral layer of the pelvic fascia, which identifies that a CME has been advised.

Most often, a conventional anastomosis follows (Fig. 6-6).

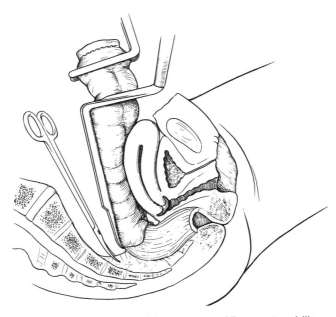

FIG. 6-3. Sharp division of the rectosacral ligament mobilizes the mesorectum without penetrating the visceral compartment and risking violation of tumor-bearing nodes, etc.

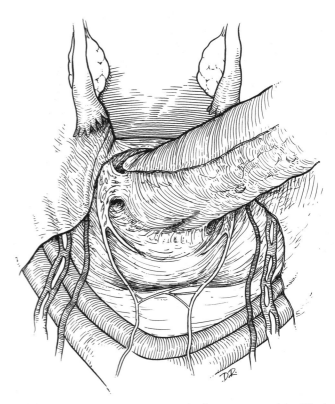

FIG. 6-4. The sacral parasympathetic nerves are identified, and dissection identifies their course from the sacral foramina to the PANP. The lateral ligament is still intact but will be divided medial to the PANP.

Anastomotic Technique

Anastomotic technique may vary with the circumstances. The surgeon embarking upon TME will face many instances in which patients who would have previously faced an APR will now be able to have a sphincter-preserving operation (SPO). Often, the anastomosis will be taking place at the lowest reaches of the rectum, i.e., the level of the pelvic floor. To accomplish these anastomoses may require new skills and a familiarity with all available anastomotic options.

These options may include (a) a standard end-to-end low anterior resection (LAR) anastomosis, between serosalized and a nonserosalized bowel; (b) a double-stapled anastomosis; (c) a coloanal anastomosis; (d) a side-to-end anastomosis between the colon and the rectum; or (e) an anastomosis between a colonic J-pouch and the lowest rectum or the anal canal. Often techniques which are taken for granted higher up, i.e., a double staple technique at the level of the rectosigmoid, must be abandoned as being either unsafe or simply not applicable in the lower reaches of the pelvis. As an example, the attempted application of a transverse linear stapler below a tumor in very tight narrow pelvic quarters may defeat the purpose of achieving safe margins of rectal and mesorectal resection in all directions.

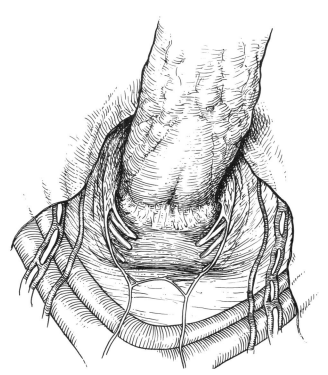

FIG. 6-5. The pelvic autonomic nerves are intact and the rectum/mesorectum has been dissected down to the pelvic floor. The smooth posterior mesorectal surface is the visceral layer of the pelvic fascia, which remains intact.

Dividing the Bowel Distal to the Tumor

Dividing the bowel distal to the tumor can be one of the more difficult parts of the operation, requiring experience and skill in order not to compromise the cancer operation. The most important factor in defining the distal margin and applying the distal purse string suture is the extent to which the rectum has been fully mobilized. The concept of the distal margin of resection is more aptly referred to as the distal margin of dissection or of mobilization. In SPO, there is no substitute for complete mobilization of the rectum from the sacral promontory to the anal hiatus within the levator ani for avoiding complications and consequences. Once the rectum is fully mobilized, two factors are operative: (a) As the rectum is held straight up, the tumor rises out of the pelvic curvature so that a 5-cm distal margin of the mesorectum in the patient is easily obtained; this is particularly true for posteriorly located tumors which were originally situated at 7 to 9 cm; since the tumor rises about 4 to 5 cm with mobilization, and the distal margin is about 4 to 5 cm, the anastomosis ends up at about the same level as the original tumor location as measured from the anal verge. (b) Placement of a transverse linear stapler or of a purse string suture is facilitated. The bulk of the tumor is up, often away from the pelvic side walls, and there is now room to manipulate either a right angle bowel clamps, a linear stapling device, or an automatic purse string applier. I often will divide the rectum between two DeBakey right

angle bowel clamps placed from either side of the rectum. With the tumor removed from the field, the automatic purse string applier or the linear stapling device can now be positioned much more easily, directly below the clamp, and fired safely without compromising the cancer operation.

In closed systems, i.e., when a transverse linear stapler is applied or when the triple stapling technique is employed, especially in laparoscopic approaches, the tumor is still in situ and the rectum should be irrigated below the clamp or the first staple line prior to firing the definitive staple line. This way, clumps of tumor cells which have been fragmented into the lumen of the rectum from the primary tumor during handling or dissection are not driven through the staple line, a potential cause of suture-line recurrence. In an open system, i.e., the rectum has been divided and opened prior to placement of the purse string suture, it makes little difference whether thorough irrigation is performed per rectum prior to dividing the bowel via the pelvis once it has been opened. In either case, the issue is one of dilution of the number of tumor cells by generous irrigation of the pelvis with multiple aliquots of saline.

For lesions which were originally situated above 10 cm from the anal verge or which are located in the intraperitoneal rectum, this author does not resect the entire mesorectum to the pelvic floor. After complete mobilization such a lesion may rise to 12 to 15 cm as the rectum is straightened by gentle upward traction. Even with the known risk of distal mesorectal deposits or nodes, a 5- to 6-cm distal margin of the mesorectum provides a very adequate regional resection of all disease (9). An anastomosis that is located 5 to 6 cm

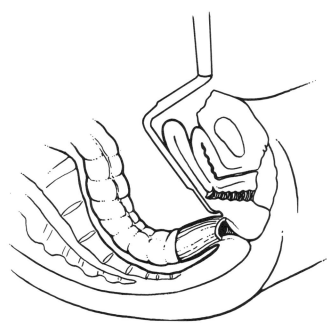

FIG. 6-6. A conventional colorectal anastomosis just proximal to the levator ani. Higher and lower (i.e., coloanal) anastomosis are possible as are straight, side-to-end or colonic J-pouch reconstructions.

below the tumor provides a safe margin of mesorectal resection, and allows the patient to retain 7 to 8 cm of distal rectum, which is most important for long-term function. To distinguish the management of the high lesion from lesions located 5 to 8 cm from the anal verge, I have emphasized the circumferential focus of the dissection by occasionally referring to this group of operations as CME, as opposed to TME. The distinction only serves the purpose of focusing on the circumferential margins and not on the distal mesorectum.

Distal Purse String

Depending upon the level at which the anastomosis will be performed, the technique of the distal purse string or rectal closure will differ. The higher the anastomosis and the wider the pelvis the easier it is to accomplish a safe anastomosis by the double-staple technique. The rectum is closed and divided above a transverse linear staple line. When a third staple line is used temporarily to allow irrigation of the rectum, the method is known as the triple-stapling technique. An end-to-end or side-to-end anastomosis is performed using the circular stapler. During open surgery, the use of an automatic purse string applying device may prove to be easier than application of the linear stapler, as the latter requires a wider pelvis to manipulate into place. A low profile, right-angled bowel clamp, i.e., the DeBakey or the Potts-Block variety, can make a difference in the successful application of either. For the most distal anastomoses, ie, those which are situated at the level of the levator ani, a hand-sewn purse string suture may be needed where the automatic staple applier or the linear stapler will have difficulty negotiating the narrow passage of the pelvis.

The position of the operating surgeon can make a major difference in the ease of applying a distal purse string suture very low in the pelvis. With the self-retaining retractor or a deep St. Marks retractor, providing as much visibility as possible, the surgeon is positioned below the pelvis on the left side of the patient for the right-handed surgeon, and vice versa for the left-handed surgeon. This position provides the surgeon with a direct line to the cut edge of the distal rectum and allows an over-and-over suture of 2-0 polypropylene to be placed with relative ease. On rare occasion, a very distal purse string suture may be placed via the anus if no other route of access can be obtained. This approach allows a uniform sutured purse-string with bites placed about 4 mm apart and 4 mm from the edge. The safety of the anastomosis is reflected in the uniformly good donuts produced by this technique.

Two or three other options exist for rare situations in which application of the distal purse string is a problem. One may sew the distal purse string suture as one cuts across the rectal wall, or one may sew over a proctoscope either before or during amputation of the specimen. Both require experience and skill, and copious irrigation both before and afterward, because the stitch is being placed while the tumor remains in situ. Again, either a bowel clamp or a transverse noncutting staple line may obviate this problem.

Anastomotic Leaks

Low anastomoses are associated with a high incidence of disruption. Heald (8) reports a 17% incidence of leakage following LAR performed in association with TME, where the anastomosis is at the level of the pelvic floor. Possible reasons for a leak are devascularization of the proximal segment, the poor blood supply of the distal segment, inadequate drainage of pelvic contents, i.e., seroma, blood or infected fluids, or the poor integrity of the rectal wall at the level of or in close proximity to the pelvic floor.

Radiation therapy and corticosteroids may also affect anastomotic healing. The distal rectal segment, long blamed for its poor blood supply, actually has quite a rich circulation. The transected rectum is often the largest source of blood loss in a rectal resection performed by the technique of TME, and few surgeons experienced with low rectal anastomoses would find fault with the distal rectal blood supply. It is much more likely that the mobilized and cleaned off sigmoid colon demarcates its blood supply some time after the anastomosis has been completed. While in many cases the line of demarcation is evident, in some cases the relative ischemia is either not evident before the anastomosis is completed, or it progresses upward, leaving an ischemic zone just proximal to the staple line. Inadequate microcirculation within the bowel wall may be associated with a history of diverticulitis, diabetes, atherosclerosis, hypertension, smoking, etc. In diverticulitis, damage may be the result of repeated attacks of sigmoid inflammation, with small vessel disease secondary to intramural fibrosis. For this, among other reasons, diverticulitis, resulting in a damaged sigmoid colon, is a contraindication to the very low colorectal or the coloanal anastomosis. These issues are among the reasons that most experienced rectal surgeons would use the descending colon for an anastomosis, avoiding the sigmoid colon in the face of such problems. When an anastomosis is performed, patients with milder cases of diverticulitis are often best served by a side-to-end colorectal anastomosis.

As indicated, a generous policy of fecal diversion is essential, if all anastomoses are to end up at the level of the pelvic floor. Too many unnecessary deaths have taken place worldwide as surgeons practicing TME have performed low rectal anastomosis without protective coverage (8). In this respect, the first author differs with Heald, who advocates that as a result of TME, all anastomoses should, at least in theory, end up at the level of the pelvic floor. In the case of upper rectal lesions, I will mobilize the entire rectum and mesorectum out of pelvis, and then take a five to six centimeter margin distal to some of the more proximal rectal lesions, without resection of the most distal mesorectum. This accomplishes a generous resection of the distal mesorectum, which may contain tumor (9) while, at the same time, leaving a longer segment of the distal rectum intact, wherever possible. Generally, this difference applies to primary cancers of the midrectum that are 9 to 12 cm from the anal verge, in which case complete mobilization of the rectum elevates the tumor by 4 to 5 cm from its location within the sacral curvature. The resulting anastomosis ends up in the midrectum where the rectal wall is often considerably thicker (i.e., integrity) than the thickness of the distal rectum at the level of the pelvic brim or the anal canal. Under these circumstances, the anastomotic leak rate is much lower, well below 5%, allowing the surgeon greater leeway in electing to avoid fecal diversion, particularly in the younger and healthier patient. Effective drainage of all potential fluid, i.e., potential abscess-forming seroma, blood, etc., is important to avoid a leak by necessity.

Diverting Colostomy or Ileostomy

Despite a relatively low leak rate (2.9%) (2), we are very liberal with the use of a temporary diverting stoma. As indicated, the incidence of anastomotic leakage is high after TME when the anastomosis is situated at or immediately proximal to the pelvic floor. In such cases, we invariably divert the fecal stream. We rarely divert anastomoses which are situated at the level of the midrectum, unless the patient has had complete preoperative radiation therapy. Factors influencing our choice to divert are a thin-walled rectum, radiation therapy, the technical difficulty or ease of the operation, the quality of the hemostasis, anemia, corticosteroids, and the risk of sepsis to the patient, especially a patient compromised by cardiac or pulmonary comorbidity.

Another factor of extreme importance is the long-term functional outcome. Sepsis causes poor long-term function due to the fibrosis and scarring associated with resolving the pelvic sepsis. Pelvic fibrosis and a distal anastomosis are a combined formula for poor long-term function. A diverting stoma allows for healing, encountering minimal consequences of a leak should a disruption take place, and long-term functional outcomes that are optimal.

Morbidity of Closure of Ileostomy or Colostomy

The colostomy or ileostomy is closed about eight to twelve weeks following a definitive resection. All diverting stomas are placed in the right lower quadrant for both functional and cosmetic reasons. Upper abdominal diverting stomas are assiduously avoided as they often create problems with appliance placement and maintenance. In the obese patient, it is much easier to construct a loop ileostomy than a loop colostomy. Since it is generally easier to close a loop colostomy, rarely requiring a resection, we prefer the loop colostomy over the ileostomy if it is possible. We would not create a colostomy if a struggle would imply the risk of skin retraction and future stoma management problems. When conducted carefully, there is minimum morbidity associated with stoma closure. Inadvertent enterotomies and the inability to reverse the stoma are virtually always the consequence of proceeding with closure too soon by allowing insufficient time for resolution of the operative inflammatory responses. Wound infection is avoided by allowing for secondary or delayed primary wound closure.

Bleeding

A transfusion requirement in association with TME is rare because the dissection is performed under direct vision along the areolar planes which are relatively bloodless, and because all hemostasis is obtained prospectively. Experience with sharp dissection leads to a knowledge of the associated pelvic anatomy, and very little likelihood of excessive bleeding. In our experience, at least 85% of patients undergoing TME according to its principles, do not require transfusion. As a proportion of the patients are anemic at the outset, the true incidence of transfusion requirement may actually be lower.

Packing the pelvis is virtually unheard of. Virtually all of the major bleeding which is commonly associated with rectal mobilization occurs when blunt dissection disrupts the presacral venous plexuses. Invariably, the need to pack the pelvis for hemostasis results in either an APR or a Hartmann's resection with abandonment of any hope of sphincter-preservation. The use of packing is decried as an example of the type of morbidity that has long been associated with blunt pelvic dissection. While the complications associated with rectal cancer surgery are still common today, they almost always occur in the setting of conventional or blunt dissection, and only rarely in the setting of sharp dissection. Bleeding which takes place in the setting of sharp dissection almost always involves a transected vessel which was inadvertently cut and may often be arrested by the standard techniques of suture, cautery, the brief application of pressure, etc.

In the event of bleeding, it is rarely massive, and simple pressure is usually the first step while everyone is organized to handle the problem together. Inadvertent venous injuries close to the midline or the parasacral region responds well to several minutes of highly localized pressure. Most often such injuries occur from pass-pointing or other classical technical mishap. When one adheres to the proper techniques of dissection (under direct vision), such events are rare.

Intraoperative Injuries

Ureters

In approximately 600 cases of TME performed by this author, there has been no single instance of ureteral injury. Ureters have been deliberately cut because of either adherence to or invasion by tumor. In these cases immediate reconstruction follows.

The ureters, especially the left ureter, are always identified prior to the onset of pelvic dissection. This is occasionally time consuming and a tedious test of one's patience, but well worth the few minutes of warranted effort. Substituting ureteral catheters for intraoperative identification of the ureter is not warranted by virtue of expense and time. Most of all, for surgeons who know the pelvic anatomy and who are qualified to perform such operations, the anatomy of the ureters should represent basic information. Ureteral catheters are, however, introduced in cases of recurrent rectal cancer, prior surgery, and radiation therapy. In such cases, where fibrosis or cancer may obscure the location of the ureter(s), time is saved and dissection is simplified by the placement of these catheters.

When the ureters are not carefully identified, the majority of ureteral injuries occur at or below the level of the pelvic brim. The key to managing the injury is its recognition. The opinion of a urologist should be sought regarding management. In the overwhelming majority of such cases, a simple and safe ureteral repair over a stent or a ureteroneocystostomy will be performed. The experienced urologist can successfully perform the repair and will make the appropriate judgements regarding such issues as a psoas hitch or the placement of a temporary indwelling ureteral stent.

Injury to the ureter can also take place at the level of the midureter, and proximally where the ureter is visible and close to the origin of the inferior mesenteric vessels. Such midureteral or proximal ureteral injuries are extremely rare and are much harder to repair. End-to-end ureteroureterotomy may be complicated by stricture and should be performed over a stent. The occasional patient will have to suffer a nephrectomy as a result of such an injury.

Vagina

The vagina may be injured in two ways: direct inadvertent entry due to loss of the operating plane, or ischemic damage due to intramural dissection. The first occurs most commonly when the patient has had a prior hysterectomy. The vagina can be identified by any of several means. Wearing a second glove, one can perform an intraoperative examination. The second assistant can place a tampon (sponge on a stick) or a device (i.e., the EEA sizer) into the vagina anteflexing the apex and holding it in place until the rectovaginal septum has been properly identified. Subsequently, or alternatively, long Allis clamps may be applied to both the left and right ends of the vaginal fornices and the vagina can be identified by lifting it away from the rectum. Where a deliberate excision of a limited portion of the vaginal wall should take place to ensure cancer-free margins, the latter technique often serves best, both for excision and for primary repair.

When the surgeon proceeds with dissection despite being uncertain about the correct plane, more often than not, the vagina is devascularized by dissecting part of the way through its wall, resulting in a delayed breakdown. The most common manifestation of such an injury is a rectovaginal fistula from the anastomosis of an LAR to the posterior vaginal wall. Generally, the fistula becomes clinically evident about two to four weeks following the operation as the ischemic injury evolves. Because of the extent of mural injury, these fistulae may be large, are difficult to repair, and rarely heal despite fecal diversion.

A third cause of vaginal injury is the inclusion of the vagina in the circular stapler during a colorectal anastomosis. This injury results from the inadequate dissection of the rectovaginal septum, allowing a portion of the vagina to be caught within the closed circular stapling device. This injury is avoided by adequate dissection and proper retraction during the anastomosis itself.

Bladder

Injuries at the dome are treatable by simple repair in layers. Complex injuries at the trigone are extremely rare. They may require repair together with ureteral transpositions (i.e., bilateral ureteroneocystostomy) and drainage.

Spleen

Splenic injury is rare and capsular injury most often results from traction. Indications for splenectomy are limited to the failure of conservative means, i.e. topical hemostatic agents to stop the bleeding.

Infections

Wound

Primary wound infection is largely beyond the scope of this chapter, and incidence of 4% to 8% is reported for operations involving the large bowel even with appropriate peri-operative antibiotic coverage. Two issues deserve serious mention: delayed primary wound closure and the handling of primary wounds after relaparotomy.

Delayed primary wound closure is a very underutilized technique which may be lifesaving and which certainly helps to avoid significant morbidity. Many cases of colorectal resections have a higher than average potential for wound abscess, associated risks of systemic sepsis, and wound dehiscence. Such circumstances include the presence of intra-abdominal or of pelvic sepsis, i.e., a perforated carcinoma or diverticular abscess, the obstructing tumor, abdominal wall or retroperitoneal involvement, fistula, etc. In many such situations, the longstanding or the undrainable nature of the sepsis raises the likelihood of wound abscess. Even a lengthy clean-contaminated case can represent a risk of wound sepsis. Delayed primary wound closure obviates the risk, allowing for a normal recovery.

It is our practice to place a series of matching horizontal-mattress dermal sutures of absorbable material on either side of the wound. The open wound is treated with moist sterile dressing changes. If the wound remains clean, beginning on or about the third or fourth day, these sutures, which up until now have been held together with adhesive strips, are separated from each other and the ends of each mattress suture are tied across the wound. One or two stitches are tied at either end of the wound daily until the wound is closed. The umbilicus will often be sutured for cosmetic reasons, and only the straight portions of the vertical wound require delayed closure. The cosmetic result is at least as good as any stapled closure and the risks of sepsis are prevented. The same is true for wounds which are opened for reexploration of the abdomen, as for example in the case of an anastomotic leak, a bowel obstruction, etc. Even in the absence of gross infection, i.e., a bowel obstruction, the likelihood of low grade infection being present is high, even without direct exposure to intestinal contents via enterostomy or to peritoneal sepsis.

Often a septic wound complication can be the difference between the death and the recovery in an older patient whose tolerance for complications may be marginal.

Bowel Obstruction

Early postoperative bowel obstruction (EPOBO) is more commonly, although not exclusively, observed following left-sided or pelvic dissections, and relatively rare after right hemicolectomy. In contrast to the traditional presentation of acute mechanical small bowel obstruction, early postoperative small bowel obstruction is frequently caused as much by an inflammatory serositis as by multiple adhesions. Most cases present with distention only after feeding commences. High-pitched bowel sounds and radiologic findings are often out of proportion to the illness of the patient. Decompression by nasogastric tube, long intestinal tube or indwelling temporary gastrostomy (placed at the time of the elective laparotomy) generally resolves the problem within the first week of treatment in 70% of patients. In the relatively quiet abdomen, it may be difficult to differentiate between a dynamic ileus and EPOBO. Both are initially treated conservatively, but ileus may be a symptom of either a gut response to opioids or of sepsis. In both cases, a CT scan may prove useful diagnostically. If the clinical picture is in question, an upper GI examination with small bowel follow-through using only 5–8 ounces of light barium is frequently helpful in expediting treatment and decision-making.

Rarely does EPOBO require a reoperation for the lysis of adhesions. If one should prove necessary it is important to avoid operating in the third to fourth postoperative weeks when tissues are exceedingly vulnerable and the bowel may be easily injured (10).

Reconstruction for Extensive Resection

Composite resections for locally advanced or recurrent disease often require pelvic reconstruction. Examples include abdominoperineal excision of the rectum with posterior vaginectomy where reconstruction via rectus myocutaneous flap or gluteal flaps may be needed. The use of intra-operative irradiation by implant or afterloading technique often benefits from separating the radiation source from the small bowel. The use of flaps or of an omental pedicle graft as a means of interposing viable healthy tissue between the radiation source and the small bowel is often beneficial in avoiding complications, i.e., a radiation injury to the intestine with fistula formation.

LONG-TERM CONSEQUENCES OF SURGERY FOR RECTAL CANCER

Pelvic Recurrence

As indicated above, pelvic recurrence is the result of a failure to circumvent all mesorectal disease. It is a direct consequence of the inadequate resection of all regional spread from the primary tumor. In a small percentage of cases, pelvic recurrence is observed despite TME and may be due to undetectable disease at the margins of dissection, even when TME has been properly performed. Other causes of local recurrence include the unresected middle rectal artery, iliac, or obturator lymph node involvement, which may be present in patients with T_3, or in N_1 lesions that are situated below the peritoneal reflection (11). The role of adjuvant therapy is under investigation for such lesions (12).

Metastases

Distant metastases are common after conventional resection for node positive lesions. Up to 65% to 70% of patients with T_3 or N_{1-2} lesions are reported to develop distant metastases after a conventional resection. TME with its complete resection of the disease bearing package, is associated with only a 23% to 25% incidence of metastases for the same stages of disease (2,13). Under the circumstances, continued high rates of failure can be viewed as consequences of the continued use of a conventional resection. The incidence of pelvic recurrence is beginning to approach 1% to 5%, where radiation or combined radiation and chemotherapy are being used prior to TME.

Sphincter-Preserving Operations

The possibility of accomplishing an SPO in conjunction with CME or TME is high. The complete mobilization and dissection of the rectum to the levator ani, referred to above, creates the opportunity for sphincter preservation. Over 90% of patients with midrectal cancers can now have an SPO. In a sense, the APR, which accompanies a conventional resection, can be viewed as a consequence or even as a complication of that technique. The opportunity to provide the patient with sphincter preservation is one of the driving forces behind the widening interest in TME (7).

Impotence and Sexual and Urinary Dysfunctions

The anatomy and the functions of the pelvic autonomic nervous system are well understood. The sympathetic hypogastric nerves originate from a preaortic nervous plexus and enter the pelvis 1 cm paramedian at the pelvic brim. The hypogastric nerve is found just anterior to the visceral fascia. When commencing the dissection medially, a step in level just anterior to the visceral fascia has to be made when the hypogastric nerves are encountered in order to leave the hypogastric nerves intact along the pelvic wall.

The parasympathetic nerves originate from the sacral foramina posterior to the parietal fascia. Approximately 3 cm laterally to the sacral foramina, the parasympathetic nerves pierce the parietal fascia and continue between a double layer of visceral fascia on their way to the pelvic viscera. Both the sympathetic hypogastric nerves and the parasympathetic sacral nerves join at the pelvic sidewall to form the PANP (14).

Avoiding injury to the pelvic autonomic nerves and plexuses preserves both sexual and urinary functions. We assessed sexual and urinary function in 175 patients who underwent TME with ANP for primary rectal cancer. Of these 175 patients, 136 (78%, 82 males and 54 females) responded to a standardized questionnaire (15). All percentages mentioned below pertain to patients with normal preoperative function. Impotence, defined as the inability to engage in intercourse, was reported by 14% of male and female patients younger than 60 years of age and by 33% of male and female patients 60 years and older. Of the male patients, inability to achieve orgasm was reported by 13%. Of the female patients, 15% reported inability to experience arousal and vaginal lubrication, and 9% could no longer achieve orgasm. Sexual dysfunction was more prevalent after abdominoperineal resection than after low anterior resection. Most patients had few or no urinary function complaints; neurogenic bladder was not seen in this group.

REFERENCES

1. Daly JM, DeCosse JJ. Complications in surgery of the colon and rectum. *Surg Clin North Am* 1983;63:121.
2. Enker WE, Thaler HT, Cranor ML, Polyak T. Total mesorectal excision in the operative treatment of rectal cancer. *J Am Coll Surg* 1995;613:69.
3. Enker WE. Designing the optimal surgery for rectal carcinoma [Editorial]. *Cancer* 1996;78:1847.
4. Quirke P, Durdey P, Dixon MF, Williams NS. Local recurrence of rectal adenocarcinoma due to inadequate surgical resection. Histopathological study of lateral tumor spread and surgical excision. *Lancet* 1986:1:996.
5. Adam IJ, McHamdee MO, Martin IG, et al. Role of circumferential margin involvement in the local recurrence of rectal cancer. *Lancet* 1994;344:707.
6. Quirke P. The pathologist's role in the evaluation of local recurrence in rectal cancer. Presented at the Surgical Workshop and Prosection Course, Royal College of Surgeons of London, April 25 and 26, 1995.
7. Enker WE. Sphincter-preserving operations for rectal cancer. *Oncology* 1996;10:1673.
8. Karanjia ND, Corder AP, Holdsworth PJ, et al. Risk of peritonitis and fatal septicaemia and the need to defunction the low anastomosis. *Br J Surg* 1991:78:196.
9. Hida J, Yasutomo M, Maruyama T, Fujimoto K, Uchida T, Okuno K. Lymph node metastases detected in the mesorectum distal to carcinoma of the rectum by the clearing method: justification of total mesorectal excision. *J Am Coll Surg* 1997;184:584.
10. Pickleman J, Lee RM. The management of patients with suspected early postoperative small bowel obstruction. *Ann Surg* 1989;210:216.
11. Sugihara K, Moriya Y, Akasu T, Fujita S. Pelvic autonomic nerve preservation for patients with rectal carcinoma: oncologic and functional outcome. *Cancer* 1996;78:1871.
12. Minsky BD. Preoperative combined modality treatment for rectal cancer. *Oncology* 1994;8:53.
13. MacFarlane JK, Ryall RD, Heald RJ. Mesorectal excision for rectal cancer. *Lancet* 1993;341:457.
14. Havenga K, de Ruiter MC, Enker WE, Welvaart K. Anatomical basis of autonomic nerve preserving total mesorectal excision for rectal cancer. *Br J Surg* 1996;83:384.
15. Havenga K, Enker WE, McDermott K, Cohen AM, Minsky BD, Guillem J. Male and female sexual and urinary function after total mesorectal excision with autonomic nerve preservation for rectal cancer. *J Am Coll Surg* 1996;182:495.
16. Enker WE, Havenga K, Polyak T, Thaler H, Cranor M. Abdominoperineal resection via total mesorectal excision and autonomic nerve preservation for low rectal cancer. *World J Surg* 1997;21:715.

CHAPTER 7

Indications and Technique of Neck Dissection for the General Surgeon

Bruce H. Campbell

GENERAL INDICATIONS

Removal of the lymphatic structures of the neck is one of the most commonly performed procedures in head and neck cancer surgery. Each side of the neck contains approximately 75 lymph nodes, and the removal of some of all of these nodes can provide important information or be a significant part of the management of an individual patient. Nevertheless, the procedure was tagged as being radical many decades ago and even today is thought of as being desperate or horrendously deforming by many physicians. When a properly selected patient undergoes the appropriate procedure, however, a neck dissection can provide symptomatic relief and survival benefit. Neck dissection can also prevent the complications and morbidity of advanced, untreatable neck metastases.

Neck dissections are performed for three basic indications. In many patients presenting with palpable cervical metastasis, neck dissection is performed primarily for therapy. The surgical resection of cervical metastasis can be curative, particularly in a patient presenting with early stage metastases. Neck dissections are also performed for diagnosis and treatment planning. A prophylactic neck dissection is used in situations where cervical lymph nodes are not palpable, yet are at significant risk for containing metastases. The histologic evaluation of these lymph nodes can direct further therapy or allow the patient and physician to gain information on expected prognosis. The third major indication for neck dissection is access. In this situation, the neck dissection is performed primarily to identify anatomic structures, either for control of blood vessels, nerves, and viscera or for safe entry into the upper areodigestive tract or central nervous system. In this setting, depending on the indications for the procedure, lymph nodes may be removed only to improve visibility.

As with other parts of the body, the cervical lymph nodes are broken down into levels (Fig. 7-1). Level I lymph nodes are in the submandibular and submental triangles. Level II lymph nodes are in the upper jugular area, both anterior and

posterior to the jugular vein and extending up above the spinal accessory nerve. Level III lymph nodes encompass the middle jugular region and extend back as far as the cervical roots. Level IV lymph nodes are found in the lower jugular area from the omohyoid muscle inferiorly to the clavicle. Level V nodes are in the posterior triangle and supraclavicular area posterior to the sternomastoid muscle and anterior to the trapezius muscle. Level VI nodes are found in the paratracheal regions. Clinically important nodes are also found in the retropharyngeal and parapharyngeal areas, in the parotid gland adjacent to the superficial temporal vein, in the retroauricular area overlying the mastoid, and in the suboccipital area adjacent to the occipital vessels.

After the initial description of the radical neck dissection by Crile (1) in 1906, the complete cervical lymphadenectomy remained the most acceptable approach to the cervical lymphatics for over 50 years. The indications were further refined by Hayes Martin during his tenure at Memorial Sloan-Kettering Cancer Center. With a comprehensive or radical neck dissection, levels I to V are removed along with the sternomastoid muscle, spinal accessory nerve and internal jugular vein. Ettore Bocca in Italy and Alando J. Ballantyne at M. D. Anderson Cancer Center each developed modifications of the radical neck dissection which preserved the sternomastoid muscle, spinal accessory nerve, and internal jugular vein while still removing the cervical lymphatics. These techniques gradually gained acceptance through the 1970s and 1980s. With the development of combined surgery and radiation therapy strategies, the modifications of the radical neck dissection became more widely utilized. This has, however, sparked an intense debate regarding the proper utilization of modified neck dissections.

The extent of a neck dissection is determined by two factors: the presence or absence of palpable lymph nodes and the site of the primary cancer. As the indications for modified neck dissections have evolved, it had become less acceptable to perform radical neck dissections in patients with N_0 necks. The use of modified neck dissections in N+ dis-

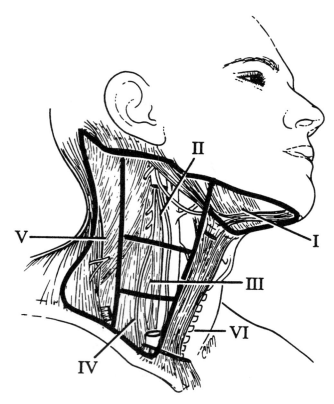

FIG. 7-1. Lymph node levels as defined for neck dissections. The diagram shows a completed radical neck dissection. (Reprinted with permission from Robbins KT, Medina JE, Wolf GT, Levine PA, Sessions RB, Pruet CW. Standardizing neck dissection terminology. *Arch Otolaryngol Head Neck Surg* 1991;117:601.)

ease has continued to evolve. In general, modified neck dissections continue to be appropriate even with multiple lymph nodes if the nodes are small, easily removed, and noninvasive. In patients with bilateral bulky nodal disease, vein-preserving modified dissections are performed on one side whenever possible.

SPECIFIC INDICATIONS

The levels dissected for therapeutic and diagnostic neck dissections vary by the primary site in patients with squamous cell carcinoma. Table 7-1 shows the nodal groups most at risk in patients with specific primary sites.

Table 7-1 reveals the most likely primary echelon nodal involvement based on the initial tumor location. Studies by Lindberg (2) revealed that palpable cervical lymphadenopathy is present in predictable distributions based on primary site. Follow-up work by Byers (3) demonstrated the same areas of initial involvement by nonpalpable occult lymphadenopathy. As nodal disease progresses, additional areas become involved. Skip metastases can occur (4), although these are based more on lymphatic drainage pattern rather than capricious nodal metastatic behavior.

Prior therapy can also affect the type of neck dissection selected. Significant doses of radiation therapy severely alter the lymphatic drainage patterns, as do prior surgical procedures that transect the cervical lymphatics. Fisch (5) showed with dye injection techniques that the lymphatic channels shrink with radiation treatments. A prior incision can alter the pattern of flow as the lymphatic drainage is reconstituted. When neck dissections are performed after high dose radiotherapy, lymph nodes can be difficult or impossible to identify. A more limited neck dissection is often performed in this setting. After previous incision, a more comprehensive neck dissection might be considered in order to take altered lymphatic drainage into account.

Histology of the primary site can also affect the extent of cervical node dissection. Squamous cell carcinomas tend to follow the nodal distributions as demonstrated in Table 7-1. Salivary malignancies tend to spread in a predictable pattern, as well. Melanoma, however, is much less predictable and often is seen at several levels, even at the time of initial discovery. Well-differentiated thyroid carcinomas tend to metastasize to resectable lymph nodes, which, even when bulky, are less likely to invade soft tissues than squamous carcinoma metastases.

Unknown primary malignancies present as a metastatic squamous cell carcinoma in the neck with no obvious source. The extent of the neck dissection depends on the size and level of the lymph node. Direct laryngoscopy is routinely performed prior to excision in order to identify a small primary. Directed biopsies are obtained, usually from the nasopharynx, tonsil, and tongue base. If no primary is seen, the node is excised through an incision which will permit further dissection. If a frozen section reveals the node to contain squamous cell carcinoma, dissection is completed, which removes at least one level surrounding the positive node. This assists in further treatment planning. A properly performed neck dis-

TABLE 7-1. *Nodal groups at highest risk*

Location	Laterality	Level
Lateral oral cavity	Ipsilateral	Levels I, II, III, ? IV
Anterior oral cavity	Bilateral	Levels I, II, III, ? IV
Oropharynx	Bilateral	Levels I, II, III, IV, V; retropharyngeal, parapharyngeal
Larynx	Bilateral	Levels II, III, IV, VI
Hypopharynx	Bilateral	Levels II, III, IV, VI; retropharyngeal, parapharyngeal
Nasopharynx	Bilateral	Levels II, III, V
Glottic larynx	Bilateral	Levels II, III, IV; paratracheal
Parotid	Ipsilateral	Level II
Facial skin and anterior scalp	Ipsilateral	Levels I, II; parotid nodes
Posterior scalp	Ipsilateral	Level II; suboccipital and postauricular nodes
Thyroid	Ipsilateral	Levels IV, V, VI
Cervical esophagus	Bilateral	Levels IV, V, VI

section might be therapeutic if histologic criteria for adjuvant radiation therapy are not met. Conversely, if a squamous metastasis is excised without proper preparation for a regional dissection, the patient will almost certainly require radiation and, possibly, further surgery.

Neck dissections performed for salvage of previously treated cancers are not neatly categorized. In general, however, a salvage neck dissection usually removes all levels at risk in addition to the recurrent nodal mass.

GENERAL TECHNIQUE

The most critical aspect of neck dissection technique is the appreciation that dissection proceeds along fascial planes until the surgeon decides to incise through the fascia and its underlying fibrofatty tissue to access the next plane. Dissection then continues in this new plane. In this way, the nodal tissue contained in the fat is included in the dissection. By keeping the tissues on-stretch, the planes are more easily identified and developed.

The general technique of neck dissection involves the elevation of subplatysmal skin flaps and the use of specific planes to effectively remove all fibrofatty tissue within the area to be cleared. For example, in a neck dissection which removes lymph nodes along the jugular vein, the dissection is begun at the anterior border of the sternomastoid muscle, developing the plane between the muscle and its deep fascia. The dissection proceeds on the deep side of the sternomastoid to its posterior border identifying the spinal accessory nerve and cervical roots. The surgeon then incises through the plane of the muscle fascia dividing the fibrofatty tissue at the posterior border of levels II and III until the deep layer of the deep cervical fascia is identified. The dissection then proceeds forward in this plane until the internal jugular vein and carotid artery are identified. Now a new plane is selected either above or below the jugular vein depending on whether the vein is to be preserved or sacrificed. By identifying and utilizing these planes, the surgeon can effectively clear the appropriate nodal levels and preserve structures with a minimum of blood loss.

Neck dissection terminology is based on the number of levels removed and the preservation or sacrifice of the sternomastoid, internal jugular vein, and the spinal accessory nerve (6). A radical neck dissection removes all five lymph node levels and all three structures (Fig. 7-2). A modified radical neck dissection (MRND) removes all five levels of lymph nodes but preserves one or more of the nonlymphatic structures. "Selective" neck dissections preserve one or more of the lymph node groups. The supraomohyoid neck dissection removes levels I, II, and III (Fig. 7-3). A lateral neck dissection removes levels II, III, and IV (Fig. 7-4). The posterior lateral neck dissection removes levels II, III, IV, and V as well as the retroauricular and suboccipital lymph nodes (Fig. 7-5). The anterior compartment neck dissection removes the pretracheal, paratracheal, and perithyroidal nodes (level VI) (Fig. 7-6). Table 7-2 provides a complete listing.

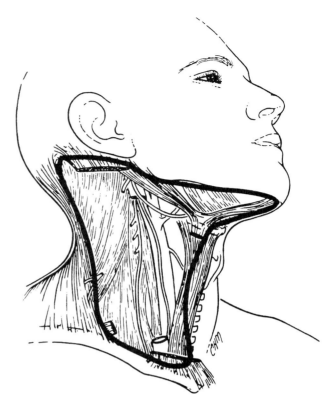

FIG. 7-2. Radical neck dissection. Levels I-V have been dissected and the sternomastoid muscle, spinal accessory nerve, and internal jugular vein have been resected. The cervical roots have been divided preserving the phrenic nerve. The cut ends of the omohyoid muscle are also visible. The hypoglossal nerve has been preserved as it crosses the carotid artery. (Reprinted with permission from Robbins KT, Medina JE, Wolf GT, Levine PA, Sessions RB, Pruet CW. Standardizing neck dissection terminology. *Arch Otolaryngol Head Neck Surg* 1991;117:601.)

Extended radical neck dissections remove additional structures not encompassed in the above described dissections. Depending on the extent of and invasion by the tumor, the dissection can include the carotid artery, hypoglossal nerve, vagus nerve, phrenic nerve, digastric muscle, or deep cervical muscles.

Skin incisions avoid trifurcations, particularly in patients who have had previous radiation therapy. Apron incisions can be placed so that trifurcations are not necessary. In patients who may subsequently require a laryngectomy, a hockey stick incision is helpful, although it is difficult to reach level I nodes unless the incision is bilateral. McFee incisions avoid trifurcations and preserve vascular supply. In patients with prior radiation therapy, they are particularly useful. They may, however, be difficult to utilize.

The superior laryngeal neurovascular pedicle should not be violated during a standard neck dissection. Fortunately, a small pad of fat with color different from subcutaneous fat overlies the area of the pedicle as it enters through the thyrohyoid membrane. By looking for this fat pat and avoiding its injury, the pedicle can be preserved.

order to preserve the intervention of the phrenic nerve. The surgeon should check frequently to make sure the deep cervical fascia is being preserved as the deep plane is developed. Dissection is carried up medially in the plane between the internal jugular vein and the common carotid artery preserving the vagus nerve. The omohyoid muscle is divided medially where it attaches to the hyoid bone. At this point, attention is directed to the level I lymph nodes. The marginal branch of the facial nerve is identified at a plane slightly deep to the platysma in the region where the facial vessels cross the mandible. This nerve is dissected gently and elevated with the flap to preserve its function. This allows the facial nodes to be included in the specimen. The facial vessels are then divided below the point when they are crossed by the marginal nerve. Dissection is carried anteriorly to the midline and the anterior belly of the digastric muscle is identified on the contralateral side. Dissection is carried down along this muscle to the hyoid bone and tissue is reflected toward the side being dissected at a plane just superficial to the mylohyoid muscle. The tissue is reflected over the ipsilateral anterior belly of the digastric muscle and the mylohyoid is then identified as the deep margin of the resection in this area. When the posterior border of the muscle has been identified, a retractor is placed and the underlying

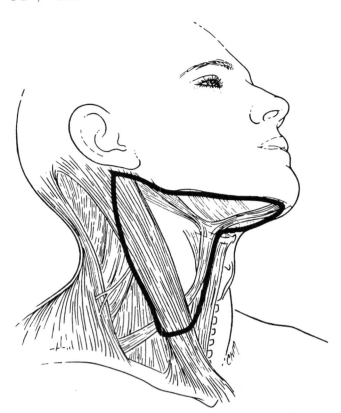

FIG. 7-3. Supraomohyoid selective neck dissection. Levels I, II, and III have been dissected, preserving the sternomastoid muscle, internal jugular vein, and spinal accessory nerve. The nerve can be seen emerging from the posterior border of the sternomastoid muscle and innervating the trapezius muscle. The omohyoid muscle has been preserved and is seen crossing under the sternomastoid muscle. This dissection is used most commonly for squamous cell carcinomas arising in the oral cavity. (Reprinted with permission from Robbins KT, Medina JE, Wolf GT, Levine PA, Sessions RB, Pruet CW. Standardizing neck dissection terminology. *Arch Otolaryngol Head Neck Surg* 1991;117:601.)

SPECIFIC TECHNIQUE

Radical Neck Dissection

Radical neck dissection technique is the most standardized of all of the neck dissections. An incision that permits exposure to all of the nodal areas is performed and a subplatysmal flap is elevated. Dissection is usually begun inferiorly with division of the heads of the sternomastoid muscle and dissection across the supraclavicular area. Usually by division of the fascia and gentle elevation of the underlying fat, the deep layer of the deep cervical fascia overlying the scalene muscles, phrenic nerve, and transverse cervical artery can be exposed. The internal jugular vein is identified, inferiorly clamped, divided, and doubly ligated. The omohyoid muscle is divided inferiorly. The tissue is then reflected superiorly and the dissection continues up the anterior border of the trapezius muscle. The spinal accessory nerve is divided. As the specimen is reflected, the cervical rootlets are divided well up onto the specimen in

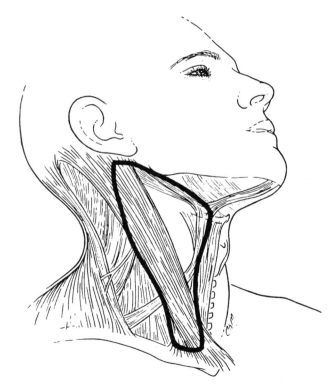

FIG. 7-4. Lateral neck dissection. Levels II, III, and IV have been dissected. The omohyoid muscle is usually sacrificed in this dissection. The spinal accessory nerve is preserved. This dissection is most commonly performed for N0 squamous cell carcinomas of the larynx and hypopharynx. (Reprinted with permission from Robbins KT, Medina JE, Wolf GT, Levine PA, Sessions RB, Pruet CW. Standardizing neck dissection terminology. *Arch Otolaryngol Head Neck Surg* 1991;117:601.)

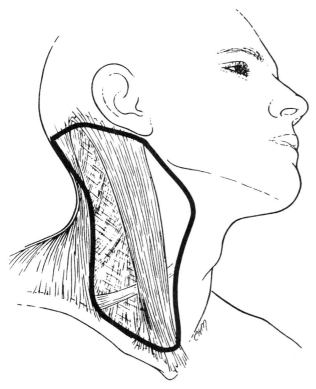

FIG. 7-5. Posterior lateral selective neck dissection. Levels II, III, IV, and V as well as the suboccipital and retroauricular lymph nodes have been dissected. It is most commonly performed for melanomas and advanced squamous cell carcinoma of the skin involving the posterior scalp. (Reprinted with permission from Robbins KT, Medina JE, Wolf GT, Levine PA, Sessions RB, Pruet CW. Standardizing neck dissection terminology. *Arch Otolaryngol Head Neck Surg* 1991;117:601.)

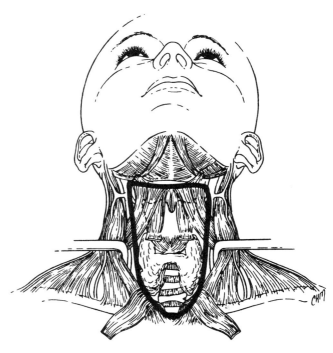

FIG. 7-6. Anterior neck dissection. Pretracheal, paratracheal, and perithyroidal lymph nodes as part of a dissection for thyroid carcinoma have been dissected. The dissection can easily be extended to include levels II, III, and IV as necessary for palpable lymphadenopathy. (Reprinted with permission from Robbins KT, Medina JE, Wolf GT, Levine PA, Sessions RB, Pruet CW. Standardizing neck dissection terminology. *Arch Otolaryngol Head Neck Surg* 1991;117:601.)

submandibular duct, lingual nerve, and hypoglossal nerve are identified. The two nerves are preserved but the duct is divided along with the chorda tympani nerve; the submandibular gland is thus elevated out of its fossa. Dissection continues along the posterior belly of the digastric muscle until the facial artery is identified and divided. This completes the level I dissection. The posterior belly of the digastric muscle is then followed to its insertion and the sternomastoid muscle is divided superiorly. Dissection is completed by dissecting inferior to superior along the carotid artery and deep layer of the deep cervical fascia. The spinal accessory nerve is divided at where it emerges underneath the digastric muscles and the upper end of the jugular vein is divided and doubly ligated. The hypoglossal nerve is preserved as it crosses the carotid artery. The specimen is removed and oriented (for a completed dissection, see Fig. 7-2). The wound is closed over suction drains.

Modified Radical Neck Dissection
Preserving Spinal Accessory Nerve

MRND follows the same basic procedures as the radical neck dissection with the exception of preservation of one or more of the nonlymphatic structures. The spinal accessory nerve is

most easily preserved by identifying it where it emerges from the posterior margin of the sternomastoid muscle and crosses the posterior triangle. The nerve is then traced up into the sternomastoid muscle toward the jugular foramen and dissected free from the surrounding tissues. It can then be reflected su-

TABLE 7–2. *Types of neck dissections*

Type	Levels removed
Radical neck dissection	I–V
Modified radical neck dissection[a]	I–V
Selective neck dissections[b]	
Supraomohyoid neck dissection	I, II, III
Posterior lateral neck dissection	II, III, IV, V; suboccipital, retroauricular
Lateral neck dissection	II, III, IV
Anterior compartment neck dissection	Pretracheal, perithyroidal, and precricoid (level VI)
Extended radical neck dissection	I–V; plus other nodes or structures (as necessary)

[a] Modified radical neck dissections preserve one or more structures, which are then listed in the procedure title.

[b] In all selective neck dissections, the spinal accessory nerve, internal jugular vein, and sternomastoid muscle are preserved. If removal is necessary, the structures removed are listed in the procedure title.

periorly as the dissection is completed. Preserving the internal jugular vein requires careful dissection within the fascial coverage of the vein. Dissection is most easily completed by working laterally to medially since there are no venous tributaries to the internal jugular vein coming in from behind. By keeping the tissues on stretch, the plane can be identified and opened using either a hemostat or scalpel. As the anterior tributaries are identified, they are dissected a short way into the specimen, divided, and ligated. The sternomastoid muscle can be preserved by dissecting the fascia around the muscle on its deep surface. The fascia is then included with the surgical specimen while the muscle itself is preserved. By preserving the sternomastoid muscle, the external jugular vein and greater auricular nerve can usually be preserved, thereby decreasing postoperative numbness and morbidity.

Supraomohyoid Selective Neck Dissection

The supraomohyoid selective neck dissection (7) removes levels I, II, and III and is most commonly utilized for patients with oral cavity cancer (Fig. 7-3). First a subplatysmal flap is elevated. The dissection usually begins with level I. The marginal branch of the facial nerve is identified, preserved, and reflect superiorly. The facial vessels are divided just inferiorly to where they cross the mandible in order to aid in the preservation of the nerve. The dissection is carried anteriorly and the fibrofatty tissue of the submandibular triangle is swept from the mandible. The submental lymph nodes are dissected free of the underlying mylohyoid muscle beginning at the contralateral anterior belly of the digastric. Blood vessels are routinely identified in the submental area and at the junction of the anterior belly of the digastric with the mandible. The submental tissue is swept over the anterior belly of the digastric and the submandiblar triangle dissection proceeds as described in the section describing the radical neck dissection. This completes the level I dissection. The omohyoid muscle is preserved, and dissection is carried down along this muscle to a point where it crosses under the sternomastoid muscle. At this point, incision is made through the fascia at the anterior margin of the sternomastoid muscle and the muscle is unwrapped by dissecting the plane between the sternomastoid muscle and its fascia. The plane is followed posteriorly toward the posterior margin of the muscle. Superiorly, the spinal accessory nerve is identified as it crosses through the plane and penetrates the muscle. The nerve is then circumferentially dissected, preserving it. When the deep sternomastoid fascia has been dissected as far posteriorly as possible, an incision is carried down through the fascia and then through the fibrofatty tissue to the deep layer of the deep cervical fascia. In order to complete this move superiorly, the fascia and fibrofatty tissue are sharply divided along the superior and posterior limbs of a triangle identified by the spinal accessory nerve, the digastric muscle, and the posterior margin of the sternomastoid muscle. By working through the fibrofatty tissue overlying the deep layer of the deep cervical fascia, the levator scapulae muscle is identified

and serves as the deep plane in this area. Working the deep fascial plane from superior to inferior, this triangle of tissue is elevated off the levator scapulae muscle until it can be passed beneath the spinal accessory nerve. The dissection then continues inferiorly along the deep cervical fascia, usually preserving the cervical roots to the point where the omohyoid muscle disappears beneath the posterior marginal of the sternomastoid. Dissection then continues anteriorly along the deep cervical fascia using traction on the specimen and counter traction on the deep cervical fascia. Once the dissection is carried to the carotid sheath, the sheath is opened and the jugular vein identified. Careful dissection between the vein and its fascia continues over the top of the vein with traction on the specimen. As the dissection is carried over the top of the internal jugular vein, branches of the ansa hypoglossi nerve are identified and preserved if possible. The facial vein is encountered and divided. The fat pad identifying the superior laryngeal neurovascular pedicle is identified and preserved. Final attachments are then divided and the specimen removed. The specimen is oriented, and the wound closed over suction drains.

Lateral Neck Dissection

The lateral neck dissection is often performed as a bilateral procedure for laryngeal of hypopharyngeal primaries (Fig. 7-4). First, a subplatysmal flap is elevated. Levels II, III, and IV are approached using dissection along the anterior border of the sternomastoid muscle to separate the muscle fascia from the overlying sternomastoid muscle. The dissection is carried posteriorly between the sternomastoid and its fascia until the internal jugular vein is fully identified. Depending on the position of the vein, the spinal accessory nerve may or may not need to be dissected as described in the section detailing the supraomohyoid selective neck dissection. The omohyoid muscle is divided over the internal jugular vein and the dissection is carried inferiorly and superiorly between the vein and its overlying fascia. The vein is fully exposed and the fibrofatty tissue dissected medially, keeping the specimen under tension. Superiorly, the dissection divides the superficial cervical fascia down to and identifying the digastric muscle so that the level II nodes can be fully dissected, but preserves the submandibular gland. The facial veins are divided. Inferiorly, the dissection can be extended to include some of the paratracheal nodes, if appropriate. The specimen is either left pedicled on the larynx if performed as part of a laryngectomy or can be removed separately. The specimen is oriented and the wound closed over suction drains.

Posterior Lateral Neck Dissection

This neck dissection (8) includes the nodal groups as described in the lateral selective neck dissection, but extends posteriorly almost to the midline to include the suboccipital nodes and retroauricular nodes (Fig. 7-5). The patient is in the lateral decubitus position and the incision extends posteriorly to allow full exposure. Thin flaps are elevated. The trapezius muscle insertion is separated, and the occipital artery is divided and included in the specimen. The specimen is swept forward and the spinal accessory nerve is identified and preserved as described above. The dissection is then completed as described in the section on the lateral neck dissection.

Modified Radical Neck Dissection Preserving Spinal Accessory Nerve, Internal Jugular Vein, and Sternomastoid Muscle

This neck dissection removes levels I to V, but preserves all structures (Fig. 7-7). This is performed using the supraomohyoid technique, but with a division of the omohyoid muscle and extension of the dissection posteriorly to the anterior border of the trapezius.

This usually requires resection of the cervical roots and may require a separate fascial incision of the posterior margin of the sternomastoid muscle in order to completely ex-

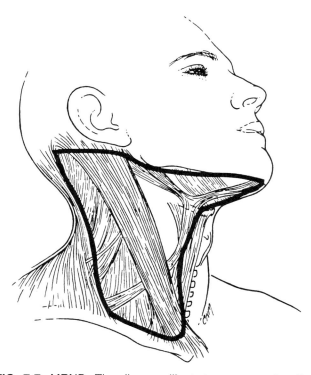

FIG. 7-7. MRND. The diagram illustrates preservation the sternomastoid muscle, spinal accessory nerve and internal jugular vein. This dissection removes levels I to V, but preserves the structures traditionally removed in a radical neck dissection. The omohyoid muscle and cervical roots are often divided in a MRND. The procedure can be varied by removing one or more of the other structures as required by the findings at the time of surgery. This procedure is appropriate for metastatic disease from any head and neck site. (Reprinted with permission from Robbins KT, Medina JE, Wolf GT, Levine PA, Sessions RB, Pruet CW. Standardizing neck dissection terminology. *Arch Otolaryngol Head Neck Surg* 1991;117:601.)

pose and remove the supraclavicular and posterior triangle lymph nodes (level V). By using these maneuvers, the inferior and posterior lymph nodes can be freed from the underlying deep layer of the deep cervical fascia and swept forward to be included in the neck dissection.

SPECIAL CONSIDERATIONS

Resectability of a neck mass can be difficult to assess. In general, tumors involving the deep layer of the deep cervical fascia carry an extremely poor prognosis. Righi and Gluckman (9) have advocated exploring this plane surgically, rather than relying on imaging studies to determine resectability. Similarly, involvement of the carotid artery does not necessarily limit resectability, but the prognosis is poor in patients with carotid replacement or ligation. Involvement of the overlying skin is not necessarily a contraindication to a procedure and satisfactory reconstruction can be accomplished. Nevertheless, invasion through the skin, particularly if there is involvement of the dermal lymphatics, carries a poor prognosis.

Incomplete resection of metastatic disease leaving gross tumor behind, is difficult to salvage. Nevertheless, if critical structures are involved or dissection cannot be completed, metal clips can be left to identify the area of persistent disease and serve as a guide for further radiation therapy. Brachytherapy catheters can be placed at the time of resection to boost high risk areas.

Bilateral neck dissections are indicated when there is bilateral risk or involvement. In situations where both internal jugular veins are involved, the neck dissections are staged with at least a 6-week interval. This allows for development of venous drainage and avoids complications of increased intracranial pressure and possible blindness from decreased flow to the retinal arteries. If it becomes necessary to take both internal jugular veins, a vein graft can be interposed to establish flow. A better alternative is usually the use of vein-preserving modified neck dissection on one side, if at all possible.

Carotid resection can be necessary in advanced invasive nodal disease. Preoperative testing can be used to predict outcome if the carotid artery is sacrificed. This is not always reliable, however. Carotid replacement can be performed either with vein or synthetic graft.

When dissecting in the left supraclavicular fossa, meticulous hemostasis permits early detection of a chyle leak. If identified, the area should be carefully searched and any potential thoracic duct injury should be gently clamped and ligated. With positive pressure ventilation, the area can be closely monitored to find other potential sites of leakage. Chyle leaks can occur on the right supraclavicular fossa as well, although they are less common.

The use of perioperative antibiotics in patients undergoing neck dissection has not been shown to be helpful. However, since many neck dissections are combined with other procedures that do involve the oral cavity or pharynx, antibiotic coverage with a cephalosporin with or without metronidazole is common.

POSTOPERATIVE CONSIDERATIONS

Immediate postoperative concerns include wound management. In general, suction drains are necessary due to the size of the dissection and the use of flaps. Drains are generally left in place for 3 days or until the drainage is less than 30 cc over a 24-h period. Depending on the use of prior radiation therapy, the sutures or staples are left in place for 7 to 10 days.

Postoperative dysphagia can occur, particularly if the vagus nerve or pharyngeal plexus nerves were manipulated. If the patient demonstrates any difficulty with swallowing or change in speech, postoperative evaluation of laryngeal function, possibly with a videofluoroscopic study of swallowing and a videostroboscopic evaluation of the larynx may be necessary to evaluate airway protection. Some patients who have had significant prior radiation therapy will have ipsilateral laryngeal edema after a radical neck dissection. These patients should be closely monitored for airway compromise. A tracheotomy is sometimes necessary.

In patients who undergo a neck dissection which injures or sacrifices the spinal accessory nerve, physical therapy should begin while in the hospital. Shoulder mobilization and stretching exercises will prevent some of the disability seen with loss of trapezius function. Despite therapy, these patients can develop painful shoulders and scapular winging. A study by Remmler (10) revealed that, in a prospective study of shoulder function after neck dissection, the preservation of the spinal accessory nerve resulted in improved shoulder function.

Numbness is always seen after a neck dissection. The area of numbness, however, varies widely. In a radical neck dissection with sacrifice of the greater auricular nerve and the cervical roots, a wide area of numbness exits from the ear to the clavicle. With modified neck dissections and nerve preservation, the area of numbness is much smaller, reflecting sacrifice of the cervical cutaneous branches only.

Handling of the specimen at the conclusion of the procedure will assure the maximum amount of information is recovered. The specimen is routinely laid out and oriented for the pathologist. This is particularly important with a modified neck dissection since many of the standard landmarks of the radical neck dissection are not included in the specimen. The nodes are identified by level, and the pathologist is encouraged to report the findings by level. Histologic evaluation looking for perineural, vascular, and capsular involvement will help determine the need for further radiation therapy in the previously untreated patient (11).

The pathology report allows the surgeon to make further recommendations regarding therapy. One lymph node with no extracapsular spread was not associated with an increase in failure within the cervical lymphatics whether or not radiation therapy was delivered (12). Conversely, the presence of extracapsular spread, i.e., soft tissue involvement, lead to a significantly higher failure rate (13). Multiple level lymph node involvement in patients receiving combined therapy was associated with higher metastatic disease rate (14). By obtaining the maximum amount of information through carefully performed neck dissection and communication with the pathologist, proper referral for postoperative radiation therapy and/or adjuvant therapy can be made.

CONCLUSIONS

Neck dissection is important in the management of the patient with head and neck cancer for therapy, for determination of prognosis, and for safer access to deeper structures of the neck. The advent of modifications of the standard radical neck dissection have decreased postoperative morbidity and deformity without any apparent compromise in oncologic safety. The properly oriented specimen allows the pathologist to identify key histologic parameters, including nodal levels, extracapsular spread, and histologic characteristics.

REFERENCES

1. Crile G. Excision of cancer of the head and neck with special reference to the plan of dissection based on one hundred and thirty-two operations. *JAMA* 1906;47:1780.
2. Lindberg R. Distribution of cervical lymph node metastases from squamous cell carcinoma of the upper respiratory and digestive tracts. *Cancer* 1972;29:1446.
3. Byers RM, Wolf PF, Ballantyne AJ. Rationale for elective modified neck dissection. *Head Neck* 1988;10:160.
4. Byers RM, Weber RS, Andrews T, McGill D, Kare R, Wolf P. Frequency and therapeutic implications of skip metastases in the neck from squamous carcinoma of the oral tongue. *Head Neck* 1997;19:14.
5. Million RR, Cassisi NJ, Mancuso AA, Stringer SP, Mendenhall WM, Parsons, JT. Management of the neck for squamous cell carcinoma. In: Million MM, Cassisi NJ, eds. *Management of head and neck cancer: a multidisciplinary approach*. 2nd ed. Philadelphia: JB Lippincott Co, 1994:75.
6. Robbins KT, Medina JE, Wolf GT, Levine PA, Sessions RB, Pruet CW. Standardizing neck dissection terminology. *Arch Otolaryngol Head Neck Surg* 1991;117:601.
7. Medina JE, Byers RM. Supraomohyoid neck dissection: rationale, indications, and surgical technique. *Head Neck* 1989;11:111.
8. Diaz EM, Austin JR, Burke LI, Goepfert H. The posterolateral neck dissection: Technique and results. *Arch Otolaryngol Head Neck* 1996; 122:477.
9. Righi PD, Kelley DJ, Ernst R, et al. Evaluation of prevertebral muscle invasion by squamous cell carcinoma: can computed tomography replace open neck exploration? *Arch Otolaryngol Head Neck Surg* 1996;122:660.
10. Remmler D, Byers RM, Scheetz J, et al. A prospective study of shoulder disability resulting from radical and modified neck dissections. *Head Neck* 1986;8:280.
11. Olsen KD, Caruso M, Foote RL, et al. Primary head and neck cancer: Histopathologic predictors of recurrence after neck dissection in patients with lymph node involvement. *Arch Otolaryngol Head Neck Surg* 1994;120:1370.
12. Byers RM. Modified neck dissection: a study of 967 cases from 1970 to 1980. *Am J Surg* 1985;150:414.
13. Johnson JT, Myers EN, Bedetti CD, Barnes EL, Schramm VL, Thearle PB. Cervical lymph node metastases: incidence and implications of extracapsular carcinoma. *Arch Otolaryngol Head Neck Surg* 1985;111:534.
14. Vikram B, Strong EW, Shah JP, Spiro R. Failure at distant sites following multimodality treatment for advanced head and neck cancer. *Head Neck* 1984;6:730.

CHAPTER 8

Salivary Gland Tumors

Ara A. Chalian and Randal S. Weber

Salivary gland tumors are uncommon, constituting less than 0.2% of malignancies overall, with less than 2% of head and neck neoplasms arising in the salivary glands (1). The treatment for these tumors has evolved over the past two decades due to advances in diagnostic imaging, needle aspiration cytologic diagnosis, a refinement in surgical techniques, and a clearer understanding of the role for adjuvant radiotherapy in treatment of malignant or recurrent benign disease. The majority or 85% of salivary gland neoplasms arise in the parotid (2). Eighty percent of these neoplasms are benign, with the most common histology being the pleomorphic adenoma (benign mixed tumor). The remaining 20% of parotid tumors are malignant. In contrast, tumors of the submandibular gland have a 50% probability of being malignant. The majority (60% to 70%) of tumors of minor salivary gland origin are malignant.

This chapter will focus on the surgical anatomy, clinical presentation, differential diagnosis, diagnostic evaluation, and treatment of tumors arising in the major and minor salivary glands.

MAJOR SALIVARY GLAND TUMORS

There are hundreds of salivary glands in the head and neck region, which are classified into the major and minor salivary glands. The parotid, submandibular, and sublingual glands constitute the major salivary glands. The glands found in the mucosa of the oral cavity, pharynx, proximal aerodigestive tract and parapharyngeal space are collectively referred to as the minor salivary glands. Enlargement or the presence of a discreet mass arising within a major salivary gland may be secondary to either a neoplastic or inflammatory process. Knowledge of the extensive differential diagnosis is important to focus the evaluation and to properly plan treatment.

Embryologically, the salivary glands are of ectodermal origin and arise through invagination of oral epithelium. During development the parotid gland becomes encapsulated and in the process lymph nodes become entrapped within the structure of the gland (3). The clinical significance is that the Warthin's tumor (papillary cystadenoma lymphomatosum) may arise within the gland and is embryologically related to

this process. The remaining tumors are of epithelial or mesenchymal origin.

Histologically, the parotid is the most complex salivary gland and is composed of secretory and excretory elements. The secretory or acinar cells drain into intercalated ducts which drain into the striated ducts. The main collecting or excretory ducts combine to form Stensen's duct which drains into the oral cavity. The histologic heterogeneity and complexity of salivary gland tumors is due to their histogenesis from the multipotential reserve cells of the intercalated ducts (4).

ANATOMY

The parotid gland is located on the lateral aspect of the face, anterior to the ear, and mostly inferior to the zygomatic arch. The major portion of the gland is posterior to the ascending ramus of the mandible but extends over the lateral aspect of the masseter muscle. The superficial lobe is defined as the portion of the gland lateral to the facial nerve. The deep lobe of the parotid is arbitrarily defined as the portion deep to the facial nerve which extends through the stylomandibular tunnel and into the lateral parapharyngeal space. The posterior aspect of the gland abuts the external auditory canal and the mastoid tip. Inferiorly it dips below the angle of the mandible to the anterior border of the sternocleidomastoid muscle. The portion of the gland lying adjacent to the sternocleidomastoid muscle and lateral to the digastric muscle constitutes the tail of the parotid. The superficial musculoaponeurotic system and platysma overlie the gland. The size of the gland is variable amongst patients. It can atrophy with age and enlarge with alcoholism, or in autoimmune derangements (i.e., Sjogren's syndrome).

The glossopharyngeal nerve (CN IX) provides the parasympathetic secretomotor innervation from the lesser petrosal nerve and otic ganglion. The postganglionic fibers reach the parotid gland via the auriculotemporal branch of the mandibular division of the trigeminal (CN V) nerve. The arterial supply to the gland is via the terminal branches of the external carotid: the internal maxillary and superficial temporal arteries. The venous drainage is to the retromandibular vein which lies deep to the marginal mandibular branch of the facial nerve. Lymphatic drainage is provided by intraparotid and extraglandular lymph nodes in the preauricular and infra-auricular region (Fig. 8-1). These nodes drain into the upper deep jugular lymph nodes.

The facial nerve is the most important structure in the parotid and provides motor innervation to the facial musculature. After exiting the skull base the nerve divides at the pes anserinus into branches supplying the platysma, depressor muscles of the lip, elevators of the lip/buccal region, muscles of eye closure, and elevator muscles of the forehead.

The paired submandibular glands are located in the submandibular triangle lying just medial to the mandible at their superior extent. The lateral aspect of the gland is superficial to the digastric and mylohyoid muscles, while a medial portion lies deep to the mylohyoid muscle. Blood supply is provided by branches of the facial artery and secretomotor innervation is by the parasympathetic fibers which travel from the chorda tympani through to the lingual nerve and submandibular ganglion. The hypoglossal nerve passes inferior to superior along the deep surface of the gland in the submandibular triangle while the lingual nerve passes from posterior to anterior along the lateral superior portion of the deep aspect of the gland. Level I or facial lymph nodes are found adjacent to the submandibular gland.

The sublingual glands reside in the submucosa of the floor of the mouth, superficial to the mylohyoid muscle. The gland is lateral to the lingual artery, vein, and nerve. These mucous producing glands drain into the submandibular duct via Bartholin's duct.

PHYSIOLOGY

The parotid gland produces a large volume of saliva, with a maximal rate of up to 1 ml/min/g of gland. Consequently, the gland is metabolically active and has a high blood flow rate, up to 10 times that of contracting muscle (5). Salivary secretions have multiple functions including lubrication, digestion of food through production of amylases, excretion of antibodies, and solubilization of food substances which is important for mediation of taste. The parotid gland salivary output is predominantly serous whereas the submandibular gland produces saliva with a higher mucous concentration.

CLINICAL PRESENTATION

Parotid Gland Tumors

The most common site of origin for salivary gland neoplasms is the parotid gland. These tumors typically present as a slow growing, asymptomatic facial mass with the majority arising in the tail of the parotid. A pertinent history for patients presenting with a mass in the parotid includes: length of time the mass has been present, growth rate, presence of pain or paresthesias, and facial weakness. Previous surgery for a mass in this region or a history of radiation therapy to the parotid area should be elicited (6). Because the parotid is a frequent site of nodal metastasis from cutaneous squamous cell carcinoma and melanoma of the ear, forehead, cheek, periauricular skin and anterior scalp, any history of prior treatment for a skin malignancy should be sought (7). Patients with a rapidly growing mass, pain, or facial weakness are more likely to have malignant processes. While acute inflammatory conditions of the parotid may present with pain, the process is usually diffuse, associated with constitutional symptoms and facial weakness is rare (the exception being uveoparotid fever).

The patient presenting with facial paralysis of unknown etiology must be evaluated with a high index of suspicion. Facial nerve dysfunction is extremely uncommon in benign salivary gland tumors but may occur in malignant ones which have a proclivity for neurotropic spread. Assessment and documentation of the facial nerve function is essential. Weakness of the facial muscles may be subtle or localized to one portion of the face; whereas, invasion of the main trunk of the nerve will produce global dysfunction of facial movement. Therefore, patients with progressive segmental or total facial paralysis must be thoroughly evaluated for a malignant parotid neoplasm. Approximately 10% to 15% of patients

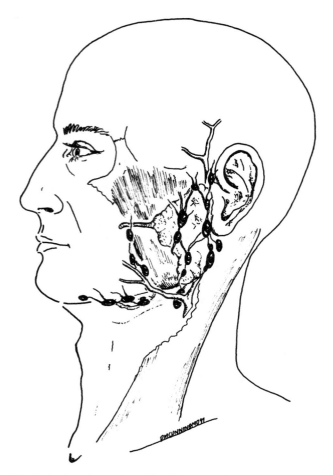

FIG. 8-1. A schematic of the intra- and periparotid lymph nodes. By performing a superficial parotidectomy the primary echelon of lymph nodes for parotid tumors are excised. The parotid lymph nodes subsequently drain to the upper deep jugular chain.

with parotid malignancies have facial nerve paralysis or paresis at the time of presentation (8,9).

Fortunately, most tumors arise in the superficial lobe of the gland and are readily palpable. Interestingly, the presentation of a mass in the tail of the parotid commonly presents a diagnostic problem that must be differentiated from an upper cervical mass. Incorrectly diagnosing a mass in the tail of the gland as an upper neck mass could result in an incorrect surgical approach leading to tumor spillage or injury to the lower branches of the facial nerve. Rupture of a parotid tumor may increase the patient's risk for tumor recurrence; therefore, differentiation between these two diagnoses is important and usually can be established with physical examination and the judicious use of diagnostic imaging studies. For tumors of the parotid gland, the physical examination should define the size of the mass, describe its physical characteristics including consistency (soft or firm), mobility, and proximity or involvement of adjacent structures. A neurological evaluation of the sensory branches of the trigeminal nerve, and assessment of the motor function of V3, is imperative. Numbness of the ear lobe suggests invasion of the great auricular nerve.

The presence of a firm mobile lobulated mass supports the presence of a pleomorphic adenoma, whereas skin invasion and fixation to the mastoid tip are more worrisome for malignancy. Trismus suggests invasion of the muscles of mastication, including the masseter or pterygoids. Salivary gland tumors of the deep lobe of the parotid or parapharyngeal space may displace the lateral wall of the oropharynx medially and present as a unilaterally enlarged tonsil, or palatal bulge/asymmetry.

A careful examination of the neck is necessary for patients with parotid masses. Regional metastasis from parotid malignancies is rare and is usually seen in the context of high-grade tumors such as mucoepidermoid carcinoma. The location (neck level) and number of suspicious lymph nodes should be documented. Metastasis from parotid cancers are usually to the subdigastric region (level II), however, once regional spread has occurred multiple nodal stations in the neck are at risk (30).

The differential diagnosis of a parotid mass broadly includes inflammatory and nonneoplastic processes versus neoplasms. Parotitis typically presents with symptoms of fever, facial pain, skin erythema and induration, and often purulent drainage from Stenson's duct. The patient with a neoplasm will typically note an asymptomatic slowly enlarging mass. Obtaining a complete history and physical exam will aid in differentiating neoplastic from inflammatory disorders. Patients with metastases to the parotid will have a history of prior head/neck cutaneous malignancy. Metastasis from a carcinoma of the kidney, prostate, lung, and breast to the parotid have been reported. Infectious and inflammatory parotid lymphadenopathy are also considerations. Patients with HIV/AIDS may present with parotid masses ranging from benign lymphoepithelial cysts of the parotid to lymphoma. The benign lymphoepithelial cysts are typically bilateral, multiple, and can be diagnosed on FNA.

Submandibular Gland

The diagnoses for enlargement of the submandibular gland include neoplasm and sialadenitis. The latter is typified by pain and fluctuating enlargement with meals while neoplasms progressively enlarge. Some patients may have palpable salivary duct stones in the floor of the mouth which supports the diagnosis of sialadenitis secondary to sialolithiasis. Submandibular gland tumors produce few symptoms but complaints of pain raise the possibility of a malignancy. Other ominous symptoms include numbness or paresthesia of the tongue due to involvement of the lingual nerve. Unilateral tongue weakness secondary to invasion of the hypoglossal nerve is rare and is usually not obvious to the patient but should be evaluated as part of the physical examination. Atrophy or fasiculations of the hemitongue in the setting of a submandibular gland tumor have a strong correlation with the presence of malignancy (10). Occasionally, lower lip weakness from invasion of the marginal mandibular branch of the facial nerve may be seen and likewise is worrisome for a malignant process.

Examination for tumors arising in the lesser major salivary glands or minor salivary glands should focus on the local extent. For tumors of the submandibular and sublingual glands fixation to the mandible, invasion of the floor of mouth or tongue, and involvement of the lingual or hypoglossal nerves should be assessed. Regional metastases are present in 25% of high-grade malignancies of the submandibular gland and the presence of any suspicious nodes should be documented (10). Similar to the parotid, skin invasion by submandibular gland tumors supports the presence of a high-grade tumor.

Minor Salivary Gland Tumors

Patients with minor salivary gland tumors usually have few symptoms and, when present, depend upon the location of the tumor. The most common site for these tumors is the palate and most present as a painless submucosal mass (11). In the absence of a prior biopsy, ulceration is rare. Minor salivary gland tumors of the base of tongue may become quite large before producing symptoms through mass effect or local infiltration. Symptomatic patients may complain of referred otalgia, dysphagia, or dysarthria. Some patients with tongue base or parapharyngeal space involvement by minor salivary gland tumors may present with symptoms of snoring and/or sleep apnea. Those arising in the larynx may produce airway impairment or voice changes, while tumors of the nose or paranasal sinuses result in unilateral nasal obstruction, epistaxis, or proptosis from secondary invasion of the orbit (12). Tumors of minor salivary gland origin have the highest rate of malignancy, in the range of 60% to 70%.

Pertinent physical findings for tumors of the minor salivary glands are dependent upon the site of origin. For those arising in the oral cavity and oropharynx, the size of the mass is noted along with the degree of fixation. For minor salivary gland tumors of the palate, fixation to the underlying mucoperiosteum raises the possibility of palatal bone invasion. Fiberoptic examination of the nose may reveal a submucosal bulge when the tumor has penetrated the hard palate and extended into the floor of the nose. Malignant palatal tumors may invade distal branches of the trigeminal nerve (e.g., greater palatine) producing hypesthesia. Therefore, examination of all three sensory divisions of the Vth nerve is necessary. For tumors of the base of the tongue, deep invasion into tongue musculature, pharyngeal wall, and epiglottis may occur. Limitation of tongue mobility is indicative of hypoglossal nerve or deep tongue muscle invasion.

When examining patients with minor salivary gland tumors of nose and paranasal sinuses, special attention is given to the presence of adjacent soft tissue invasion of the cheek and orbit. Limitation of extraocular eye movement is the hallmark of orbital adnexal invasion. The presence of decreased sensation in the distribution of the trigeminal cranial nerve should be sought in patients with tumors of the paranasal sinuses. Tumors arising in the larynx may produce airway impairment due to mass effect or voice change from vocal cord fixation.

PEDIATRIC NEOPLASMS

Salivary gland tumors are encountered in the pediatric population as well (13). A parotid mass in a newborn or infant will most often be an hemangioma (the most common cause for a parotid mass in infancy), which classically will increase in size during the first six months of life. This mass will then decrease in size over months to years and often spontaneously disappears. Patients may have other concomitant cutaneous vascular malformations. Pediatric patients may develop parotid neoplasms as well. The retrospective data on this entity suggest the spectrum of benign and malignant neoplasms of the major salivary glands in children mirrors that of adults. The surgical treatment of parotid neoplasms in the pediatric patient is identical to that of adults.

HISTOLOGIC SPECTRUM

Because salivary gland tumors are rare, the treating physician should seek out the consultation of a pathologist experienced with the broad histologic spectrum that comprises these tumors. Errors in diagnosis are not uncommon and may lead to inadequate treatment and local recurrences. The common benign and malignant neoplasms of the salivary glands are shown in Table 8-1.

Of the malignant parotid tumors, the mucoepidermoid carcinoma is the most common histologic type followed by adenoid cystic carcinoma. For minor salivary gland tumors, the adenoid cystic, mucoepidermoid carcinoma, and low-grade polymorphous adenocarcinoma (terminal duct carcinoma) predominate (14). The malignant tumors have a variable behavior based upon tumor histology. For example, adenoid cystic carcinoma has significant propensity to invade adjacent nerves and progress in a retrograde fashion to the central nervous system. Cranial nerves frequently involved by this tumor are the VII, V, and XII. With complete tumor removal and adjuvant radiotherapy, local recurrence is decreased; nevertheless, distant metastatic spread is common. Distant metastases from adenoid cystic carcinoma may develop years after initial treatment and tend to progress slowly and can be initially noted decades after treatment of the primary tumor. Survival following onset of distant spread is in the range of 10 to 20 years. Low-grade mucoepidermoid carcinoma behaves in a benign fashion and is usually cured with complete local excision. In contrast, high-grade mucoepidermoid carcinoma is associated with a significant incidence of regional spread and local recurrence despite aggressive surgical resection and postoperative radiotherapy. The survival for low-grade, intermediate grade, and high-grade mucoepidermoid carcinoma have been reported in the ranges of 92%, 63%, and 0%, respectively, at 5 years (15). This tumor frequently metastasizes to distant sites which can be rapidly progressive.

The polymorphous low-grade adenocarcinoma most frequently arises in minor salivary glands and often invades adjacent nerves. Despite this ominous mode of spread, the prognosis for this tumor is favorable.

Squamous cell carcinoma of the major salivary glands, though rare, is occasionally encountered. This is a high-grade salivary gland malignancy; however, certain criteria are necessary to establish the diagnosis. There must be no previous

---

TABLE 8–1. *Neoplasms of the parotid*

Benign neoplasms	Malignant neoplasms
Pleomorphic adenoma (benign mixed tumor)	Mucoepidermoid carcinoma 　High-grade 　Intermediate grade 　Low-grade
Papillary cystadenoma lymphomatosum (Warthin's tumor)	Adenoid cystic carcinoma
Monomorphic adenoma	Acinic cell carcinoma
Sebaceous lymphadenoma	Adenocarcinoma
Oncocytoma	Squamous cell carcinoma
Myoepithelioma	Low-grade polymorphous adenocarcinoma
Vascular tumors	Lymphoma
Lymphangioma	
Hemangioma	
	Metastases

history of a cutaneous or upper aerodigestive tract squamous cell carcinoma. The carcinoma usually arises in the parotid or submandibular gland and histologic examination of the adjacent salivary gland tissue demonstrates ductal metaplasia progressing to dysplasia and frank invasive carcinoma (16). Regional nodal metastases is frequent with primary squamous carcinoma of salivary gland origin.

DIAGNOSTIC EVALUATION

In addition to the history and physical examination, diagnostic imaging and fine-needle aspiration biopsy (FNAB) may provide additional information for proper treatment planning. For the usual patient with a mobile mass in the lateral lobe of the parotid gland and intact facial nerve function, no further ancillary diagnostic procedures are indicated. The most cost-effective approach is to perform a superficial parotidectomy for establishing the diagnosis and treating the neoplasm. In contrast, for the patient with an aggressive tumor associated with facial weakness, fixation, clinically positive lymph nodes, or extension into the deep lobe or parapharyngeal space, additional diagnostic evaluation is indicated.

The computed tomography (CT) scan and magnetic resonance image (MRI) are useful adjuncts to delineate the extent of disease and to assess the regional lymph nodes for metastatic spread. MR scan is probably the most useful imaging modality available for salivary gland tumors. This modality provides superior soft tissue detail, multiplanar images and an absence of radiation exposure (17). Tumors with well delineated borders are generally benign or are low-grade malignancies. Those with irregular margins or a permeative appearance on MRI are more likely to be malignant or inflammatory. However, the sensitivity, specificity, and accuracy of this modality for differentiating a benign from a malignant process is between 50% and 80% (18,19).

MRI is very useful for evaluating salivary gland tumors of the parapharyngeal space. Differentiating a salivary gland tumor of the deep lobe of the parotid from a benign salivary gland tumor of the parapharyngeal space is very critical for surgical planning. The latter arises from either congenital rests of salivary gland tissue or from minor salivary glands in the parapharyngeal space.

Tumors of the parapharyngeal space not involving the deep lobe of the parotid can be removed without identifying or dissecting the facial nerve. On MRI imaging, when the fat plane between the deep lobe of the parotid and the parapharyngeal mass is preserved, the neoplasm is not originating from the parotid gland (20). Armed with this knowledge the surgeon may proceed with a transcervical resection of the tumor and without dissection of the facial nerve. In contrast tumors of the deep lobe of the parotid which secondarily extend into the parapharyngeal space are best managed with dissection of the facial nerve and total parotidectomy.

Sialography currently has no role in the evaluation of tumors of major salivary gland origin, and, in fact, the contrast material produces an intense inflammatory response, making surgery more difficult and increasing the risk of nerve injury in the surgical field.

While not providing the same degree of soft tissue detail as MRI, CT nevertheless yields important information with regard to invasion of the mandible, temporal bone, or skull base and the presence of regional lymph node metastasis. For extensive tumors that involve the skull base, both modalities are complementary and should be obtained. These modalities provide valuable definition of the relationship between neoplasm and the internal carotid artery. Imaging is necessary in the evaluation of most patients with neoplasms of the sublingual, submandibular, and minor salivary glands. These tumors are more commonly malignant and determining the extent of disease is important for surgical planning and complete extirpation.

Incisional biopsy of parotid neoplasms should be avoided due to the risk of seeding the wound with tumor. The need to obtain a cytologic diagnosis in patients with parotid gland tumors remains controversial. The FNAB will differentiate benign from malignant tumors in approximately 70% to 80% of cases (21); however, accurate interpretation of FNAB requires an experienced cytologist. An adverse effect of FNAB is necrosis in parotid tumors which were aspirated preoperatively. These findings have prompted significant discussion between pathologists and head and neck surgeons as to the exact role and indications for FNAB in the evaluation of salivary gland tumors. The routine use of FNAB should be discouraged for the straightforward clinical situation. However, when lymphoma or metastasis from a cutaneous or noncutaneous primary tumor is suspected, FNAB is helpful for treatment planning. For deep lobe parotid tumors preoperative FNAB may be useful, allowing the surgeon to better inform the patient of the extent of the procedure and the possibility that a malignant tumor is present. The facial nerve is never resected based upon the cytologic diagnosis alone due to false positives with this modality. The need for facial nerve resection is determined by the findings at the time of surgery. FNAB is useful for evaluating masses in the submandibular gland and will differentiate inflammatory from malignant processes. For tumors of minor salivary gland origin, an incisional biopsy is always obtained prior to definitive treatment. Excisional biopsy for minor salivary gland tumors is unnecessary and may make subsequent surgery more difficult.

STAGING

The tumors of the salivary glands are staged according to the American Joint Committee on Cancer (AJCC) system (Table 8-2). Stage is dependent upon size of the primary tumor, local extension, involvement of regional lymph nodes, and the presence or absence of distant metastases. Data from the clinical examination and diagnostic imaging (CT or MRI) are used to assign a TNM stage. Pathological staging should be obtained on all resected specimens.

Other factors negatively impacting upon survival in patients with salivary gland cancer include cranial nerve invasion, lymph node metastasis, involvement of the skin, ad-

TABLE 8–2. *AJCC staging for major salivary glands*

T stage
    TX: primary tumor cannot be assessed
    T0: no evidence of primary tumor
    T1: tumor ≤2 cm in greatest dimension without extraparenchymal extension
    T2: tumor >2 cm but not >4 cm in greatest dimension without extraparenchymal extension
    T3: tumor having extraparenchymal extension without seventh nerve involvement and/or >4 cm but not >6 cm in greatest dimension
    T4: tumor invades base of skull, seventh nerve, and/or >6 cm in greatest dimension

N stage
    NX: regional lymph nodes cannot be assessed
    N0: no regional lymph node metastasis
    N1: metastasis in a single ipsilateral lymph node, ≤3 cm in greatest dimension
    N2: metastasis in a single ipsilateral lymph node >3 cm but not >6 cm in greatest dimension, or in multiple ipsilateral lymph nodes, none >6 cm in greatest dimension, or in bilateral or contralateral lymph nodes, none >6 cm in greatest dimension
        N2a: metastasis in a single ipsilateral lymph node >3 cm but not >6 cm in greatest dimension
        N2b: metastasis in multiple ipsilateral lymph nodes, none >6 cm in greatest dimension
        N2c: metastasis in bilateral or contralateral lymph nodes, none >6 cm in greatest dimension
    N3: Metastasis in a lymph node >6 cm in greatest dimension

Adapted from American Joint Committee on Cancer. *AJCC cancer staging manual.* 5th ed. Philadelphia: Lippincott–Raven Publishers, 1997:53.

vanced disease stage, location of the primary tumor, recurrence following prior therapy, and distant metastases.

SURGICAL MANAGEMENT

Few procedures in the head and neck require a more thorough knowledge of the regional anatomy and meticulous surgical technique than parotidectomy. Surgical misadventure may result in injury to the facial nerve, tumor spillage, or incomplete tumor removal. Prior to the surgery, the patient is informed of the risks in particular facial weakness or paralysis. Though postoperative weakness of one or more branches may occur, provided the integrity of the nerve has not been disrupted, complete recovery is expected. The technique of superficial parotidectomy can be summarized as identification and dissection of the facial nerve with removal of the lateral lobe. The patient is placed supine on the operating table and the neck is slightly hyperextended by the placement of a transverse shoulder role at the level of the scapulae. Neuromuscular blockade is usually avoided so that the facial nerve may be stimulated as necessary. The corner of the mouth and eye should remain exposed in the surgical field to observe facial movement as the nerve is dissected. Some surgeons prefer constant nerve monitoring during the procedure and use intraoperative facial nerve electromyography. The nerve integrity monitor and stimulator (NIMS) alerts the surgeon when the facial nerve is stimulated through surgical manipulation. For a routine parotidectomy the use of the NIMS is probably unnecessary and adds additional expense. For reoperation where the facial nerve has been previously dissected this device may greatly aid in the identification and dissection of the nerve.

The parotidectomy is typically performed through a modified Blair incision that is placed in the preauricular skin crease (Fig. 8-2). The incision extends from the root of the helix to the lobule of the ear. At this point, the incision is

curved posteriorly toward the mastoid bone then extends anteriorly into the neck approximately two fingerbreadths below the angle of the mandible. The inferior limb of the incision may be extended more inferiorly if a lymphadenectomy is necessary. If the tumor lies at the anterior aspect of the parotid, the incision may be extended anteriorly from the root of the helix into the sideburn where it is well hidden.

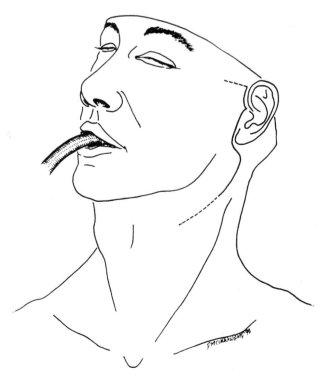

FIG. 8-2. The modified Blair incision. The *broken lines* demonstrate the extensions of the incision both superiorly and inferiorly if additional anterior exposure is necessary.

Next, the parotid flap is elevated in the subcutaneous plane and superficial to the platysma muscle. A thinner flap may be necessary when the tumor approaches or penetrates the parotid fascia. If the overlying skin is invaded it should be left attached to the parotid and resected with the specimen. Once the flap is secured, the great auricular nerve is identified and divided (it should be tagged with a suture if the possibility exists for nerve grafting since this is an ideal nerve for this purpose). Next, the sternocleidomastoid muscle is reflected posteriorly while the parotid gland is retracted anteriorly. The tragal pointer is skeletonized and the dissection is deepened until the posterior belly of the digastric muscle is identified. Careful hemostasis with the bipolar cautery is important to prevent obscuration of the surgical landmarks.

The facial nerve must be identified using the standard landmarks of the tragal pointer, tympanomastoid suture line, styloid process, and the posterior belly of the digastric muscle. Illumination of the surgical field with a head light and magnification with surgical loupes are useful to facilitate identification and dissection of the nerve. The nerve exits the skull base from the stylomastoid foramen, which is posterior to the attachment of the styloid process. The nerve is anteroinferior and approximately 1 cm deep to the tragal pointer (Fig. 8-3). It exits approximately 6 to 8 mm deep to the tympanomastoid suture line. The nerve is identified between the bony ear canal posteriorly and the parotid gland anteriorly.

Once the main trunk is identified the overlying parotid gland is incised. As the nerve is dissected into the body of the parotid gland, it branches into an upper and lower division also known as the pes anserinus or ducks foot. The branching patterns of

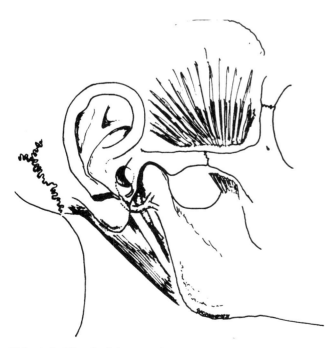

FIG. 8-3. The facial nerve is seen exiting from the stylomastoid foramen. Note the proximity of the nerve to the tympanomastoid suture, bony ear canal, and posterior belly of the digastric muscle.

the facial nerve are variable, but the dissection is guided by direct visualization of the nerve regardless of the arborization pattern. The dissection may proceed with the upper or lower division, and each branch is followed distally until it exits the gland. The branches are dissected sequentially until the lateral lobe containing the tumor is removed. Adherence to the nerve by benign tumors is rare and despite close proximity the nerve can be dissected away safely. With large pleomorphic adenomas, the nerve is at times quite attenuated over the capsule of the neoplasm; however, with meticulous dissection the nerve can be safely separated from the tumor and preserved.

Management of the facial nerve in the setting of malignancy has evolved and the guiding principle currently is to preserve this structure whenever possible (22). Twenty-five years ago, the facial nerve was routinely sacrificed when parotid malignancy was encountered (23). More recent data supports preservation of the nerve provided no gross residual disease is left behind. With malignant tumors, major or minor branches of the nerve may become adherent or even encased. If a plane between the nerve and tumor can be established and the dissection can be performed without leaving gross disease, the nerve is spared (9,24). If the nerve is encased and preservation would result in gross tumor remaining, the nerve is resected. Though microscopic disease may remain at the margin between the nerve and the tumor, several series have shown when postoperative radiotherapy is added the recurrence in the parotid region is less than 10% (25,26).

Patients presenting with facial muscle fasiculations or paralysis preoperatively will have tumor involving the nerve. The patient should be counseled preoperatively that resection of a part or all of the facial nerve may be necessary. If preoperative facial paralysis is present, grafting of the resected nerve will not result in functional recovery and should be avoided. Provided facial nerve function is present preoperatively, immediate grafting should be performed if the nerve is sacrificed. Proximal and distal margins of the resected facial nerve are always examined by frozen section to insure complete tumor resection prior to nerve grafting. If the great auricular nerve or cervical sensory nerves are not involved with tumor they can be successfully used for nerve grafting, thus avoiding a second donor site (27). If greater lengths of nerve are necessary the sural nerve has been extensively used for facial nerve grafting as well.

Once the procedure is completed, the Blair incision is closed with fine suture. Most surgeons use closed suction drains with or without a pressure dressing. Perioperative antibiotics are optional but if administered one preoperative dose is adequate.

MANAGEMENT OF THE REGIONAL LYMPHATICS

The potential for cervical metastases exists in patients with salivary gland malignancies. Traditionally, the neck is treated electively in patients with greater than a 20% to 25% possibility of occult metastasis. Fortunately, regional metastasis from parotid gland malignancies is rare. Notable exceptions include squamous cell and high-grade mucoepidermoid carcinomas which are associated with a high incidence of occult metastasis. Frankenthaler et al. (9) found regional metastasis occurred among patients with high-grade tumors, preoperative facial nerve dysfunction, and extensive soft tissue spread. Spiro et al. (28) noted that advanced primary stage was also predictive of cervical metastasis. Regional metastasis occurred in 1% of stage I, 14% of stage II, and 67% of stage III tumors in their series. Other studies have noted a high incidence of cervical metastases in patients with preoperative facial nerve dysfunction. Conley and Hamaker (29) and Eneroth (8) noted positive lymph nodes in 66% and 77% of patients with preoperative facial nerve paralysis. The authors advocated either elective neck dissection or radiotherapy to treat occult disease in lymphatics. When metastases are identified either by clinical examination or by imaging studies, a comprehensive neck dissection is indicated (levels I to V). The pattern of regional metastasis from salivary gland tumors does not always follow an orderly progression; therefore, a comprehensive neck dissection is advocated. The sternocleidomastoid muscle, spinal accessory nerve, and internal jugular vein are spared unless directly invaded by tumor. At the time of parotidectomy the first echelon of upper cervical lymph nodes can be identified below the posterior belly of the digastric muscle and biopsied if suspicious for metastasis. If frozen section identifies metastatic disease, a neck dissection is performed.

SURGICAL MANAGEMENT OF SUBMANDIBULAR AND SUBLINGUAL GLAND TUMORS

Surgical management of tumors arising in the sublingual and submandibular glands follows similar principles. All gross disease must be resected and regional nerves are preserved unless directly invaded by tumor. Direct invasion of the mandible or muscles of mastication require an extended resection. The minimal surgical procedure for tumors of the submandibular gland is a level I dissection, which removes the gland, adjacent soft tissue, and lymph nodes in the submental and submandibular triangles. Approximately 25% of malignant tumors arising in this gland will have metastasized at the time of diagnosis (10); therefore, a neck dissection is indicated for management of the regional lymphatics. The sternocleidomastoid muscle, spinal accessory nerve, and internal jugular vein are preserved unless they are directly involved with tumor.

Surgical management of minor salivary gland tumors is dependent upon location, size, and tumor grade. Surgical treatment of these rare neoplasms is beyond the scope of this chapter and may be found in textbooks or references addressing these rare neoplasms.

ADJUVANT TREATMENT

Indications for postoperative radiotherapy depend upon several factors. For parotid malignancies postoperative radiotherapy is administered to patients with high-grade tumors, close or positive margins, perineural spread, and lymph node metastasis. Soft tissue extension beyond the gland is another relative indication for postoperative radiotherapy. In clinical practice, most malignant salivary gland tumors of the parotid require postoperative radiotherapy. Similar indications apply to malignant tumors of the lesser major salivary glands and the minor salivary glands. When postoperative radiotherapy is indicated for treatment of the primary tumor for parotid, submandibular, and sublingual gland tumors, the ipsilateral neck is included in the treatment portals. The incidence of lymphatic spread in minor salivary gland tumors is sufficiently low that elective treatment to the regional lymphatics is unnecessary.

FOLLOW-UP

Follow-up for the patient with a salivary gland neoplasm is prolonged due to the delayed appearance of recurrent disease years after initial treatment. The primary site and regional nodes are visually assessed and palpated. Relevant neurologic evaluation is performed to detect new onset of motor weakness or paresthesias. For patients with malignant tumors an annual chest x-ray is obtained to screen for distant metastases. Development of sensory nerve symptoms or motor weakness of the facial or hypoglossal nerve are indicators of recurrent disease and are evaluated by CT or MRI scans.

CONCLUSIONS

Salivary gland tumors comprise a heterogeneous group of neoplasms of varying histology, biologic behavior, and site of origin. As the size of the salivary gland decreases, the incidence of malignancy for neoplasms arising in these glands increases. Knowledge of the differential diagnoses and patterns of progression are instrumental in establishing the correct diagnosis and instituting appropriate treatment. Surgical resection is the mainstay of treatment, and for malignant tumors, a combination of surgical resection and postoperative radiotherapy has been shown to decrease local regional recurrence. Although extremely radical surgery was once advocated, a more conservative complete resection in combination with radiation therapy has been shown to provide good local regional control with preservation of form and function.

REFERENCES

1. Miller BA, Gloeckler LA, Hankey BF, et al. *SEER cancer statistics review 1973–1990.* NIH publication no. 93-2789. Bethesda: National Cancer Institute, NIH, Department of Health and Human Services, Public Health Service, 1990:1.
2. Laccourreye H, Laccourreye O, Cauchois R, Jouffre V, Menard M, Brasnu D. Total conservation parotidectomy for primary benign pleomorphic adenoma of the parotid gland: a 25-year experience with 229 patients. *Laryngoscope* 1994;104:1487.
3. Johns ME, Kaplan MJ. Surgical therapy of tumors of the salivary glands. In: Thawley SE, Panje WR, eds. *Comprehensive management of head and neck tumors.* Philadelphia: WB Saunders, 1987:1104.
4. Regezi JA, Batsakis JG. Histogenesis of salivary gland neoplasms. *Otolaryngol Clin North Am* 1977;10:297.

5. Batsakis JG. Physiology. In: Cummings CW, ed. *Otolaryngology: head and neck surgery.* 2nd ed. St. Louis: Mosby–Year Book, 1993:986.

6. Schneider AR, Favus MJ, Stachura ME, Arnold MJ, Frohman LA. Salivary gland neoplasms as a late consequence of head and neck irradiation. *Ann Intern Med* 1977;87:160.

7. Jackson GL, Ballantyne AJ. Role of parotidectomy for skin cancer of the head and neck. *Am J Surg* 1981;142:464.

8. Eneroth CM. Facial nerve paralysis: a criterion of malignancy in parotid tumors. *Arch Otolaryngol* 1972;95:300.

9. Frankenthaler RA, Luna MA, Lee SS, et al. Prognostic variables in parotid gland cancer. *Arch Otolaryngol Head Neck Surg* 1991;117:1251.

10. Weber RS, Byers RM, Petit B, Wolf P, Ang K, Luna M. Submandibular gland tumors. Adverse histologic factors and therapeutic implications. *Arch Otolaryngol Head Neck Surg* 1990;116:1055.

11. Beckhardt RN, Weber RS, Zane R, et al. Minor salivary gland tumors of the palate: clinical and pathologic correlates of outcome. *Laryngoscope* 1995;105:1155.

12. Cohen J, Guillamondegui OM, Batsakis JG, Medina JE. Cancer of the minor salivary glands of the larynx. *Am J Surg* 1985;150:513.

13. Schuller DE, McCabe BF. Salivary gland neoplasms in children. *Otolaryngol Clin North Am* 1977;10:399.

14. Perzin KH. Pathology. In: Conley J, Casler JD, eds. *Adenoid cystic cancer of the head and neck.* Stuttgart: Thieme Medical Publishers, 1991:5.

15. Nascimento AG, Amaral AL, Prado LA, Kligerman J, Silveira TR. Mucoepidermoid carcinoma of salivary glands: a clinicopathologic study of 46 cases. *Head Neck Surg* 1986;8:409.

16. Gaughan RK, Olsen KD, Lewis JE. Primary squamous cell carcinoma of the parotid gland. *Arch Otolaryngol Head Neck Surg* 1992;118:798.

17. Tabor EK, Curtin HD. MR of the salivary glands [Review]. *Radiol Clin North Am* 1989;27:379.

18. Byrne MN, Spector JG, Garvin CF, Gado MH. Preoperative assessment of parotid masses: a comparative evaluation of radiologic techniques to histopathologic diagnosis. *Laryngoscope* 1989;99:284.

19. Casselman JW, Mancuso AA. Major salivary gland masses: comparison of MR imaging and CT. *Radiology* 1987;165:183.

20. Miller FR, Wanamaker JR, Lavertu P, Wood BG. Magnetic resonance imaging and the management of parapharyngeal space tumors. *Head Neck* 1996;18:67.

21. Sismanis A, Merriam JM, Kline TS, Davis RK, Shapshay SM, Strong MS. Diagnosis of salivary gland tumors by fine needle aspiration biopsy. *Head Neck Surg* 1981;3:482.

22. Johnson J. Salivary glands. In: Gluckman J, Gullane P, Johnson J, eds. *Practical approach to head and neck tumors.* New York: Raven Press, 1994:17.

23. Beahrs OH, Chong GC. Management of the facial nerve in parotid gland surgery. *Am J Surg* 1972;124:473.

24. O'Brien CJ, Soong SJ, Herrera GA, Urist MM. Malignant salivary tumors: analysis of prognostic factors and survival. *Head Neck Surg* 1986;9:82.

25. McNaney D, McNeese MD, Guillamondegui OM, Fletcher GH, Oswald MJ. Postoperative irradiation in malignant epithelial tumors of the parotid. *Int J Radiat Oncol Biol Phys* 1983;9:1289.

26. Boles R, Raines J, Lebovits M, Fu KK. Malignant tumors of salivary glands. A university experience. *Laryngoscope* 1980;90:729.

27. Cueva RA, Robbins KT, Martin PJ. Lower cervical cutaneous sensory nerves: an alternative for facial nerve cable grafting. *Otolaryngol Head Neck Surg* 1996;114:479.

28. Spiro RH, Huvos AG, Strong EW. Cancer of the parotid gland. A clinicopathologic study of 288 primary cases. *Am J Surg* 1975;130:452.

29. Conley J, Hamaker RC. Prognosis of malignant tumors of the parotid gland with facial paralysis. *Arch Otolaryngol* 1975;101:39.

30. Pocket Guide to Neck Dissection, Classification and TNM Staging of Head and Neck Cancer. Edited by K. Thomas Robbins, M.D. AAO-HNS Foundation Inc. 1991.

CHAPTER 9

Thyroid Cancer

Jeffrey A. Norton and Scott A. Hundahl

EPIDEMIOLOGY

For 1998, the estimated number of new cases of thyroid cancer in the United States is 17,200 with nearly 12,500 occurring in women (1). Thyroid cancer is the most common endocrine malignancy. If ovarian cancer is excluded, thyroid cancer accounts for nearly 92% of all estimated endocrine cancer. It also accounts for the majority of endocrine cancer deaths. For 1998, thyroid cancer deaths are estimated at 1,200, which is 60% of the deaths estimated from endocrine cancer (1). Recent data suggest that the incidence of thyroid cancer is increasing while the death rate is decreasing. Thyroid cancer generally affects women between the ages of 25 and 65 years, but it also occurs in children and the elderly. For well-differentiated thyroid cancers, age at diagnosis is an important prognostic variable (2). Older patients have a poorer prognosis. Survival rates of patients younger than 45 years are better than those seen in older patients (2,3). Thyroid cancer can be one of the most indolent tumors and one of the most aggressive (3). Patients with papillary thyroid cancer (PTC) are usually cured, whereas patients with anaplastic thyroid cancer seldom live longer than 24 months (4).

PATHOLOGY OF THYROID CANCER
PATHOLOGICAL TYPES

Thyroid cancer is divided into four types: papillary, follicular, medullary, and anaplastic (Table 9-1). Lymphoma, sarcoma, and renal cell cancer may also present as a thyroid mass. The pathologic classification of thyroid cancer is based primarily on the cell of origin and the degree of differentiation. Most thyroid cancers are well differentiated (approximately 90%), and the cell of origin is the follicular cell for papillary, follicular, Hurthle cell, and anaplastic thyroid carcinoma. However, the parafollicular calcitonin secreting c-cell may also become cancerous, the so-called medullary thyroid carcinoma (MTC). Well-differentiated thyroid cancer includes both papillary and follicular thyroid cancer. The degree of malignancy can vary greatly among differentiated tumors and some have categorized them further based on the degree of differentiation. There is well dif-

ferentiated (papillary carcinoma, follicular carcinoma), intermediate differentiation (Hurthle cell carcinoma, tall cell variant of papillary carcinoma, insular carcinoma), and undifferentiated (anaplastic carcinoma).

RISK FACTORS

PTC is associated with neck irradiation. Thyroid exposure to irradiation can occur by either external sources or ingestion. The former is generally medically mediated, the later is environmental exposure from nuclear weapons or nuclear power plant accidents. PTC was seen associated with the atomic bombing of Japan and more recently with the nuclear accident in Chernobyl (5). Younger individuals exposed to irradiation are at greater risk for the development of papillary carcinoma. The risk of development PTC following neck irradiation increases with the dose of radiation up to 2,000 cGy, and the interval of time from radiation exposure. Radiation-induced PTC has the same prognosis as PTC not associated with irradiation (6).

Iodine deficient diets or vegetable diets that may significantly reduce the absorption of iodine may be associated with elevated serum levels of TSH and the development of goiter. People from countries such as Switzerland, in which thyroid goiter is common, have an increased incidence of follicular and anaplastic thyroid carcinoma. However, a causal relationship has not been proven. Conversely, people with excessive iodine intake from seafood (in countries such as Iceland and Norway) have a greater incidence of papillary carcinoma of the thyroid (4). MTC may occur as part of an autosomal dominant familial endocrine syndrome in the setting of multiple endocrine neoplasia (MEN) type 2A or B and familial MTC. These patients have inherited a missense mutation in the RET gene which can be identified by genetic analysis of the peripheral leukocytes (7,8). Individuals with this mutation have a 100% chance of developing MTC.

PAPILLARY THYROID CARCINOMA

PTC comprises about 80% of thyroid malignancies in developed countries with adequate iodine in the diet. Grossly, PTC

TABLE 9–1. *Incidence, risk factors, and long-term survival of thyroid cancers*

Type	n	Irradiation	Family history	10-year survival (%)
Papillary	42,686	+	–	93
Follicular	6,746	–	–	85
Hurthle cell	1,585	–	–	76
Medullary	1,928	–	+	75
Anaplastic	893	–	–	14

has a variable appearance from cicatrizing whitish scars to large tumors (5 to 6 cm in size) that invade into surrounding tissues. Most tumors are solid, 2 to 3 cm in size, firm to palpation, and lie within the capsule of the thyroid. Cystic change, cystic-solid tumors, necrosis, calcification, and ossification may also occur. Microscopically, papillary carcinomas generally have papillary fronds but may appear like follicles and are then termed the follicular variant of PTC. The former terminology of mixed papillary-follicular carcinoma is no longer used since most tumors will have some follicular appearance. Biologically, all PTCs, regardless of the follicular appearance, have similar behavior (9).

PTCs have specific nuclear features that define the neoplasm. The nuclei are enlarged and ovoid with thick nuclear membranes and intranuclear grooves. These nuclei can appear clear, the so-called "Orphan Annie" nuclei. The nuclei frequently overlap each other, which may be a helpful clue to the diagnosis. PTC has a propensity to spread throughout the thyroid gland via lymphatics (thus, it is multifocal in a significant proportion of patients) and to spread early to regional lymph nodes. Occasionally, microscopic or small papillary carcinomas may present with palpable regional lymph node metastases. Abnormalities of the RET oncogene have been found in approximately 25% of papillary tumors and may be associated with a poorer prognosis. Certain types of papillary carcinomas are clearly more aggressive and malignant, including the following 3 variants: tall cell, clear cell, and sclerosing cell (3). In terms of differentiation, these three variants would each be placed in the intermediate category.

Insular thyroid carcinoma is a new subvariant of well differentiated tumors that are more aggressive and fit into an intermediate grade category of malignancy. It is derived from the follicular cells and stains positively for thyroglobulin. It has a nested growth pattern with markedly increased vascularity. Insular carcinomas invade both lymphatics and veins and are associated with lymph node and distant metastases. This tumor may occur as a dedifferentiation of PTC. Its prognosis is poor with a 5-year survival of 40% (3).

FOLLICULAR THYROID CARCINOMA

Follicular thyroid carcinoma is a rarer form of thyroid cancer (10). It is more common in goitrous areas of the world, but in America, it represents only 5% to 10% of thyroid malignancies (Table 9-1). Follicular thyroid carcinoma is generally large (3 to 5cm), unifocal, and encapsulated. The hallmark for

the diagnosis is the detection of capsular or vascular invasion. Tumors are generally follicular, trabecular, or solid, and most cases show combinations of all three (9). Follicular carcinomas invade veins and not lymphatics such that distant metastases and death are more commonly associated with this type of thyroid malignancy. However, in the absence of distant metastases most patients do extremely well with this tumor and the long-term survival is between 85% and 100%. Hurthle cell tumors are actually a subgroup of follicular tumors and the criteria for malignancy are similar, namely capsular and vascular invasion. Older studies suggest that all large Hurthle cell tumors are malignant and that the pathologist is unable to distinguish benign from malignant tumors. However, recent data suggest that the pathologist can reliably determine the presence of malignancy in these tumors and only 30% are cancerous (4).

MEDULLARY THYROID CARCINOMA

MTC arises from the parafollicular c-cells. It comprises approximately 5% to 9% of all thyroid cancers, depending on different series (Table 9-1). It is also inherited in an autosomal dominant fashion in the setting of MEN-2. Parafollicular c-cells arise from the neural crest and share characteristics with other cells from the neuroendocrine system. These cells are located at the junction of the upper and middle third of the thyroid lobes with an increased density posteriorly. This feature is important for surgeons because the locus of primary MTC is generally near the ligament of Berry where the recurrent laryngeal nerve enters the larynx. This is a portion of the thyroid that is commonly left intact during near-total or subtotal thyroidectomies; obviously this should not be done if the patient has MTC.

Grossly, MTC appears either tan or yellow in color, is firm, and locally infiltrative and aggressive. Cytologically, the cells are dyscohesive and variable with small, round, spindle shapes with elongated nuclei. Plasmacytoid cells with moderate cytoplasm, and large cells with well defined cytoplasm, are also seen. Histologically, the cells are described as glandular, solid, clear-cell, small cell, and giant cell. Approximately, 75% of MTC stain positive for amyloid, which is procalcitonin (9). Because of considerable variability in the cellular appearance and shape, the best method to diagnose MTC is to stain the tumor with antibodies to calcitonin. The presence of immunoreactive calcitonin within tumor tissue is diagnostic of MTC. Tumors generally originate as part of a progression from c-cell hyperplasia to in situ MTC and invasive, MTC. Tumors that are confined to the thyroid are cured with surgery. It is important to remember that 30% to 40% of cases are familial and these cases are always bilateral and require a total thyroidectomy. Tumors that occur sporadically and present as thyroid nodules (more than 1 cm) often have lymph node metastases at diagnosis and require central lymph node dissection. Patients with lymph node metastases may still be cured, but the chance of cure is much less in these cases.

ANAPLASTIC THYROID CARCINOMA

Anaplastic or undifferentiated thyroid cancer is rare in that it is less than 1% to 2% of all thyroid malignancies (Table 9-1). It is one of the most malignant human neoplasms as the median survival is less than 24 months. Anaplastic thyroid cancer is more common in endogenous goitrous regions and it may be associated with long-standing untreated PTC. Its incidence is decreasing as iodine deficient diets and untreated PTC are less common. Grossly, anaplastic thyroid carcinomas present as large neck masses with respiratory stridor or difficulty swallowing secondary to local invasion by tumor. Cytologically, the cells are large with pleomorphic nuclei, irregularly distributed chromatin, and evidence of mitoses. Two main patterns have been identified: spindle cell and giant cell. In either case, the spindle or giant cell, the tumor is aggressive and almost always rapidly fatal. Leukocyte common antigen should be obtained to exclude lymphoma. Most anaplastic thyroid cancer express cytokeratin, which can be used to help diagnose it. Anaplastic thyroid carcinoma is commonly unresectable at presentation. It commonly extends outside the capsule of the thyroid with direct extension and invasion into adjacent structures and the muscles of the neck. Bulky lymph node metastases may occur and distant metastases at diagnosis are common. Death may be caused by uncontrolled local disease or widespread dissemination. The median survival is 6 months.

THYROID NODULE

The occurrence of thyroid nodules in the general population is between 4% and 7%. There are approximately 250,000 new nodules per year in the United States. Most patients with thyroid cancer present with a thyroid nodule that is palpable on physical examination. However, only about 5% to 10% of thyroid nodules are cancerous. The goal of the evaluation is to select cancerous nodules for surgery and to avoid surgery in benign nodules that are not causing symptoms. Previously, thyroid scan and ultrasound were recommended as the initial part of the work-up of most patients with thyroid nodules. Currently, however, neither are recommended because studies have demonstrated that neither are able to discriminate between benign and malignant disease. Ultrasound is able to accurately determine the size of a nodule and whether or not it is solid or cystic. Most cancerous nodules are solid and large; however, occasionally a small cystic and solid nodule may

still be malignant. In individuals who are referred for a possible thyroid nodule in whom the examiner is uncertain whether or not one exists because of size or location of the nodule or habitus of the patient, a thyroid ultrasound may be indicated to precisely image the size and location of the nodule. Further, in instances like this, ultrasound guided fine-needle aspiration (FNA) of the nodule is the method of choice to be certain that the nodule has been aspirated for diagnosis.

Thyroid scan is able to determine whether or not a nodule is functional or nonfunctional (hot or cold). Most malignant nodules are cold. Hot nodules are generally benign, and only rarely are malignant. Currently, thyroid function studies are recommended in all patients with thyroid nodules. If the thyroid function studies suggest hyperthyroidism (low level of TSH and elevated level of T4), a thyroid scan is indicated to determine if the nodule is functional.

The single best, most cost-effective test to select patients for surgery is FNA of the nodule for cytology (12–14). Palpable nodules should simply be aspirated with tactile control. Nonpalpable or difficult to palpate nodules are aspirated with ultrasound guidance. The procedure is best performed by individuals with experience in FNA. The procedure is safe and there are few contraindications. The thyroid is carefully palpated and the nodule is localized between two fingers. The patient is generally positioned supine with the neck hyperextended. The nodule is immobilized with the nonaspirating hand and a 25- or 23-gauge needle is fitted to either a 10-ml syringe holder or a 3-ml syringe if no suction is desired. The needle is placed within the nodule and moved back and forth in a straight line in order to loosen cellular material. If suction is used, the suction must be released before removing the needle from the lesion. "Preloading" the syringe with a few milliliters of air will facilitate expulsion of the specimen from the needle after the nodule is sampled. Nodules are generally sampled from multiple areas within the lesion, including the periphery. Both air-dried and alcohol-fixed smears are made from each pass and stained with the Papanicolaou staining procedure. Adequacy of the specimen is defined as the presence of 6 to 10 well-preserved follicular cell groups present on two different aspiration attempts.

Results of FNA can be divided into benign, atypical, suspicious, or malignant (Fig. 9-1). If a nodule appears benign on FNA, there is only a low probability that it is cancerous (3%), so surgery can be safely avoided. A total of 75% of fine-needle aspirates are benign, and most require only simple clinical follow-up. False-negative results (cancer with a benign FNA) may uncommonly occur because of sampling error. Therefore, in order to ensure the best possible results, it is important to obtain multiple aspirates. In some instances, the aspirates show atypical cells or suspicious cells in which some abnormalities are present but the findings are not diagnostic for cancer. In these instances, it is important to assess the cellularity of the specimen. If the diagnosis is based on adequate sampling with adequate numbers of cells, surgical lobectomy is warranted for diagnosis. If not, repeat FNA is the best procedure to further evaluate the nodule. If the result of the FNA

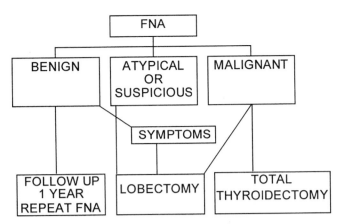

FIG. 9-1. Flow diagram for the management of thyroid nodule by FNA (fine-needle aspiration).

is malignant, there is a high probability of malignancy (80% to 90%), so definitive surgery can be planned. FNA is especially useful for diagnosing PTC because characteristic cytologic features are commonly obtained in this setting. These include papillary fronds, psammoma bodies, intranuclear cytoplasmic pseudoinclusions, nuclear grooves, and oval nuclei with granular chromatin. If the diagnosis is PTC on FNA, most experts proceed to definitive surgery without frozen section. MTC and anaplastic thyroid carcinoma can also be accurately diagnosed on FNA. However, follicular or Hurthle cell tumors are usually within the suspicious or atypical category and require thyroid lobectomy and permanent sectioning for diagnosis. Definitive surgery should be avoided for these tumors until an unequivocal tissue diagnosis is obtained (Fig. 9-1).

SYMPTOMS

Most patients with thyroid nodules are asymptomatic, but there are some signs and symptoms that must be considered in the evaluation of patients for possible surgery. Size of the nodule is an important consideration. Larger nodules (>4cm) have a greater incidence of false negative results on FNA and have a greater propensity to cause symptoms. Nodules that are both cystic and solid may also have a false negative aspiration result. In these instances, sampling of the fluid may inhibit the ability to sample the malignant cells that are present.

Nodules may cause symptoms by pressure or local encroachment on vital neck structures. For example, a large nodule may cause compression or narrowing of the airway or esophagus that leads to difficulty breathing or dysphagia. A benign or malignant mass can either compress or invade directly into neck muscles causing neck pain. It may affect the voice either by temporarily or permanently inhibiting the function of the recurrent laryngeal nerve. Patients may be concerned or apprehensive about the appearance or presence of a neck mass. This constant concern leads to anxiety that affects the patient's overall well-being.

Patients may have signs or symptoms of hyperthyroidism or hypothyroidism. Signs and symptoms of hyperthyroidism include anxiety, tremulousness, tachycardia, atrial fibrillation, weight loss, diarrhea, hyperphagia, exophthalmos, hyperactivity, tiredness, increased deep tendon reflexes, and irritability. Hypothyroidism is associated with tiredness, deep voice, weight gain, slow pulse, depression, sleepiness, constipation, decreased appetite, and decreased deep tendon reflexes. Careful questioning for the signs and symptoms of both hyper- and hypothyroidism should be performed. Thyroid function studies including a serum level of thyroid stimulating hormone (TSH), T3, and T4 should be obtained. Patients with hyperthyroidism need a thyroid scan to ascertain whether or not the thyroid nodule is functional. Toxic hot nodules are seldom malignant but warrant thyroid lobectomy to control the signs and symptoms of hyperthyroidism.

Each patient with a thyroid mass should be carefully questioned for the presence of symptoms. Airway compression, pressure on the trachea, neck pain, and difficulty swallowing are all indications for a thyroid lobectomy. Rapid or definite enlargement of an existing neck mass are also relative indications for surgery. The three indications for thyroid surgery are cancer, symptoms related to the nodule, and hyperfunction of the nodule. Symptoms and hyperfunction are less common. The usual indication for surgery is a suspicious or malignant FNA result.

THYROID SURGERY

Patients with thyroid nodules are selected for surgery based on the results of FNA and the size or symptoms related to the nodule. In general, total thyroidectomy is recommended for most types of thyroid cancer and ipsilateral thyroid lobectomy is recommended for definitive diagnosis of a suspicious nodule. Frozen section analysis at the time of surgery following the lobectomy may not be able to determine the presence of cancer and select patients for total thyroidectomy. Most experts now rely on the results of FNA for cytology or the final pathological analysis.

Thyroid surgery is performed with the patient supine and the neck hyperextended. Generally, a rolled towel is placed between the shoulders to better expose the neck. The patient should be positioned such that the anesthesiologist can have adequate control of the airway, but the surgeon needs access and space in order to perform the surgery. A transverse cervical collar incision is fashioned approximately 1 cm above the sternal notch. The incision should be as short as possible (4–6 cm) as this is a cosmetically noticeable area and thyroid surgery generally occurs in women who are concerned about appearance. The incision is carried through the skin, subcutaneous tissue, and platysma muscle. Flaps are then raised both cephalad and caudad. The flaps extend cephalad to the thyroid notch and caudad to the sternal notch. A self-retaining retractor is inserted for adequate exposure. The strap muscles are then opened in the midline and the lobe of the thyroid with the nodule is exposed. An accurate assessment of the size of the thyroid nodule should be obtained as well as determination of the presence of direct invasion into the strap muscles or other contiguous structures. Further, lymph nodes in the area should also be assessed both visually and by biopsy in order to determine the presence or absence of lymph node metastases. As the lobe is mobilized, the surgeon should identify two parathyroid glands, the recurrent laryngeal nerve, and the superior laryngeal nerve on the ipsilateral side of the neck. These structures should be able to be preserved as the dissection progresses. The inferior thyroid artery and the recurrent laryngeal nerve have a clear relationship to each other. The nerve generally lies posterior to the artery (60% of the time) and at right angles to it. The nerve can most easily be identified in the trachea-esophageal groove as it courses from the chest to the point where it enters the larynx, which is 1 cm medial to the inferior horn of the thyroid cartilage. Both parathyroid glands also have a relationship to these two structures.

The inferior parathyroid gland is inferior to the inferior thyroid artery and anteromedial to the recurrent laryngeal nerve, while the superior gland is superior to the inferior thyroid artery and posterolateral to the recurrent laryngeal nerve. The surgeon tries to preserve the blood flow to the parathyroid glands by ligating the inferior thyroid artery close to the thyroid gland. However, in some instances it is impossible to preserve the parathyroid glands with intact blood flow. In those instances it is best to remove the involved parathyroid gland and place it in sterile iced saline solution which should be present on the back table. A small biopsy of it is sent for frozen section to confirm that it is, in fact, parathyroid tissue and then the gland is sliced into 2 x 1 mm fragments which are transplanted into the sternocleidomastoid muscle. Approximately 20 fragments are needed for an effective transplant. The thyroid lobe and any suspicious lymph nodes are removed. As mentioned previously, frozen section may not be able to determine the difference between a benign and malignant thyroid tumor. If the frozen section and the aspiration biopsy are not diagnostic of thyroid malignancy, the procedure performed should be terminated. Suspicious lymph nodes should be removed. If no nodes appear suspicious, normal lymph nodes should be sampled. If the final pathologic diagnosis is cancer, it may be necessary to perform a second operative procedure to complete the thyroidectomy.

TREATMENT OF THYROID CANCER

Papillary Thyroid Cancer

PTC is the most common type of thyroid cancer. It occurs approximately 80% of the time (Table 9-1). In general, it has an excellent prognosis and therefore it is critical for the surgery and other therapy to be nonmorbid. PTC tends to be bilateral and metastasize early to regional lymph nodes. However, nodal metastases do not portend a worse prognosis (Table 9-2). In fact, for younger women with small primary tumors and cervical lymph node metastases, studies suggest that thy-

roid lobectomy (removing the involved lobe and adjacent lymph nodes) is adequate surgery (15). Generally, these patients have also been treated with 1-thyroxine to suppress serum levels of thyroid stimulating hormone. Patients treated in this manner have similar survival to patients treated with total thyroidectomy (15).

A minority of patients with PTC will have more malignant disease that will require more extensive surgery and additional treatment. For patients with PTC, a combination of surgery, radioactive iodine (RAI) treatment, and thyroid suppression therapy is indicated depending on the type, size, and extent of PTC and the age of the patient (16). Retrospective studies done by Mazzaferri (17) have demonstrated that each of these modalities are safe and able to decrease the rate of recurrence. PTC is bilateral in approximately 40% of instances and frequently spreads to cervical lymph nodes. Poor prognosis variables associated with mortality from PTC include the tall cell, insular and sclerosing type, tumor size greater than 3 to 4 cm, direct invasion of tumor into strap muscles and other contiguous structures, tumor outside the capsule of the thyroid, distant metastases, and older patient age (greater than 45 years). Experts agree that patients with these criteria warrant more aggressive treatment (2,3). Interestingly, cervical lymph node metastases, multifocal disease, younger patient age (less than 18 years), and history of neck irradiation are not associated with decreased survival, but are associated with a greater propensity of local recurrence (4,15). Patients with these findings may also warrant more extensive treatment with the caveat that it is administered without morbidity.

The use of total thyroidectomy in patients with PTC has been controversial (2,4,15–17). Only one study has convincingly suggested that the general use of total thyroidectomy prolongs survival (17). Several studies have demonstrated that it decreases local recurrence rates. The major issue is that total thyroidectomy is associated with more complications than thyroid lobectomy or subtotal thyroidectomy. Both re-

TABLE 9-2. *Staging for papillary and follicular thyroid cancer*

Stage	Age (years)	
	<45	≥45
I	AnyT, AnyN, M_0	T_1, N_0, M_0
II	AnyT, AnyN, M_1	T_2 T_3, N_0, M_0
III		T_4, N_0, M_0 AnyT, N_1, M_0
IV		AnyT, AnyN, M_1

T_0, no evidence of primary tumor; T_1, tumor ≤ 1 cm, limited to thyroid; T_2, tumor >1 cm to 4 cm, limited to thyroid; T_3, tumor > 4 cm, limited to thyroid; T_4, tumor of any size extending beyond the thyroid capsule.
N_0, no regional lymph node metastasis; N_1, regional lymph node metastasis; N_{1a}, metastasis in ipsilateral cervical lymph node(s); N_{1b}, metastasis in bilateral, midline, or contralateral cervical or mediastinal lymph node(s).
M_0, no distant metastasis; M_1, distant metastasis.
Adapted from Sobin LH, Wittekind C, eds. *TNM classification of malignant tumours.* 5th ed. New York: Wiley-Liss, 1997:47.

current and superior laryngeal nerves are at risk for injury during total thyroidectomy, while only one side is at risk during lesser procedures. There is a risk of hypoparathyroidism during total thyroidectomy while there is no risk during lesser procedures. Therefore, many argue that since total thyroidectomy is associated with a higher complication rate and most studies have suggested no survival benefit associated with it, total thyroidectomy is not indicated in most patients with thyroid cancer (15). However, recent studies have indicated that total thyroidectomy can be performed with low complication rates, a recurrent laryngeal nerve injury rate, and a hypoparathyroidism rate of 1% (3,4,10). Total thyroidectomy is clearly indicated in patients with the poorer prognostic forms of PTC. Total thyroidectomy allows more accurate staging of the true extent of disease since such a high proportion is bilateral. Total thyroidectomy facilitates the postoperative use of RAI. When the entire thyroid has been removed, the RAI will be taken up by any remaining thyroid or tumor cells that are present in lymph nodes or distant sites. Total thyroidectomy allows a lesser dose of RAI and thus potentially improves the efficacy and reduces side effects of RAI treatment. Retrospective studies have demonstrated a reduced incidence of local recurrence and improved survival with total thyroidectomy (16,17). Finally, the combination of total thyroidectomy and RAI should result in an undetectable serum level of thyroglobulin which can be used to follow the patient and assess recurrence. Concerning thyroidectomy, the major issue is safety. If total thyroidectomy can be performed with the same morbidity and mortality as lobectomy, everyone agrees that it is indicated in patients with PTC. Most recent data suggest that endocrine surgeons (surgeons with a special interest in the thyroid) can perform total thyroidectomy with very minimal morbidity and no mortality. These data further emphasize total thyroidectomy as the procedure of choice for patients with PTC (16,17). While total thyroidectomy or near-total thyroidectomy is favored for most types of PTC, treatment by unilateral lobectomy or isthmusectomy for a low-risk lesion (e.g., a less than 1.5-cm intracapsular papillary carcinoma in a patient without risk factors for recurrence) remains valid (18,19).

Following thyroidectomy, RAI is generally administered when the patient is hypothyroid as documented by a serum TSH level of 50 UIU/ml. RAI is used to obliterate any possible remaining thyroid tissue and eradicate any tumor that may have spread to lymph nodes or distant sites (16). Following RAI, a whole body scan is performed to assess the distribution of the isotope. This will also image the extent of disease. RAI is usually given in doses between 25 and 100 mCi and has minimal side effects up to a maximum dose of 300 to 600 mCi. Following RAI, 1-thyroxine is started at doses designed to keep the serum level of T3 and T4 in the normal range while keeping the serum TSH level suppressed less than 1 UIU/ml (16). PTC is known to have TSH receptors and suppression of serum TSH levels decreases the tumor growth rate. Serum levels of thyroglobulin both during 1-thyroxine and after withdrawal of 1-thyroxine in preparation for a follow-up thyroid scan or treatment with RAI are used to assess recurrent or persistent PTC. In general, if levels are elevated or if disease can be imaged on thyroid scan, more RAI is administered.

There are some special clinical circumstances with PTC that merit special attention. First, some patients present with PTC in lymph nodes, usually in the lateral compartment of the neck. These individuals may not have an apparent mass on palpation of the thyroid gland or even ultrasound. The pathologists can reliably diagnose PTC that has metastasized to lymph nodes. In this instance, total thyroidectomy or at least thyroid lobectomy is indicated to identify and remove the primary tumor. These individuals will always have a primary PTC in the ipsilateral thyroid lobe. Second, the next special situation occurs after the surgeon has removed a thyroid lobe for a nodule which, on final pathology, is benign but there is a microscopic focus of PTC. It is important to remember that approximately 3% to 6% of the autopsies will demonstrate a microscopic focus of PTC that is of no clinical significance (9). It is fairly clear that PTCs that are less than 3 to 5 cm in size are inconsequential. Therefore, the individual presented with microscopic PTC does not need any additional surgery or treatment. The final case scenario is the patient who presents with multiple pulmonary metastases from PTC and a large primary tumor within the thyroid that has not been treated (3). Despite the presence of pulmonary metastases, total thyroidectomy is still indicated and necessary in this patient to provide local control for the primary tumor and to facilitate the use of RAI to treat the pulmonary metastases.

Data from the National Cancer Data Bureau for PTC treated with surgery, RAI, and 1-thyroxin suggest that stage of disease at presentation is an important determinant of subsequent survival. Patients with stage I, II, or III—disease localized to the neck (Table 9-3)—have similar excellent 5-year survival of about 90% (Fig. 9-3). However, patients who present with distant metastases (stage IV disease), primarily to the lung, have significantly decreased 5-year survival of 50% (Fig. 9-3). Other reports have similar data with 10-year survival rates for all patients with PTC in the range of 80% to 90%.

Follicular Thyroid Cancer

Both follicular and Hurthle cell thyroid cancer are considered as the same diagnosis: that is, Hurthle cell tumors are really a variant of follicular tumors and require the same treatment and have the same prognosis as follicular tumors. Some individuals caution that all large (4 cm) Hurthle cell tumors should be considered malignant. Although others suggest that pathologists can reliably determine malignancy of Hurthle cell tumors, by using the same criteria as follicular tumors.

Although the incidence of follicular thyroid cancer is less than PTC, the death rate is greater for follicular thyroid cancer than papillary (3). A major issue with follicular tumors of the thyroid is accurate diagnosis. Patients generally present with a large thyroid mass that is found to have atypical follicular or Hurthle cells on FNA. Surgery (thyroid lobectomy) is indicated to ascertain the correct diagnosis (Fig. 9-1). Unfortu-

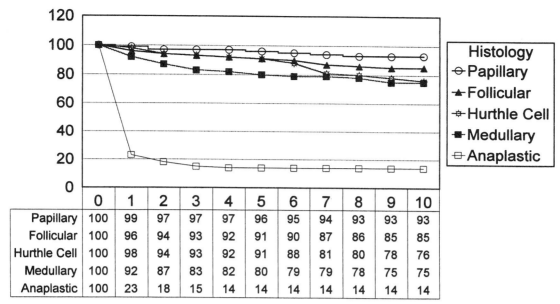

FIG. 9-2. Ten-year overall survival, by histology. Based on 53,856 cases of thyroid cancer accessioned by the National Cancer Data Base, 1985–1995. (Reprinted with permission from Hundahl SA, Fremgen A, Fleming ID, Menck H. 53,856 cases of thyroid carcinoma treated in the United States, 1985–1995: a National Data Base report. *Cancer, in press.*)

nately, frozen sections have been unreliable for follicular tumors. The pathologist relies on evidence of capsular or vascular invasion that usually requires multiple sections and permanent pathologic analysis (9). Since follicular or Hurthle cell cancers of the thyroid have a poorer prognosis than papillary cancers, treatment always involves total thyroidectomy, RAI, and suppression therapy. This aggressive treatment is recommended even if the patient has distant metastases. Despite the fact that this tumor causes the most deaths of any thyroid tumor, most patients still do reasonably well and can live for long periods even in the presence of distant metastases.

Overall, the 10-year survival for these patients is approximately 75% to 80%, which is significantly less than the 80% to 90% reported for PTC (3). Further, survival does decrease with extent of disease (Table 9-2) and patient with stage III and IV disease have reduced survival (Figs. 9-2 and 9-3). The 5-year survival for stage III and IV follicular thyroid cancer is 70% and 40%, respectively (Fig. 9-4). Hurthle cell cancers are less common and are, therefore divided between local and distant disease. Patients with local disease have a 5-year survival of 80%, while patients with distant metastases have a 5-year survival of 80%, while patients with distant metastases have a 5-year survival of 60% (Fig. 9-5).

Medullary Thyroid Cancer

MTC may occur in a sporadic form like all other thyroid tumors, and it may occur in multiple familial forms, MEN types 2A (MEN-2A) and 2B (MEN-2B) as well as familial MTC (FMTC) (4,7,8,20). MEN-2A is an autosomal dominant in-

herited endocrine syndrome that is characterized by MTC, adrenal pheochromocytoma(s), and parathyroid hyperplasia. MEN-2B is an autosomal dominant inherited endocrine syndrome that is characterized by MTC, adrenal pheochromocytoma(s), and a characteristic phenotype that includes mucosal neuromas, puffy lips, bony abnormalities, marfanoid habitus, intestinal ganglioneuroma, and corneal nerve hypertrophy. Unlike MEN-2A, parathyroid disease is not associated with MEN-2B. FMTC is characterized by an autosomal dominant inheritance of only MTC without any other endocrine abnormalities. The gene for all the familial forms of MTC has been localized to the pericentromeric region of chromosome 10. The responsible gene is called RET, which is a transmembrane protein kinase receptor. Mutations of RET enhance cellular growth. Recent studies have demonstrated missense mutations of RET in all individuals with the familial forms of MTC. MEN-2A and familial MTC mutations have been identified in the extracellular portion of the RET gene, while MEN-2B mutations have been identified in the intracellular domain (7,8).

In patients with MEN-2A, MTC generally appears between the ages of 5 and 25 years, prior to the development of pheochromocytoma or primary hyperparathyroidism. Recently, detection of RET mutations in the peripheral white blood cells of patients from kindreds with MEN-2A has been used as a screening procedure to diagnose an affected individual (7,8). Since 100% of individuals with MEN-2A will develop MTC, total thyroidectomy has been performed when RET mutations are detected. Prior to thyroid surgery, it is important to rule out the presence of a pheochromocytoma

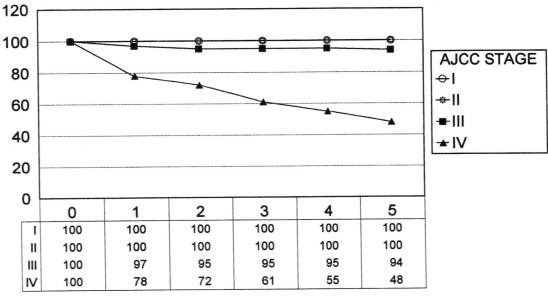

	0	1	2	3	4	5
I	100	100	100	100	100	100
II	100	100	100	100	100	100
III	100	97	95	95	95	94
IV	100	78	72	61	55	48

Years after Diagnosis

FIG. 9-3. Five-year stage-stratified survival (AJCC 3rd/4th edition staging) of papillary carcinoma cases accessioned to the National Cancer Data base, 1985–1995. (Reprinted with permission from Hundahl SA, Fremgen A, Fleming ID, Menck H. 53,856 cases of thyroid carcinoma treated in the United States, 1985–1995: a National Data Base report. *Cancer, in press.*)

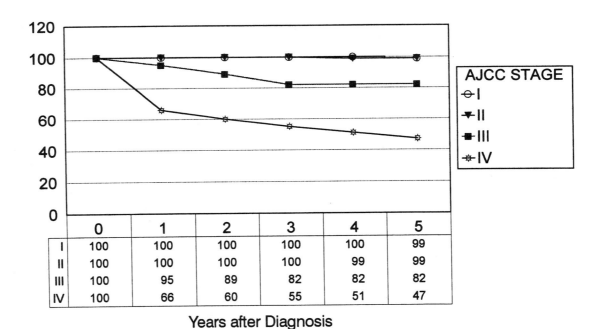

	0	1	2	3	4	5
I	100	100	100	100	100	99
II	100	100	100	100	99	99
III	100	95	89	82	82	82
IV	100	66	60	55	51	47

Years after Diagnosis

FIG. 9-4. Five-year stage-stratified survival (AJCC 3rd/4th edition staging) of follicular carcinoma cases accessioned to the National Cancer Data Base, 1985–1995. (Reprinted with permission from Hundahl SA, Fremgen A, Flemin ID, Menck H. 53,856 cases of thyroid carcinoma treated in the United States, 1985–1995: a National Cancer Data Base report. *Cancer, in press.*)

by measuring normal 24h urine levels of vanyl mandelic acid (VMA), metanephrines, and total catecholamines. When total thyroidectomy has been performed on these patients based solely on genetic testing, either premalignant C-cell hyperplasia or in situ MTC has been identified in each patient (7). These patients are generally cured of the MTC by thyroidectomy in this setting. Previously, patients from kindreds with MEN-2A were diagnosed by abnormal plasma levels of calcitonin in response to provocative testing with either calcium or pentagastrin. Calcitonin is a sensitive and specific hormone marker which can be used to establish the presence of MTC. Patients with clinically occult familial forms of MTC diagnosed either by genetic testing or provocative testing for calcitonin are generally cured of MTC by thyroidectomy.

Individuals with MEN-2B have a characteristic phenotype. These individuals have prognathism, puffy lips, poor dentition, mucosal neuromas, comeal nerve hypertrophy, and multiple bony abnormalities. These patients usually have a palpable thyroid mass or lymph node metastases at the time of diagnosis. The presence of MEN-2B can be ascertained clinically by the observation of corneal nerve hypertrophy on slit light examination, but the current key to diagnosis is the measurement of RET mutation in peripheral leukocytes. Patients with MEN-2B usually have locally advanced MTC at presentation. These patients are seldom cured by thyroidectomy and usually die of the MTC.

Individuals with FMTC have the most indolent form of MTC (20). In these patients, the MTC may occur at an older age, but despite the fact that they usually present with a large thyroid mass and more advanced local disease, they seldom die from MTC. Thus, in the three different familial settings, although the same oncogene is affected, the virulence of the MTC is different. The most virulent form is MEN-2B, the intermediate form is MEN-2A, and the least virulent is familial MTC. Total thyroidectomy is indicated for each of the familial types of MTC as each involves both lobes of the gland.

In the sporadic setting, patients with MTC typically present with a thyroid nodule or mass. FNA can reliably ascertain the diagnosis of MTC. FNA diagnosis of MTC requires a total thyroidectomy. MTC is usually bilateral in the familial forms and unilateral in the sporadic form. Therefore, pathologic analysis of the entire thyroid can help determine whether or not it is familial. However, genetic testing is required to unequivocally confirm familial disease. MTC may spread to regional lymph nodes. Central compartment lymph node excision and jugular lymph node sampling are indicated to exclude nodal metastases. The staging for patients with MTC is given in Table 9-3. The detection of modal metastases (stage III disease) is important, as few are cured stage III disease. Additional therapies including RAI, external beam irradiation, and doxorubicin, have been used in patients with MTC without success. Surgery is the only potentially curative treatment. l-Thyroxine is prescribed to replace normal thyroid function, but not as an antitumor treatment.

TABLE 9–3. *Staging for medullary thyroid carcinoma*

Stage	Description
I	T_1, N_0, M_0
II	T_2, T_3 or T_4, N_0, M_0
III	Any T, N_1, M_0
IV	Any T, Any N, M_1

T_0, no evidence of primary tumor; T_1, tumor ≤ 1 cm, limited to thyroid; T_2, tumor >1 cm to 4 cm, limited to thyroid; T_3, tumor > 4 cm, limited to thyroid; T_4, tumor of any size extending beyond the thyroid capsule.

N_0, no regional lymph node metastasis, N_1, regional lymph node metastasis; N_1, regional lymph node metastasis; N_{1a}, metastasis in ipsilateral cervical lymph node(s); N_{1b}, metastasis in bilateral, midline, or contralateral cervical or mediastinal lymph node(s).

M_0, no distant metastasis; M_1, distant metastasis.

Adapted from Sobin LH, Wittekind C, eds. *TNM classification of malignant tumours.* 5th ed. New York: Wiley-Liss, 1997:47.

Serum TSH levels for these patients should be maintained in the normal range between 1 and 5 UIU/ml.

Postoperatively, plasma levels of calcitonin can be used as a marker to detect recurrent disease (21). Patients with elevated basal or pentagastrin-calcium stimulated levels of calcitonin have MTC. Recent studies demonstrate that approximately one third of these patients can be rendered disease-free by modern techniques of neck dissection called microdissection (22). Experience has shown that prior to this repeat surgery, venous sampling for calcitonin should be used to indicate which side of the neck has disease and laparoscopy of the liver should be performed to exclude small liver metastases which may be present and undetectable on imaging studies (22).

Overall, approximately 80% of patients with MTC will have the sporadic form of the disease. Survival of patients following surgery is dependent on the extent of disease. In general, patients without lymph node metastases (stage I and II) are cured by total thyroidectomy. However, survival is significantly reduced as the stage of disease progresses, with stage III disease having a 4-year survival of 80% and stage IV disease having a 5-year survival of 40% (Fig. 9-6).

Anaplastic Thyroid Cancer

Anaplastic, or undifferentiated, thyroid carcinoma is one of the most difficult of human malignancies to treat. Fortunately, the incidence appears to be decreasing and it accounts for only 1% to 2% of thyroid cancers (Table 9-1). It is more common in iodine deficient regions like Switzerland. This leads some persons to hypothesize that long-standing goiters or PTCs may dedifferentiate into anaplastic thyroid carcinoma. Anaplastic thyroid cancer rarely occurs in individuals younger than age 60. Prognosis is so grave that all patients with this diagnosis are termed stage IV. The median survival in some series is only 4 to 5 months, with long-term

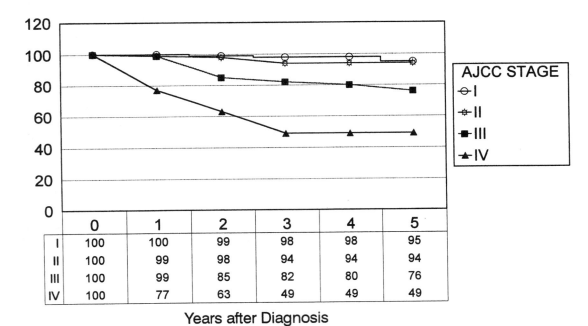

	0	1	2	3	4	5
I	100	100	99	98	98	95
II	100	99	98	94	94	94
III	100	99	85	82	80	76
IV	100	77	63	49	49	49

Years after Diagnosis

FIG. 9-5. Five-year stage-stratified survival (AJCC 3rd/4th edition staging) of Hurthle cell carcinoma cases accessioned to the National Cancer Data base, 1985–1995. (Reprinted with permission from Hundahl SA, Fremgen A, Fleming ID, Menck H. 53,856 cases of thyroid carcinoma treated in the United States, 1985–1995: a National Cancer Data Base report. *Cancer, in press.*)

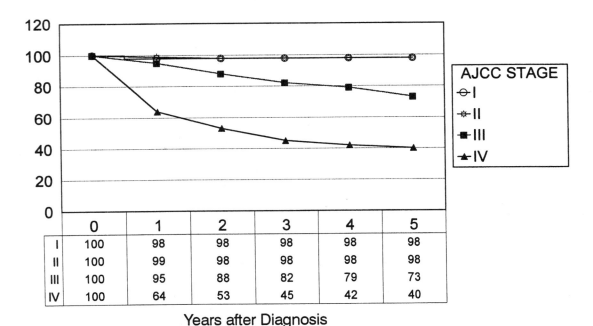

	0	1	2	3	4	5
I	100	98	98	98	98	98
II	100	99	98	98	98	98
III	100	95	88	82	79	73
IV	100	64	53	45	42	40

Years after Diagnosis

FIG. 9-6. Five-year stage-stratified survival (AJCC 3rd/4th edition staging) of medullary carcinoma cases accessioned to the National Cancer Data Base, 1985–1995. (Reprinted with permission from Hundahl SA, Fremgen A, Fleming ID, Menck H. 53,856 cases of thyroid carcinoma treated in the United States, 1985–19995: a National Cancer Data Base report. *Cancer, in press.*)

survival rare. Patients present with two problems: first is local control of the tumor. These tumors are usually quite large and locally invasive. Patients may develop vocal cord paralysis and airway obstruction secondary to the mass of tumor. The second problem is early pulmonary and distant metastases that decrease subsequent survival. Therapies must be designed to address both problems.

Surgery is not generally indicated in the management of patients with anaplastic thyroid carcinoma, unless the primary tumor is less than 4 cm. Surgical debulking is generally not useful because the tumor bulk tends to regrow rapidly. Total thyroidectomy is the initial procedure for patients with small (less than 4 cm) anaplastic thyroid cancer. Certainly in this instance, additional treatment will be necessary as the tumor may rapidly recur locally. For larger tumors (more than 5 cm), trucut needle biopsy or FNA will provide the diagnosis and thyroidectomy should not be attempted as it will not improve local control rates or subsequent outcome.

RAI is ineffective against anaplastic thyroid cancer. External beam radiotherapy has dramatically improved local control rates and is indicated in all patients with this diagnosis. Hyperifractionated radiotherapy appears to be more effective than conventional radiotherapy (23). Best results have been obtained when doxorubicin is also administered in low doses to serve as a radiation sensitizer (23). The combination has improved local control rates. Doxorubicin at more conventional doses has been used as a chemotherapy drug in an attempt to control systemic tumor. Recently, several series have reported long-term survival of a few patients with tumors less than 4 cm in size who were treated with a combination of surgery, chemotherapy, and radiation therapy. Thus the treatment is evolving, but requires multimodalities. Recent survival curves with the combination treatments are improved. The median survival is now approximately 18 months, and the 5-year survival is 10% (Fig. 9-2). Improved long-term survival will depend on enhanced effects of chemotherapy. Preliminary studies indicate that both cisplatin and taxol may also be useful.

ACKNOWLEDGMENT

The authors acknowledge the assistance of Amy Fremgen in preparing the data.

REFERENCES

1. Landis SH, Murray T, Bolden S, Wingo PA. Cancer statistics, 1998. *CA Cancer J Clin* 1998;46:6.
2. Jossart GH, Clark OH. Well-differentiated thyroid cancer. *Curr Probl Surg* 1994;31:937.
3. Robbins J, Merino MJ, Boice JD Jr, et al. Thyroid cancer: a lethal endocrine neoplasm. *Ann Intern Med* 1991;115:133.
4. Norton JA, Levin B, Jensen RT. Cancer of the endocrine system. In: DeVita VT Jr, Hellman S, Rosenberg SA, eds. *Cancer: principles and practice of oncology.* 4th ed. Philadelphia: JB Lippincott, 1993:1333.
5. Nikiforov Y, Gnepp DR. Pediatric thyroid cancer after the Chernobyl disaster. *Cancer* 1994;74:748.
6. Schneider AB, Shore-Freedman E, Ryo JY, et al. Radiation-induced tumors of the head and neck following childhood irradiation. *Medicine* 1985;64:1.
7. Wells SA Jr, Chi DD, Toshima K, et al. Predictive testing and prophylactic thyroidectomy in patients at risk for multiple endocrine neoplasia type 2a. *Ann Surg* 1994;220:237.
8. Lips CJ, Landsvater RM, Hoppener JW, et al. Clinical screening as compared with DNA analysis in families with multiple endocrine neoplasia type 2A. *N Engl J Med* 1994;331:828.
9. LiVolsi VA. *Surgical pathology of the thyroid.* Philadelphia: WB Saunders, 1990.
10. Brennan MD, Bergstralh EJ, van Heerden JA, McConahey WM. Follicular thyroid cancer treated at the Mayo Clinic 1946–1970: initial manifestations, pathology findings, therapy and outcome. *Mayo Clin Proc* 1991;66:11.
11. Brander A, Viikinoski P, Nickels J, Kivisaari L. Thyroid gland: U.S. screening in an adult population. *Radiology* 1991;181:683.
12. Mazzaferi EL. Thyroid cancer in thyroid nodules: finding a needle in a haystack. *Am J Med* 1992;93:359.
13. Gharib H, Goellner JR. Fine-needle aspiration biopsy of the thyroid: an appraisal. *Ann Intern Med* 1993;118:282.
14. Mazzaferri EL. Management of a solitary thyroid nodule. *N Engl J Med* 1993;328:553.
15. Cady B, Rossi R, Silverman M, Wool M. Further evidence of the validity of risk group definition in differentiated thyroid carcinoma. *Surgery* 1985;98:1171.
16. Mazzaferri EL, Young RL, Oertel JE, Kemmerer WT, Page CP. Papillary thyroid carcinoma: the impact of therapy in 576 patients. *Medicine* 1977;56:171.
17. Mazzaferri EL, Jhiang SM. Long-term impact of initial surgical and medical therapy on papillary and follicular thyroid cancer. *Am J Med* 1994;97:418.
18. Shah JP, Loree TR, Dharker D, et al. Lobectomy versus total thyroidectomy for differentiated carcinoma of the thyroid: a matched-pair analysis. *Am J Surg* 1993;166:331.
19. Gagel RF, Goepfert H, Callender DL. Changing concepts in the pathogenesis and management of thyroid carcinoma. *CA Cancer J Clin* 1996;46:261.
20. Farndon JR, Leight CS, Dilley WG, et al. Familial medullary thyroid carcinoma without associated endocrinopathies: a distinct clinical entity. *Br J Surg* 1986;73:278–282.
21. van Heerden JA, Grant CS, Gharib H, Hay, ID, Ilstrup DM. Long-term course of patients with persistent hypercalcitoninemia after apparent curative primary surgery for medullary thyroid cancer. *Ann Surg* 1990; 212:395.
22. Moley JF, Dilley WG, DeBenedetti MK. Improved results of cervical reoperation for medullary thyroid carcinoma. *Ann Surg* 1997;225:7
23. Kim, JH, Leeper RD. Treatment of anaplastic giant and spindle cell carcinoma of the thyroid gland with combination adriamycin and radiation therapy: a new approach. *Cancer* 1983;52:954.

CHAPTER 10

Nonmelanoma Skin Cancer

Mark David Gendleman, Thomas A. Victor, and Tianna Tsitsis

The incidence of nonmelanoma skin cancer in the United States is approximately 1,200,000 new cases per year, similar in magnitude to the incidence of noncutaneous cancers (1,2). Nonmelanoma skin cancers may be associated with morbidity, scarring, and financial burden. On occasion, they may be fatal due to local or distant metastasis. Early detection is essential in reducing these serious consequences. A comprehensive total body cutaneous examination should be performed regularly on susceptible patients. Biopsies should be obtained on any potentially malignant lesion.

Basal cell and squamous cell carcinomas are the most common malignant tumors in the Caucasian population (3,4). They usually occur on sun-exposed areas. Squamous cell carcinoma (SCC) may also occur on sites protected from the sun such as the mucous membranes, lower extremities, and genitalia, where other factors play a role. In the Black population, SCC presents more commonly than basal cell carcinoma (BCC). These tumors usually occur in sites not exposed to sunlight and are often more aggressive. Mortality from nonmelanoma skin cancer is rare, with SCC accounting for most of these deaths. Overall, less than one in 500 patients diagnosed with SCCs will die, amounting to approximately 1,500 deaths each year in the United States (5).

Host risk factors in the White population that are associated with a higher incidence of nonmelanoma skin cancer are listed in Table 10-1 (5). The main etiological factors are the susceptibility of the skin to ultraviolet (UV) light and the amount of sunlight exposure. The incidence of skin cancer increases as people spend more time outdoors for work or recreation. Sun exposure before the age of 20 years old appears to be of critical importance (2). The effects of the UV rays are cumulative (6). This process is irreversible and unfortunately may not manifest itself for many years (2). Together with individuals' hair color (blond or red), eye shade (blue or green), and hereditary descendants (Celtic), UV light can instigate and propagate extensive skin damage (7). Living close to the equator or at high altitudes may accentuate these effects. UVB causes damage to DNA and its repair mechanism and can alter the immune system. UVA damages DNA in a similar way acting as a cocarcinogen.

Other environmental and medical conditions associated with an increased risk of skin cancer are listed in Table 10-2 (5). There is a greater incidence of SCC in organ transplant patients on immunosuppressive therapy (8). SCCs in these patients occur on sun exposed areas, often are multiple and more aggressive, and have an increased risk of metastasis. These tumors increase in frequency with time after transplantation. Arsenic, which was used years ago for medicinal purposes and can be found today in well water, can induce cutaneous carcinogenesis: SCC, BCC, and squamous carcinoma *in situ* (Bowen's disease) (3,8). Cigarette smokers have an increased incidence of SCCs of the lip and mouth. Human papillomavirus has been demonstrated in many SCCs. The association of the human immunodeficiency virus (HIV) with skin cancer [Kaposi's sarcoma (KS), BCC, SCC] has been recently established. Ionizing radiation for benign and malignant skin disease can also have carcinogenic effects on the skin years later (9). PUVA phototherapy for the treatment of skin diseases can also lead to the development of skin cancer (8). The risk is dose dependent with a preponderance of SCC over BCC (8).

There are several cutaneous cancers about which the general surgeon should have some knowledge. These include KS and extramammary Paget's disease (EMP), both often serving as cutaneous markers for systemic disease such as AIDS, immunosuppression, and malignancy. Angiosarcoma (AS), Merkel cell carcinoma, and microcystic adnexal carcinoma (MAC) are all aggressive biologically, difficult to diagnose, and very problematic to treat. Dermatofibrosarcoma protuberans (DFSP), atypical fibroxanthoma (AFX), and cutaneous leiomyosarcoma are soft tissue sarcomas (STS) that occur in the skin and have a high recurrence rate with standard surgery. Finally, there is the keratoacanthoma (KA), a common distinctive tumor of the skin that exhibits very rapid growth with a clinical and histopathologic picture similar to SCC.

BASAL CELL CARCINOMA

BCC has become the most common human malignancy (3). This slow-growing tumor arises from the basal layers of the

TABLE 10–1. *Host factors associated with an increased risk of skin cancer*

Fair skin
Older age
Skin that burns easily or tans poorly
Freckles
Male sex
Celtic ancestry
Red, blond, or light hair
Blue or light-colored eyes
History of previous skin cancer

Adapted from Preston and Stern (5).

epidermis and its adnexal structures, such as hair follicles and sebaceous glands (7,10). Typically, BCC is found in older White men on sun-exposed and hair-bearing areas (3,10). Common locations include the face (especially the nasolabial folds, cheek, and nose), the head (especially the scalp and helix of the ear), and the neck (7,11). It is rarely found on the dorsa of the hands where SCC is more common (7).

There are five clinical types of BCCs: (a) noduloulcerative BCC, including rodent ulcer; (b) superficial BCC; (c) pigmented BCC; (d) morphea-like or fibrosing BCC; and (e) fibro-epithelioma.

Noduloulcerative BCC is by far the most common type of BCC (11). It begins as a small, smooth, waxy papule in actinically damaged skin. There are often small telangiectatic blood vessels on the surface (3). The papule usually increases in size slowly and often undergoes ulceration centrally (2,3). The typical lesion then consists of a slowly enlarging ulcerated nodule surrounded by a rolled, pearly, translucent border (3). The differential diagnosis of BCC includes sebaceous hyperplasia, adnexal tumors, ruptured hair follicle, and SCC. Most BCCs have a limited growth potential. Sometimes they may be aggressive and infiltrate and invade deeply, reaching considerable size. They may destroy the nose or eye and even penetrate the skull and invade the brain. The "rodent ulcer" historically refers to these enlarging destructive ulcerating ragged tumors with relentless behavior (Figs. 10-1 and 10-2).

Superficial BCC begins as an erythematous, scaly, slightly infiltrative patch (3). The patches are often surrounded by a fine, subtle, threadlike, pearly border (2). The central portion may be atrophic or show areas of crusting or ulceration (3).

TABLE 10–2. *Environmental and medical conditions associated with an increased risk of nonmelanoma skin cancer*

Ionizing radiation
Immunosuppression
Chronic ulceration or inflammation
Scars
Viral carcinogens
Chemical carcinogens (arsenic)
Cigarette smoking
Phototherapy

Adapted from Preston and Stern (5).

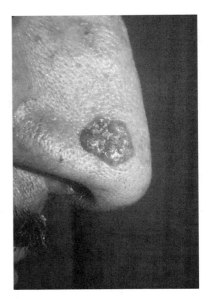

FIG. 10-1. Basal cell carcinoma, nodular type. It is shiny and translucent with surface telangiectasias. (Reprinted with permission from the American Academy of Dermatology.)

Lesions enlarge by peripheral extension causing centrifugal growth (2). Superficial basal cells resemble inflammatory dermatoses, but they persist in spite of topical therapy (3). Over time, dermal invasion may occur, giving the appearance of discrete nodules within the red plaque. The superficial BCC commonly occurs on the trunk but can also occur on the face (3) (Fig. 10-3).

Pigmented BCC looks like a noduloulcerative basal cell with pigment (3). The pigment is due to melanocytes within the tumor. It may resemble a nevus, melanoma, or other pigmented lesion. Pigmented BCCs have the same biological behavior and should receive the same treatment as the other BCCs (Fig. 10-4).

Morphea-like or fibrosing (sclerotic) BCC manifests as a solitary, indurated, whitish plaque (3). The surface is smooth

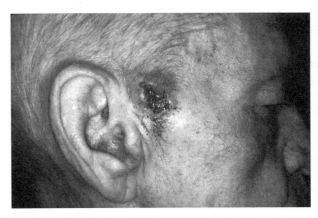

FIG. 10-2. Basal cell carcinoma, noduloulcerative type.

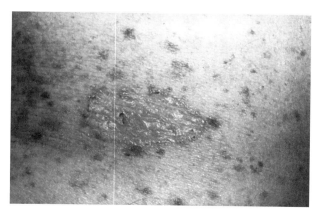

FIG. 10-3. Superficial basal cell carcinoma. A pink patch with a fine papular thread-like border.

and shiny, and the border is ill-defined (3). It resembles a scar or small patch of localized cutaneous scleroderma. In contrast to the nodular type, it rarely ulcerates or has telangiectasias (2,10). The morphea-type BCC often goes undetected for many years and may result in a large ill-defined, infiltrating aggressive tumor (3). Consequently, it is more likely to recur following therapy (3,11).

Fibroepithelioma (of Pinkus) is the rarest of the types of BCC. It consists of one or several raised, firm, slightly pedunculated nodules. The surface is smooth or red. They most commonly resemble fibromas. The back is the most common location.

The biopsy of a suspected skin cancer can provide essential information to assess the proper treatment of any BCC (2). In each case, the technique selected should yield the optimal histopathologic information. There are four biopsy types: shave biopsy, punch biopsy, incisional biopsy, and excisional biopsy. The shave biopsy is where a superficial portion of the tumor is elevated and a portion of the tumor

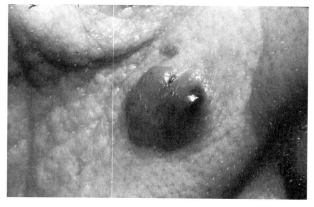

FIG. 10-4. Pigmented basal cell carcinoma. Shiny translucent nodule with small amount of pigment. It resembles a typical basal cell carcinoma except for the pigment. (Reprinted with permission from the American Academy of Dermatology.)

is removed with a scalpel or scissors. It is adequate to evaluate most noduloulcerative or superficial BCCs. The punch biopsy is done with a cylindrical metal "punch," allowing deeper penetration into the deep dermis or subcutaneous tissue. This is best for deeper types such as the morphea or sclerotic BCC. Extreme care should be taken with biopsy specimens to avoid crush artifact by use of the forceps. The incisional biopsy allows a portion of the tumor to be incised with a scalpel. The excisional biopsy provides the most information because the entire lesion is excised and sent for pathological analysis. This biopsy is conducted when the clinical diagnosis is certain or when time is important. In pigmented BCCs, where melanomas and other pigmented lesions are in the differential diagnosis, an excisional biopsy is best. Biopsies of suspected malignancies are performed under local anesthesia with 1% or 2% xylocaine either with or without epinephrine in a concentration of 1:100,000. Sutures may be used to decrease the morbidity of bleeding and infection.

The histopathologic features of BCC are important in the management of this disease. These neoplasms can be classified by their degree of differentiation as well as by the pattern in which they grow. The latter approach includes not only the appearance of the epithelial component, but it encompasses the manner in which the epithelial aspect relates to the fibrous stroma and to the manner in which the tumors behave. The patterns are nodular (tend to be circumscribed), superficial multicentric (tend to be localized at the junction, but not well circumscribed), and morpheic (tend to be diffuse and fibrosing).

A combined classification scheme has been suggested that incorporates features of differentiation and pattern (12). Two major classes include circumscribed and diffuse tumors. The circumscribed group includes solid (undifferentiated, basosquamous, adamantinoid, granular, and sebaceous), adenoid, cystic, keratotic, follicular, and fibroepithelioma. A circumscribed growth pattern is correlated with a high cure rate because the margins can be easily determined clinically and complete removal with a narrow margin is possible. At times, a solid type may have a diffuse component, usually at the deep margin, and these tumors behave like the diffuse types and recur more frequently. A technique that employs margin control at the time of removal is crucial for complete excision of these types. Diffuse types include the superficial multicentric, morpheic, infiltrating, micronodular, eccrine epitheliomatous, and apocrine epitheliomatous BCCs. As opposed to the solid types, which grow expansively and have defined margins, the diffuse types consist of small islands and strands of basaloid cells that infiltrate insidiously with a fibrous stroma. As a result of this growth pattern, these tumors are ill-defined and extend beyond the clinically palpable lesion. Without careful control of margins, the lesions are incompletely excised and will recur.

The most aggressive types are the basosquamous, infiltrating, morpheic (morpheaform), and micronodular BCCs.

Basosquamous carcinomas show squamoid differentiation, but they have the appearance of a BCC. These tumors tend to recur more frequently, are more aggressive and destructive, and have a higher incidence of metastasis than other BCCs (13). Infiltrating BCCs have no central cohesive mass as do the solid, nodular, well-circumscribed carcinomas. They consist of islands and cords of cells which are widely separated and spike down deeply into dermis and subcutis. These tumors show less peripheral palisading and usually have a fibrotic stroma. The margins of these forms are poorly defined. Morpheic BCCs extend insidiously, radially, and deeply with ill-defined edges. Thin cords and strands of tumor only 1 or 2 cells thick are seen in a dense collagenous stroma. These features make margin definition extremely difficult clinically. Micronodular BCCs consist of small, rounded nests of basaloid cells. Again, these tumors grow radially in an ill-defined manner and invade deeply, often without a dense stroma in the deep regions of the neoplasm. A large central component does not occur, and some of the larger nests may show peripheral palisading. The aggressive dispersed growth pattern again makes margin control difficult.

The majority of BCCs are slow growing and are not a significant cause of morbidity or mortality. There is, however, a small percentage of basal cells that are at a higher risk for recurrence or metastasis (14) (Table 10-3). Size is one of the most important risk factors. Recurrence rate increases with increasing tumor diameter (11,15). BCCs larger than 2 cm that are treated with electrodesiccation and curettage have a 5-year recurrence rate of more than 26% (14). The nose is the most common anatomic site for recurrence (11). The ear, periorbital area, and posterior auricular area are also common areas of recurrence (16). Previously treated BCCs are more likely to recur than primary tumors. Signs of recurrence include erythema, nodularity, ulceration, or hemorrhage at the site of a previously treated lesion (2). Positive postoperative margins increase the risk of recurrence. Radiation after surgical excision (with positive margins) decreases the risk of recurrence but does not eliminate it (15). Fortunately, even if positive margins are noted, only 33% recur (2,16,17). The reasons for this observation are unclear.

Metastatic BCC is rare. Only 300 cases have been noted in the worldwide literature (10). Most commonly, the cancer travels to regional lymph nodes, but may spread through the lymphatics or blood stream to the lungs, bone, or liver. When diagnosed, survival is usually only 8 to 12 months (11). The scalp is the most likely site to metastasize (14). Perineural invasion is an area of less resistance for tumor spread, which can lead to central nervous system involvement. Rare complications may include stroke, blindness, ophthalmoplegia, paranasal sinus involvement, and cavernous sinus involvement (14).

Throughout the years, clinical syndromes associated with BCC have been recognized. The most widely known is the basal cell nevus syndrome or "Gorlin's syndrome" (2,3). This is an autosomal dominant disorder in which dozens of BCCs develop on non–sun-exposed areas. The genetic abnormality has been traced to the ninth chromosome and has complete penetrance with variable expression for future generations (10). Small papules or nodules appear at an early age, resembling nevi. There may be hundreds of them by adulthood (2). They slowly increase in size and occur anywhere on the face and body. During adulthood, many of these BCCs ulcerate. Later in life, the disease may enter a neoplastic stage in which some of the BCCs, especially those on the face, become destructive and mutilating. Occasionally, even death occurs as a result of invasion of the orbit or brain or from pulmonary metastasis (18). Other characteristic findings of the syndrome include palmar and plantar pits, odontogenic keratocysts of the jaw, skeletal abnormalities (such as bifid ribs) and large occipitofrontal head circumference, cataracts and colobomas, and an increased risk of ovarian sarcoma, medulloblastoma, and meningioma (2,3,10).

Xeroderma pigmentosum is another genetic disorder that represents an autosomal recessive abnormality of the DNA repair mechanism (10). UV light is a prerequisite to developing the characteristic findings of severe sun sensitivity at a very early age, photophobia, cutaneous pigmentary alteration, ocular and neurological abnormalities, and multiple skin tumors of both basal and squamous cell types (3). In about 3% of the patients with xeroderma pigmentosum, malignant melanoma occurs. In some patients the melanomas show no tendency to metastasize while in others they may be aggressive and metastasize rapidly. Early diagnosis is essential to recommend complete photoprotection early in life.

The Muir-Torre syndrome is a third genetic disorder (autosomal dominant) in which sebaceous adenomas and carcinomas are seen in association with KAs and BCCs (3). Its significance lies in the fact that it is often accompanied by an internal gastrointestinal malignancy, most commonly colon cancer. Basex disease is a rare autosomal dominant disorder with follicular atrophoderma, anhidrosis, and hypotrichosis (3). In this disease, small BCCs usually arise on the face during childhood or adolescence (3). Albinism, in which one's skin does not contain melanin, predisposes the individual to cutaneous carcinoma. Both BCC and SCC can occur, with SCC presenting more often.

Nevus sebaceous (of Jadassohn) presents at birth with a single lesion on the scalp or face. In childhood it occurs as a localized, slightly raised hairless plaque. It is usually linear but may

TABLE 10–3. *Profile of the high-risk basal cell carcinoma*

Size greater than 2 cm
Anatomic location
    Mid-face
    Ear
    Scalp
Aggressive histological subtype
    Infiltrative pattern
    Sclerotic stroma
    Basosquamous (metatypical)
    Micronodular
Perineural invasion
Previously treated lesion
History of radiation exposure

Adapted from Barrett (14).

be round or irregularly shaped. During puberty, the lesion may become nodular or verrucous. Some patients with extensive nevus sebaceous may have a neurocutaneous syndrome consisting of skeletal deformities, epilepsy, and mental retardation. In adulthood, various types of appendageal tumors may develop within lesions of nevus sebaceous (18,19). BCC may also occur in 5% to 7% of cases of nevus sebaceous. These basal cells are usually small and not aggressive. Surgical excision before puberty is the treatment of choice. For patients who decline surgery (before puberty), it is important that they observe the nevus sebaceous and report any change to the physician.

Treatment goals for BCC should be to obtain a cure with good cosmetic results. Any treatment strategy should take into account the location and size of the tumor, age of the patient, nature of the cancer (whether it is a primary or recurrent tumor), type of cancer (clinically and histologically), cost, and the patient's symptoms, medical status, and preference. The common therapeutic modalities include excisional (scalpel) surgery, Mohs microscopically controlled surgery, electrosurgery, cryosurgery, and radiation. Less common therapy includes intralesional interferon or 5-fluorouracil (5-FU), topical fluorouracil, oral retinoids, phototherapy, and systemic chemotherapy (Tables 10-4 and 10-5).

Electrodesiccation with curettage is a simple outpatient procedure. It is done under local anesthesia and is efficient and cost effective (2). A small metal object, called a "curette," is used to debulk or shell out the soft tumor along with 1 to 5 mm of normal tissue surrounding the area. The residual tumor is electrodesiccated. This curettage and electrodesiccation is repeated two to three times and done more often with large tumors (7). The depth and lateral margins of the tumor can usually be determined with the curette by the sound or feel of the difference in consistency of the tumor from normal dermal connective tissue. This method of treatment is effective for small primary BCCs of the noduloulcerative or superficial type in low-risk locations (17). These tumors should have clearly defined borders. It is also very useful for tumors on the lower extremities or trunk or when cosmetic result is not essential. Considerable expertise is necessary to acquire proper technique. The risk of recurrence is

related to the site and size of the tumor (20). Low-risk locations are the neck, trunk, and extremities (20). High-risk sites are the nose, paranasal and nasolabial areas, preauricular and postauricular areas, scalp, and perioral and periocular areas (20). Treating recurrent BCCs with this procedure leads to a 40% recurrence rate (20).

Cryosurgery is a second alternative destructive modality that is a simple outpatient procedure (20). The tumor cells are frozen with liquid nitrogen applied via a cotton swab or spray. It is effective for superficial BCCs and can be used on small noduloulcerative types. This technique is simple, requires no local anesthetic, and is relatively free of postoperative complications. It can be used on tumors fixed to underlying structures. Successful treatment depends on adequate freezing after properly estimating the width and depth of the tumor. The disadvantages include no specimen for pathology, slow healing due to blister formation, and a hypopigmented scar (2).

Simple surgical excision is effective for all types of BCCs (15). It is a quick, relatively inexpensive outpatient procedure that provides a specimen for pathology (15,21). It is very appropriate for large tumors, aggressive subtypes, recurrent tumors, and tumors in high-risk areas. The disadvantages include bleeding in patients receiving anticoagulation therapy and the lack of tissue sparing (15). Frozen-section control technique is very useful, but there is loss of operating room time while the sections are processed. The cure rate approaches 99% when the histological margins are clear (2). If the margins are positive, only one third of basal cell tumors will recur (2,16,17). Should the final pathology indicate positive margins, some surgeons prefer to simply observe the area, while others will reexcise or radiate the field. Recurrence is more prevalent when the lesion is located on the head, when less than 4 mm margins are taken, or when the patient is male (20). Treating recurrent lesions with excision leads to a 17.4% recurrence rate (20).

Mohs micrographic surgery is the most successful mode of treatment, approaching a 99.6% cure rate in primary as well as recurrent lesions less than 10 mm, and 92.2% in those greater than 50 mm (20). First described by Frederick Mohs in the 1930s, only a limited number of physicians perform this painstaking procedure (7). The surgery involves initially debulking the cancer with a curette and then marking the skin in order to preserve orientation of the lesion (22). The tumor is excised in thin layers so that the lateral and deep margins can be examined and the 2- to 3-mm-thick specimens are prepared for frozen sectioning (22,23). Multiple dyes are used to map the skin and the lesion to retain orientation to each other while sections are cut (22). The surgeon also serves as the pathologist in the operating room and uses the microscope to determine if the margins are free of tumor. If the margins are not free of tumor, the surgeon returns to the site appropriately marked, and continues to excise tissue until this goal is accomplished (22). The physician may decide to suture the defect left in the skin or allow it to heal by secondary intention. This may take 4 to 8 weeks to close and another 6 to 8 months to completely heal. A plastic surgeon can perform reconstructive surgery should the

TABLE 10–4. *Treatments for basal cell carcinoma*

Common treatments
  Curettage and desiccation
  Simple excision
  Excision with frozen-section control
  Mohs surgery
  Cryosurgery (liquid nitrogen)
  Radiation therapy
Less common treatments
  Intralesional injection with interferon-α
  Topical and intralesional 5-fluorouracil
  Oral retinoids
  Photodynamic therapy
  Systemic chemotherapy

Adapted from Goldberg (2).

TABLE 10–5. *Treatments of basal cell carcinoma*

Characteristic	Excisional surgery	Mohs surgery	Radiation therapy	Electrodisiccation and curettage	Cryosurgery
Number of visits	2	2–3	3–9	1	1
Operative time (hours)	$\frac{1}{2}$–2	2–3	NA	$\frac{1}{4}$–$\frac{1}{2}$	$\frac{1}{4}$
Tissue sparing	No	Yes	Yes	No	Yes
Verification of margins	Yes	Yes	No	No	No
Time to heal (weeks)	1–2	1–2	NA	3–6	3–6
Scar	Linear	Variable	Atrophic, hypopigmented, telangiectatic	Round atrophic, hypertrophic, telangiectatic	Round hypopigmented
Most appropriate application					
Tumors > 1.5 cm	Yes	Yes	Yes	No	No
Aggressive subtypes	Yes	Yes	No	No	No
Recurrent tumors	Yes	Yes	Yes	No	No
Tumor in high-risk area	Yes	Yes	Yes	No	No
Tumor in patient on anticoagulants	No	No	Yes	No	Yes
Five-year recurrence rates (%) (rates vary with age, location, subtype)	1.2–23.4	0.7–1.8	4.1–31	1.3–18.8	0–12.9

Adapted from Preston and Stern (5).

size and location of the residual defect warrant this approach. Despite the technical challenges of Mohs, the advantages are numerous. These include the ability to cure recurrent lesions or those located in high-risk areas (20,22). It is also advantageous where tissue conservation is imperative (e.g., eyelids, digits, penis, perioral area, ear, and nose), for those tumors with ill-defined borders (e.g., morpheaform type), in previously irradiated skin and burn scars, and for tumors with diameters greater than 2 cm (20,22). Although this multistaged and multifaceted approach can be time consuming and expensive, the excellent cure rates are impressive.

Radiation therapy is also used in the treatment of BCC. It carries a 90% to 95% cure rate despite its lack of popularity today (2,15). Radiation therapy is useful in patients with complicated medical or surgical problems (2,21). It is painless with little postoperative scarring. It maximizes tissue preservation, but it is also time consuming and costly (21). Fractionated standardized doses are given over 2 to 3 weeks. It does require multiple visits to the doctor's office, and carries possible side effects of postradiation fibrosis/dermatitis, alopecia, and carcinogenesis (thyroid and breast cancer). Radiation is useful in elderly patients, those on anticoagulants, or for keloid formers (2,21). It should not be used in young patients, lesions previously treated with radiation, morpheaform BCCs, or lesions in the inner canthus or poorly defined tumors. Difficult areas where tissue preservation is important, such as on the eyelid, nose, and lip, can be treated with this modality (21). Recurrence is related to the size and histology of the lesion (20,21). It is also effective as an adjuvant therapy for large tumors. Treatment of recurrent tumors with radiation leads to a 9.8% recurrence rate (20).

Numerous reports and studies of different recurrence rates with different surgical modalities have been reported. In a systematic review of all the studies (1947 to 1987) on recur-

rence rates for primary BCC, the following 5-year recurrence rates were determined. Mohs micrographic surgery 1.0%, surgical excision 10.1%, radiation therapy 8.7%, curettage and electrodesiccation 7.7%, and cryosurgery 7.5% (24).

New and innovative nonsurgical techniques are being developed. Topical and oral retinoids are being used. They cause regression of some tumors, but complete remission occurs in less than 20% and therapy must be continued (20). Immuno-therapy is becoming popular, but it is still in its infancy with interferon-2-alpha and gamma, interleukin 1 and 2, primary recall antigens, and antibodies against tumor angiogenesis factor (8). Long-term studies are forthcoming. Photodynamic therapy uses a porphyrin or D-ALA chemical to seek out tumor cells and is followed by laser treatment to the area (2). Theoretically, the preselected cells are killed while the normal cells are unharmed. The major disadvantage of this treatment is severe generalized photosensitivity lasting as long as 1 month. Chemotherapy with topical 5-FU is useful in superficial BCC, but it is not appropriate for deeper tumors (11). Intralesional 5-FU is being tested but it has a cure rate of only 20% to 50% (20). Systemic chemotherapy with cisplatin or doxorubicin has demonstrated a complete response in only 14% of cases and is considered purely palliative for metastatic disease (20).

Overall, the principles of treatment are to identify the high-risk patients and lesions, completely remove the tumor, and perform careful follow-up (15). The best cosmetic results are obtained with excision or radiation. Electrosurgery and cryosurgery are more destructive and less definitive, therefore yielding less satisfying cosmetic results. However, they are efficient and inexpensive. Mohs surgery produces excellent results, but it is time consuming and requires specialty training and expertise. Mohs is the best modality for recurrent BCC, as well as for those occurring in the nasolabial fold, inner canthi, or posterior auricular folds. Reducing exposure to sunlight is key for prevention.

SQUAMOUS CELL CARCINOMA

SCC is a malignant tumor that originates in the keratinocytes of the epidermis. It may occur anywhere on the skin or mucous membranes lined by squamous epithelium. It most commonly appears on sun-damaged skin, but it may arise in the precursor lesions of actinic keratoses, Bowen's disease (carcinoma *in situ*), or leukoplakia, or from scars or chronic ulcers.

Actinic or solar keratoses are small, pink or white, discrete, adherent, keratotic or crusty lesions which may vary in size from 2 to 10 mm. They may coalesce into large lesions. They are extremely common in elderly or middle-aged, fair-skinned individuals living in sunny climates. In many cases there are a number of lesions. The most common sites are the face, scalp, and the back of the hands and forearms. The forehead, cheeks, and temples are more commonly affected than the lower face. The ears, sides of the neck, and upper lip are often sites of predilection. The lesions are usually asymptomatic, but they may be painful, pruritic, or become irritated. Malignant transformation of actinic keratosis into SCC fortunately is very infrequent (approximately less than one per 1,000 per year) (5,6). Some actinic keratoses improve spontaneously or with topical steroids. Therefore, predicting which lesion will involute or degenerate is difficult. A change in an actinic keratosis such as tenderness, erythema, erosion, nodularity, or the development of a cutaneous horn may all indicate malignant degeneration (Fig. 10-5).

Leukoplakia is a white patch or plaque that cannot be rubbed off. It occurs on the oral, genital, or anal mucosa. Leukoplakia and actinic keratoses may exhibit little evidence of cellular atypia for much of their history. The point at which the lesion degenerates into an invasive tumor is determined histologically by the breaching of the basement membrane.

Bowen's disease (SCC *in situ*) is a well-demarcated, erythematous, scaly plaque. It can be difficult to differentiate from eczema or psoriasis. Persistence of the plaque in spite of topical therapy is often a helpful clinical sign. Bowen's disease usually occurs singly, but it can be multiple. Location is usually on the trunk or legs and women are affected more frequently. Slow-growing and asymptomatic, the lesions may persist for years before becoming invasive. Ulceration is often a clinical sign of invasion.

SCC usually begins as a small, firm, skin-colored or slightly erythematous nodule. The margins of the nodule are indistinct and often indurated. The induration is frequently irregular and often extends beyond the visible margins of the lesion. Resistance to palpation is greater than that seen with inflammation. The area around the growth is often erythematous. Many times, early lesions are covered by a keratotic or verrucous crust. Removal of this crust may reveal an ulcer or erosion with a red, granular, bleeding base. Sometimes raised, verrucous, fungating lesions occur (5,18). Typically, the carcinoma enlarges both in elevation and diameter. Progressive invasion beyond the skin eventually fixes the tumor to the structures below and may invade along peripheral nerves. Ulceration, which is usually central, may occur early or late, but often it occurs earlier in fast-growing tumors (Figs. 10-6 and 10-7).

Marjolin's ulcer is a SCC that arises at the periphery of a chronic scar or ulcer. The scar may be due to a burn, radiation, or a vaccination. Stasis ulcers or decubitus ulcers may also be underlying causes. Any chronic inflammatory process (osteomyelitis, pilonidal sinus, or chronic lupus erythematosus) may also degenerate into SCC (2,18,25).

Verrucous carcinoma is a low-grade SCC. There are three forms, all occurring in areas of maceration. Verrucous carcinoma of the oral cavity is also called "oral florid papillomatosis." It presents as white cauliflower-like areas on the

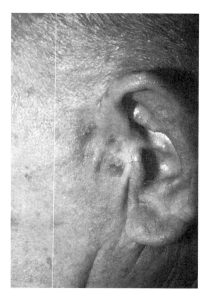

FIG. 10-5. Actinic keratosis. A discrete pink scaly papule on the face. There is generalized actinic degeneration. (Reprinted with permission from the American Academy of Dermatology.)

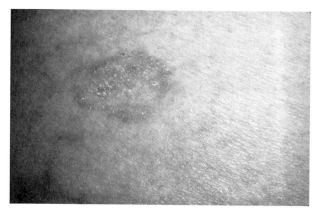

FIG. 10-6. Bowen's disease. Eczematous, well-demarcated plaque. (Reprinted with permission from the American Academy of Dermatology.)

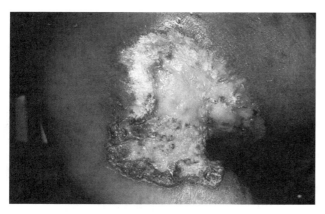

FIG. 10-7. Squamous cell carcinoma. This is an ulcerative lesion with a verrucous border.

oral mucosa. Verrucous carcinoma of the anogenital region is also called "giant condylomata of Buschke and Loewenstein." It most commonly is seen on the glans of the penis or foreskin of uncircumcised men. It may develop in the anal region or in the vulva of women. Plantar verrucous carcinoma initially presents like an intractable large wart. It grows as a protruding verrucous mass which evolves into a large cyst-like area filled with keratotic, horny material and pus. Verrucous carcinoma has been described on other areas of the body (18). Although a viral cause of verrucous carcinoma has been suspected, there have been only a few cases where the viral particles have been detected by electron microscopy (EM).

Anaplastic SCC may arise from normal skin and is very difficult to recognize. The lesion is a fast-growing, red papule or nodule, and inflammatory rather than neoplastic in appearance. It tends to ulcerate early in the course of development. It resembles a KA, but the central core of keratin is absent. Induration is less pronounced. It can infiltrate deeply and metastasize early.

The differential diagnosis of SCC includes KA, other cutaneous malignancies, and infectious granulomas (either deep fungal or atypical mycobacterial). KAs are very difficult to distinguish from SCCs and will be discussed below. However, the very rapid growth phase as well as the classic morphology of a dome-shaped nodule filled with central horny material typically suggest KA. A helpful clinical distinguishing sign between BCCs and SCCs is the lack of verrucous or keratotic surface in a BCC. This is because the cells of BCC do not keratinize. Also, the growth phase of BCCs is much slower.

The histologic hallmark of actinic keratosis is the atypical keratinocyte (26). The disease begins in the basal and lower layers of the epidermis and consists of keratinocytes with large, irregular, hyperchromatic nuclei with prominent nucleoli. Dyskeratotic cells or cells with eosinophilic cytoplasm may be seen. With time these cells may proliferate downward to form buds or may migrate upward into the epidermis. Coarse parakeratosis of the stratum corneum is an important clue to the diagnosis, especially in cases with subtle cytologic

features and clinically correlates with a scaly appearance. In the dermis a superficial perivascular dermatitis is usually present and associated with erythema clinically. The lesions are usually well-circumscribed and do not extend below the follicular infundibulum. This feature allows more superficial treatment of the lesion to be successful. The major problems in assessing these lesions are distinguishing actinic keratosis from early SCC, differentiating hypertrophic actinic keratosis from verrucae and seborrheic keratoses, distinguishing lichenoid actinic keratosis from lichen planus or carcinoma, and recognizing actinic keratosis with minimal atypia. Clinical correlation and corroboration are extremely important in these instances.

In contrast to actinic keratosis, Bowen's disease consists of full-thickness epidermal keratinocytic atypia with dyskeratotic cells and mitotic figures at all levels. The mitotic figures may be abnormal. Multinucleated atypical cells may also be seen. The differential diagnosis includes Paget's disease (extramammary) and melanoma in situ. Immunohistochemistry may be necessary to make the distinction. Keratinocytes will be cytokeratin positive as might the Paget cells, but the latter will be epithelial membrane antigen (EMA) and CEA positive. Melanoma cells will be S100 and HMB 45 positive. The lesions may be circumscribed or ill-defined and can extend down into follicular epithelium, which may affect choice of treatment. SCC arising in Bowen's disease has a higher rate of metastasis.

SCC can be classified into four main histologic patterns: the conventional or differentiated pattern, spindle cell growth, an acantholytic type, and verrucous carcinoma (27). In the conventional pattern, the neoplasm recapitulates keratinocytes by producing keratin, which corresponds to an eosinophilic cytoplasm and keratinous material usually seen in keratin whorls or pearls. The conventional type is further subclassified by its degree of differentiation. The more differentiated neoplasms have keratin production and intercellular bridges. The Broder system is used to grade the degree of differentiation and the grade correlates directly with biologic behavior (recurrence, invasiveness, and metastasis) (28). Grade 1 carcinomas are well differentiated and have abundant keratinization with little nuclear anaplasia, and less than 25% of the tumor is not differentiated. Grade 2 carcinomas are moderately differentiated, and at least 50% are keratinizing. Nuclear anaplasia is present, and less than 50% of the tumor is undifferentiated. Grade 3 carcinomas are moderately to poorly differentiated, with less than 25% keratinizing. Nuclear anaplasia is extensive, and less than 75% of the tumor is undifferentiated. Grade 4 carcinoma is poorly differentiated with little or no keratinization, extensive nuclear anaplasia, and more than 75% of the tumor is undifferentiated.

In the spindle cell variant of SCC, the neoplasm is completely undifferentiated. The differential diagnosis includes malignant melanoma, leiomyosarcoma, and atypical fibroxanthoma (AFX). Immunohistochemistry helps again and is critical because the treatment and prognosis for these tumors differ greatly. The SCC is often cytokeratin positive. Melanoma will stain with vimentin, S100, and HMB 45. Leiomyosarcoma stains with desmin and muscle specific actin. AFX is negative for these antigens and will often stain for histiocytic markers. Acantholytic carcinomas consist of varying sized nests of tumor with acantholysis. This feature gives a resemblance to an adenocarcinoma. Here, the cytokeratin stain and lack of other antigens typical of adenocarcinoma are helpful. The latter two variants tend to be more aggressive tumors and treatment should take this into account. Verrucous carcinomas histologically may be deceptively benign and resemble a condyloma or pseudoepitheliomatous hyperplasia. The diagnosis may require clinicopathological correlation in such cases. The neoplasms may be locally aggressive, but metastasis is rare. Radiation therapy may cause dedifferentiation.

Pathologic features associated with risk of metastasis include the site (ear, lip, genitalia), the size (larger than 4 cm), grade (grade 2 to 4), Clark's level (IV or V), Breslow depth (larger than 2 mm), perineural invasion, and margin status. All of these elements should be in the pathology report and form the basis for treatment selection.

A primary goal of the clinician is to identify the high-risk tumors. Several variables have been identified as prognostic risk factors for SCC of the skin (Table 10-6) These include (a) size (diameter), (b) depth of invasion, (c) anatomic location, (d) histologic differentiation, (e) rapid growth, (f) etiology (scar, ulcer), (g) perineural invasion, (h) recurrence, and (i) immunosuppression (14). All high-risk patients should be followed closely, since 75% of local recurrence and 80% of metastatic disease occur within the first 2 years.

SCC of the skin has an overall rate of metastasis between 2% and 10%, although rates as high as 30% have been reported (5,18). Carcinomas arising in sun-damaged skin or in actinic keratoses have a low propensity to metastasize. Carcinomas that are thicker than 4 mm, longer than 2 cm, or less well-differentiated have a higher risk of metastasis. Tumors occurring on the lip or ear, in immunocompromised hosts, or in sites of radiation dermatitis, chronic inflammatory dermatosis, or scars all have a greater chance to metastasize. The thickness of the tumor and the depth of invasion are greater predictors of the risk of metastasis than the degree of differentiation. Regional lymph nodes are the most common sites of metastasis. The liver, lung, brain, and bone are less frequent sites of spread.

TABLE 10-6. *Profile of the high-risk squamous cell carcinoma*

Size greater than 2 cm
Depth of invasion 4 mm or greater (at or below the reticular dermis)
Anatomic location (ear or lip)
Rapid growth
Immunosuppression
Etiology (scar, ulcer, sinus tract, radiation)
Histologic subtype (poorly differentiated)
Perineural invasion
Recurrence

Adapted from Barrett (14).

Cutaneous SCCs may spread by infiltration and expansion, shelving or skating, conduit spread, or metastasis (9). Expansion and infiltration refer to the local invasion, not unlike a tree with roots. Shelving and skating represent the way SCCs may extend along fascial planes, muscle, periosteum, or perichondrium. The tumor may shelve or skate laterally underneath clinically visible normal skin when it contacts a hard surface such as a bone, cartilage, or muscle. This is especially important when dealing with tumors in areas with little subcutaneous adipose tissue such as the upper lip, ear, nose, or temple. Conduit spread occurs as SCCs extend through areas of least resistance in the perineural or perivascular space in a pipeline or conduit manner. This must always be remembered in dealing with SCCs overlying major nerves, especially in the head and neck (9).

Treatment planning should include a consideration of the same factors as in BCC: location and size of the tumor, histopathological type, primary or recurrent tumor, age of the patient, associated symptoms, general medical status of the patient, patient's input, and cost. An adequate biopsy should be obtained before definitive therapy can be recommended. Biopsy specimens can then be processed for routine histological staining as well as special stains. Blood tests can be performed to determine the patient's hematologic, hepatic, and coagulation status. An anergy panel and tests for cell-mediated immunity, including subsets of T-lymphocytes, may be helpful in determining the patient's immune surveillance. Chest x-ray, computed tomography (CT), magnetic resonance imaging (MRI), and lymphangiography all can be performed to determine local, regional, or distant metastasis. Patients with a high-risk profile should be staged, using the TNM classification. A less formal classification might include palpation of all regional lymph nodes since SCCs metastasize to regional lymph nodes first in 85% of cases (14). Patients with high-risk tumors of the face and no detectable cervical nodes may benefit from a CT scan of the neck. Patients with palpable nodes should have a chest x-ray to determine if there is pulmonary metastasis.

There are three different classical approaches to the cure of SCC: surgery, radiation, and local destruction. Excisional therapy is the mainstay of therapy. Simple primary closure, flap, skin graft, or secondary intention can all be used to repair the defect. The palpable margin of the tumor should be outlined before any local anesthesia is injected. There is no uniform recommendation for the excisional margins, but a 3- to 5-mm border for small tumors with at least a 1-cm margin for larger more aggressive tumors is recommended (5). Even the most harmless SCCs may extend beyond the palpable margins. Therefore, the surgical margins should be examined histologically. Surgery is also the best treatment for tumors which have invaded bone or cartilage or when lymph node metastasis has occurred. It is also best for recurrent tumors resulting from other treatment modalities or tumors with poorly defined margins. Excisional surgery has the advantage of being able to assess margins and optimize cosmetic results. These wounds heal rapidly and require very little postoperative care. The resultant scar is often cosmetically acceptable.

Mohs microscopically controlled surgery is done under local anesthesia. It allows the surgeon to examine the margin of the tumor microscopically and serially. This allows the entire tumor to be removed with minimal loss of normal tissue. It is best for high-risk or recurrent tumors, or when the primary excision was inadequate (6).

Radiation therapy is used primarily in poorly differentiated SCC of the head and neck that has not spread to cartilage or bone and has not metastasized. It is also useful in primary tumors where there is concern about preserving function or the patient's appearance (6). Slightly less successful than surgery, there is a higher recurrence rate, especially in large tumors (6). Tissue necrosis and wound breakdown are potential short-term complications. Chronic problems include radiation dermatitis and carcinogenesis. For the latter reason, it should not be used in young patients. Adjuvant radiotherapy may be combined with surgery for high-risk tumors or for deeply invasive lesions in high-risk areas (e.g., lip or ear). It may also be indicated after regional lymph node dissection where there is concern over extracapsular extension or evidence of residual disease microscopically (6). Radiotherapy can also be helpful in palliation.

Local destruction with curettage and electrodesiccation may be appropriate for small, primary, well-defined SCCs of the head and neck. It may be the method of choice for tumors of the extremities which are too large for simple excision and primary closure. The cosmetic results may be superior to surgery or radiation. Cryosurgery can be effective treatment for some SCCs. It allows the local destruction of tissue to a considerable depth. Collagen, cartilage, and bone are less sensitive to freezing. Scar formation and necrosis are greatly reduced. Success depends on adequate freezing to the proper width and depth and the experience of the clinician. Both cryosurgery and electrodesiccation with curettage can be effective and efficient therapy for actinic keratosis, Bowen's disease, or leukoplakia.

Other treatment options are available to treat SCCs. Topical fluorouracil can be used to treat carcinoma *in situ* (Bowen's disease). Intralesional interferon alpha is an experimental therapy being studied. Side effects include an influenza-like syndrome, local pain, and necrosis of the skin. Lasers, particularly the carbon dioxide laser, can be used in place of electrodesiccation and curettage. It offers a bloodless field, but has few advantages over electrosurgery and is more costly. Photodynamic therapy can be helpful in patients with multiple lesions, in transplant recipients or immunocompromised individuals, or in patients with solitary lesions in difficult to reach locations. Chemotherapy is reserved for metastatic disease. It seldom results in eradication of the tumor. Choosing the correct treatment requires a high degree of skill and clinical judgment. Physicians should take into account the wishes of the patient as well as their own.

KERATOACANTHOMA

Perhaps one of the most controversial dermatologic tumors is the KA, initially described in 1889 as a "crateriform ulcer of the face, a form of acute epithelial cancer" (29). Traditionally believed to be a benign, self-limited epithelial lesion derived from hair follicles, some feel it represents an early SCC and demand it be treated as such. Others argue that it is an "abortive malignancy that rarely progresses into invasive SCC" and ought to be conservatively managed (29).

The cause of KA is unknown. Definite risk factors have been identified that contribute to its pathogenesis and include the following: UV light, antecedent radiation, PUVA, trauma, immunosuppressed states, viral infections with HPV, light skin color, and chemical exposure to tar, pitch, machine oil, and topical podophyllin (29,30).

Two types of KA exist: solitary and multiple. The typical solitary KA is seen in elderly or middle-aged persons on sun-exposed areas (29,30). Although lesions can occur anywhere on the body, the most common locations are on the head and neck, especially the nose, cheeks, and eyebrow area, the dorsum of the hands, and the forearms (10,29). KA progresses through three stages in its development. In the proliferative stage that lasts 1 to 2 months, an initial small, red, papule rapidly enlarges to become a firm, smooth, dome-shaped nodule 1.0 to 2.5 cm in diameter (29,30). In the mature, quiescent stage, an umbilicated keratinous plug develops in the center and the nodule remains stagnant in size and freely moveable over underlying tissue (29,30). If the keratotic core is removed, it appears crateriform. In the involutional stage, regression begins (29,30). The keratinous plug is expelled and the area becomes a thin, hypopigmented, atrophic, puckered scar. The entire process occurs over 2 to 8 months, but it has been noted to take as long as 1 year (29,30) (Fig. 10-8).

There are two variants of multiple KAs (29). Both types are rare. The first variant is the Ferguson-Smith type or multiple self healing epitheliomas of the skin (29). An autosomal dominant disorder, dozens of red macules present simultaneously or in rapid succession on sun-exposed as well as covered areas; they become papular and develop into typical KA lesions. The process can start as early as childhood or adolescence, but it typically occurs around 25 years of age. Men are

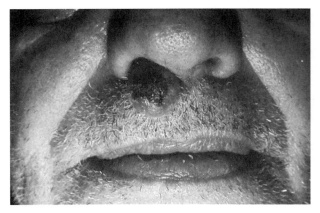

FIG. 10-8. Keratoacanthoma. Rapidly growing nodule with keratotic core of material in the center. (Reprinted with permission from the American Academy of Dermatology.)

affected more frequently than women. The tumors regress only to reappear, often over a lifetime. The second variant is termed "generalized eruptive KA of Grzybowski" (29). Hundreds of minute 2- to 3-mm KAs develop over the entire body, including the mucous membranes, typically in middle-aged White patients. Unlike the previous syndrome, there is no familial association and cases are sporadic. The lesions usually resolve within 6 months, but they may coalesce and become quite pruritic. There is an increased incidence of female genital tract carcinoma in these patients (29). KAs can also be seen in the Muir-Torre syndrome, which typically is a problem of sebaceous neoplasms and internal malignancy (29). There is also an increased incidence in immunosuppressed patients, in xeroderma pigmentosum, and nevus sebaceous.

There are three rare clinical variants of solitary KAs (29). In two types, giant KA and KA centrifugum marginatum, the KA can reach a very large size. In giant KA, the lesion rapidly attains a size of 5 cm or more, often resulting in destruction of underlying structures. The most common sites are the nose and eyelids. Usually, spontaneous resolution occurs after several months. In the KA centrifugum marginatum, the lesion may reach a size of 20 cm in diameter. Common locations include the legs and the dorsum of the hand. There is no tendency for spontaneous involution. There is a third variant: subungual KA. Here, a destructive crateriform lesion develops under the distal portion of the fingernail. It is tender, fails to regress spontaneously, and eventually may cause pressure erosion of the underlying bone (18).

The most important lesion to differentiate from KA is a *de novo* SCC. Clinically, the rapid development of a nodular lesion with a central keratotic horn-filled crater favors the diagnosis of KA (29). Microscopically, the architecture of a crater surrounded by buttresses with a glassy histologic appearance of many of the cells favors KA. This differentiation is much more difficult in early lesions because cellular atypia may be found in KA and a horn-filled invagination may be seen in SCC.

An adequate biopsy of the suspicious area is imperative and must include the lateral border and central core, delving deep into subcutaneous fat as well. This is achieved by either total excision or by a fusiform partial excision through the entire KA, including the center and both sides. This allows analysis of both the architecture of the tumor and the presence or absence of invasion into the underlying tissue. The presence of deep invasion mandates therapy for a *de novo* SCC (29). Shave and punch techniques are unacceptable. Multiple staining and immunohistochemical techniques are available to differentiate the disease states, although much overlap exists. Other conditions that present similarly to KA include verrucous carcinoma, BCC, giant condyloma, hypertrophic actinic keratosis, cutaneous horns, metastatic cancer, deep fungal infections, large molluscum contagiosum, and adnexal tumors (29).

The solitary types of KA have a distinctive morphology despite the varying clinical appearances, but the histologic features vary depending on the stage of the lesion. In the early rapid growth stage there is an exoendophytic, dome-shaped lesion which consists of a horn-filled (ortho- and parakeratosis) invagination of the epidermis formed by proliferating joined follicular infundibula (29). The proliferating cells extend outward and downward into the dermis. There may not be a central depression and at the edges the cells may form strands, have nuclear atypia, and display multiple mitotic figures which resemble carcinoma. Less keratinization is seen than at later stages although cells with glassy eosinophilic keratinized cytoplasm may be observed. A sparse inflammatory infiltrate may be present at the dermal interface. Vascular, perineural, and lymphatic invasion have been described. Although other authors ignore this finding, it should not be dismissed without careful consideration of the possibility that the lesion could represent a SCC. Invasion deeper than the sweat gland is probably an indication of a SCC (29).

The second stage or fully developed lesion is larger, exoendophytic or cone-shaped with the V pointing toward the subcutis. The central crater now has an epidermal lip and irregular papillary epidermal protrusions as well as cornified cells and inflammatory debris. Keratinization is now marked as evidenced by cytoplasm which is eosinophilic and glassy. Microabscesses and trapped collagen may be seen in the epithelium. At the edges, broad columns or tongues of squamous proliferation push outward or between dermal collagen bundles. Inflammatory cells at the interface include lymphocytes, histiocytes, eosinophils, neutrophils, and plasma cells. If there is desmoplasia and angulated, thin columns of atypical squamous cells splaying collagen, then the possibility of SCC should be seriously considered.

In the third or involutional stage, the lesion becomes less craterform and thinned. At the base, the inflammatory infiltrate now includes multinucleated giant cells, and there is degeneration and necrosis of the neoplastic cells, which are extruded upward. A lichenoid infiltrate with granulation tissue is also present at the base. The lesion heals with a fibrous scar.

Subungual KA may not have a prominent crater, and its lobular proliferation may be difficult to distinguish from SCC histologically. Clinical features such as younger age of onset, rapid initial growth, and destruction of underlying bone rather than invasion are helpful (31). KA dyskeratoticum and segregans may also closely resemble a SCC due to its dyskeratosis and acantholysis. Multiple KAs generally demonstrate the histologic features of solitary KAs. In eruptive variants such as Gryzbowski's type smaller lesions may show less crater formation and may appear to be pseudoepitheliomatous hyperplasia or well-differentiated carcinoma. In the Ferguson-Smith type the KAs tend to have a typical morphology, although in different stages.

The major problem with KAs is their distinction from SCC. Based on metastasis in cases where the morphology is typical of KAs, some authors think that all KAs should be considered SCCs (32). Other authors think that there is a regressing squamous neoplasm which can be recognized in typical cases with a proper biopsy and represents an entity distinct from SCC. Unfortunately, the problem of differentiating a KA from SCC is a common one as both can have similar histological and clinical findings. In some cases, the distinction may not be possible and a diagnosis of KA-like carcinoma or KA, which cannot rule out SCC, may be necessary. KAs left untreated should be followed to confirm the diagnosis and complete involution.

There are multiple modalities of treatment available for KAs (29,30). In many cases, the acceptable course may be close observation of the lesion and frequent follow up visits. Many clinicians will follow this plan when the clinical and or histopathological examination are typical of KA. Allowing KA to take its natural course of spontaneous involution in ill patients, in patients where surgery is difficult, or where excision will yield a poor cosmetic result, appears sensible. Even large lesions less amenable to surgery usually regress within a short time (33). Most KAs are easily removed surgically without complications. Lesions for which the histological diagnosis is unclear, lesions that cause the patient pain or distress, or those adjacent to vital structures (e.g., the eyelid) should be excised (33). Surgery creates cure or resolution, prevents rapid enlargement, and allows improvement cosmetically. Mohs surgery is used for lesions in difficult locations, for recurrent disease, or for tissue sparing. Curettage with electrodesiccation is an option for solitary, small, superficial lesions. Two disadvantages here include an 8% recurrence rate secondary to insufficient shaving and the possibility of leaving a hypopigmented residual scar (29). Cryosurgery is also available for small, early lesions or as an adjunct to surgery or curettage with electrodesiccation. Radiation therapy can be employed in elderly or debilitated patients unable to undergo a surgical procedure, with large lesions in difficult locations, or in recurrence. Sometimes, radiation can induce a rapid regression, resulting in a superior cosmetic outcome. The same radioactive doses are used as for SCC. Intralesional 5-FU, bleomycin, methotrexate, triamcinolone, and interferon alpha have been employed. Topical podophyllin and 5-FU are noninvasive alternatives. Oral retinoids, such as isotretinoin, for multiple and recurrent KAs and etretinate for solitary, multiple, eruptive, and atypically aggressive KAs have been effective in both treatment as well as prophylaxis. Systemic methotrexate is even being used in multiple, large, aggressive KAs with some response noted.

In general, recurrence is rare (0% to 8%) and metastasis even more so, with individuals who have lesions on the fingers, hands, or lips, giant KAs, or lesions only partially excised at a higher risk (29). In cases of recurrence or metastasis, the biopsy ought to be reexamined and the diagnosis of SCC entertained more seriously. Because most authorities agree that SCC can mimic KAs, it is best, when histological and clinical findings are inconclusive, to treat the lesion as a SCC.

OTHER CUTANEOUS CARCINOMAS

Additional cutaneous carcinomas include Merkel cell carcinoma, microcystic adnexal carcinoma (MAC), sebaceous gland carcinoma (SGC), and extramammary Paget's disease (EMP).

Merkel Cell Carcinoma

The Merkel cell carcinoma, or cutaneous small cell carcinoma, was initially described in 1972 as a "trabecular carcinoma" based on its cellular architecture (34). Further research has shown it to be a neuroendocrine carcinoma arising from an epidermal basal cell known as the Merkel cell (10,34). The exact function of this specialized cell is unknown, but it is felt to be a mechanoreceptor that has the capacity to release neuropeptides and influence the nervous system (34–36). Regardless of etiology, Merkel cell tumors are rare and have only been reported approximately 600 times since their initial description (37). They are often seen in association with SCC, BCC, Bowen's disease or actinic keratoses, which implies a role for UV light in their pathogenesis (34,36,37). Other conditions occasionally concurrently found with Merkel cell carcinoma include Cowden's disease (multiple hamartoma syndrome), Hodgkin's lymphoma, and various solid tumors (breast, pancreas, colon, prostate, bronchus) (34,37). This implies a role for immunosuppression in their pathogenesis.

Clinically, elderly White men and women in their sixth or seventh decade of life notice a rapidly enlarging single nodule or indurated plaque (35–37). The 0.5- to 2-cm intracutaneous lesion is firm and painless, often with a red, blue, or purple color. The surface is shiny and smooth and rarely ulcerates (10,34,35–37). Overlying telangiectasias may be present. Sometimes, satellite nodules form around the primary site. Occasionally they may become pedunculated. The head and neck area is the most common site, especially the eyelid (34, 35,37). Lesions may also occur on the extremities. Merkel cell carcinoma is usually solitary, but occasionally multiple tumors may arise. The differential diagnosis includes SCC, BCC, melanoma, pyogenic granuloma, KA, cysts, clear cell acanthoma, lymphoma, adnexal tumors, and cutaneous metastasis (34–36). Biologically aggressive, Merkel cell carcinoma is difficult to diagnose and treat effectively. Over the past several years, electron microscopic and immunocytochemistry advances have made early and accurate diagnosis possible.

Histologically, Merkel cell carcinoma can be grouped into one of three different patterns (37). These include the trabecular type, an intermediate cell type, and a diffuse small cell type. The trabecular type is the least frequent and consists of polygonal cells arranged compactly in trabeculae separated by a connective tissue stromal. There is a Grenz zone and the tumor is seen next to adnexal structures. Mitotic figures are seen. The intermediate cell type has a solid growth pattern with some trabeculae near the edges. The tumor cells are less compact than in the trabecular type and have less cytoplasm. These tumors may connect with the epidermis. This is the most frequent type in some series and is more aggressive than the trabecular form. The third pattern is the diffuse small cell type. It resembles the small cell or oat cell carcinoma of the lung. A ribbon or rosette pattern may be present in this type. Chromatolytic crush artifact and necrosis similar to oat cell carcinoma occur and may be associated with the Azzopardi effect (deposition of chromatin in blood vessel walls). These cells are small and round or fusiform. The major problem with this tumor is its distinction from metastatic small cell carcinoma of lung, small cell melanoma, lymphoma, and undifferentiated carcinoma, which influences selection of therapy. EM and special stains for neuropeptides make it possible to identify the nature of this carcinoma and distinguish it from other lesions of the skin which have similar appearance (38).

Immunohistochemistry is very useful in identifying Merkel cell carcinoma. Merkel cell carcinomas show neuroendocrine differentiation and thus tend to stain positively for neuron-specific enolase, chromagranin, and synaptophysin. In addition, 100% of these tumors stain positively for low molecular weight cytokeratin in a characteristic manner consisting of an inclusion-like paranuclear button or dot. This pattern by EM corresponds to a whorl of paranuclear keratin filaments. Metastatic small cell carcinoma does not usually stain with this pattern, nor do lymphoma, melanoma, and undifferentiated carcinoma.

Merkel cell carcinoma is difficult to manage due to its biologic aggressiveness, and this problem is compounded by the difficulty in making a certain diagnosis. If immunohistochemistry is not useful, a clinical search for another primary site is necessary. Histologic features which predict a more aggressive course include small cell morphology, a mitotic rate greater than 10 per high power field, angiolymphatic invasion, and distant metastasis.

Treatment is dependent upon the stage of the disease. Stage I is solely a primary lesion (37). Stage II includes regional node involvement, and stage III, systemic metastasis (37). Wide surgical excision with 2- to 5-cm margins is the mainstay of therapy in stage I (34,35,37). Some recommend lymph node dissection in all cases, while others recommend it only if lymph nodes are clinically palpable. A third group recommends lymph node dissection in tumors located on the head and neck, size greater than 2 cm, histologic evidence of invasion into lymphatic or blood vessels, in patients less than 40 years old, males, or when the onset of disease is greater than 6 weeks (35,37). Mohs microscopically controlled surgery may be considered for the management of localized disease as a tissue-sparing technique. However, the lymphatic and vascular invasion that Merkel cells exhibit dictate that a wide tumor-free margin should be taken when Mohs surgery is performed. The margins must be carefully examined for tumor extension.

Radiation has a role as primary therapy in poor surgical candidates (37). More often, radiation therapy is used as an adjunct to surgery (34,37). Its field typically includes the primary site, 5-cm margins, and lymph node drainage channels (34,37). Radiation is recommended in stage I disease when lesions are greater than 1.5 cm or are close to the surgical margins (37). It may also be considered for unresectable or bulky lesions, those invading lymphatic vessels or nodes, or encroaching on vital structures, or after lymph node dissection in head and neck tumors (37). Most authorities recommend wide local excision of the primary tumor, regional lymph node resection if nodes are palpable, and then radiotherapy of both the postsurgical bed and the lymph node basin.

Chemotherapy can be used for stage I tumors when there is extensive local disease, small cell histology, or difficulties with resection and radiation (37). Stage II tumors are treated with wide surgical excision and radiation and, occasionally, chemotherapy (37). Stage III disease has the worst prognosis and is treated primarily with chemotherapy, with protection against tumor lysis syndrome an important consideration (34,37). Various combinations include cyclophosphamide and doxorubicin or cisplatin and etoposide (34). Although 50% to 75% of the cases respond, they do so only for a transient 6 to 12 months (34,37). Overall survival remains unchanged (34,37). Interferon and hyperthermia are two therapies that are currently being studied (34,37). Optimal treatment regimens are difficult to establish because of Merkel cell carcinoma's rarity. Most evidence for success or failure comes from anecdotal experiences.

The long-term prognosis of patients with Merkel cell carcinomas is relatively unfavorable. Frequent follow-up examination after the initial excision is essential. From 26% to 44% of tumors recur postoperatively within 4 months (37). Regional lymph nodes become involved in 50% to 75%, especially in head and neck lesions (34,35,37). There is a 60% salvage rate if local recurrence or regional lymph node metastasis is treated aggressively with immediate reexcision, lymph node dissection and radiation (34–36). Distant metastasis occurs in 30% to 50% within 2 years of the initial diagnosis; death follows closely within 6 months (34–37). The most common sites for dissemination include the lymph nodes, liver, bone, brain, lung, and skin (34–37). Survival in years 1, 2, and 3 after discovery is 88%, 72%, and 55%, respectively (34). There have been rare cases of spontaneous regression (10). Realistically, death is imminent in Merkel cell carcinoma, especially if it is not treated early and aggressively (37). Careful follow-up is imperative after any therapy is undertaken. History and physical exam with particular attention paid to the lymph nodes, liver and spleen, chest x-ray, laboratory tests (CBC, LFTs), and possibly CT scans of the chest, abdomen, and/or pelvis if lymph node dissection is being considered are essential in the search for recurrent disease (34,36,37). The recommended schedule for follow-up is monthly for 6 months, then every 3 months for 2 years, and then every 6 months thereafter for life (34,37).

Microcystic Adnexal Carcinoma

Another aggressive carcinoma of the skin is the MAC. Since its discovery in 1982, it has received a plethora of names, such as sclerosing sweat gland carcinoma, malignant syringoma, sweat gland carcinoma with syringomatous features, aggressive trichofolliculoma, and combined adnexal tumor of the skin (39,40). A pluripotential keratinocyte that has the ability to differentiate along both eccrine and follicular lines is believed to be the cell of origin (40). Besides a slight tendency for these tumors to develop in areas that were radiated 30 to 40 years before, there do not appear to be other risk factors contributing to its development (39,40).

Clinically, MAC presents in 40- to 60-year-old men or women on the head and neck (39,40). The upper and lower lips constitute most of the cases, but it can occasionally occur on the chin, cheeks, or nasolabial folds (39). Often present for years prior to diagnosis, the lesions typically grow slowly as firm, solitary nodules or plaques, with a yellow hue and induration (39,40). Usually asymptomatic, a fullness in the area may be its only presenting sign (39,40). The tumor usually ranges in size from 0.25 to 2.5 cm in diameter (39,40). Paresthesias, stinging, pain, or burning are the consequences of the tumor's aggression and its tendency towards perineural invasion (39,40). Despite a benign appearance, MAC has a relentless destructive nature, spreading along nerves and vasculature into the subcutaneous muscle, cartilage, and blood vessel adventitia (39). One case demonstrated its ability to infiltrate bone and replace bone marrow elements (39,40). Differentiating between cysts, BCC, SCC, and other adnexal tumors is important because of MAC's potential for aggressive behavior (40). When a neoplasm presents in the nasolabial region and has the features of a syringoma, trichoadenoma, or a desmoplastic trichoepithelioma, the possibility of MAC must be considered. The tumor can of course occur in other areas of the head and neck region and, more rarely, elsewhere. A deep biopsy is necessary to study the base to ascertain an accurate diagnosis and should be requested if necessary.

Histologically, the neoplasm tends to be asymmetric and is broad rather than narrow (41). Typically, the tumor extends deep into the subcutis, which distinguishes it from syringoma and desmoplastic trichoepithelioma. There may or may not be contiguity with the epidermis. The tumor invades the perineural space, blood vessel walls, perichondrium, and periosteum. Characteristically, the tumor in the upper dermis forms squamoid cysts with central cornifying cells. In the mid-portion the tumor forms solid nests with central cells having pink cytoplasm and peripheral cells having clear cytoplasm. Near the base of the lesion tubules or duct-like structures are seen. These ducts contain eosinophilic secretion and are lined by dark cells which may have decapitation-like lining. The outer cells are pale. Atypia is not a feature of this lesion. Mitotic figures are not seen. The stroma is desmoplastic. The histogenesis of this neoplasm has not been established. Initially, it was thought to be eccrine and follicular in origin. The lesion is most likely a tumor showing apocrine differentiation and, as such, is pilosebaceous in origin.

The mainstay of treatment presently is wide surgical excision with histologically controlled 5-cm margins (39,40). Sixteen of 27 cases thus managed showed evidence of recurrence (40). With the Mohs technique, only one of six cases managed this way displayed evidence of recurrence (40). Adjuvant radiotherapy is being used; however, the overall cure rate has been unaffected (39). Radiation therapy is not effective alone (39). Recurrence develops in 59% of lesions, typically around 3 years postoperatively, but can occur from 5 months to 29 years later (39,40). Direct invasion is MAC's mode of recurrence. No lymphatic or distant metastasis has been reported (40).

Sebaceous Gland Carcinoma

Reported as early as 1865, SGC is a rare, aggressive malignancy that comprises 0.2% of all skin cancers (35,42). The etiologic basis for the tumor's development is unclear. A few reports of antecedent radiation therapy and arsenical skin cancers have been noted, while a stronger association is found between SGC and the Muir-Torre syndrome (see previous description of the latter) (35,42).

As its name implies, this tumor arises from various sebaceous glands throughout the body (43). Because of the density of sebaceous glands in the eyelid, 75% of cases are found there (42). SGC often originates in the Meibomian glands of the tarsus, the Zeis glands of the lid margin, or the pilosebaceous glands of the caruncle, eyebrow, and eyelid (35,42–44). Extraocular SGC does occur (43). The head and neck area is involved 75% of the time with 29% of these involving the parotid gland (43,45). Other, less common locations include the external genitalia, external auditory canal, trunk, and upper extremities (35,42,43,45). Clinically, 60- to 80-year-old Asian women are the prototype patients (42,43). They present with small (less than 6 mm), solitary, painless, pink to yellow nodules that slowly enlarge, sometimes up to 20 cm in the extraocular locations (42,43). The epidermis is usually intact, only occasionally becoming verrucous or ulcerated (35). Symptoms of tenderness, facial weakness, or bleeding may be present (43). The lesions can closely resemble conditions such as benign chalazions, blepharoconjunctivitis, keratoconjunctivitis, BCC, or SCC (35,42).

The tumors of the sebaceous gland have been divided into sebaceous adenomas, BCC with sebaceous differentiation (rare), and SGC. SGC has been classified on the basis of growth pattern into lobular, comedocarcinoma, papillary, and mixed types (42). It has also been classified on the basis of differentiation into squamoid, basaloid, adenoid, spindle cell, and differentiated types. Clearly, the diagnosis can be difficult. Malignancy can be recognized due to the lack of encapsulation, a vertical growth orientation, asymmetry, lack of cell cohesion, and a jagged outline. The tumor is often lobulated.

The diagnosis is based on evidence of sebaceous differentiation. The presence of cytoplasmic lipid supports the diagnosis. The tumor cells are arranged in varying sized nests and show septate vacuolization, which is evidence of sebaceous differentiation. The vacuoles impinge on the nucleus, which tends to be central. In undifferentiated areas the nuclei are crowded and atypical with mitotic figures. A clue in the absence of mature sebaceous cells is the presence of spaces in single cells. Necrosis en masse is another important feature.

This carcinoma begins in preexisting sebaceous glands and moves up the ducts into the epidermis, eventually invading the dermis. It is therefore analogous to mammary Paget's disease. Pagetoid spread is a feature of this disease in the ocular location and is helpful in the diagnosis. The cells tend to be vacuolated, have hyperchromatic nuclei, and splay singly through the epidermis. This pattern must be distinguished from melanosis, melanoma, Bowen's disease, and primary conjunctival carcinoma *in situ*. S-100 and HMB-45 immunohistochemical stains identify melanocytic cells. Mucin stains identify conjunctival carcinomas. Human milk fat globule stains help identify SGC as does a negative CEA (46). In extraocular sites the intraepidermal component of SGC has a bowenoid appearance. SGC must be distinguished from metastatic renal cell carcinoma, clear cell eccrine carcinomas, melanoma, clear cell sarcoma, and clear cell SCC.

Treatment of SGC in all locations involves wide surgical excision with 5- to 6-mm, histologically clear margins (35, 42,43,45). The rarity of this tumor, as with the Merkel cell carcinoma, has precluded extensive studies of optimal adjunctive treatment (42). Lymph node dissection is indicated in clinically suspicious or histologically proven lymphatic involvement (43). Radiation should not be employed alone in surgically accessible lesions, but it may be useful in recurrent, unresectable areas (42,43,45). Chemotherapy with intralesional 5-FU and doxorubicin is being studied, as is cryotherapy (42).

Recurrence, metastasis, and mortality are related to the site, duration, size, and histology of the tumor (35). For the ocular malignancies, 9% to 36% locally recur and 14% to 25% metastasize (42). Some 50% to 67% patients die within 5 years of the original diagnosis (43). Lymphatics, blood vessels, and the lacrimal secretory and excretory systems provide the means for metastasis (42). Most frequently, the preauricular, submandibular, and cervical lymph nodes are affected first, followed by distant dissemination to the lung, liver, bone, brain, and parotid gland (42). Mortality is highest in lesions found on the upper eyelids, duration longer than 6 months, size larger than 6 mm, and a histology showing multicentricity, poor differentiation or high grade, Pagetoid intraepithelial spread, infiltrative growth pattern, or angiolymphatic invasion (35,42). Extraocular SGC is less aggressive (42). Local recurrence is seen in 18% to 39%, with regional lymph node involvement in 13%, and distant dissemination in 10% to 15% (35,42).

Should the diagnosis of SGC be made, the initial and follow-up evaluations of the patient need to include a history and physical examination, especially of the lymph nodes. Chest x-ray, chemistries for electrolyte and liver function abnormalities, and a CBC should be obtained (42). Inquiring about and searching for Muir-Torre manifestations in the patient's personal and family history is critical (42). Because of Muir-Torre's strong association with internal malignancies, particularly with proximal colon cancer, full colonoscopy should be undertaken should the situation warrant (42). The sebaceous carcinomas that may occur among the multiple sebaceous neoplasms of the Muir-Torre syndrome do not metastasize, although the visceral malignancies may. Sometimes, a sebaceous carcinoma represents the only cutaneous manifestation of the syndrome.

Extramammary Paget's Disease

EMP was first described in 1889 (47). The cell of origin is felt to be from an apocrine gland (10,47). At an incidence of 0.2% per 100,000 per year, 62- to 65-year-old women are most commonly affected on their vulva (65%), perianal region (20%), or groin (47,48). Men can also develop the disease perianally, or on their penis, scrotum, or groin (47). Additional locations include mucous membranes, the buttocks, thighs, or axilla (47). In cases with axillary involvement, the genital area also may be affected (47).

Extramammary Paget's disease has the same clinical features as mammary Paget's disease except for its location (47). It typically presents as an erythematous, slightly elevated, eczematous patch that may crust, scale, ooze, ulcerate or bleed (10,47,48). In contrast to mammary Paget's, intense pruritus and pain are not uncommon (47,48). The average time from the appearance of the lesion to diagnosis may range from 1 month to 30 years (47). The appearance of an eczematous rash often leads to a delay in diagnosis resulting in more advanced lesions at the time of treatment. A typical patient's history would be a chronic, weepy eruption for months that has been unresponsive to multiple topical agents from several physicians. Conditions that clinically mimic EMP are fungal or candidal infections, eczematous dermatitis, lichen sclerosis et atrophicus, Bowen's disease, psoriasis, and seborrheic dermatitis (10,47,48) (Fig. 10-9).

Histologically, EMP is an intraepidermal malignancy with apocrine differentiation and has the ability to extend into underlying adnexal and dermal structures as an adenocarcinoma. This progression is associated with a poor prognosis. Microscopically, the involved epidermis is acanthotic and hyperkeratotic due to rubbing instigated by pruritus. The characteristic feature is the presence of Paget cells infiltrating singly or in groups throughout the epidermis. The cells are large, round, and have abundant cytoplasm which is clear,

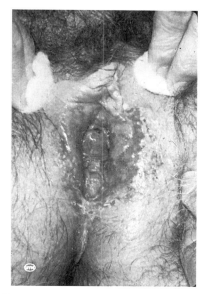

FIG. 10-9. Extramammary Paget's disease. A weepy inflammatory eruption of the vulva. The eruption is chronic, pruritic, and unresponsive to topical therapy. (Reprinted with permission from the American Academy of Dermatology.)

granular, or basophilic. The nuclei are hyperchromatic and have vesicular chromatin. A polymorphic inflammatory infiltrate is seen in the upper dermis. The cells contain mucin which can be stained by mucicarmine, PAS, Alcian blue at pH 2.5, or colloidal iron. Immunohistochemical stains are CEA, low molecular weight cytokeratin, and gross cystic disease fluid protein positive, which is indicative of glandular and apocrine differentiation (49).

The differential diagnosis for a Pagetoid growth pattern includes Pagetoid malignant melanoma and Bowen's disease. S-100 and HMB-45 positive stains help to identify melanoma, and high molecular weight cytokeratin with the presence of dyskeratotic cells helps to identify Bowen's disease. Early and accurate diagnosis of this disease should lower the mortality.

The standard of care for the cutaneous lesions of EMP is either Mohs micrographic surgery or wide surgical excision with 3-cm, pathologically evaluated margins (48). Because of its multifocality and occult peripheral extensions, some advocate that numerous punch biopsies be obtained from the nearby areas (47). Despite these practices, 12% to 61% of cases recur within 45 months (50). Lymph node dissection is a debatable issue. Generally, it is not done if there is evidence of epidermal and/or adnexal involvement alone (47). The contrary is true when the dermis is affected or lymph nodes are palpable on physical examination. Prophylactic dissection is of questionable value (47). Topical 5-FU is helpful in delineating the extent of the cutaneous disease and evaluating its recurrence (47,48). This chemical selectively produces necroses of tumor cells and leaves a visible area of inflammation which the physician can use to guide the scalpel. Systemic 5-FU is not a treatment option because of its inability to penetrate through to the neoplastic cells (47). Topical bleomycin, however, can and has resulted in a response in four of seven cases thus far (47). Radiation therapy has recently been found effective in five of five cases studied; yet, previous investigations indicated a high-risk of recurrence and 100% mortality when used alone (47). Furthermore, no chemotherapy has proven to be of benefit.

EMP is associated with underlying cutaneous adnexal adenocarcinomas such as apocrine, eccrine, Molls, and sebaceous and ceruminous gland carcinomas (48). In addition, 12% to 29% of cases are associated with regional internal carcinoma (with and without metastasis), mostly of GI and GU origin (47,48). Interestingly, the location of the EMP is closely related to the underlying cancer (47). For example, perianal EMP is seen with adenocarcinoma of the rectum; penile, scrotal and groin EMP are seen with male GU cancer (e.g., of the prostate, urethra or bladder) (47). Vulvar EMP is seen with female GU cancer (e.g., of the cervix, urethra, bladder, Bartholin's glands, or squamous cell of the vulva) (47). Rarely, EMP may occur as an extension of an adenocarcinoma either of the rectum to the perianal region, of the cervix to the vulva, or of the urinary bladder to the urethra, glans penis, or groin. Sometimes the Paget's disease, if chronic, can invade inward to the urinary tract or cervix.

An essential component of the treatment for EMP is the search for regional spread and underlying malignancy with thorough GI and GU evaluations (47,51). This includes pelvic and rectal examinations, barium enema, colonoscopy, IVP, and even cystoscopy if warranted. Prognosis is related to the underlying processes rather than to the EMP itself. When the lesion is confined to the epidermis and adnexal tissues alone, mortality is around 18% (47). When adjacent adnexal carcinoma or regionally proximate internal malignancy is evident, mortality ranges from 46% to 83%. When invasive carcinoma is present, mortality approaches 80% (47). Of note, perianal EMP carries a particularly grave prognosis, probably due to its rich lymphatic system and the ease of spread via this route (47). Regional internal cancer is found in 78% to 86% of perianal EMP, and 75% of these patients die (47). In contrast, those without perianal EMP have an overall 33% mortality (47).

ANGIOSARCOMA

AS is a malignant neoplasm composed of cells that show the morphological and functional properties of endothelium (35,51). Vascular neoplasms have been classified as angiomas that are benign variants, ASs that are malignant variants, and hemangioendotheliomas that are intermediate in their biologic behavior and in their appearance. Since it is not possible to distinguish the tumor cells as capillary or lymphatic endothelial in origin, the less definitive term of "angiosarcoma" is used by convention. Associated etiologic factors seem to be radiation, chronic lymphedema, long-standing A-V fistula, and foreign bodies (51).

Most ASs of the skin occur in three clinical settings: (a) AS of the face and scalp in the elderly, (b) AS secondary to chronic lymphedema, and (c) AS as a complication of radiation dermatitis:

a. AS can occur on the scalp or face of elderly White men (35). It is less common in Asians and rare in Blacks. It usually begins insidiously as an erythematous or bruise-like patch (51). The lesion quickly expands into a large ill-defined ecchymotic area (51). Induration, plaque formation, nodularity, or ulceration may subsequently develop (30,35,51–54). Satellite lesions and a surrounding erythema may occur (30,52–54). Sometimes pain, hemorrhage, edema, or secondary infection become a problem (30,35,51,54). Rapid, relentless infiltration results. Most patients die as a result of extensive aggressive local disease. Metastasis to lymph nodes or internal organs usually occurs as a very late complication. The differential diagnosis would include benign hemangiomas, KS, malignant melanoma, metastatic tumors, inflammatory dermatoses, trauma, and elder abuse (35,54). Usually, the very rapid progression of an ecchymotic area in an older White man on the upper face or scalp alerts the clinician to the diagnosis of AS. Early recognition is paramount since only a very small percentage of patients with lesions (usually less than 5 cm at presentation) can be successfully treated (55).

b. AS may follow chronic lymphedema (51). The most typical presentation is in women who have had long standing lymphedema of the arm following breast cancer (postmastectomy lymphangiosarcoma or the Stewart-Treves syndrome) (35,53,54). The tumor arises on the inner portion of the upper arm after lymphedema has been present for 10 years or more (52). The AS usually presents beyond the area of chronic radiation dermatitis, therefore excluding radiotherapy as an etiologic factor. Lymphedema-induced AS can also arise on the lower extremity from other causes besides cancer surgery such as congenital lymphedema or acquired tropical lymphedema from filariasis.

c. AS may occur postradiotherapy for internal cancer. The most common sites are the chest wall, breast, or lower abdomen following therapy for breast or gynecologic surgery. This type of AS may occur after severe trauma or ulceration. There are also reports of previous radiotherapy being an etiological factor in the AS of the head and neck region (52,53).

Histologically, ASs show variable differentiation and may tend to either extreme (56). The ASs encountered in each of the clinical settings described above are similar in appearance. In well-differentiated areas the tumor consists of irregular, anastomosing channels which dissect between collagen bundles of the dermis, adipocytes of the subcutis, or elements of the fascia. The channels are lined by a single layer of cells, some of which have large, hyperchromatic nuclei. The channels are usually bloodless, but they may contain extravasated erythrocytes.

In less differentiated areas, the endothelial cells tend to pile up and form intraluminal papillations. The vessels may form bizarre shapes and cribriform structures without fibrous stroma. In poorly differentiated areas the tumor forms solid sheets of pleomorphic epithelioid or spindle-shaped cells which have higher mitotic activity. Some more poorly differentiated tumors may have more differentiated areas which give a clue to the diagnosis. Very poorly differentiated tumors exist in which differentiation of the tumor may not be apparent. Tumors such as SCC, malignant melanoma, and fibrosarcomas may be confused with these variants.

In this situation, immunohistochemistry and EM may be useful in making the distinction. Endothelial cell differentiation may be evident by positive staining for factor VIII related antigen, CD 34 (human hematopoietic progenitor cell antigen), and, more specifically, CD 31 (platelet-endothelial cell adhesion molecule). Other stains such as S-100, HMB-45, and cytokeratin may help to distinguish other similar-appearing tumors.

Treatment is challenging because of the extremely aggressive behavior of the tumor, the occult invasion of surrounding tissue, and the tumor's multicentricity (35,51,52). Wide local surgery with margin control in combination with wide-field radiotherapy is the current recommendation (35,51, 52,54). Either option by itself portends a high recurrence rate (51). Some studies advocate a new surgical approach where the lesion is excised along with taking multiple punch biopsies of the surrounding tissue in an attempt to discover the clinically undetectable multifocal nests of cancer cells that are somewhat removed from the primary site (35,53). Prophylactic lymph node dissection is usually not advised since AS spreads directly or hematogenously (51,53). Radiation alone can be useful for palliation in patients who have advanced disease or for those who are unable to undergo surgery (35,52,54). Chemotherapy is not a viable option; doxorubicin, dactinomycin, and cisplatinum have all proven to be ineffective (35,51,54).

Despite treatment, AS has a very high rate of recurrence with 33% to 66% of patients with face and scalp tumors developing metastasis (35). Common destinations of dissemination include (in order of frequency): cervical lymph nodes, lung, liver, spleen, bone, kidney, and heart (30,35,53,54). Prognosis is dependent upon the cell type, grade, size, and site of origin (35,51). Tumors less than 5 cm or those located on the head, neck, or extremities fare better (35,51,53,54). Histologically, those displaying a lymphocytic infiltrate with only a mild degree of appendageal destruction have a slight advantage (35,54). Disappointingly, the overall survival rate for all ASs is 12% at 5 years, with over 50% of the patients dying within 15 months (51,53,54). Close follow-up is very important in the survivors (35). Recurrences as well as metastasis have been reported even years later (35).

KAPOSI'S SARCOMA

Described in 1872 by Moritz K. Kaposi as an "idiopathic multiple pigmented sarcoma of the skin," the origin of KS is still being debated today (53). Possible derivation from endothelial, lymphatic, or pluripotential mesenchymal cells are popular theories (54). Genetically, HLA type may be important (30,57). Infection with various viruses such as herpes, HPV, or mycoplasma has been proposed, yet the studies are inconsistent (30,54,57). Several recent cases have shown HSV type 8 in lesions (58). The evidence supporting an association of KS with other tumors is stronger, implying that immunosuppression plays a role (54). One third of patients with KS have or will develop a second primary cancer, and more than 50% of these are of lymphoreticular origin (e.g., lymphoma, leukemia, myeloma, mycosis fungoides, angioimmunoblastic lymphadenopathy) (30,54,57). Autoimmune diseases are also common in this population (59).

Until the late 1960s, KS occurred as an uncommon, slowly progressive, multifocal, vascular tumor arising in elderly White male patients of Mediterranean or Eastern European descent. This clinical pattern is now referred to as the "classic" form of the disease. Currently we recognize that KS is a very common tumor in tropical Africa and that it also is a hallmark of the acquired immunodeficiency syndrome (AIDS). In addition, the sarcoma can arise in association with other immunodeficiencies, especially drug-induced. Several unexplained features of KS still remain: genetic, epidemiologic, transmission, and pathogenesis.

There are four clinical subtypes of KS that differ in terms of the patients affected, clinical presentation, course, prognosis, and treatment options, as seen in Table 10-7 (57). The

TABLE 10–7. *Clinical characteristics of Kaposi sarcoma*

Type	Age (years)	Male/female ratio	Cutaneous lesions	Mucosal lesions	Lymph node involvement	Visceral involvement	Course	Survival
Classical	50–80	8–17:1	Plaques/nodules on distal legs/feet	Rare	Rare	Occasional	Slowly progressive over 10 to 15 years	10–15 years
Endemic (African) Nodular	25–40	17:1	Plaques/nodules, lower extremities	Rare	Rare	Rare	Slowly progressive	8–10 years
Florid	25–40	17:1	Nodules, widespread		Occasional	Occasional	Rapidly progressive	3–5 years
Infiltrating/ aggressive	25–50	17:1	Infiltrating exophytic nodules, lower extremities		Rare	Occasional	Locally invasive, destructive	5–8 years
Lymphadenopathic	1–10	1–3:1	None to few	None	Always	Usual	Rapid dissemination	1–3 years
Iatrogenic-immunosuppressed	12–83	2:1	Patches/plaques/ nodules, extremities	Frequent	Occasional	Occasional	Localized or rarely disseminate	Often improves after discontinuing immunosuppressant
Epidemic (AIDS)	18–65	50–100:1	Patches/plaques/ nodules anywhere	Frequent	Common	Common	Rapidly progressive	Depends on underlying disease

Adapted from Martin et al. (59).

classic form is an indolent, slow-growing vascular tumor seen in men aged 50 to 80 years old of Mediterranean or Eastern European origin (52–54,57). Ashkenazi Jews have a much higher incidence than the general population (52–54,57). This form presents as a single or multiple pink, red, purple, or blue-black macule on the lower extremity, with a predilection for the ankle and the plantar surface (30,52,53,57). These lesions enlarge and coalesce into thick angiomatous plaques or nodules which can become quite painful (30,52,53,57). Late in the course edema, ulceration, hemorrhage, or secondary infection may occur (53,57). Chronic edema and induration result in hyperkeratotic fibrotic plaques. The upper extremities may become involved as well; however, the head, neck, and mucosal membranes are rarely affected (30,52,57). Interestingly, spontaneous involution may ensue (52). Affected patients may survive 10 to 20 years, even when presenting at later stages with widespread cutaneous nodules. Visceral disease may occur, most commonly in the gastrointestinal tract (30,52,57). Suggestive suspicious symptoms include abdominal pain, GI bleeding, or diarrhea (59). Other areas that can become involved include the lungs (usually as a solitary pulmonary nodule seen radiographically), liver, conjunctiva, heart, adrenals, lymph nodes, and bone (52,57). These sites are often not discovered until autopsy.

The endemic form, found in sub-Saharan central African populations residing near the equator, represents 3% to 10% of all malignancies in this geographic location (57). There are five subtypes recognized: florid KS, nodular KS, lymphadenopathic KS, African cutaneous KS, and AIDS-associated African KS (57). Florid KS is seen in 25- to 40-year-old men and presents as disseminated nodules (57). The course is one of rapid deterioration and death within 3 to 5 years (57). Nodular KS is also seen in 25- to 40-year-old men and clinically resembles the classic form with lower extremity plaques and nodules that progress over 8 to 10 years (57). Lymphadenopathic KS is different. An aggressive tumor found in children less than 10 years old, the only evidence of disease may be located within the lymph nodes, sparing the skin (52,53,57). Occasionally, eyelids, conjunctiva, and salivary glands are affected, causing extreme morbidity to the individuals (57). Life expectancy is less than 2 years (52). African cutaneous KS is a locally invasive and destructive tumor of 20- to 50-year-old men. Lower extremity infiltrating, exophytic nodules, or vascular lesions are the hallmarks (57). Although extensive leg edema and bony erosion can occur, visceral involvement is uncommon (57). Survival ranges from 5 to 8 years (57). AIDS-associated African KS has only recently been recognized and resembles the epidemic form that will be described below (57).

Epidemic or AIDS-associated KS is seen in HIV+ males and represents the most common neoplasm in the AIDS population of the United States and Europe (57). KS is the AIDS defining manifestation in 15% of HIV patients (57). Specific groups within this population are at a higher risk for the tumor. Homosexual males, IV drug abusers, African-Americans who have received blood transfusions, and individuals with con-

current lymphoma seem to be prone to KS (57). The lesions begin as solitary to multiple, red to blue macules with asymmetric borders and surrounding white halos on the trunk, head, neck, or mucous membranes (particularly, the palate and gingiva) (30,35,53,57). Thicker patches evolve into plaques, papules and nodules with diameters of less than 1 cm (30,53). Local pruritus, burning, pain, edema, and ulceration may develop as may systemic symptoms of fever, anorexia, lymphadenopathy, and splenomegaly. Twenty-five percent of the sarcomas manifest solely within the skin, while 29% manifest solely within the viscera, commonly the GI tract (50%), lymph nodes (50%), and lungs (37%) (52,57). Pulmonary nodules can occlude the airways causing respiratory distress, failure, and death (57). The clinical features of the AIDS-related KS differ from the classic disease in their appearance (the former are smaller and flatter), the rapid evolution of the lesions, truncal distribution, and mucosal involvement. Visceral involvement is often not apparent clinically during life, but it is very common at autopsy. Visceral lesions can occur without cutaneous lesions. Death is usually secondary to AIDS-related complications (i.e., opportunistic infections) rather than to the direct effect of the KS itself (52) (Figs. 10-10 and 10-11).

The iatrogenic immunocompromised form of KS is seen in patients taking immunosuppressants, especially renal transplant patients using prednisone, azathioprine, or cyclosporin, and in individuals who have received radiation therapy (53, 57). The age range is wide, and the usual lesions are patches, plaques or nodules found on the extremities or mucous membranes with occasional lymph node or visceral involvement (57). Typically occurring 10 to 22 months postsurgery, 0.4% to 4% of renal transplant patients develop KS (57). Fifty percent of their deaths are attributable to the tumor, in contrast to the AIDS-related KS (57). A longer onset of disease is characteristic in the chronically immunosuppressed or irradiated subgroups, commonly around 41 months later. A peculiarity of this type of KS is the frequent regression or apparent cure on discontinuation of the immunosuppressant therapy (57). Also, the male-dominant ratio is much smaller.

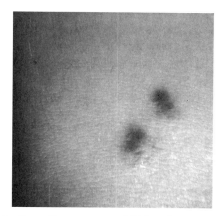

FIG. 10-10. Kaposi's sarcoma in AIDS patient. Purple soft nodules on the trunk.

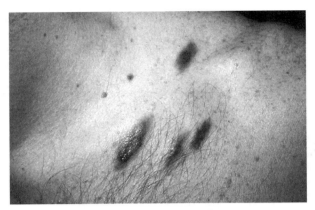

FIG. 10-11. Kaposi's sarcoma. Hemorrhagic nodules on the chest of a patient with AIDS. (Reprinted with permission from the American Academy of Dermatology.)

A wide differential must be considered when viewing the suspicious lesions of KS, which includes pyogenic granulomas, melanoma, hemangioma, glomus tumors, lymphoma, dermatofibroma, inflammatory dermatoses, ecchymosis, insect bites, AS, and trauma (35,54). Staging is important when considering treatment (57). Stage I includes cutaneous, locally indolent lesions, typical of classical KS (57). Stage II designates cutaneous, locally aggressive lesions with or without lymph node involvement (57). Stage III refers to mucocutaneous, generalized lesions with or without lymph node involvement, and in stage IV are found visceral lesions (57). A and B indicate constitutional symptomatology; A implies none, while B implies weight loss, night sweats, fever, etc. (57).

There is no difference in the histological appearance of KS in each of the clinical groups (56). The macular stage is perhaps seen more frequently in the AIDS-associated variant. The macular, plaque, and nodular stages all have corresponding histological characteristics. Early in the macular stage there is a proliferation of small capillary-like vessels surrounding larger, dilated postcapillary-like venular structures. A loose ramifying network of jagged vessels then appears and tends to separate collagen bundles. When preexisting vessels protrude into these ectatic new vessels, the pattern is termed the "promontory sign." A sparse infiltrate of lymphocytes with plasma cells is a helpful clue to the diagnosis. This stage may resemble well-differentiated AS, but the cytologic atypia is absent. This stage is difficult to recognize and may be overlooked or misdiagnosed.

The plaque stage is characterized by a more extensive proliferation of vessels that now pervade the dermis and extend into the subcutis. This lesion is slightly elevated above the skin surface. Cord-like vascular structures and a bland spindled cell component now appear in the vicinity of the proliferating vessels. PAS-positive diastase-resistant intracytoplasmic hyaline globules are now seen in areas of dense infiltrate. These globules are characteristic and are probably derived from effete erythrocytes. The globules are seen more frequently in AIDS-associated KS.

With time, the spindle cell foci coalesce to form fascicles and create the diagnostic nodular stage of KS. The spindle cell fascicles arc and intersect in the manner of a fibrosarcoma. A honeycombed network of endothelial-lined slitlike spaces containing erythrocytes separate the spindle cells, a diagnostic feature not seen in fibrosarcoma. Extavasated erythrocytes are also seen. The spindle cells shown by marker studies are endothelial-derived. CD 34 and 31 stains highlight the honeycomb pattern of vascular structures, which is an important diagnostic feature not seen in most angiomas. Dilated vessels, hemosiderin pigment, and inflammatory cells are seen at the periphery of the nodules. The hyaline globules are more frequent at this stage. In aggressive late stage lesions, tumor cells may be more pleomorphic and cytologically atypical with frequent mitotic figures.

Multiple treatment options are available. Due to the multifocal, aggressive, and recurrent nature of KS, no treatment has been curative. Local control can be achieved in classical, endemic, or epidemic KS if the lesions are unsightly, painful, or invasive (57). Local therapy includes radiation, excisional surgery, cryotherapy, or intralesional chemotherapy (35,53,57,58). Sclerosing agents, interferon alpha or recombinant granulocyte macrophage colony stimulating factor, or topical ointment applications with tretinoin or bleomycin also have been tried (58). Local excision can be beneficial for selected troublesome lesions at selected sites (oral, eyelid, penis) or very painful lesions. KS is radiosensitive (30). Radiotherapy has been successful in attaining 85% remission for 10 to 92 months (30). Radiation appears best suited for problems caused by mass effects such as large intraoral lesions or localized lymphedema of the extremities or penis, and can aid in palliation of pain, limiting edema and cosmetic disfigurement (57). However, the skin may become blistered, inflammatory, or desquamative while mucous membrane treatments may result in mucositis with candidal or herpetic superinfections (58). Cryotherapy has an 85% complete or partial response rate lasting up to 6 months for the majority of patients (60).

Systemic or perfusion chemotherapy has also been used successfully with the vinca alkaloids actinomycin and doxorubicin (30,35,52). Ninety percent of classical KS has a complete response, while only 15% of epidemic KS does (30). Combination chemotherapy has produced better short-term results, but overall survival is unchanged (57). Interferon alpha is becoming popular by inducing remission in 40% of cases by unknown mechanisms—perhaps via immune modulation or antiviral effects (35,52,57). Classic and endemic KS have shown the best responses to interferon alpha; however, the doses required in the epidemic form are too high to be considered safe (58). Frequent side effects include a flu-like syndrome, anorexia, nausea, depression, anemia, and laboratory abnormalities (57,58). Future possibilities for treatment include targeted drug delivery in which chemotherapeutic agents are encapsulated liposomally for superior tissue penetration, anti-angiogenesis factors that inhibit neovascularization, Paclitaxel chemotherapy that inhibits microtubule assembly within neoplastic cells, cytokine inhibitors and autologous CD8 T cells, and IL2 (58). Spontaneous remission has been reported in 2% of the patients (30,35).

Prognosis is related more to the clinical picture than to the staging. Cutaneous plaques or nodules appearing quickly, lymph node or visceral involvement, patient age less than 45 years old, CD4 counts less than 300, opportunistic infections, hematologic abnormalities, clinical symptoms, and an elevated sedimentation rate all portend a poor prognosis (57). If KS directly contributes to death, it is usually secondary to its visceral complications, with GI and pulmonary obstructions being the most common (59).

SOFT TISSUE SARCOMAS

Although rare, cutaneous soft tissue sarcomas (STS) form an important category of malignancies in the skin. Examples include dermatofibrosarcoma protuberans (DFSP), atypical fibroxanthoma (AFX), malignant fibrous histiocytoma (MFH), and cutaneous leiomyosarcoma. All these tumors have a high recurrence rate when removed with standard excisional surgery and may metastasize. All STS are staged according to grade, size, and evidence of metastatic disease by the American Joint Committee on Cancer Staging (53). Local STS are stage I if well differentiated, stage II if moderately differentiated, and stage III if poorly differentiated. A and B designations within each stage denote size: A is less than or equal to 5 cm, while B is greater than 5 cm. Stage IVA signifies regional lymph node metastasis, and stage IVB distant metastasis. All these characteristics are important prognostically as is the location of the tumor and the depth of invasion (53). Wide excision and surgical techniques involving meticulous surgical margin control appear to be the most effective treatments (61).

Dermatofibrosarcoma Protuberans

DFSP begins as a solitary, indurated plaque of variable color (ranging from fleshy to violet), usually on the trunk (chest and shoulders) of young adults (35,53,61–63). Other common locations include the proximal extremities and the head and neck (35,62). The tumor's nonspecific features and indolent behavior often cause it to be overlooked by the patient or physician. Over a time frame of months to years, the lesion enlarges to 1 to 5 cm in diameter, and multiple firm nodules can form within the original plaque (30,61,62). At this point, the once asymptomatic area may ulcerate, bleed, or become quite painful (35,62). Although it remains free from underlying subcutaneous tissue, it is commonly fixed to the overlying layers (30,62). Beneath the skin, the cancerous cells spread like tentacles, projecting centrifugally, invading between collagen bundles and into fat, fascia, muscle, nerves, blood vessels, and even bone (61–63). It is this occult infiltration that accounts for DFSP's high rate of recurrence and is the reason that differentiating it from benign dermatofibromas and keloids is important. Other entities that can appear similar include morpheaform BCC, fibrosarcoma, localized scleroderma, and nodular fasciitis (35,61,63).

DFSP is a spindle cell neoplasm of intermediate malignancy. Despite the clinical appearance of a circumscribed lesion, dermatofibrosarcoma diffusely infiltrates the dermis and subcutis. In the plaque-like areas the neoplasm consists of slender, monotonous-appearing, fibroblast-like, spindle cells which spread between and replace preexisting collagen bundles. The cells proliferate in a multilayered fashion parallel to the skin surface. There is usually a Grenz zone and the epidermis may be atrophic. There is little pleomorphism and mitotic activity is low. The infiltration extends into the subcutis in an intimate pattern between adipocytes, giving a lacy or honeycomb pattern. There is a multilayered orientation of cells parallel to the skin surface as well as in the dermis. Secondary cells such as giant cells, xanthoma cells, and inflammatory cells are rare.

In the nodular areas of the tumor, the cells grow in a more storiform pattern centered around inconspicuous vessels. The cells in these areas are also bland and slender or neural-like. The cells are CD 34 positive and factor XIIIa negative, which distinguishes them from dermatofibromas or fibrous histiocytomas. The latter tumors have the reverse staining properties. These staining characteristics and EM studies suggest that the cells of DSFP are derived from perineurial cells. Another helpful distinction is that dermatofibromas and cellular dermatofibromas either have a pushing margin at the dermal-subcuticular interface or have a radial or wedge-shaped extension into the subcutis along fibrous septae which define the lobular architecture of the subcutis. There is frequently a lymphocytic infiltrate as well. In contrast, DFSP infiltrates the subcuticular lobule diffusely.

A most important aspect of the tumor is its tendency to infiltrate at its margins in a deceptively bland manner. This is because the cells are attenuated and not as plentiful. This makes evaluation of the margin difficult, and if the tumor cells are not recognized as such, incomplete excision may result with eventual recurrence. There are variants of DFSP which have cells containing melanin pigment known as the Bednar tumor, and tumors which have a myxoid appearance due to the presence of abundant mucopolysaccharides. The latter tumor may be mistaken for a myxoid liposarcoma. The absence of chicken-wire vessels and lipoblasts helps to make the distinction. Rarely, DFSP may have fibrosarcomatous areas or areas typical of MFH characterized by pleomorphism, necrosis, and high mitotic activity in the latter case. If these areas exceed 10% of the tumor mass, the lesions are more likely to behave like the more malignant tumors, particularly with regard to metastasis.

Treatment of DFSP has been constantly evolving as the aggressive nature of the tumor has been elucidated. The growth pattern of DFSP supports the need for resection of skeletal muscle fascia to remove the deep tumor mass. Mohs microscopic surgery allows the surgeon to trace out the multiple finger-like tumor extensions (63). This modality ensures complete margin examination and opportunity to discover neoplastic projections beyond the surgical site (63). In addition, excising only tumor-involved tissue spares healthy tissue, allowing simpler reconstruction and less disfigurement. Wide excision with a 3-cm margin was found to be inferior to Mohs in multiple trials (61,62). In worldwide studies, the average recurrence rate following Mohs was 0.6%, with a total recurrence rate of 1.6% (62). In comparison, when treated with wide surgical excision, the average recurrence rate was 18%, with the total recurrence rate of 20% (62). Furthermore, when treated with excision of undefined or conservative margins, the average recurrence rate was 43%, with the total recurrence rate of 44% (62). Radiation therapy can play an adjunctive role to surgery when residual disease is evident or when excision is impractical because of the severe functional or cosmetic loss that would ensue on areas that are difficult to treat, such as the face (35,53,61). Chemotherapy is not useful, even in metastatic disease (53,61,62).

Dissemination is rare and is found in less than 5% of cases (35,53,62). The primary mode of spread is hematogenous and the primary site for spread is to the lungs (in 75% of patients with metastatic disease) (30,35,53,61,62). The lymph nodes are the second most common destination (in 25% of patients with metastatic disease) (30,35,53,61). Typically, multiple recurrences are evident preceding the development of distant metastasis (35,62). Once metastasis is present, death is imminent within 2 to 4 years (53,62).

Careful follow-up is of utmost importance in this aggressive and potentially fatal tumor (30). Current recommendations include frequent office visits every 3 to 6 months after surgery, and then annually for life (62).

Atypical Fibroxanthoma

AFX is identical in appearance to the pleomorphic variant of MFH and is considered to be a superficial form of this tumor (53,61,64). Due to its low grade malignant behavior as a superficial tumor, the name AFX has been retained for this subtype of the neoplasm. The tumor is seen in two clinical settings: on the head and neck (particularly the nose, ear, and cheek) of elderly people and on the limbs and trunk of young people (30,53,61). MFH occurs more typically in the retroperitoneum and in the deep tissues of the thigh and buttock. Solar radiation is believed to be the predisposing factor for AFX (53,61). As the lesion grows, it may erode the skin and cause hemorrhage. Important to differentiate clinically here are SCC, BCC, epidermoid cyst, and ulcerating pyogenic granuloma (30,61,64).

Histologically, AFX is an exophytic, unencapsulated, densely cellular tumor that can ulcerate the epidermis by pressure atrophy and can invade the subcutis (65). It does not invade muscle and fascia. It is composed of unusual appearing cells that can be haphazard or fascicular in arrangement. Generally, a storiform pattern is not seen. The cells are spindle-shaped fibroblasts, or round to polygonal histiocyte-like cells. They are usually pleomorphic and some multinucleated forms are seen. The cells may be vacuolated and contain lipid or hemosiderin. The nuclei can be atypical and numerous mitotic figures are evident. Inflammatory cells and blood vessels are also components of the tumor. EM indicates the tumor is composed of histiocytic, fibroblastic, and myofibroblastic cells.

The major problem with this tumor is distinguishing it from MFH and other malignant tumors such as spindle SCC,

leiomyosarcoma, metastatic renal cell carcinoma, malignant schwannoma, and malignant melanoma. MFH is diagnosed when tumors involve the subcutis extensively, involve the fascia and deep muscle, undergo necrosis, or invade vascular structures. Melanoma is recognized by display of S-100 and/or HMB-45 antigens. Cytokeratin is useful in recognizing SCC. Morphology, actin, and desmin stains are used to distinguish leiomyosarcoma.

The treatment of AFX is surgical excision with 1-cm margins and dissection into the subcutaneous tissue (30,53,61). Mohs surgery is gaining popularity and may soon become the standard of care (53,61). Full pathologic evaluation must be conducted due to the resemblance of AFX to MFH (53). The latter is a much more aggressive tumor and must be dealt with differently, as will be explained below. Because of the need for treatment to extend into deeper layers of skin, electrodesiccation with curettage is not recommended (53).

The risk of recurrence and metastasis in AFX is low, ranging from 5% to 7%, due to its superficial location (30). Reports of lymph node involvement and dissemination have been noted, especially in those tumors that demonstrate recurrence, vascular or deep tissue invasion, necrosis on biopsy, or inadequate surgical margins (53).

Malignant Fibrous Histiocytoma

As its name implies, both fibroblastic and histiocytic differentiation are evident microscopically, implying that this tumor is derived from a primitive mesenchymal stem cell (63). Despite its being the most common STS of adulthood, risk factors for its development are minimal (35). UV light does not play a significant role, although radiation exposure may (53).

Clinically, MFH is found in White males between 50 and 70 years old (35). It arises in the skeletal muscle of the extremities, especially the thigh and buttock (30). Some 10% of cases are located in the head and neck region (53). Frequently asymptomatic, the lesion may be multinodular and fleshy and may grow to 4 to 10 cm within months (53,63). Fever and leukocytosis may be present (35,53,63). Patients with retroperitoneal tumors can experience additional systemic manifestations, such as weight loss, fatigue, and abdominal pain (35,53,63). DFSP, AFX, other sarcomas (such as liposarcomas and rhabdomyosarcomas), hemangiomas, hematomas, and venous thrombosis need to be excluded from the differential diagnosis (30,35,63).

The tumors can be classified into four subtypes. These include the storiform-pleomorphic type, the myxoid type, the giant cell type, and the inflammatory type. The morphology of the storiform-pleomorphic type has been described in the section on AFX, and the criteria for distinguishing primary cutaneous MFH from AFX were discussed. In MFH, by comparison, a storiform pattern is almost always present and is not typically seen in AFX. This can also be an important distinguishing factor.

The myxoid variant can be very problematic as it can arise deeply on the extremities and mimic a cutaneous neoplasm or myxomatous lesion. The key features include a tendency for the spindle tumor cells to anchor to the potentially numerous curvilinear blood vessels. Typically, there will be cellular, pleomorphic foci with a storiform pattern which help make the diagnosis. The giant cell variant contains numerous osteoclast-like giant cells with vesicular nuclei and cellular areas resembling the pleomorphic variant of MFH. The inflammatory type is characterized by sheets of neutrophils and benign and malignant xanthoma cells phagocytosing neutrophils. Areas with very few tumor cells make the diagnosis difficult. Identifying areas with spindle cells and storiform pattern help to establish the diagnosis.

Current treatment recommendations include Mohs surgery in only the most superficial lesions and wide, deep surgical excision with margins of at least 3 to 5 cm in all other tumors. Unless clinically indicated, lymph node dissection is not routine. Amputation has even been used, albeit rarely, without prognostic significance. Pre- and postoperative radiation therapy has been employed in the treatment since STS are relatively radioresponsive (35,53). Adjuvant chemotherapy with doxorubicin has shown some promise in a National Cancer Institute study; whether this becomes widely accepted is yet to be seen (53).

Despite these aggressive therapies, local recurrence and metastatic dissemination rates of 40% to 45% are seen (35,53). Clinically, the tumors appear localized. However, the microscopic pattern is often infiltrative along fascial planes and between muscle fibers, causing the high rate of local recurrence. These complications are usually evident within 24 months following surgery, with a 2-year survival of 60% for all cases (30,53). The most common site for distant disease is the lung, followed by the lymph nodes, liver, and bone (30,53). The most important factor in morbidity and mortality is the depth of the tumor. Those superficially limited recur in 30% and metastasize in less than 10%; tumors extending to the fascia metastasize in 30% (35,63). MFH that is deep-seated and invades muscle recurs in 54% and metastasizes in 40% to 50% of patients (35,63). The size and location are also important; the smaller, more distal tumors are prognostically more favorable (53,63). Five-year survival rates of 28% are seen in the proximal, usually deeper lesions versus 73% in the distal, usually superficial ones (63). Surprisingly, histologic features, such as the number of mitoses and degree of anaplasia, add little predictive value (53,63). The myxoid and angiomatoid subtypes do fare somewhat better, particularly if there is a significant inflammatory response surrounding the area (35,53,63). Clinical evaluation of the lymphatics as well as a chest x-ray, sometimes even a CT scan of the chest in high-risk MFH, are warranted both preoperatively and during follow-up (53).

Leiomyosarcoma

Cutaneous leiomyosarcoma has its origin in smooth muscle. It can be divided into two groups: tumors arising from arrector pili muscles confined to the dermis and tumors arising from blood vessels in the subcutis (61,63,66). Those confined

to the dermis have a good prognosis with metastasis occuring very rarely. Subcutaneous leiomyosarcomas, on the other hand, have a guarded prognosis with a higher rate of metastasis. This distinction is important when deciding upon therapy and assessing prognosis (66). The etiologic basis for this disease is unknown; however, possible risk factors contributing to its development include antecedent trauma or radiation (53,66).

Clinically, these tumors present in middle-aged (40 to 60 years old) White men as solitary, round to oval nodules that gradually enlarge (61,63,66). Up to 80% to 90% of patients have complaints of pain in the area, especially when pressure is applied (63). Other symptoms include pruritus, burning, and even bleeding (66). The hair bearing extensor surface of the proximal lower extremities (i.e., the thigh) is the most common location for cutaneous leiomyosarcoma (53,61, 66). Some 50% to 75% of lesions are found on the legs; 20% to 30% on the arms; 10% to 15% on the trunk; 1% to 5% on the face (66). The skin overlying the cutaneous tumors can be erythematous and frequently adherent to the underlying (less than 2 cm) mass (66). In subcutaneous leiomyosarcomas, the skin can be umbilicated or discolored, but is often nonadherent to the underlying, typically 5-cm mass (53,61). The differential diagnosis of cutaneous leiomyosarcoma may include many entities: BCC, SCC, dermatofibromas, lipomas, neurofibromas, cysts, fibrosarcomas, schwannomas, and MFH (61,63,66). Biopsy with specific staining techniques is very useful.

Cutaneous leiomyosarcomas tend to consist of nodular aggregates of spindle cells arranged in interlacing fascicles. At the edge of the tumor, the cells infiltrate between collagen bundles (67). The cells have eosinophilic, fibrillar cytoplasm corresponding myofilaments which stain positively for smooth muscle specific actin and desmin. The nuclei tend to be elongated and have blunt ends. Giant cells may be seen, but pleomorphism is not common, and the tumors are usually well- to moderately well-differentiated. Hemorrhage, necrosis, and hyalinization are not encountered. The histologic criteria used to diagnose malignancy include high cellularity, some atypism with plump, hyperchromatic nuclei, a mitotic rate of at least 2 mitotic figures per 10 high-power fields, and depth of invasion.

Subcutaneous leiomyosarcomas have a similar appearance to cutaneous variants. There may be more pleomorphism. These tumors tend to have dilated, thin-walled blood vessels which are surrounded by smooth muscle cells. The depth of invasion is important, and when the fascia or muscle is invaded, the potential for recurrence and metastasis is high.

Treatment and prognosis are closely related to the depth of the neoplastic process, its size, grade, and DNA content (63,66). Dermal leiomyosarcoma can be treated conservatively with local excision (63). Up to 30% to 40% will recur locally, at which time wide excision needs to be undertaken (53,63,66). Recurrence usually follows within 36 months of the initial surgery (66). Less than 10% of cutaneous tumors metastasize (53,66). Subcutaneous leiomyosarcoma, however, has a more aggressive and infiltrating nature which requires wide excision initially with 3- to 5-cm lateral margins and extension vertically into the underlying fascia (53,61, 63,66). Up to 40% to 50% of these will recur, while 30% to 40% metastasize (53,66). Dissemination is hematogenous, frequently involving the lungs (53,63). Radiation and chemotherapy results have not been studied adequately due to the rarity of this disease (63,53). At this time, these forms of treatment are not felt to be useful, even as adjuncts. Death is not uncommon in cutaneous leiomyosarcoma. Overall, the 5-year survival rate is 64% (53).

REFERENCES

1. Miller DL, Weinstock MA. Nonmelanoma skin cancer in the United States: incidence. *J Am Acad Dermatol* 1994;30:774.
2. Goldberg LH. Basal cell carcinoma [Review]. *Lancet* 1996;347:663.
3. Grande DJ, Ratner D, Stadecker MJ. Basal cell carcinoma. In: Roenigk RK, Roenigk HH Jr, eds. *Roenigk and Roenigk's dermatologic surgery.* 2nd ed. New York: Marcel Dekker, 1996:489.
4. Melton JL, Hanke CW. Squamous cell carcinoma. In: Roenigk RK, Roenigk HH Jr, eds. *Roenigk and Roenigk's dermatologic surgery.* 2nd ed. New York: Marcel Dekker, 1996:503.
5. Preston DS, Stern RS. Nonmelanoma cancers of the skin [Review]. *N Engl J Med* 1992;327:1649.
6. Marks R. Squamous cell carcinoma [Review]. *Lancet* 1996;347:735.
7. Hacker SM, Browder JF, Ramos-Caro FA. Basal cell carcinoma [Review]. *Postgrad Med* 1993;93:101.
8. Miller SJ. Biology of basal cell carcinoma (Part II) [Review]. *J Am Acad Dermatol* 1991;24:161.
9. Johnson TM, Rowe DE, Nelson BR, Swanson NA. Squamous cell carcinoma of the skin (excluding skin and oral mucosa) [Review]. *J Am Acad Dermatol* 1992;26:467.
10. Safai B. Cancers of the skin. In: De Vita VT, Hellman S, Rosenberg SA, eds. *Cancer: principles and practices of oncology.* 4th ed. Philadelphia: Lippincott–Raven Publishers, 1993:1567.
11. Miller, SJ. Biology of basal cell carcinoma (Part I) [Review]. *J Am Acad Dermatol* 1991;24:1.
12. Lang PG Jr, Maize JC. Basal cell carcinoma. In: Friedman RJ, Rigel D, Kopf AW, Harris MN, Baker D, eds. *Cancer of the skin.* Philadelphia: WB Saunders, 1991:46.
13. Farmer ER, Helwig EB. Metastatic basal cell carcinoma: a clinicopathologic study of seventeen cases. *Cancer* 1980;46:748.
14. Barrett, Terry. High risk tumors—clinical and histopathological considerations. Presented at the American Academy of Dermatology Focus Session, San Diego, March 23–24, 1997.
15. Fleming ID, Amonette R, Monaghan T, Fleming MD. Principles of management of basal and squamous cell carcinoma of the skin [Review]. *Cancer* 1995;75[Suppl 2]:669.
16. Luce EA. Oncologic considerations in nonmelanotic skin cancer [Review]. *Clin Plast Surg* 1995;22:39.
17. Lawrence CM. Mohs surgery of basal cell carcinoma—a critical review. *Br J Plast Surg* 1993;46:599.
18. Kirkham N. Tumors and cysts of the epidermis. In: Elder D, Elenitsas E, Jaworsky C, et al., eds. *Lever's histopathology of the skin.* 8th ed. Philadelphia: Lippincott–Raven Publishers, 1997:685.
19. Sober AJ, Burstein JM. Precursors to skin cancer [Review]. *Cancer* 1995;75[Suppl 2]:645.
20. Otley CC, Lim KK, Roenigk RK. Cure rates for cancer of the skin: basal cell carcinoma, squamous cell carcinoma, melanoma and soft tissue sarcoma. In: Roenigk RK, Roenigk HH Jr, eds. *Roenigk and Roenigk's dermatologic surgery.* 2nd ed. New York: Marcel Dekker, 1996:745.
21. Goldschmidt H, Breneman JC, Breneman DL. Ionizing radiation therapy in dermatology [Review]. *J Am Acad Dermatol* 1994;30:157.
22. Robinson JK. Mohs micrographic surgery [Review]. *Clin Plast Surg* 1993;20:149.
23. Rapini RP. Pitfalls of Mohs micrographic surgery [Review]. *J Am Acad Dermatol* 1990;22:681.
24. Carter DM, Lin An. Basal cell carcinoma. In: Fitzpatrick TB, et al., eds. *Dermatology in general medicine.* 4th ed. New York: McGraw-Hill, 1993:840.
25. Patterson JA, Geronemus RG. Cancers of the skin. In: De Vita VT, Hellman S, Rosenberg SA, eds. *Cancer: principles and practices of oncology.* 4th ed. Philadelphia: Lippincott–Raven Publishers, 1993:1469.
26. Callen JP. Possible precursors to epidermal malignancies. In: Friedman RJ, Rigel D, Kopf AW, Harris MN, Baker D, eds. *Cancer of the skin.* Philadelphia: WB Saunders, 1991:27.
27. Kwa RE, Campana K, Moy RL. Biology of cutaneous squamous cell carcinoma [Review]. *J Am Acad Dermatol* 1992;26:1.
28. Broders AC. Squamous epithelioma of the skin. *Ann Surg* 1921;73:141.
29. Schwartz R. Keratoacanthoma. *J Am Acad Dermatol* 1994;30:1.
30. Caro WA, Bronstein BR. Tumors of the skin. In: Moschella SL, Hurley HJ, eds. *Dermatology.* 2nd ed. Philadelphia: WB Saunders, 1985:1533.
31. Allen CA, Stephens M, Steel WM. Subungual keratoacanthoma. *Histopathology* 1994;25:181–183.
32. Hodak E, Jones RE, Ackerman AB. Solitary keratoacanthoma is a squamous cell carcinoma: three examples with metastasis [Review]. *Am J Dermatopathol* 1993;15:332.
33. Netscher DT, Wigoda P, Green LK, Spira M. Keratoacanthoma: when to observe and when to operate and the importance of accurate diagnosis. *South Med J* 1994;87:1272.
34. O'Connor WJ, Brodland DG. Markel cell carcinoma [Review]. *Dermatol Surg* 1996;22:262.
35. Marenda SA, Otto RA. Adnexal carcinomas of the skin [Review]. *Otolaryngol Clin North Am* 1993;26:87.
36. Andrew JE, Silvers DN, Lattes R. Merkel cell carcinoma. In: Friedman RJ, Rigel D, Kopf AW, Harris MN, Baker D, eds. *Cancer of the skin.* Philadelphia: WB Saunders, 1991:288.
37. Haag ML, Glass LF, Fenske NA. Merkel cell carcinoma. Diagnosis and treatment [Review]. *Dermatol Surg* 1995;21:669.
38. Ratner D, Nelson BR, Brown MD, Johnson TM. Merkel cell carcinoma [Review]. *J Am Acad Dermatol* 1993;29:143.
39. Sebastien TS, Nelson BR, Lowe L, Baker S, Johnson TM. Microcystic adnexal carcinoma [Review]. *J Am Acad Dermatol* 1993;29:840.
40. Billingsley EM, Fedok Fred, Maloney ME. Microcystic adnexal carcinoma: case report and review of the literature [Review]. *Arch Otolaryngol Head Neck Surg* 1996;122:179.
41. LeBoit PE, Sexton M. Microcystic adnexal carcinoma of the skin. A reappraisal of the differentiation and differential diagnosis of an underrecognized neoplasm. *J Am Acad Dermatol* 1993;29:609.
42. Nelson BR, Hamlet KR, Gillard M, Railan D, Johnson TM. Sebaceous carcinoma [Review]. *J Am Acad Dermatol* 1995;33:1.
43. Barlet JW, Zimmerman MC, Arnstein DP, Wollman JS, Mickel RA. Sebaceous carcinoma of the head and neck. Case report and literature review [Review]. *Arch Otolaryngol Head Neck Surg* 1992;118:1245.
44. Hashimoto K. Adnexal carcinoma of the skin. In: Friedman RJ, Rigel D, Kopf AW, Harris MN, Baker D, eds. *Cancer of the skin.* Philadelphia: WB Saunders, 1991:209.
45. Fitzpatrick JE, Golitz LE. Unusual tumors. In: Roenigk RK, Roenigk HH Jr, eds. *Roenigk and Roenigk's dermatologic surgery.* 2nd ed. New York: Marcel Dekker, 1996:585.
46. Ansai S, Hashimoto H, Aoki T, Hozumi Y, Aso K. A histochemical and immunohistochemical study of extra-ocular sebaceous carcinoma. *Histopathology* 1993;22:127.
47. Lupton GP, Graham JH. Mammary and extramammary Paget's desease. In: Friedman RJ, Rigel D, Kopf AW, Harris MN, Baker D, eds. *Cancer of the skin.* Philadelphia: WB Saunders, 1991:217.
48. Epidermal nevi, neoplasms, and cysts. In: Arnold HL Jr, Odom RB, James WD, eds. *Andrews' diseases of the skin: clinical dermatology.* 8th ed. Philadelphia: WB Saunders, 1990:745.
49. Helm KF, Goellner JR, Peters MS. Immunohistochemical stains in extramammary Paget's disease. *Am J Dermatopathol* 1992;14:402.
50. Gibson LE, Perry HO. Male and female genitalia. In: Roenigk RK, Roenigk HH Jr, eds. *Roenigk and Roenigk's dermatologic surgery.* 2nd ed. New York: Marcel Dekker, 1996:371.
51. Mark RJ, Poen JC, Tran LM, Fu YS, Julliard GF. Angiosarcoma: a report of 67 patients and a review of the literature [Review]. *Cancer* 1996;77:2400.
52. Dermal and subcutaneous tumors. In: Arnold HL Jr, Odom RB, James WD, eds. *Andrews' diseases of the skin: clinical dermatology.* 8th ed. Philadelphia: WB Saunders, 1990:682.
53. Brown MD. Cutaneous soft tissue sarcomas. In: Roenigk RK, Roenigk HH Jr, eds. *Roenigk and Roenigk's dermatologic surgery.* 2nd ed. New York: Marcel Dekker, 1996:565.
54. Waldo E, Colen S. Vascular neoplasms of the skin. In: Friedman RJ, Rigel D, Kopf AW, Harris MN, Baker D, eds. *Cancer of the skin.* Philadelphia: WB Saunders, 1991:296.

55. Calonje E, Wilson-Jones E. Tumors and tumor-like conditions of blood vessels and lymphatics. In: Elder D, Elenitsas E, Jaworsky C, et al., eds. *Lever's histopathology of the skin.* 8th ed. Philadelphia: Lippincott–Raven Publishers, 1997:889.

56. Malignant vascular tumors. In: Enzinger FM, Weiss SW. *Soft tissue tumors.* St. Louis: Mosby–Year Book, 1995:641.

57. Martin RW 3d, Hood AF, Farmer ER. Kaposi sarcoma [Review]. *Medicine* 1993;72:245.

58. Tur E, Brenner S. Treatment of Kaposi's sarcoma [Review]. *Arch Dermatol* 1996;132:327.

59. Krizek TJ, Foster RS Jr. Skin and soft tissue. In: Davis JH, ed. *Clinical surgery.* St Louis: Mosby, 1987:2369.

60. Tappero JW, Conant MA, Wolfe SF, Berger TG. Kaposi's sarcoma: epidemiology, pathogenesis, histology, clinical spectrum, staging criteria, and therapy [Review]. *J Am Acad Dermatol* 1992;28:371.

61. Fish, Frederick S. Soft tissue sarcomas in dermatology [Review]. *Dermatol Surg* 1996;22:268.

62. Gloster HM Jr. Dermatofibrosarcoma protuberans [Review]. *J Am Acad Dermatol* 1996;35:355. [For erratum, see *J Am Acad Dermatol* 1997;36:526.]

63. Andrew JE, Silvers DN, Lattes R. Sarcomas involving the skin and superficial tissues. In: Friedman RJ, Rigel D, Kopf AW, Harris MN, Baker D, eds. *Cancer of the skin.* Philadelphia: WB Saunders, 1991:263.

64. Andrew JE, Silvers DN, Lattes R. Pseudosarcomatous lesions (neoplastic and non-neoplastic) of the skin and superficial tissues. In: Friedman RJ, Rigel D, Kopf AW, Harris MN, Baker D, eds. *Cancer of the skin.* Philadelphia: WB Saunders, 1991:237.

65. Malignant fibrohistiocytic tumors. In: Enzinger FM, Weiss SW. *Soft tissue tumors.* St. Louis: Mosby–Year Book, 1995:351.

66. Bernstein SC, Roenigk RK. Leiomyosarcoma of the skin. Treatment of 34 cases [Review]. *Dermatol Surg* 1996;22:631.

67. Leiomyosarcoma. In: Enzinger FM, Weiss SW. *Soft tissue tumors.* St. Louis: Mosby–Year Book, 1995:491.

CHAPTER 11

Melanoma

Harry D. Bear

Melanoma is a malignancy arising from the pigment cells or melanocytes and may occur anywhere in the skin or, less often, the mucous membranes. Melanocytes and their malignant counterparts have the capacity to produce the black pigment melanin. Derived from the amino acid tyrosine by a series of enzymatic reactions, melanin is normally released from dendritic processes of the melanocyte and is taken up by other cells in the skin and skin appendages, providing the pigmentation or coloring of the skin. Melanomas have a reputation for being particularly aggressive and unpredictable, but as we shall see, the behavior of these cancers can be reasonably well predicted, at least statistically, based on a number of prognostic factors, and most are cured by simple surgical excision. Surgeons play a key role in the diagnosis, staging, and curative treatment of this malignancy and, therefore, should be thoroughly familiar with its biology and treatment. Despite some recent evidence of benefit from adjuvant therapy with interferon-α (IFN-α), surgery remains the mainstay for treatment of this disease. As a result of several key studies and new surgical techniques, both our understanding of melanoma and current management guidelines have undergone major changes in the last 5 years, and this chapter will include much of this new information to update the practicing surgeon.

EPIDEMIOLOGY

The incidence of melanoma has been steadily increasing over the past three decades, with more than 40,000 new cases expected in the United States in 1997 (1). Melanoma accounts for 3% of all cancers, but only 7,300 deaths are expected in the same year. The 5-year survival for patients with this cancer has been increasing; compared to only 60% for white patients with melanoma in 1960 to 1963, the 5-year survival for the same subset of patients diagnosed in 1986 to 1992 was 88% (1). This improvement almost certainly results from increased public awareness and earlier diagnosis. Most melanomas found in this country are "thin" lesions, requiring only surgical treatment and having a high likelihood of cure. The rising incidence of melanoma in recent years has been attributed to

the increasing amount of exposure to ultraviolet light, the increasing population of fair-skinned people in tropical and semitropical climates and, perhaps, to gradual depletion of ozone in the upper atmosphere. However, sun exposure is not as clearly related to the occurrence of this cancer as it is to other skin cancers, such as squamous cell and basal cell cancers, which occur almost exclusively in sun-exposed areas of the skin. Whatever its underlying causes, it is estimated that by the year 2000, 1 in 90 white individuals living in the United States will develop a melanoma during his or her lifetime (2).

PRECURSOR LESIONS

Considerable controversy exists as to whether melanoma usually arises from benign pigmented lesions or is more likely to arise *de novo* from individual melanocytes. Clearly, both occur, and it has been variously estimated that 18% to 85% of melanomas arise at the site of a previously noted nevus or mole (3–5). Among the common benign nevi, the junctional nevus is considered to be the type from which a melanoma is most likely to arise. A junctional nevus presents as a flat, well-circumscribed mole with homogeneous pigmentation and is composed of melanocytes located at the basal layer of the epidermis (i.e., at the junction of epidermis with dermis). Compound nevi, having melanocytes both at the epidermal-dermal junction and within the dermis, only rarely give rise to melanomas. The intradermal nevus is also an unlikely source for melanomas, but the giant progressive nevus, or "bathing trunk" nevus, which has a similar microscopic pattern, was once thought to give rise to melanomas in up to 10% of cases. Although this is probably an overestimate of the risk, it is generally not possible to excise these lesions entirely, and they should be followed closely for any suspicious changes. The Spitz nevus, also known as benign juvenile melanoma, occurs mainly in young children. It is heterogeneous in color and is generally 1 to 2 cm in size. These lesions are actually a type of compound nevus, but, because of their high cellularity, they may be mistaken histologically for melanomas. Despite their appearance, they are benign. Because melanoma is actually very uncommon in children, the distinction may be facilitated, but the diagnosis can be treacherous. Although removal of any and all nevi is neither practical nor useful, any change should prompt biopsy or removal of a nevus to rule out melanoma. Particularly worrisome are the atypical or dysplastic nevi found in patients with the familial syndromes discussed below.

RISK FACTORS AND SCREENING

Based on a multivariate analysis of 200 melanoma patients, six significant risk factors were shown to predict the occurrence of melanoma (6). These are the first six factors listed in Table 11-1. The presence of one or two of these factors conferred a 3.5-fold increased risk for melanoma; three or more factors imparted a 20-fold risk compared to the general population. Other factors associated with the occurrence of melanoma are also listed in Table 11-1 (seventh through fifteenth in the list). Patients with a previous history of melanoma have a lifetime risk of about 5% of developing a second primary melanoma (2).

Of particular importance, identifying a group of individuals who need particularly close surveillance, is the familial atypical multiple mole-melanoma (FAMMM) syndrome, previously known as familial dysplastic nevus syndrome (7). The typical syndrome is characterized by the presence of numerous moles or nevi (over 100), one or more nevi 8 mm or larger in diameter, and at least one mole with atypical or melanoma-like features. A patient with multiple dysplastic nevi is shown in Fig. 11-1. The risk of melanoma among families with this syndrome varies, but in affected individuals within FAMMM kindreds in which other affected family members have had melanoma, the risk is approximately 150-fold greater than that for the general population (5). Figure 11-2 shows a melanoma that has developed from a dysplastic nevus in such a patient.

Melanoma of the skin can be detected by visual inspection of the skin by physician or patient, and early or thin melanomas have very high cure rates, approaching 100%. Therefore, melanoma is in some ways an ideal disease for large-

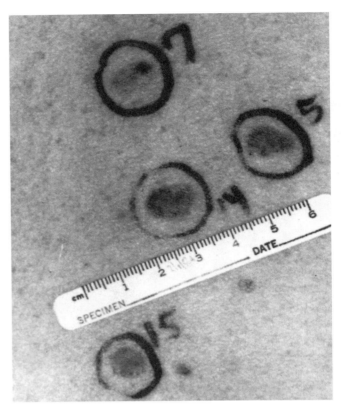

FIG. 11-1. Dysplastic nevi in a patient with dysplastic nevus syndrome or FAMMM. (Reprinted with permission from Greene MH, Clark Jr WH, Tucker MA, et al. Current concepts: Acquired precursors of cutaneous malignant melanoma. The familial dysplastic nevus syndrome. *N Engl J Med* 312:91–97, 1985.)

TABLE 11–1. *Risk factors for melanoma*

Family history
Blond or red hair
Multiple freckles on the upper back
≥3 severe sunburns before age 20
≥3 summers with outdoor jobs as a teenager
Actinic keratosis
Adulthood
One or more large or irregularly pigmented nevi
Congenital mole
Caucasian race
Immunosuppression
Previous melanoma
Sun sensitivity
Latitude
Familial atypical multiple mole melanoma (dysplastic nevus) syndrome

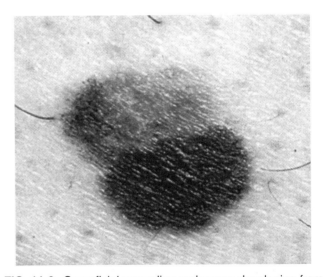

FIG. 11-2. Superficial spreading melanoma developing from a dysplastic nevus. (Reprinted with permission from Rhodes AR, Weinstock MA, Fitzpatrick TB, Mihm MC, Sober AJ. Risk factors for cutaneous melanoma. A practical method of recognizing predisposed individuals. *JAMA* 1987;258:3146–3154.)

scale screening programs. Techniques for thorough self-examination, involving use of a few simple tools (good light, a full-length mirror, hair dryer, and chairs) have been well-described (6). Whether mass screening by self-examination or physician examination for the entire adult population would be cost-effective is unknown, but the cost should not be excessive, assuming that it would not result in a large number of benign biopsies. At the very least, it is apparent that routine screening (once or twice each year) should be made available to individuals with recognized risk factors for this cancer, especially for individuals with dysplastic nevi in FAMMM kindreds. Such screening requires clear documentation, including photographs, of all dysplastic nevi, and excisional biopsy of any moles that change. Newer techniques, including epiluminescence microscopy and computerized image analysis, along with increasingly sophisticated genetic analysis, may increase the efficacy of screening for melanoma and further decrease the death rate from this disease.

DIAGNOSIS

Recognition of melanoma on clinical grounds is the first step in the success of any screening program and for early diagnosis in all individuals. Particularly useful are the so-called "ABCD's" of melanoma recognition. This acronym denotes the clinical features of *A*symmetry, *B*order irregularity (e.g., notching or scalloping of the edges), *C*olor variegation, and *D*iameter greater than 6 mm. The first three are illustrated in Figs. 11-3 to 11-6. Other features that may be clues to the malignant nature of a skin lesion include recent changes in color, shape, size or elevation, scaling, erosion, ulceration, bleeding, satellite pigmented lesions, itching, pain, or friability.

Of course, regardless of the level of clinical suspicion, definitive diagnosis depends on surgical biopsy and histopathology. Whenever feasible, excisional biopsy with a minimal

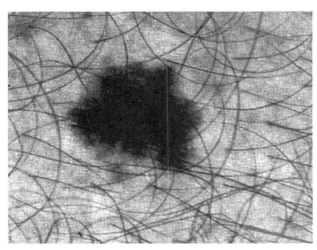

FIG. 11-4. Melanoma illustrating irregular borders.

margin is the preferred approach to diagnosis, and should provide adequate tissue for microstaging. The tissue obtained should include the full thickness of the gross lesion and extend into the subcutaneous fat. For small lesions, this biopsy can be most easily performed using a punch biopsy and local anesthesia. If the lesion is so large that complete excision would be a major procedure, then an incisional biopsy can be performed. If possible, it should include the most raised portion of the lesion and should also include a small sample of adjacent normal-appearing skin. Attention to these details enables the pathologist to measure the thickness accurately; this, in turn, profoundly affects the plan of definitive treatment. Other techniques, such as shave biopsies, curetting, and coagulation, are to be avoided.

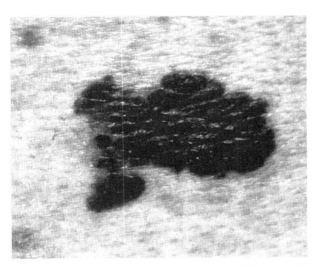

FIG. 11-3. Superficial spreading melanoma, demonstrating asymmetry.

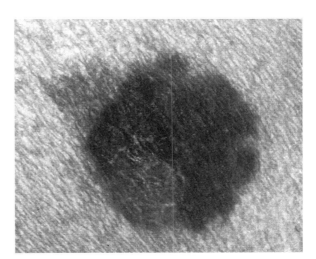

FIG. 11-5. Melanoma illustrating color variegation. (Reprinted with permission from Friedman RJ, Rigel DS, Silverman MK, Kopf AW, Vossaert KA. Malignant melanoma in the 1990's: the continued importance of early detection and the role of physician examination and self-examination of the skin. *CA Cancer J Clin* 1991;41:201–226.)

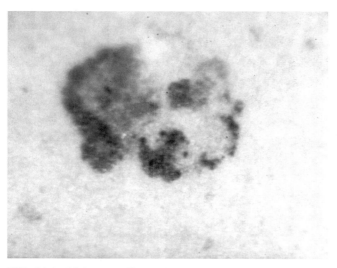

FIG. 11-6. Melanoma illustrating color variegation as well as areas of regression.

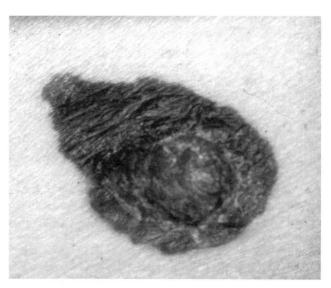

FIG. 11-7. Nodular melanoma.

CLASSIFICATION (TYPES) AND MICROSTAGING

Melanomas have been classified into several categories according to their gross morphology, location, and histologic growth pattern. Superficial spreading melanomas account for roughly 70% of all cases and are flat, slightly elevated in configuration, and may be variegated in color (Figs. 11-2 to 11-5). Microscopically, this corresponds to a predominantly radial or horizontal growth pattern, with spread of the process along the junctional layer. Nodular melanomas, which have more prominent vertical growth patterns, account for approximately 15% to 20% of all melanomas. These lesions tend to be darker and more "heaped up" in appearance (Fig. 11-7) and tend to occur in middle-aged patients. Correlating with their

deeper invasiveness, nodular melanomas have a poorer prognosis than the other types. Lentigo maligna melanoma accounts for only 5% to 10% of melanomas. These are found in elderly patients, particularly men, and are characteristically large flat lesions on the face (Fig. 11-8). Lentigo maligna, or "Hutchinson's freckle," may be present for many years as an *in situ* or thin lesion, but may become more invasive, with the development of nodularity (Fig. 11-9). Despite their reputation for being fairly innocuous, these melanomas can sometimes become more aggressive. The patient shown in Fig. 11-9, despite the thin level described histologically, developed liver metastases within a few years of primary excision. Melanomas found on the palms of the hands, soles of the feet, and under the nail beds (Fig. 11-10) are classified as

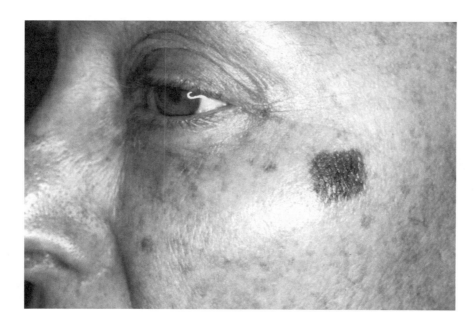

FIG. 11-8. Lentigo maligna of the cheek.

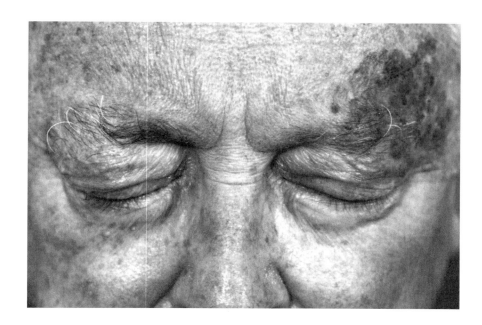

FIG. 11-9. Lentigo maligna of the forehead, with the development of nodularity. Despite being a thin lesion (Clark's level II), this patient eventually died of melanoma metastatic to the liver.

acral lentiginous melanomas. These are quite uncommon in Whites, accounting for approximately 5% of melanomas overall. However, among Blacks, acral lentiginous lesions account for up to 60% of all melanomas (7). The lesions on the palms and soles tend to be large and deeply invasive, with a correspondingly poor prognosis.

STAGING

Although the categorization described above has some prognostic implications, the introduction of microstaging according to the depth of invasion, introduced by Clark in 1969, has markedly improved our ability to predict the clinical behav-

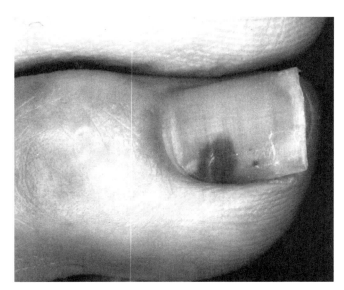

FIG. 11-10. Subungual melanoma; falls within the acral lentiginous subtype.

ior of melanomas (8). This schema, based on the depth of invasion relative to defined objective "landmarks," is illustrated in Fig. 11-11, and has been widely adopted, forming one basis for the current staging system. Not long after introduction of Clark's levels, Breslow correlated the prognosis of melanoma with the measured depth of invasion (9). The reproducibility of this method depends on measuring from the granular layer of the epidermis to the deepest point of invasion of the tumor. Breslow's thickness, because of the variable thickness of different layers of the skin at different anatomic sites and in different individuals, does not correlate precisely with Clark's levels, although corresponding depths for the two systems are occasionally shown. Breslow's thickness is a more precise predictor of nodal metastasis and overall prognosis than Clark's levels (Table 11-2), but both are used in the currently accepted staging system. If only one in-

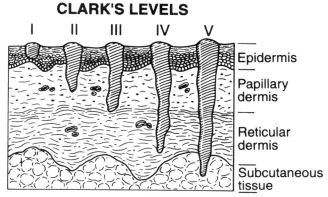

FIG. 11-11. Diagram of Clark's levels. Level I, noninvasive or *in situ* melanoma; level II, invades the papillary dermis; level III, invades to the papillary/reticular dermis interface; level IV, invades the reticular dermis; level V, invades the subcutaneous tissue.

TABLE 11–2. *Prognostic significance of melanoma thickness*

Breslow's thickness	Likelihood of nodal metastases	Five-year survival (with clinically negative nodes)
In situ	0	100%
≤0.75 mm	5%	96%
0.75–1.5 mm	10–20%	87%
1.51–4.00 mm	25–30%	70%
>4 mm	70%	47%

dicator of depth is used, Breslow's thickness should be preferred.

The current American Joint Committee on Cancer (AJCC) staging system, based on assessment of tumor, nodes, and metastases (TNM) is shown in Table 11-3 (10). The T assessment is based mostly on the prognostic significance of the microscopically assessed depth of invasion, preferably Breslow's thickness. Nodal assessment may be either clinical or pathologic, but patients with clinically detectable nodal metastases have a much worse prognosis than patients with occult nodal involvement found only histologically. The prognostic significance of TNM stage is shown in Table 11-4 and profoundly affects the recommended extent of additional staging work-up and the predicted likelihood of survival.

OTHER PROGNOSTIC FACTORS

In addition to the measured tumor thickness and TNM staging, other factors have also been shown to have prognostic significance for patients with melanoma. One of these, satellosis, is actually a component of the AJCC staging system (Fig. 11-12). Other factors shown to be independent predictors of outcome include ulceration, sex (females fare better than males), anatomic location (extremities better than trunk or head and neck; cutaneous sites better than mucosal lesions), and number of involved nodes. Whether the better prognosis for females is related to estrogen influence on tumor cell behavior is controversial (11). At one time, melanomas in the so-called "BANS" regions (upper back, posterior arm, posterior neck, and scalp) were thought to have poorer prognoses than other sites, but more recent multivariate analysis has shown

TABLE 11–3. *AJCC staging for cutaneous melanoma*

Primary tumor (pT) (for definitions of Clark's levels, see Fig. 11-11)
pTX	Primary tumor cannot be assessed
pT0	No evidence of primary tumor (unknown primary tumor)
pTis	Melanoma in situ, not an invasive lesion (Clark's level I)
pT1	Tumor 0.75 mm or less in thickness and/or Clark's level II
pT2	Tumor more than 0.75 mm but not more than 1.5 mm in thickness and/or Clark's level III
pT3	Tumor more than 1.5 mm but not more than 4 mm in thickness and/or Clark's level IV
pT3a	Tumor more than 1.5 mm but not more than 3 mm in thickness
pT3b	Tumor more than 3 mm but not more than 4 mm in thickness
pT4	
pT4a	Tumor more than 4 mm in thickness and/or Clark's level V
pT4b	Satellite(s) within 2 cm of the primary tumor

Regional lymph nodes (N)
NX	Regional lymph nodes cannot be assessed
N0	No regional lymph node metastasis
N1	Metastasis 3 cm or less in greatest dimension in any regional lymph node(s)
N2	
N2a	Metastasis more than 3 cm in greatest dimension in any regional lymph node(s)
N2b	In-transit metastasis[a]
N2c	Both (N2a and N2b)

Distant metastasis
MX	Presence of distant metastasis cannot be assessed
M0	No distant metastasis
M1	Distant metastasis
M1a	Metastasis in skin, subcutaneous tissue, or lymph node(s) beyond the regional lymph nodes
M1b	Visceral metastasis

Stage grouping
Stage 0	pTis	N0	M0
Stage I	pT1	N0	M0
	PT2	N0	M0
Stage II	pT3	N0	M0
	pT4	N0	M0
Stage III	Any pT	N1	M0
	Any pT	N2	M0
Stage IV	Any pT	Any N	M1

[a] In-transit metastasis involves skin or subcutaneous tissue more than 2 cm from the primary tumor, but not beyond the regional lymph nodes.

TABLE 11–4. *Prognosis for melanoma according to AJCC/UICC TNM stage*

TNM Stage	Estimated 5-Year Survival
I	75%–85%
II	60%–70%
III	35%–45%
IV	5%–15%

that this is not an independent prognostic factor when thickness of the lesions is taken into account (12). A number of other prognostic factors, based on genetic or immunologic analysis of melanomas have also been described, and are summarized in two recent reviews (2,13).

STAGING WORK-UP AFTER DIAGNOSIS

Because the risk of metastasis is closely linked to the TNM stage, the extent of evaluation looking for clinically occult distant metastases will depend on tumor thickness, nodal involvement, and cost considerations. All patients should have a thorough history and physical exam. Review of systems should focus on symptoms of spread to the lungs (cough, dyspnea, pleuritic pain), CNS (headache, seizures, motor or sensory defects), or gastrointestinal (GI) tract (cramping, bleeding, anemia). The examiner should look for related findings and should also include careful inspection of the entire skin surface and all node-bearing areas. For patients with early melanomas (*in situ* or less than 0.76 mm without clinically evident nodal metastases), no additional tests are indicated. For patients with stage I and II disease, only chest x-rays and routine blood chemistries (including liver function tests) are needed. More sophisticated and costly testing, such as computed tomography (CT) scans of the chest, abdomen, and CNS are indicated *only* in patients with symptoms suggestive of distant disease. Whether these are needed in patients with stage

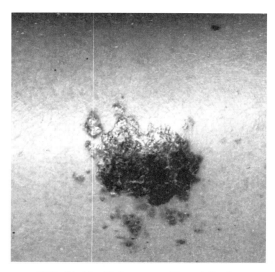

FIG. 11-12. Melanoma with satellosis.

III disease is less clear. These are unlikely to be useful in patients with microscopic nodal involvement, but may have a higher yield in patients with gross nodal involvement. Although extensive radiologic staging has been advocated for patients with stage III disease, a recent study of the experience at Memorial-Sloan Kettering Cancer Center demonstrated that the yield from such studies is too low to justify the expense (7,14). CT of the pelvis and abdomen, however, is indicated in patients with clinical groin node involvement in whom a superficial and deep ilioinguinal node dissection is planned. This study may identify patients who would derive little benefit from the planned operation, which does carry some morbidity. Similar considerations apply to patients with recurrent or extensive disease in an extremity in whom amputation or isolated limb perfusion is being considered (see below).

SURGICAL MANAGEMENT OF THE PRIMARY LESION

Adequate surgery is the key to the cure and survival of patients with melanoma, so the surgeon is still the most important provider of care for this disease. Until quite recently, the extent of excision of the primary lesion had been dictated by autopsy observations made in 1907 on a single patient by William S. Handley (15,16). Based on microscopic examination of a fairly advanced tumor, he recommended removal of all skin within one inch of the lesion and removal of two inches of subcutaneous tissue in all directions. This description led to the standard approach for excision of melanomas, with 5-cm margins in all directions, which almost always led to the need for skin grafting to close the resulting defect. Most surgeons practicing today learned this approach during their training. It was said that if the wound could be closed without a skin graft, then the excision was not wide enough. It has taken almost 90 years to put this dogma aside; it is more accurate to say, for most melanomas seen today, that the need for a skin graft indicates *too radical* an excision. Breslow's description of the relationship of depth to risk for recurrence led some to question the need for very wide excision, and two prospective randomized trials have now shown that narrower excision margins are just as effective as wider ones for most lesions. The World Health Organization (WHO) trial demonstrated no significant difference in recurrence or survival for patients with melanomas 2 mm or less in thickness for 1- versus 3-cm excision margins (17). When narrow excision was used, the dissection was carried laterally 1 to 2 cm wider in the subcutaneous tissue (Fig. 11-13). No local recurrences were observed for lesions less than 1 mm in depth. Although not statistically worse than the wider excision, four local recurrences were observed in the narrow margin group with melanomas 1.1 to 2 mm deep. The results of a large trial comparing wide (4 cm) versus narrow (2 cm) margins for melanomas 1 to 4 mm in depth were reported in 1993 (18). With analysis of results in 486 randomized patients at a median 8 years of follow-up, no significant difference in overall survival or local recurrence rates was found. Thus, except for very deep and/or wide lesions or lesions with satellosis, the

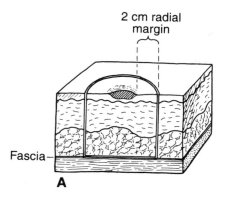

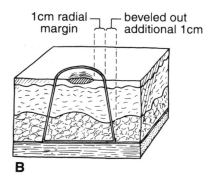

FIG. 11-13. Wide excision of melanomas. **A:** When a 2-cm or greater margin is used at the skin level, the incisions should extend perpendicularly straight down to the depth of excision at the fascia. Care should be taken not to bevel the incisions inward under the lesion. **B:** When narrower skin margins are necessary, then wider excision of the deeper tissues should be achieved by beveling the incisions outward away from the lesion.

traditional radical excision is clearly too aggressive and morbid. A recent NIH Consensus Conference on early melanoma made the following recommendations: for *in situ* melanoma, the lesion or biopsy site should be excised with 0.5-cm margins; for "thin" invasive melanomas (less than 1-mm thick), the excision should include 1 cm of normal skin and subcutaneous tissues in all directions (19). From the data available, 2-cm margins appear adequate for lesions 1 to 4 mm in thickness (see Table 11-5). Care should be taken to extend the incisions perpendicularly down to the fascia, without undermining beneath the lesion (Fig. 11-13A). In locations where even these margins would result in significant morbidity (e.g., on the face, particularly near the eye), narrower margins may be considered. When narrower skin margins are used, the excision should extend out more widely as one goes deeper (Fig. 11-13B). For more aggressive or advanced lesions, wider excision may be appropriate. Obviously, the specimen needs to be carefully assessed by a pathologist, and there should be no tumor at the margins. The depth of excision should generally extend to the deep fascia, but there does not seem to be any advantage to removing the fascia.

With the use of the narrower margins than in the past, closure of the defect after excision should only rarely require skin grafting, perhaps in 5% to 10% of all cases. For most excisions, after mobilizing the skin, the defect can be closed primarily without tension. In some instances, especially on narrow parts of the extremities or on the face, simple advancement or rotational flaps can be employed by the general surgeon per-

forming the excision. As shown in Fig. 11-14, use of double M-plasties instead of excision of a large ellipse of skin may allow closure without "dog ears" or excess tension. The simple rhomboid flap technique shown in Fig. 11-15 is especially useful for distal extremity lesions. Occasionally, more complex flaps are required, especially for more extensive lesions involving the face, such as the one illustrated in Fig. 11-9.

If necessary, consultation and assistance by a plastic surgeon can be very helpful in such situations. For acral lentiginous melanoma of the palmar and plantar surfaces, complex flaps may be needed, but skin grafts actually perform surprisingly well, even on weight-bearing surfaces. More complex reconstructions can be reserved for instances in which these simpler methods fail. For subungual lesions and lesions of the skin of the digits, conservative amputation at the distal interphalangeal or proximal interphalangeal joint is the best approach, with removal of at least 1 cm of normal skin above

TABLE 11–5. *Guidelines for excision of primary cutaneous melanoma*

Breslow thickness of primary	Margins of excision
In situ	Minimal, to obtain negative margins
≤1.0 mm	1 cm
1.1–4.0 mm	2 cm
≥4.0 mm	2 cm or greater

Decisions regarding margins should also take into account factors such as ulceration, satellosis, or regression, which would necessitate wider margins. Conversely, cosmetic and functional considerations in the absence of particularly aggressive melanomas may lead to use of narrower margins.

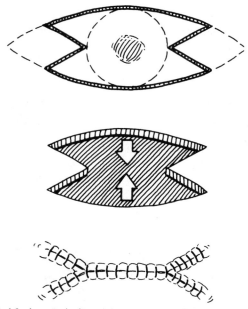

FIG. 11-14. Instead of excising the long ellipse shown at top, bilateral M-plasties can be used, still achieving excision with the same margins. Closure as shown results in less tension and no "dog ears," as would result from closure of the elliptical excision.

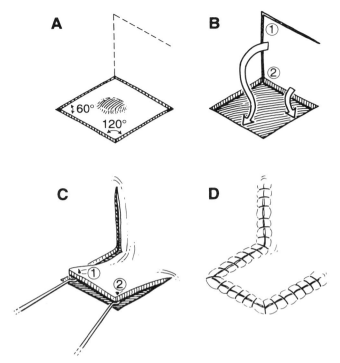

FIG. 11-15. Rhomboid flap closure of excision wound. **A:** Excision of the lesion as a rhomboid or diamond, with the wider angles where excess skin is available (determined by pinching tissue between skin and forefinger). **B:** Additional incisions are made as shown, by extending a line from the wider angle that bisects that angle and extends the same length as one side of the rhomboid. A second line is incised at 60° to the first line and parallel to the side of the rhomboid defect. **C:** The flap is rotated into the defect. **D:** All incisions are closed as shown.

the lesion. More proximal amputations are more debilitating and have not been shown to decrease local or systemic recurrences (20,21).

MANAGEMENT OF MUCOSAL MELANOMAS

Primary melanomas arising in mucosal surfaces (as opposed to metastases to these sites) account for less than 3% of melanomas but present unique problems in management. Mucosal melanomas have been found in the anorectum, vulva, vagina, head and neck region, and, rarely, the esophagus. The prognosis for these lesions tends to be much worse than for cutaneous lesions, perhaps because of late diagnosis. Although patients with very thin lesions tend to do well, most mucosal melanomas are quite deep, and overall 5-year survivals are in the range of 20% to 35% (22,23). The most common presenting symptom for these melanomas is bleeding, usually a sign of a deeply invasive lesion. As for cutaneous lesions, complete surgical excision, if possible, is the best treatment, but the location of these tumors often makes this problematic. Wide local excision may be possible in the oral cavity. Anorectal lesions should be treated with local excision, if possible, or by ab-

dominoperineal resection (APR), if necessary. APR does not appear to provide a survival advantage over local excision, but of course those patients treated with APR are likely to be those with more advanced disease. Survival of patients with anorectal lesions is particularly low, being approximately 5% to 28% at 5 years (22–24). Vulvar and vaginal melanomas should also be treated with local excision if possible; radical vulvectomy or vaginectomy are reserved for large, very advanced lesions. Similar to the situation with cutaneous melanoma, the value of prophylactic inguinal node dissection remains unproven. Because of the difficulty in achieving complete resection of mucosal melanomas, radiation is used in some patients but has not been proven to increase the cure rates.

MANAGEMENT OF THE REGIONAL LYMPH NODES

Therapeutic Lymph Node Dissection

For patients with clinically involved lymph nodes (clinical stage III disease), the prognosis is definitely worse than for patients without gross nodal involvement, including those with microscopic nodal metastases. These patients are at high risk for the presence of distant metastatic disease. Nevertheless, if distant metastases are not evident at the time of nodal involvement, 5-year survival rates may vary from 15% to 40% (2,4,25,26). This, along with the fact that there is no other particularly effective modality for eradication of gross melanoma, leads to a consensus on the surgical treatment of palpable lymph node metastases. A minority of patients may actually be rendered disease-free by surgical resection, and an additional fraction may achieve long-term survival with the addition of IFN-α. Even if the patient eventually succumbs to distant disease at some time in the future, radical lymphadenectomy may also provide significant palliative benefit to the patient, avoiding problems of pain, ulceration, bleeding, and nerve involvement. For patients with axillary node involvement, a chest CT may be justifiable, in addition to more routine staging studies. If distant metastases are not found, then a standard axillary node dissection should be performed. In contrast to the more limited axillary node sampling becoming more common in the management of breast cancer, the axillary dissection for melanoma-involved lymph nodes should include levels I, II, and III. The pectoralis minor muscle should be removed, or at least divided, to achieve an adequate dissection.

For patients with clinically positive inguinal-femoral nodes, it has been recommended that a laparotomy should precede the node dissection, in order to rule out the presence of incurable intraabdominal or retroperitoneal metastases. With modern computerized tomography (CT), magnetic resonance imaging (MRI), and positron emission tomography (PET) available, this is probably unnecessary today. For therapeutic ilioinguinal lymph node dissection, both the deep and superficial nodes are usually removed. This procedure can be performed through a number of incisions, shown in Fig. 11-16. Either the

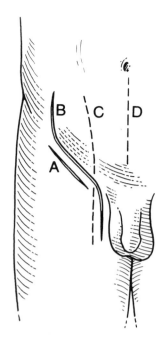

FIG. 11-16. Choices of incisions for inguinal node dissection. **A:** Oblique, parallel to the inguinal ligament. **B:** S-shaped for superficial and deep dissection. **C:** Vertical. **D:** Lower midline can be combined with oblique incision (A or transverse part of B) for deep dissection combined with superficial dissection.

S-shaped or oblique incision is used most often. Another acceptable approach is to use a transverse groin incision for the superficial inguinal-femoral dissection combined with a lower midline incision to access the iliac nodes. At one time it was considered standard to remove a large triangular segment of skin overlying the inguinal and femoral nodes. Unless this defect is closed with a skin graft, as originally described, this leads to excess tension on the closure and skin necrosis, and it does not add to the oncologic goals of the procedure unless the

skin is directly involved by the underlying nodal metastases. A number of good descriptions of the surgical procedure are available (27–29). The block of tissue to be removed below the inguinal ligament is demarcated by the anterior superior iliac spine at the superior lateral corner, a point 2 cm above the pubic tubercle superior and medially, the beginning of the femoral canal (at the point where the sartorius and adductor longus muscles meet) inferior and medially, and a point directly lateral to this and directly inferior to the anterior superior iliac spine. All of the fat and lymphatic tissue in this area should be removed, stripping the femoral artery and vein. At the conclusion of the dissection, the sartorius muscle should be detached from its origin, transposed medially and sutured to the inguinal ligament and surrounding muscles to cover the femoral vessels (Fig. 11-17). This helps to prevent exposure of the vessels and vessel rupture if wound breakdown and/or infection should develop. The deep portion of the dissection should strip the nodes and fat from the superficial and deep iliac vessels down to the inguinal ligament. In all instances, it is best to drain the dead space under the flaps to avoid seroma formation. We generally confine patients who have had inguinal node dissections to bed rest for several days postoperatively to reduce lymphatic flow.

Elective or Prophylactic Lymph Node Dissection

Although there is general agreement about how to manage the melanoma patient who has clinically positive lymph nodes, there has been considerable controversy about whether clinically negative lymph node basins should be surgically resected. Several arguments have been made to support the routine use of prophylactic or elective lymph node dissection (ELND) for some melanomas, particularly those of intermediate thickness (1.1 to 4.0 mm). Certainly, the pathologic examination of lymph nodes provides prognostic information that separates patients into groups at greater or lesser risk of distant recurrence. Patients with clinically negative but patho-

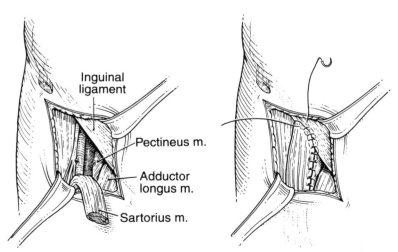

Inguinal ligament

Pectineus m.

Adductor longus m.

Sartorius m.

FIG. 11-17. Transposition of the sartorius muscle to cover the femoral vessels after removal of the fat and lymph nodes. A suction drain (not shown) is always used under the flaps.

logically positive nodes have 5-year survivals in the range of 50% (13,25). This may provide information that the patients find useful (or frightening), but until recently this had little practical value, since there was no adjuvant therapy that was proven to reduce the risk of death in these patients. Even with the recent "breakthrough" using IFN-α as an adjuvant, it is not clear that the benefit to the subset of patients with occult nodal metastases is worth the morbidity of the procedure.

Although the trend in recent years has been a decline in the therapeutic importance attributed to lymph node dissection for other cancers, most of the impetus to perform ELND for melanoma has been a presumed therapeutic value. This has been extrapolated in part from the prognosis for patients who undergo ELND and are found to have micrometastases in the nodes. In contrast to the 50% 5-year survival estimates for these patients, patients who present with or later develop clinically positive nodes have only a 20% to 35% chance of surviving 5 years (25). The difference, it has been argued, reflects the beneficial effect of ELND. This conclusion certainly contradicts recent paradigm shifts in how other malignancies are managed, but there is no *a priori* reason to assume that all cancers manifest similar behavior. It certainly is possible that some patients harbor melanoma metastases in the regional nodes for a period of time before systemic spread. If so, then removal of these nodes before they become clinically enlarged (and perhaps before dissemination) may benefit some patients. This may or may not be the case; not all patients with nodal micrometastases would necessarily have developed gross nodal disease or distant metastases if observed. Conversely, some patients will develop distant metastases without manifesting clinical node involvement. The latter has been the principal argument for not offering ELND to patients with clinically negative nodes and primary melanomas deeper than 4.0 mm (13,30). These patients have a 60% chance of regional node involvement, but also have a 70% or greater chance of distant metastases. For this reason, ELND probably would not benefit these patients. Data supporting this conclusion have been published from Duke University (31,32). Interestingly, they also reported 5-year survival in 56% of these patients, similar to our own experience with level V lesions (33). At the other end of the spectrum, most experts agree that patients with thin melanomas (variously defined as less than 0.76, 1.0, or 1.5 mm) have too low a likelihood of occult node involvement or distant metastases to derive any benefit from ELND (32).

Most of the controversy surrounding ELND has been centered on the population of patients with intermediate thickness melanomas, 1.1 to 4.0 mm in depth. A number of retrospective analyses have suggested that the prophylactic removal of lymph nodes harboring micrometastases in this subset of patients has therapeutic benefit (7,13,34). Some of these reports indicated rather remarkable improvements in outcome with ELND, resulting in increased survival of more than 40% in absolute terms at 10 years (34). Another large retrospective study from Duke University, however, did not confirm the therapeutic value of this procedure (35).

Three prospective randomized trials, two sponsored in Europe by the WHO and one at the Mayo Clinic in the United States, failed to confirm a benefit for ELND (36–38). Because these trials had several methodologic and statistical flaws, the issue of whether ELND was worthwhile was not considered to be settled. In the WHO trials, many of the primary lesions were not microstaged in advance, and retrospective analysis suggests that the results were "diluted out" by a large number of favorable, thin lesions. Other factors, such as a predominance of female patients, have also been cited as problems. In the second WHO trial, for patients with trunk lesions, the lack of lymphoscintigraphy may have led to surgical treatment of the wrong lymph node basin (13,37). The major flaw of the Mayo Clinic study was the small sample size, with 171 patients divided into three groups. Because of the persistent uncertainty, a "definitive" multicenter prospective randomized trial was therefore carried out under the direction of Dr. Charles Balch and sponsored by the National Cancer Institute. The first results of this trial were reported in 1996 (39). With 740 patients enrolled in the trial and a median follow-up of 7.4 years, there was no statistically significant survival advantage for patients treated with ELND over those who were observed and only underwent LND for clinical recurrence. However, by analyzing subsets of patients, improved survival in patients treated with ELND could be demonstrated for certain groups. Patients under the age of 60 years, particularly those with lesions 1.0 to 2.0 mm in depth and without ulceration, were found to have a statistically significant improvement in survival with ELND. The magnitude of this benefit in terms of an increase in 5-year survival, however, was only about 10% in absolute terms, and was not comparable to the benefit indicated by retrospective analyses. The propriety of analyzing subsets of patients in this trial according to criteria that were not part of the stratification variables prior to randomization is certainly questionable, leading some to conclude from this study only that ELND does not have an overall benefit. Others, however, have reached the conclusion that this study proves the value of ELND in certain patients (13).

Along with the conflicting data on the benefits of ELND in certain patients with melanoma, the decision of whether to perform ELND must also take into account the potential morbidity of the procedure. This was not considered as an endpoint in the recently reported randomized trial from the Intergoup Melanoma Surgical Program (39). For all of these procedures, there is a fairly low incidence of minor acute complications, such as seromas, infections, and skin necrosis, and major morbidity is uncommon. For axillary dissection, general anesthetic is generally required, but hospitalization should usually be 1 day or less. The incidence of lymphedema of the upper extremity is fairly low, on the order of 10%. For inguinal node dissection, hospitalization is generally longer, but the most significant morbidity is the occurrence of leg edema, which is reported in approximately 25% of patients with long-term follow-up. This complication, along with the associated risks for repeated infections and significant disability, cannot be reliably predicted or prevented. Moreover, once it develops, there is no effective cure. Treatments are available that palliate the symptoms, but these must be continued for the patient's lifetime. It is difficult to justify this problem to a patient who has undergone ELND with no histologically positive nodes.

Role of Lymphoscintigraphy in Melanoma

Once a decision has been made to perform ELND, then the surgeon must decide which nodes should be targeted. For melanomas of the distal extremities, this will be either the axillary or inguinal nodes. For melanomas of the head and neck region, a partial radical neck dissection was usually performed, sometimes including the superficial parotid gland to remove the nodes within it. For lesions of the trunk, classical descriptions based on anatomic dissections of cadavers were used to choose the appropriate nodal basin, either axilla, neck, or groin and to decide which side was at risk. However, lymphoscintigraphic studies, performed by injecting a radio-labeled colloid that is taken up by the lymphatics and then imaging the patient, has shown that dependence on these classical descriptions will frequently lead to incorrect choices (13,40). The ambiguous areas that can drain across the midline or across Sappey's line to the "unexpected" nodal basins are much wider than previously thought. The classical descriptions, therefore, should not be relied upon to determine which lymph node basins to stage surgically. Radionuclide imaging may also identify in-transit nodes that are distal to standard nodal basins. Indeed, it has been suggested that the omission of lymphoscintigraphy for trunk lesions in the WHO trials may have lead to ELND of irrelevant basins and may have contributed to apparent lack of benefit for this procedure. Lymphoscintigraphy can be performed either as a separate procedure to determine which nodal basin(s) should be dissected or as part of a mapping procedure to identify a "sentinel" lymph node (SLN) on the day of surgery. Utilized in conjunction with SLN mapping, lymphoscintigraphy also aids in identifying the location and number of sentinel nodes.

Sentinel Lymph Node Mapping and Biopsy

The arguments for and against ELND may well have been rendered moot with the emergence of lymphatic mapping and SLN biopsy, introduced by Donald Morton (41). This procedure is based on the premise that the lymphatic drainage of skin neoplasms is more organized and "sequential" than had been generally assumed. If this is true, then one might be able to predict whether any nodes in the appropriate drainage basin contain metastases by determining whether the first lymph node in the sequential drainage pattern, the so-called "sentinel node," contains melanoma cells. In initial and subsequent trials, they showed that certain vital blue dyes drain into dermal lymphatics and then to one or a few lymph nodes after being injected into the skin around the lesion or biopsy site. With experience, a blue-stained sentinel node could be

identified in most patients. Moreover, by performing complete lymph node dissection on a large number of patients, Morton's group demonstrated that histologic examination of the sentinel node was highly accurate at predicting the complete nodal status determined by examination of all of the draining nodes (41). This is particularly advantageous for the patients with negative sentinel nodes, since it appears that they can be spared the morbidity of full lymph node dissection. At present, the standard of care for patients with positive sentinel nodes is to proceed with a full dissection, although this may change with the completion of trials currently under way. In fact, nonsentinel nodes were the only nodes with metastases in only 2 of 3,079 nodes in Morton's series, and even in the presence of positive SLN, only a small number of nonsentinel nodes were positive. The accuracy of this technique is also reflected in the recent finding that only 2% to 3% of patients with negative SLN have developed recurrences in the undissected node basin, although follow-up is still fairly short (13,42).

Because of the significant learning curve for mastery of the SLN mapping technique with vital blue dye, Krag and others (43–45) devised a technique for detecting the SLN using radionuclide-based mapping and based on previous experience with lymphoscintigraphy. Technetium-99m-sulfur colloid is injected around the lesion, usually 2 to 4 h before surgery. Using both lymphoscintigraphic imaging, as described above, and intraoperative localization with a hand-held gamma probe (Neoprobe, Columbus, OH or C-Trak from Care Wise Medical Products, Morgan Hill, CA), the SLN can be identified as a "hot" spot prior to incision and then as the "hot" node during surgery (Fig. 11-18). There is some controversy as to whether the radionuclide should be filtered or unfiltered; the unfiltered material, which contains larger particles, may migrate more slowly, but tends to remain "trapped" in the sentinel node for a longer period of time without migrating on to other nodes. If multiple nodes become "hot," then the selectivity of the procedure would be lost. The advantage of the radiolymphoscintigraphic technique, using imaging and the hand-held probe, is the ability to localize the SLN through the skin, making it possible to identify and remove the SLN through a limited incision, often under local anesthesia. With the vital blue dye technique alone, a more extensive incision may be required to identify the blue lymphatics leading to the SLN. In fact, as suggested by several groups at the forefront of this field, combining both techniques may be best, combining the advantages of radiolymphoscintigraphy with the visual confirmation of the blue staining.

The following technique is suggested, although there are many variations that appear to work as well:

Approximately 2 to 4 h prior to planned surgery, approximately 500 µCi of unfiltered technetium-99m-sulfur colloid in 1 cc total volume is injected intradermally (*not* subcutaneously) around the periphery of the lesion or the biopsy scar. Importantly, this technique may not be accurate after wide excision has already been performed, since this may alter the lymphatic drainage pattern. We perform the injection in the should be less than 1.5 times background after removal of the SLN's. If residual counts are higher than this level, a search should be made for additional "hot" nodes. After completion of the SLN biopsies, the wound is closed, and the surgeon can proceed with wide excision of the primary site. Occasionally, if the primary site is too close to the draining lymph node basin (e.g., in the skin overlying the scapula), it may be necessary to excise the primary before proceeding to SLN biopsy in order to reduce the background counts sufficiently to identify the "hot" node.

Pathologic examination of the SLN should be done on fixed tissue. Some groups have described performing frozen section examination of the SLN intraoperatively, with complete node dissection if metastases are found (41). However, this is not compatible with an outpatient procedure performed under local anesthesia, and more detailed examination of the SLN will increase the rate of finding positive nodes. Because the radionuclide has a short half-life, the specimens should contain very little radioactivity after 24 to 48 h, and our pathologists prefer to wait a day or two before handling the specimens. The SLN should not be handled as a "routine" pathologic specimen, with only one face of the node being examined. The node should be serially sectioned for H&E staining, and additional sections should be examined by immunohistochemistry for the S-100 and HMB-45 antigens that identify most melanoma cells. Even greater sensitivity (1 tumor cell out of one million lymph node cells) may be achievable by using reverse transcriptase polymerase chain reaction (RT-PCR) assays for melanoma-specific mRNA's, such as tyrosinase (13,46). However, the clinical significance of finding such low-level nodal involvement is unclear, and this should be considered experimental. At this point, standard management after SLN biopsy would be observation if the SLN is negative and full regional lymph node dissection if the node is positive. A recent report found that among a large number of melanoma patients with negative SLN's (by routine histologic examination), less than 3% had a regional node recurrence at 20 months of follow-up (42). In 75% of this small group, reexamination of the SLN by more sophisticated techniques revealed the presence of metastases, indicating that the actual false negative rate for SLN biopsy can be made very low by highly sensitive examination of the node. It will be interesting to learn whether this low false negative rate for SLN biopsy will hold up over longer follow-up. Whether or not a full regional lymph node dissection is beneficial in patients with positive SLN, especially for nodes that are only found to be positive by meticulous examination using immunohistochemistry or RT-PCR, is currently unknown and is under study. A current management algorithm that incorporates the use of lymphatic mapping and SLN biopsy is shown (Fig. 11-19).

Successful use of the SLN mapping technique depends upon cooperation between the departments of surgery, nuclear medicine, and pathology. As described, lymphoscintigraphic imaging certainly synergizes with use of the hand-held gamma probe and the use of blue dye to localize the sentinel

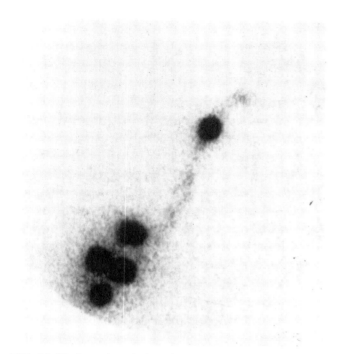

FIG. 11-18. Lymphoscintigraphy performed as part of a SLN mapping procedure. Radionuclide was injected at four points around the biopsy site of a melanoma on the distal thigh (four hot spots in lower part of the figure). This image, taken 5 min after injection, shows a lymphatic channel leading to a single lymph node in the inguinal region. This was identified with a gamma probe intraoperatively and excised. Histologically, this node was negative for metastases, and the patient was disease-free 2 years later.

Nuclear Medicine suite, thus avoiding any problems with transport of radionuclides through the hospital. In addition, it allows for early lymphoscintigraphic images to be obtained, as described above, for delineating ambiguous lymphatic drainage. In general, a lymphatic channel can be visualized within a few minutes (Fig. 11-18), which leads to the first lymph node, or SLN. Images are repeated for 30 to 60 min, until a clear picture of the location of the SLN is obtained. This "hot spot" is marked on the skin by the Nuclear Medicine team, and the patient is then transported to the surgical area, usually an outpatient facility.

With the patient appropriately positioned on the operating table, the hand-held probe is used to obtain background counts and to confirm the "hot spot" identified preoperatively. After prepping and draping the patient for surgery, 0.5 to 1.0 cc of 1% aqueous solution of Isosulfan blue dye (Lymphazurin, Hirsch Industries, Inc., Richmond, VA) is injected intradermally around the melanoma or biopsy site. The area is massaged to encourage uptake of the dye into the lymphatics. After local anesthetic block, a small (2- to 4-cm) incision is made over the previously identified hot spot. Using a combination of visual inspection and the hand-held probe, blue-stained and "hot" nodes are excised. Generally, one to three such nodes are found, and the radioactivity in the field

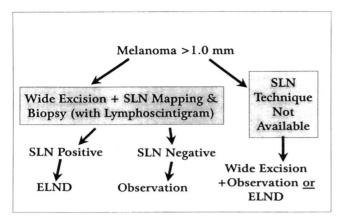

FIG. 11-19. Algorithm for management of regional lymph nodes in patients with melanoma. Some might consider pathologic examination of SLN or regional lymph nodes only for lesions 1.5 mm or larger in depth. If SLN mapping and biopsy are not available, one may consider ELND for patients less than 60 years of age, especially with lesions 1 to 2 mm and without ulceration. This subset appeared to benefit from ELND in a randomized trial (39). Observation would also be considered appropriate for all patients not undergoing SLN biopsy, especially for melanomas of the lower extremity.

node and facilitates planning of the operative procedure. Careful pathologic examination, including multiple sections and immunohistochemistry, are also essential to the successful application of SLN technology. Although this may initially seem excessive to the pathologist, this detailed examination of a single or even a few nodes is no more difficult than cursory examination of numerous nodes from a complete node dissection, as currently practiced. In fact, it would be impossible to perform the type of detailed examination recommended for a SLN on many nodes. This constitutes a major potential advantage to the SLN technique. Given the decreased morbidity and apparent accuracy of SLN biopsy, this appears to be the best approach to the patient with clinically negative nodes. It has been suggested that if the SLN is not available, then one should perform ELND using the guidelines from the recent Intergroup Melanoma Surgical Trial (13). However, given the morbidity of ELND, especially in the groin region, it may be more appropriate to recommend referral of these patients to centers where SLN mapping is available. With the rapid proliferation of this technology, this should soon be readily available to most patients in the United States.

ADJUVANT THERAPY

The purpose of adjuvant systemic treatment is to reduce the likelihood of cancer recurrence and cancer-related death. Until recently, however, the discussion of effective adjuvant therapies for melanoma would have been extremely brief. Randomized trials of multiple drugs and biologic agents (singly or in combinations) had shown no benefit in the adjuvant setting. In 1996, however, the Eastern Cooperative Oncology Group (ECOG) completed and reported on a prospec-

tive randomized trial in which patients at high risk for systemic metastases from melanoma were randomly allocated to either observation or 1 year of therapy with high-dose IFN-α-2b (47). This trial demonstrated a statistically significant increase in survival in the treated group. Median overall survival was increased by 1 year (3.8 versus 2.8 years, p = 0.047), and 5-year survival was increased from 36% to 47%. The Food and Drug Administration has now approved IFN-α-2b for this indication. It should be noted, however, that the treatment was associated with significant toxicity, especially flu-like symptoms and fatigue, for the entire year of treatment. Moreover, the vast majority of the patients in this trial had clinically positive nodes, either simultaneously with the primary lesion or as a regional recurrence. Thus, despite renewed enthusiasm for ELND as a staging procedure on which to base adjuvant treatment decisions, it is not yet clear that patients with occult microscopic nodal metastases, especially those with only one node (e.g., the SLN) involved, will actually benefit from this treatment. This question is currently being addressed in a prospective trial. Other adjuvant treatments, especially immunologic stimulants and vaccines are also under investigation in both the advanced disease and adjuvant settings (see below).

Melanoma has generally been considered resistant to radiotherapy, but newer techniques and fractionation schemes have demonstrated efficacy against this disease (48). Using larger doses per fraction may increase the response rates. These findings have led to some renewed interest in the use of radiotherapy as adjuvant treatment after resection of bulky nodal disease and as palliative treatment for unresectable tumors. As with regional chemotherapy perfusion (see below), local hyperthermia may also increase the responsiveness of melanoma to radiotherapy (48).

FOLLOW-UP

As is the case for initial staging work-up of patients with melanoma, the recommendations for follow-up after primary treatment vary according to initial stage and are usually arbitrary. To some degree, the intensity and frequency of follow-up after surgery will be dictated by the nodal status and the depth of invasion of the primary lesion. The majority of patients who will develop a recurrence will do so in the first 2 years, and 80% to 90% of recurrences will occur in the first 5 years. In all patients who have had a melanoma, especially those with a family history, routine annual or semiannual screening examinations of the entire skin surface are important to detect new primaries. In patients with melanomas deeper than 0.75 mm, regular examinations for local or regional recurrence, especially in those who have not had ELND, are important. As time passes, the frequency of examinations can be decreased. Although no definitive studies of follow-up testing have been done, several studies indicate fairly clearly that routine x-rays, CT scans, and blood tests are not worthwhile. In one series from the Mayo Clinic, 94% of melanoma recurrences were evident on the basis of symp-

TABLE 11–6. *Suggested follow-up schedule for melanoma (intervals between follow-up visits, in months)*

Years postsurgery	1	2	3	4	≥5
Tumor staging					
Tumor ≤1.0 mm	6	6	12	12	12
Tumor >1.0 mm, no SLN biopsy or ELND	3	3	6	12	12
Tumor >1.0 mm, nodes pathologically negative	3	6	6	12	12
Nodes positive	3	3	6	6	12

At each visit, review of systems, with particular attention to symptoms of likely sites of metastases and physical examination, with particular attention to skin, lymph nodes, nervous system, chest, and abdominal exams.

toms or on routine physical examination (49). Only 6% were detected by chest x-ray, and none were manifested solely as abnormalities in laboratory tests. Similarly, at the University of Alabama, more than 90% of patients with recurrent melanoma presented with symptoms of their disease (50). Although treatment of local or regional recurrence may result in long-term survival, the same cannot be said for distant metastases. If the latter occurs, there is no truly effective treatment other than metastectomy for a small number of patients with resectable disease, and only a tiny minority (around 1%) of patients with distant metastases will survive long-term. Thus, the routine use of blood tests, expensive nuclear medicine studies, CT scans, or even chest x-rays cannot be justified. Having said that, there is current research interest in the use of highly sensitive PET scanning to detect and follow recurrent melanoma. A suggested follow-up routine for thin and deeper (or node-positive) melanomas after curative surgery is outlined in Table 11-6.

ISOLATED LIMB PERFUSION FOR RECURRENCE OR AS AN ADJUVANT

First described by Creech et al. four decades ago, isolated limb perfusion (ILP) with chemotherapeutic agents offers the advantage of selective exposure of the perfused extremity to high doses of drug with limited systemic toxicity (51). ILP has been used for recurrent melanoma of the limbs, principally for extensive local recurrences and in-transit metastases (52). Interest in this technique has increased over the last 5 years, with the addition of hyperthermia and cytokines, particularly tumor necrosis factor (TNF) and interferon-γ (IFN-γ). This is now a reasonable alternative in patients for whom the only other real chance for a complete eradication of tumor would be extensive surgery, often an amputation. To date, no chemotherapeutic agent has been shown to be superior to melphalan, an alkylating agent. The addition of increased limb temperature, using heat exchangers to warm the perfusate and warming blankets applied externally, can be used to raise the temperature in the extremity to 40°C, which results in increased response rates. TNF, which is too toxic to give systemically at doses that have antitumor effects in humans, is ideal for regional perfusion, since this technique largely restricts exposure to the treated extremity and protects the rest of the patient from toxicity. TNF also appears to in-

crease the response rate to ILP with melphalan and hyperthermia. Overall response rates in the range of 90% have been observed with this approach, and the proportion of complete responses is quite high, 50% to 90%. Despite these impressive response rates, most of the patients who are candidates for this treatment will succumb to distant metastases within a few years. Nevertheless, a few will experience extended survival and many will be spared the need for amputation. It has also been argued that this treatment may have benefit in the adjuvant setting, but this has not been convincingly demonstrated. One study was stopped prematurely when the ILP group had a significantly improved disease-free survival compared to the controls (53). However, the control group had a much higher than expected recurrence rate, and the early cessation of the trial left the study with very small numbers of patients. At present, the significant logistic effort, expense, and toxicity do not seem to be justified in this setting.

Technically, the ILP procedure requires sophisticated equipment and a dedicated team of physicians, perfusionists, and other personnel. For the lower extremity, the external iliac vessels are cannulated through a retroperitoneal approach, and the root of the extremity is tourniqueted, usually with the use of a Steinman pin placed in the anterior superior iliac spine. Venous tributaries must be ligated to eliminate "leak" of the perfusate into the systemic circulation. An extracorporeal circuit, consisting of a roller pump, oxygenator, and heat exchanger is used. By a combination of heating the perfusate and the extremity, the tissue temperature is kept between 38.5°C and 40°C. The melphalan dose can be based on body weight (0.5 to 1.5 mg/kg) or on volume of the extremity being treated (10 to 13 mg/L). The optimal TNF dose appears to be 4 mg (54). The limb is perfused at flow rates of 50 mL/L limb volume/min for 90 min. Safety is achieved by monitoring the leak of perfusate into the systemic circulation. Either ^{131}I-labeled albumin or [99]Technetium-labeled erythrocytes are added to the perfusate, and the degree of leak is monitored with a gamma detector positioned over the heart. Monitoring the leak rate and keeping it to a minimum is critical to limiting the systemic toxicity, which is the major advantage of this technique. It is evident from even this very abbreviated description that the labor intensity and costs associated with ILP limit the number of facilities that can effectively administer this treatment. Given the estimates of the small proportion of all melanoma patients who are likely to benefit from ILP, referral of such patients to those few centers would be the most efficient approach.

TREATMENT OF METASTASES

Melanoma can metastasize to almost any site; the lungs, skin and subcutaneous tissues, distant lymph nodes, liver, CNS, and GI tract are commonly affected. No consistently effective systemic treatment is available for metastatic melanoma, and 5-year survival after distant recurrence is uncommon (10% to 15%). Dacarbazine, the only chemotherapeutic agent approved by the FDA for use in melanoma, produces objective responses in only 20% of patients, and few if any patients have long-term freedom from disease (55). Trials of a number of different drug combinations have made little impact (55). Much of the excitement in this area is related to a number of immunologic approaches summarized briefly below. At present, however, these should all be considered experimental and should only be administered in the context of a clinical trial.

Some patients with limited metastases may be significantly palliated, and a few may achieve long-term survival after surgical resection of metastases to certain sites. Based on the experience with sarcomas metastatic to the lungs, resection of solitary or limited metastases of melanoma to the lungs has been reported. However, most of these patients have undetected disease in the remaining lung tissue or at other sites and will succumb to their disease in a fairly short time. Median survival after pulmonary metastectomy is 9 to 16 months (55). Most of these patients are not symptomatic, so that the procedure cannot be justified on palliative grounds. However, because many such patients are young and because systemic treatment results are so abysmal, it is not unreasonable to attempt complete metastectomy in the rare patient who presents with limited pulmonary metastases from melanoma.

GI metastases, in contrast, are usually resected to relieve symptoms. Although metastases to the GI tract only rarely present clinically, metastases to the stomach, duodenum, small bowel, or colon are found in nearly 60% of patients who die of melanoma (55,56). In the few patients in whom these lesions become clinically manifest, the presenting symptoms are usually anemia secondary to GI bleeding, acute or intermittent obstruction (often a result of intussusception), or abdominal pain. Most patients are treated by resection of the involved bowel segments, and most are well palliated, with minimal operative morbidity or mortality. Overall survival is poor in most series, with median survivals of 4 to 10 months in patients undergoing palliative resection (56–58). Some patients, however, present with limited GI tract metastases and no other disease. If all of the known disease is resected, some of these patients may experience prolonged survival (56,57). Thus, it is important to consider GI metastases in patients with a history of melanoma who present with intermittent crampy abdominal pain or anemia with heme-positive stools. The diagnosis can usually be made with upper GI series, upper endoscopy, or colonoscopy. Since the small bowel is the most

common site for melanoma metastases in the GI tract, an upper GI series with small bowel follow-through should be the initial study. Occasionally, distal small-bowel metastases can be appreciated only on an enteroclysis study. CT scans may identify concomitant hepatic or intraabdominal metastases; however, if the patient is symptomatic and otherwise in good condition, one should proceed to abdominal exploration for palliative resection without these additional studies.

Metastases to the CNS occur frequently in patients with metastatic melanoma, and may account for 20% of the deaths from this disease (55,59). They may present as motor dysfunction, seizures, headaches, personality changes, or other more subtle findings. Diagnosis and "staging" of the extent of CNS involvement is best achieved by CT scan or MRI. The latter has the significant advantage of greater sensitivity and is more likely to detect additional lesions beyond those causing symptoms; the finding of multiple rather than solitary lesions will impact on the choice of treatment. Therefore, patients with a prior history of melanoma and any significant neurological symptoms should have an MRI of the brain, if available. In virtually all patients with CNS metastases, the treatment should be considered palliative, as almost all of these patients will die of their disease in an average of 3 to 6 months. Most patients with brain involvement by melanoma present with multiple lesions, and the treatment of symptoms includes steroids, anticonvulsive medication, and brain irradiation. In approximately a quarter of patients with brain metastases, a solitary lesion will be found. In these patients, craniotomy and resection of the metastasis, if feasible, followed by irradiation may result in slightly longer survival than irradiation alone (59,60).

NEW APPROACHES—BIOLOGIC THERAPY

Immunologically active cytokines have been tested extensively in the treatment of melanoma, alone, in combination with chemotherapy or with adoptive transfer of activated lymphocytes. The different types of interferons have all been studied in the treatment of metastatic disease. Other than the adjuvant effect of IFN-α described earlier, none has proven more than moderately effective. Interleukin-2 (IL-2) has produced response rates in the range of 20%, but only a few of these have been complete responses, and the costs in terms of toxicity are considerable (61). Interestingly, some of the complete responses were quite durable, lasting several years. The toxicity has been reduced somewhat by modifications of dosing and schedule, but response rates have remained low. Several groups have reported higher response rates using combinations of IL-2, IFN-α, and chemotherapy, but no single regimen has been found that can be considered for standard treatment of either advanced disease or in the adjuvant setting (62). Combining tumor-specific T lymphocytes [derived from tumor-infiltrating lymphocytes (TIL) or from lymph nodes draining the sites of vaccination with autologous tumor] with IL-2, has produced higher response rates than with IL-2 alone, but these therapies should also be considered experimental (62).

For almost three decades, active specific immunotherapy (ASI) or vaccine therapy for melanoma has been explored. The different vaccines tested have ranged from autologous tumor cells mixed with bacterial adjuvants to genetically modified tumor cells to small synthetic peptides identified as relevant melanoma antigens. As immunologic methodology has become more sophisticated, it has been possible to identify a number of melanoma-associated antigens and peptide epitopes that are recognized by T lymphocytes or can induce antibody responses. Donald Morton's group has reported use of a polyvalent vaccine made up of several melanoma cell lines with a broad spectrum of antigens represented. Compared to a matched set of historical controls, they have shown significantly improved survival in stage III and IV patients treated with this vaccine (63). Controlled trials to confirm the efficacy of this vaccine are currently underway. Defined ganglioside vaccines and viral lysates of melanoma cells can induce immune responses in patients with melanoma, but have yet to demonstrate clinical efficacy in controlled trials (64,65). Despite the limited success of vaccine approaches, the identification of well-defined peptide epitopes that are recognized by T lymphocytes from melanoma patients in HLA-restricted fashion has generated new enthusiasm for research and clinical testing in this area (66). One of the major advantages of this approach is its minimal toxicity. In addition, genetically engineered tumor cells and dendritic cells have been shown in animal models to have markedly increased immunogenicity compared to wild-type tumor cells. In some animal models, these vaccines can induce regression of established tumors. This promising approach is now being tested in several independent clinical trials.

CONCLUSION

Melanoma incidence is rapidly accelerating, to a point approaching an epidemic in developed countries. Fortunately, the vast majority of patients with this disease can be cured, and the most effective therapy remains surgery. With a high index of suspicion, a timely diagnosis can be made, and appropriate surgical management of the primary lesion no longer needs to be mutilating. The long-standing controversy over ELND, with its attendant risks and long-term morbidity, seems to be coming to a close. New technology and inventive surgical investigators have given us a less morbid and apparently accurate alternative—SLN mapping and biopsy. Finally, an effective adjuvant therapy, IFN-α, is now available for patients at high risk for recurrence. Hopefully, with continued research on the biology of melanoma and host immune responses to this tumor, more effective and less toxic systemic treatments will become available in the near future.

REFERENCES

1. Landis SH, Murray T, Bolden S, Wingo PA. Cancer statistics, 1998. *CA Cancer J Clin* 1998;48:6.
2. Lee JE. Factors associated with melanoma incidence and prognosis. *Semin Surg Oncol* 1996;12:379.
3. Goldsmith HS. Melanoma: an overview. *CA Cancer J Clin* 1979;29:194.
4. Adam YG, Efron G. Cutaneous malignant melanoma: current views on pathogenesis, diagnosis, and surgical management. *Surgery* 1983;93:481.
5. Rhodes AR, Weinstock MA, Fitzpatrick TB, Mihm MC, Sober AJ. Risk factors for cutaneous melanoma. A practical method of recognizing predisposed individuals. *JAMA* 1987;258:3146.
6. Friedman RJ, Rigel DS, Silverman MK, Kopf AW, Vossaert KA. Malignant melanoma in the 1990s: the continued importance of early detection and the role of physician examination and self-examination of the skin. *CA Cancer J Clin* 1991;41:201.
7. Evans GR, Manson PN. Review and current perspectives of cutaneous malignant melanoma. *JAMA* 1994;178:523.
8. Clark WH, From L, Bernardino EA, Mihm MC. The histogenesis and biologic behavior of primary human malignant melanomas of the skin. *Cancer Res* 1969;29:705.
9. Breslow A. Thickness, cross-sectional area and depth of invasion in the prognosis of cutaneous melanoma. *Ann Surg* 1970;172:902.
10. Beahrs OH, Henson DE, Hutter RVP, Kennedy BJ, eds. Malignant melanoma of the skin. In: *American Joint Committee on Cancer Manual for Staging of Cancer.* 4th ed. Philadelphia: JB Lippincott Co, 1992:143.
11. Neifeld JP. Endocrinology of melanoma. *Semin Surg Oncol* 1996;12:402.
12. Cascinelli N. BANS: a cutaneous region with no prognostic significance in patients with melanoma. *Cancer* 1986;57:441.
13. Reintgen D, Balch CM, Kirkwood J, Ross M. Recent advances in the care of the patient with malignant melanoma. *Ann Surg* 1997;225:1.
14. Kuvshinoff B, Kurtz C, Coit DG. Computed tomography in evaluation of patients with stage III melanoma. *Ann Surg Oncol* 1997;4:252.
15. Handley WS. The pathology of melanotic growths in relation to their operative treatment. Lecture I. *Lancet* 1907;1:927.
16. Handley WS. The pathology of melanotic growths in relation to their operative treatment. Lecture II. *Lancet* 1907;1:966.
17. Veronesi U, Cascinelli N. Narrow excision (1-cm margin). A safe procedure for thin cutaneous melanoma. *Arch Surg* 1991;126:438.
18. Balch CM, Urist MM, Karakousis CP, et al. Efficacy of 2-cm surgical margins for intermediate-thickness melanomas (1 to 4 mm): results of a multi-institutional randomized surgical trial. *Ann Surg* 1993;218:262.
19. NIH Consensus Conference. Diagnosis and treatment of early melanoma [Review]. *JAMA* 1992;268:1314.
20. Park KG, Blessing K, Kernohan NM. Surgical aspects of subungual malignant melanomas. *Ann Surg* 1992;216:692.
21. Finley RK, Driscoll DL, Blumenson LE, Karakousis CP. Subungual melanoma: an eighteen-year review. *Surgery* 1994;116:96.
22. McKinnon JG, Kokal WA, Neifeld JP, Kay S. Natural history and treatment of mucosal melanoma. *J Surg Oncol* 1989;41:222.
23. Sutherland CM, Chmiel JS, Henson DE, Winchester DP. Patient characteristics, methods of diagnosis, and treatment of mucous membrane melanoma in the United States of America. *JAMA* 1994;179:561.
24. Ben-Izhak O, Levy R, Weill S, et al. Anorectal malignant melanoma, a clinicopathologic study, indluding immunohistochemistry and DNA flow cytometry. *Cancer* 1997;79:18.
25. Harris MN, Shapiro RL, Roses DF. Malignant Melanoma, primary surgical management (excision and node dissection) based on pathology and staging. *Cancer* 1995;75:715.
26. Karakousis CP, Emrich LJ, Driscoll DL, Rao U. Survival after groin dissection for malignant melanoma. *Surgery* 1991;109:119.
27. Pearlman NW, Robinson WA, Dreiling LK, McIntyre RC Jr, Gonzales R. Modified ilioinguinal node dissection for metastatic melanoma. *Am J Surg* 1995;170:647.
28. Devereux DF. Regional node dissection. In: Daly JM, Cady B, Low DW, eds. *Atlas of surgical oncology.* St. Louis, MO: Mosby, 1993:705.
29. Balch CM, Urist MM, Maddox WA, Milton GW, McCarthy WH. Management of regional metastatic melanoma. In: Balch CM, Milton GW, eds. *Cutaneous melanoma: clinical management and treatment results worldwide.* Philadelphia: JB Lippincott Co, 1985:93.
30. Balch CM, Soong S, Milton GW, et al. A comparison of prognostic factors and surgical results in 1,786 patients with localized (stage I) melanoma treated in Alabama, USA, and New South Wales, Australia. *Ann Surg* 1982;196:677.
31. Crowley NJ, Seigler HF. The role of elective lymph node dissection in the management of patients with thick cutaneous melanoma. *Cancer* 1990;66:2522.

32. Reintgen DS, Cox EB, McCarty KS, Vollmer RT, Seigler HF. Efficacy of elective lymph node dissection in patients with intermediate thickness primary melanoma. *Ann Surg* 1983;198:379.

33. Bear HD, Neifeld JP, Kay S. Prognosis of level V malignant melanoma. *Cancer* 1985;55:1167.

34. Balch CM. The role of elective lymph node dissection in melanoma: rationale, results and controversies. *J Clin Oncol* 1988;6:163.

35. Slingluff CL Jr, Stidham KR, Ricci WM, Stanley WE, Seigler HF. Surgical management of regional lymph nodes in patients with melanoma: experience with 4682 patients. *Ann Surg* 1994;219:120.

36. Veronesi U, Adamus J, Bandiera DC, et al. Inefficacy of immediate node dissection in Sage I melanoma of the limbs. *N Engl J Med* 1977;297:627.

37. Veronesi U, Adamus J, Bandiera DC, et al. Delayed regional lymph node dissection in stage I melanoma of the skin of the lower extremities. *Cancer* 1982;49:2420.

38. Sim FH, Taylor WF, Pritchard DJ, Soule EH. Lymphadenectomy in the management of stage I malignant melanoma: a prospective randomized study. *Mayo Clin Proc* 1986;61:697.

39. Balch CM, Soong S, Bartolucci AA, et al. Efficacy of an elective regional lymph node dissection of 1 to 4 mm thick melanomas for patients 60 years of age or younger. *Ann Surg* 1996;224:266.

40. Norman J, Cruse CW, Espinosa C, et al. Redefinition of cutaneous lymphatic drainage with the use of lymphoscintigraphy for malignant melanoma. *Am J Surg* 1991;162:432.

41. Morton DL, Wen D-R, Wong JH, et al. Technical details of intraoperative lymphatic mapping for early stage melanoma. *Arch Surg* 1992;127:392.

42. Ross MI. Surgical management of stage I and II melanoma patients: approach to the regional lymph node basin. *Semin Surg Oncol* 1996;12:394.

43. Reintgen D, Cruse CW, Wells K, et al. The orderly progression of melanoma nodal metastases. *Ann Surg* 1994;220:759.

44. Krag DN, Meijer SJ, Weaver DL, et al. Minimal-access surgery for staging of malignant melanoma. *Arch Surg* 1995;130:654.

45. Albertini JJ, Cruse CW, Rapaport D, et al. Intraoperative radiolymphoscintigraphy improves sentinel lymph node identification for patients with melanoma. *Ann Surg* 1996;223:217.

46. Wang X, Heller R, VanVoorhis N, et al. Detection of submicroscopic lymph node metastases with polymerase chain reaction in patients with malignant melanoma. *Ann Surg* 1994;220:768.

47. Kirkwood JM, Strawderman MH, Ernstoff MS, Smith TJ, Borden EC, Blum RH. Interferon alfa-2b adjuvant therapy of high-risk resected cutaneous melanoma: the Eastern Cooperative Oncology Group trial EST 1684. *J Clin Oncol* 1996;14:7.

48. Schmidt-Ullrich RK, Johnson CR. Role of radiotherapy and hyperthermia in the management of malignant melanoma. *Semin Surg Oncol* 1966;12:407.

49. Weiss M, Loprinzi CL, Creagan ET, Dalton RJ, Novotny P, O'Fallon JR. Utility of follow-up tests for detecting recurrent disease in patients with malignant melanomas. *JAMA* 1995;274:1703.

50. Shumate CR, Urist MM, Maddox WA. Melanoma recurrence surveillance patient or physician based? *Ann Surg* 1995;221:566.

51. Creech OJ Jr, Krementz ET, Ryan RF, Winblad JN. Chemotherapy of cancer: regional perfusion utilizing an extracorporeal circuit. *Ann Surg* 1958;148:616.

52. Alexander HR Jr, Fraker DL, Bartlett DL. Isolated limb perfusion for malignant melanoma. *Semin Surg Oncol* 1996;12:416.

53. Ghussen F, Nagel K, Groth W, Müller JM, Stützer H. A prospective randomized study of regional extremity perfusion in patients with malignant melanoma. *Ann Surg* 1984;200:764–768.

54. Fraker DL, Alexander HR, Andrich M, Rosenberg SA. Treatment of patients with melanoma of the extremity using hyperthermic isolated limb perfusion with melphalan, tumor necrosis factor, and interferon gamma: results of a tumor necrosis factor dose-escalation study. *J Clin Oncol* 1996;14:479.

55. Yeung RS. Management of recurrent cutaneous melanoma. *Curr Probl Cancer* 1994;18:143.

56. Ollila DW, Essner R, Wanek LA, Morton DL. Surgical resection for melanoma metastatic to the gastrointestinal tract. *Arch Surg* 1996; 131:975.

57. Ihde JK, Coit DG. Melanoma metastatic to stomach, small bowel, or colon. *Am J Surg* 1991;162:208.

58. Khadra MH, Thompson JF, Milton GW, McCarthy WH. The justification for surgical treatment of metastatic melanoma of the gastrointestinal tract. *Surg Gynecol Obstet* 1990;171:413.

59. Ewend MG, Carey LA, Brem H. Treatment of melanoma metastases in the brain. *Semin Surg Oncol* 1996;12:429.

60. Patchell RA, Tibbs PA, Walsh JW, et al. A randomized trial of surgery in the treatment of single metastases to the brain. *N Engl J Med* 1990; 322:494.

61. Rosenberg SA, Yang JC, Topalian SL, et al. Treatment of 283 consecutive patients with metastatic melanoma or renal cell cancer using high-dose bolus interleukin 2. *JAMA* 1994;271:907.

62. Bear HD, Hamad GG, Kostuchenko PJ. Biologic therapy of melanoma with cytokines and lymphocytes. *Semin Surg Oncol* 1996;12:436.

63. Morton DL, Foshag LJ, Hoon DSB, et al. Prolongation of survival in metastatic melanoma after active specific immunotherapy with a new polyvalent melanoma vaccine. *Ann Surg* 1992;216:463.

64. Livingston PO, Wong GY, Adluri S, et al. Improved survival in stage III melanoma patients with GM2 antibodies: a randomized trial of adjuvant vaccination with GM2 ganglioside. *J Clin Oncol* 1994; 12:1036.

65. Wallack MK, Sivanandham M, Balch CM, et al. A phase III randomized, double-blind, multiinstitutional trial of vaccinia melanoma oncolysate-active specific immunotherapy for patients with stage II melanoma. *Cancer* 1995;75:34.

66. Slinghuff CL Jr. Tumor antigens and tumor vaccines: peptides as immunogens. *Semin Surg Oncol* 1996;12:446.

CHAPTER 12

Esophageal Cancer

Robert J. Korst and Nasser K. Altorki

Carcinoma of the esophagus is a devastating disease, which is uncommon except in endemic areas throughout the world. Unfortunately, symptoms usually do not become apparent until the disease is in its advanced stages, which contributes to the poor outcome. Squamous cell carcinoma has historically been the most common histologic type of esophageal carcinoma. However, a recent increase in the incidence of esophageal adenocarcinoma is well documented in the Western world. Due to the advanced nature of esophageal carcinoma at the time of diagnosis, palliation of symptoms plays a critical role in the treatment of this disease. In the uncommon situation where earlier, localized esophageal carcinoma is detected, cure can be obtained by esophagectomy utilizing a number of different approaches. The surgical approach and extent of resection remain controversial issues in the treatment of this type of solid tumor. The technique of esophagectomy has evolved extensively throughout the 20th century and what was once a procedure with a prohibitive mortality rate can now be performed safely in the vast majority of cases.

INCIDENCE

Carcinoma of the esophagus is estimated to be the seventh most common malignancy worldwide. The incidence of squamous cell carcinoma of the esophagus varies widely based on geographic location. Areas associated with a higher incidence include China, Japan, Iran, France, southern Africa and central South America. Low risk areas include North and Central America, North and Central Africa and western Asia.

Even more striking are localized pockets within the above areas where the incidence of squamous cell esophageal cancer approaches almost epidemic proportions. Examples include several Northern Chinese provinces, areas immediately adjacent to the Caspian Sea, the mountainous regions of Japan, and the Transkei district in South Africa. Severe geographic variations in incidence rates suggest that environmental factors play a significant role in esophageal carcinogenesis. Unfortunately, no single environmental factor seems to be a universal etiologic agent, implying that squamous cell

carcinoma of the esophagus is the result of a multistep carcinogenic process.

In North America squamous cell carcinoma of the esophagus is an uncommon disease. The average incidence is thought to be five to 10 per year per 100,000 population. As with other industrialized countries, such as those in western Europe, the rates are higher in the urban, rather than rural, areas. The coastal southeastern states seem to have the highest incidence of squamous cell esophageal cancer, with age adjusted rates of greater than 20 per year per 100,000 population in some counties.

Adenocarcinoma of the esophagus is mainly a disease of the industrialized, western countries of Europe and North America. The typical patient is a middle-aged to elderly White male with a history of gastroesophageal reflux. Many epidemiological studies demonstrate the rise in incidence of adenocarcinoma of the esophagus in this setting (1), although the actual incidence is difficult to determine since it is unclear if adenocarcinoma of the gastroesophageal junction is gastric or esophageal in origin.

ETIOLOGY AND RISK FACTORS

Genetic and Familial Factors

Historically, both squamous cell and adenocarcinoma of the esophagus are diseases of the elderly. Infrequent prior to age forty, the incidence rises with each progressive decade of life. Males are generally more affected than females, but in high prevalence areas of squamous cell carcinoma, the percentage of females is higher. Squamous cell carcinoma is more common in Blacks, while adenocarcinoma is more common in Whites.

The only genetic disease associated with the development of esophageal cancer is tylosis, a condition characterized by hyperkeratosis of the palms and soles. An autosomal dominant disease, it is estimated that patients afflicted with tylosis have a 90% chance of developing squamous cell carcinoma of the esophagus by age 65 (2).

Scattered reports of esophageal cancer running in families from China and Iran and the strong family history of esophageal carcinoma in patients from these areas support that there may be other undefined genetic factors present in the etiology of esophageal cancer (3). In addition, molecular analysis of tumor specimens reveals activation of oncogenes and/or mutations in tumor suppressor genes in a significant percentage of both adenocarcinomas and squamous cell carcinomas of the esophagus (4).

Environmental Factors

Heavy alcohol consumption is thought to predispose to the development of squamous cell carcinoma of the esophagus. The relationship between drinking and adenocarcinoma, however, is much more vague, with some studies suggesting a predisposition (5) and others finding no relationship at all (6). Most of these data suggest that hard liquor carries the highest risk, although some studies amongst beer drinkers are also incriminating (7). The smoking of tobacco in its multiple forms (cigar, cigarette, pipe) has also been shown to increase the risk of developing esophageal cancer in several prospective and retrospective studies (8). This increased risk seems to apply mainly to squamous cell carcinoma; however, recent studies suggest an association with adenocarcinoma as well (5).

Much more impressive is the striking increase in risk when heavy alcohol consumption is combined with cigarette smoking. This combination has been reported to increase the risk of developing esophageal cancer by more than 100-fold in some studies (8). Confounding this information, however, is the observation that in some of the geographic areas (Iran) where esophageal cancer reaches almost epidemic proportions, alcohol use is rare, and even forbidden. This fact reiterates that multiple environmental factors can act as carcinogens in the esophagus, and suggests that no one agent is necessary for tumor development.

In those cultures where alcohol and tobacco may not be used, other recreational activities are thought to predispose to esophageal cancer development. Examples include the chewing of betel nut and betel leaf in India, the swallowing of silica-laden soil in southern Africa, the chewing of opium residue in Iran, and the chronic ingestion of hot liquids in South America.

Diet and nutrition are considered to play a major environmental role in the development of carcinoma of the esophagus. Intuitively this is not surprising since the esophageal mucosa contacts ingested carcinogens immediately following their consumption. Common findings in areas with a high incidence of esophageal cancer are poverty and malnutrition. Although overt clinical malnutrition may not be seen, specific deficiencies are present which have been shown to promote carcinogenesis in the esophagus. Diets in these areas are characteristically low in animal protein, vitamins A and C, riboflavin and trace elements. Epidemiologic as well as experimental studies suggest that deficiencies in these substances may play a role in esophageal tumorigenesis (9). Large-scale nutritional replacement trials are currently underway in

China to further evaluate the role of nutritional deficiencies in the etiology of esophageal cancer (10).

Diets consisting of large amounts of nitrates, nitrites, and nitrosamines are thought to increase the risk of esophageal cancer. Again, epidemiologic and experimental studies suggest that these substances are carcinogenic to the esophagus in humans as well as animals (11). Increased exposure to these substances has been reported in regions where the incidence of esophageal cancer is high, including southern Africa, Iran, and China.

Preexisting Esophageal Diseases

Conditions of the esophagus that have been reported to predispose to the development of carcinoma are multiple and include the presence of Plummer-Vinson syndrome, lye strictures, and achalasia. Scattered case reports of carcinoma arising in esophageal diverticulae have suggested that these may predispose to cancer as well (12).

The most important preexisting condition of the esophagus with regard to cancer formation in the Western world, however, is the columnar-lined (or Barrett's) esophagus. It is universally accepted that this condition results from chronic gastroesophageal reflux, and numerous studies show a high prevalence of adenocarcinoma in the metaplastic esophagus (13). In addition, animal models of gastroduodenal reflux result in a significant incidence of intestinal metaplasia and esophageal carcinoma (14). The relative risk of developing adenocarcinoma in Barrett's esophagus is thought to be 30 to 40 times higher than the general population (13). Due to aggressive endoscopic screening protocols in patients with Barrett's esophagus, a significant number of these cancers are being detected at an early stage, when esophagectomy offers the best chance for cure.

PATHOLOGY
Cell Types

The vast majority of esophageal carcinomas are either squamous cell carcinoma or adenocarcinoma. Historically, the most common histologic type has been squamous cell carcinoma, but multiple studies are reporting an increasing percentage of adenocarcinoma (1). This change is mainly occurring in North America and western Europe and the majority of cases involve White males.

In less than 2% of cases of primary esophageal malignancies, a cell type other than squamous cell carcinoma or adenocarcinoma is encountered (15). These include sarcomas, choriocarcinoma, malignant melanoma, lymphomas, and rare carcinomas (small cell, carcinoid, mucoepidermoid, adenoid cystic). These tumors are very rare and the majority of the literature addressing them consists of isolated case reports. They will not be considered further in this chapter.

Squamous cell carcinoma arises from the squamous epithelium that lines the majority of the esophagus. Adenocarcinoma, on the other hand, may arise from the superficial or submucosal glands of the esophagus, islands of ectopic gastric mucosa, or from columnar metaplasia in the distal esophagus (Barrett's). The most common site of origin of esophageal adenocarcinoma seems to be the Barrett's esophagus.

Tumor Location

The majority of squamous cell carcinomas arise in the middle third of the esophagus. This region is defined as ranging from the carina superiorly to the level of the inferior pulmonary veins inferiorly. Most large studies confirm that approximately 50% to 60% of these tumors originate in this region, 20% to 30% arise in the distal third, and only 10% to 20% in the proximal third (16).

Adenocarcinomas, on the other hand, arise mainly in the distal third of the esophagus, and at the gastroesophageal junction. This observation reiterates the fact that most of these tumors originate in dysplastic Barrett's mucosa. Even short segment Barrett's (less than 3 cm) is currently thought to predispose to the development of cancer. Adenocarcinomas located at the gastroesophageal junction, however, are less likely to be associated with Barrett's metaplasia since the tumor may completely overgrow any associated metaplastic areas, resulting in the absence of Barrett's mucosa on pathologic examination (17). Additionally, some of the tumors involving the lower esophagus may be the result of cephalad extension of a primary gastric cancer. In our clinical practice, the tumor is considered esophageal in origin if 75% or more of the tumor mass is within the tubular esophagus.

Macroscopic Appearance

The gross, morphologic appearance of esophageal cancer has been reported by multiple authors. Akiyama et al. (18) described esophageal cancers as being exophytic protuberant, ulcerative with a regular border, ulcerative with an irregular border, superficial, endophytic, and endophytic with protuberance. The significance of this classification lies in the incidence of lymph node metastases with the varying types—the former two having a low incidence of metastatic lymph nodes and the latter four having a high incidence. In Akiyama's studies, the morphological appearance translated into a significant difference in survival.

Other reports classify esophageal cancer using similar gross descriptive terms, but it seems unnecessary to discuss the gross appearance since the depth of wall penetration and degree of lymph node metastases are the important determinants of survival.

Patterns of Spread

Esophageal cancer, regardless of the histologic type, can spread via four mechanisms. These include intraesophageal spread, wall penetration with direct extension into surrounding structures, lymphatic spread, and hematologic dissemination.

Intraesophageal spread of esophageal cancer occurs far beyond the extent of the gross tumor that is visualized in the esophagus. Microscopic tumor is often present several centimeters proximal to the gross margin of the tumor and clinicopathologic studies have also demonstrated that anastomotic recurrences are more common as the extent of the proximal resection gets shorter (19). This type of spread occurs in the submucosa and is facilitated by the extensive lymphatics present in this layer. Skip lesions and satellite nodules are frequent occurrences as a result of submucosal microscopic spread. Distal submucosal spread, however, is not as extensive as proximal spread for reasons that are not known. Both squamous cell and adenocarcinomas tend to spread in this fashion.

Tumor invasion and penetration through the esophageal wall into surrounding structures is another mechanism of spread. Midesophageal lesions can easily invade into the bronchi whereas distal third lesions tend to invade the diaphragm, stomach, and liver. Upper third tumors can involve the trachea or great vessels, the spine or recurrent laryngeal nerves. The earliest type of esophageal carcinoma is that which is confined to the muscularis mucosa (intramucosal) and submucosa. These early lesions, however, are rare in regions where routine screening for esophageal cancer is not practiced.

Lymphatic spread is common in patients with esophageal cancer. Patterns of lymphatic spread have been extensively studied, especially in Japan. Lymphoscintigraphy has demonstrated that lymphatic flow in the esophagus proceeds mainly in a longitudinal, not transverse, fashion. In general, lymphatic spread of esophageal cancer is most likely to proceed in a caudad direction; however, flow in either direction from a lesion anywhere in the esophagus can be observed.

The incidence of lymph node metastases in large series of patients who underwent resection of squamous cell carcinoma of the esophagus has been reported to be 59% (16), but this figure is highly dependent on the depth of wall penetration of the primary tumor (Table 12-1). In addition, the incidence of lymph node metastases also depends on the extent of lymphadenectomy performed. The data in Table 12-1 confirm that the more radical the lymphadenectomy, the higher the rate of lymph node metastases. Nodal metastases in adenocarcinoma, however, are thought to be more common, with multiple studies reporting an incidence of around 75% (20). This higher rate for adenocarcinoma may reflect the tendency of this histologic type to invade submucosal lymphatics at a very early stage.

As alluded to previously, lymphatic spread from esophageal cancer can occur to nodal stations in the abdomen, chest, and neck. The most commonly involved lymph nodes, regardless of the location of the primary tumor, tend to be lower mediastinal (periesophageal, diaphragmatic) and upper abdominal (paracardiac, lesser curve). An example of a complete lymph node map for esophageal cancer has been proposed and is shown in Fig. 12-1. The corresponding nodal stations are listed in Table 12-2. It should be noted that this map is an adaptation of the lung cancer lymph node staging

TABLE 12–1. *Incidence of lymph node metastases according to tumor depth in patients undergoing esophagectomy for carcinoma*

Reference (first author)	No. of patients	Extent of lymphadenectomy	Nodal metastases[a]			
			T1	T2	T3	T4
Lu (61)	504	Nonradical	0[b]	29.7	43.2	69.1
Kato (38)	79	Radical	50	72.7	88.6	75
Nishimaki (62)	141	Radical	51.9	65	70.8	76.2

[a] Incidence of nodal metastases in the surgical specimens displayed as percent of total cases
[b] Only one patient had a T1 tumor in this study

map, and that some nodal stations reported to be particularly relevant to the spread of esophageal cancer (e.g., recurrent laryngeal nodes) are not clearly delineated on this map. Cervical and supraclavicular lymph nodes have been reported to be involved in 15% to 30%; however, one large autopsy series placed this figure at only 6.9% (21). One recent prospective study demonstrated cervical lymph node metastases in 30% of patients with lower third tumors who underwent a three-field lymph node dissection (22).

Distant metastases (visceral) are seen in approximately 15% to 30% of patients with esophageal cancer at the time of presentation, with one recent report placing this figure at 18% (23). The most commonly involved areas, in decreasing order of frequency, are lung, liver, pleura, bone, kidney, and adrenal glands. The presence of visceral metastases indicates advanced, unresectable disease.

CLINICAL MANIFESTATIONS

The clinical manifestations of esophageal carcinoma are, unfortunately, usually indicators of advanced disease. Table 12-3 demonstrates the relative frequencies of symptoms in a large series of patients with esophageal cancer.

The most common symptom is dysphagia which results from obstruction of the esophageal lumen. Dysphagia first begins to solids, and progresses to soft foods and finally liquids, as opposed to the dysphagia associated with motor disturbances of the esophagus, which typically do not show a clear progression of this kind. Unfortunately, at least two-thirds of the esophageal lumen must be obliterated before dysphagia becomes significant, and this indicates advanced local disease.

Early carcinoma of the esophagus is usually asymptomatic. Dyspepsia and symptoms of regurgitation may be present but are not due to the malignancy itself. Instead, they may reflect the underlying gastroesophageal reflux that is present in a significant number of patients with esophageal cancer. Early lesions may also present with gastrointestinal bleeding, although this is more uncommon. Most early lesions are diagnosed as a result of screening endoscopy in regions where squamous cell carcinoma is common, or in patients with Barrett's esophagus.

As the tumor penetrates the esophageal wall, symptoms that may occur include hoarseness due to involvement of the recurrent laryngeal nerve (usually left-sided), back pain due to invasion of the prevertebral fascia, and cough and pneumonia as the airway structures are invaded.

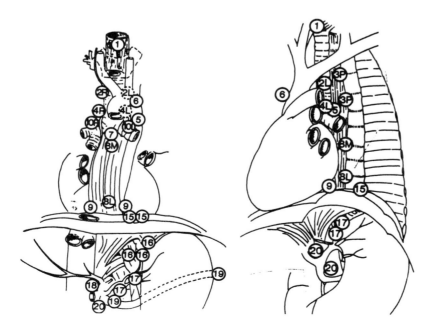

FIG. 12-1. Lymph node staging map for esophageal cancer. For description of nodal stations, see Table 12-2. (Reprinted with permission from Bristol-Myers Oncology Division.)

TABLE 12–2. *Nodal stations*[a]

Station no.	Description
1	Cervical
2R, 2L	High paratracheal
3P	Upper paraesophageal
4R, 4L	Lower paratracheal
5	Aortopulmonary window
6	Preaortic
7	Subcarinal
8M, 8L	Middle, lower paraesophageal
9	Inferior pulmonary ligament
10R, 10L	Tracheobronchial
15	Diaphragmatic (posterior crural)
16	Paracardial
17	Left gastric (lesser curve)
18	Common hepatic
19	Splenic and splenic artery
20	Celiac axis

[a] Nodal stations as depicted in Fig. 12-1.

Physical examination findings are usually absent in patients with early lesions. Palpable supraclavicular adenopathy, hepatomegaly and jaundice, and cachexia indicate far advanced disease. Laboratory investigation can reveal signs of malnutrition, as well as anemia and hypercalcemia. Again, significant laboratory abnormalities usually indicate advanced disease.

DIAGNOSIS

As mentioned previously, early carcinomas of the esophagus are infrequently discovered since these tumors do not become symptomatic until their late stages. In regions where squamous cell carcinoma is endemic, however, screening protocols have diagnosed these early lesions more readily. In China, cytologic screening performed by brushing the esoph-

ageal wall with an abrasive balloon catheter has diagnosed esophageal cancer in asymptomatic patients. Screening flexible esophagoscopy with biopsies has been shown to be useful as well.

In North America and western Europe, aggressive screening endoscopy is advocated for patients with Barrett's esophagus. In addition to the diagnosis of early Barrett's cancer, the finding of high grade dysplasia (carcinoma *in situ*) on systematic biopsies is thought by most to be an indication for esophagectomy, since approximately 40% of these patients will be found to have invasive adenocarcinoma in the resected specimen (24).

In symptomatic patients a barium swallow is usually the first diagnostic maneuver. Carcinoma is usually seen as a filling defect on these studies (Fig. 12-2), which can be fairly easily distinguished from benign masses based on its appearance. Lesions can be polypoid, ulcerative, or stricture-forming and usually some degree of obstruction to barium flow is noted. In the years prior to the use of computed tomography (CT) and endoscopic ultrasound (EUS), barium swallow was useful for determining which tumors were unresectable based on invasion of neighboring structures. Akiyama et al. (25) determined that 74% of esophageal tumors that penetrated the wall were associated with abnormalities of the normal axis of the esophagus. Axis abnormalities are caused by tethering of the esophagus in the region of the tumor. This tethering causes angulation and tortuosity of the normally concave, smooth barium column.

TABLE 12–3. *Presenting symptoms in 820 patients with squamous cell carcinoma of the esophagus*

Symptom	Percentage of patients
Dysphagia	94.4
Regurgitation	45.5
Weight loss	41.3
Cough	26.5
Pain	18.8
Hoarseness	16.8
Anorexia	15.2
Cough on swallowing	7.4
Dyspnea	5.0
Malaise	4.0
Constipation	3.9
Neck mass	3.5
Hemoptysis	3.3
Tarry stool	3.2
Hematemesis	2.8
Other	2.4

Adapted from Fok and Wong (63).

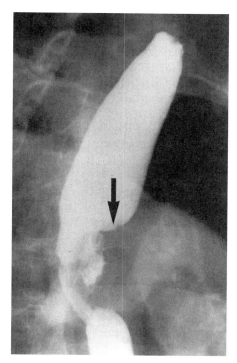

FIG. 12-2. Barium esophagram from a 77-year-old man with dysphagia. A protuberant mass *(arrow)* is seen at the level of the carina. Biopsy revealed squamous cell carcinoma.

The majority of esophageal cancers are diagnosed with flexible esophagoscopy. A positive tissue diagnosis can be made in most cases by either biopsy or brushings. In addition, endoscopy allows for visualization of the entire esophagus, which is important in the determination of tumor extent and the extent of Barrett's mucosa, if present. The distance between the tumor and landmark structures such as the aortic arch and lower esophageal sphincter can be measured, which aids in operative strategy. Skip lesions can also be diagnosed in this fashion. Staining of the esophageal mucosa with toluidine blue or Lugol's solution with endoscopic visualization has also been reported to diagnose early cancers that do not present with an obvious mass (26). Additionally, flexible endoscopy allows for a full examination of the stomach and duodenum for associated abnormalities, such as duodenal ulceration, that may influence operative strategy.

PREOPERATIVE STAGING

Once the diagnosis of esophageal carcinoma is made, the tumor must be staged as accurately as possible, because treatment for this disease is stage dependent. Although multiple modalities exist for the staging of esophageal cancer, none is entirely accurate.

Computed Tomography/Magnetic Resonance Imaging

CT is presently the most utilized imaging study in the workup and staging of esophageal carcinoma. Information obtainable from a CT scan in a patient with esophageal cancer pertains to the local invasion of the primary tumor, the extent of lymph node metastases, and the presence or absence of visceral metastases.

The least controversial aspect of the CT scan in the staging of esophageal carcinoma is its ability to detect visceral metastases. Liver and lung metastases are readily visualized using this modality; however, as the sensitivity of newer generation scanners increases, the specificity may fall because many small lesions in the lungs prove to be benign. It is for this reason that histologic proof of metastases must be obtained prior to basing therapeutic decisions on the results of a CT scan.

CT is also useful for predicting invasion of mediastinal structures by the primary tumor (T4). The depth of tumor invasion into the esophageal wall (T1-2), however, is not accurately predicted by the CT scan. Invasion of surrounding structures is predicted by looking for mass effect and loss of normal fat planes in the mediastinum. The accuracy of CT scan for detecting tracheobronchial invasion has been reported to be as high as 97% based on deformation of these structures by the tumor (27) (Fig. 12-3). Loss of normal fat planes in the mediastinum is used to detect invasion of the aorta and pericardium. If the paravertebral triangular fat space normally present between the aorta, vertebral column, and the esophagus is lost, invasion of the aorta is usually present (Fig. 12-4). Others have based the probability of aortic in-

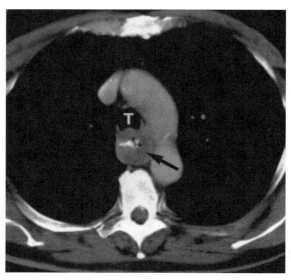

FIG. 12-3. CT scan of the chest with intravenous and oral contrast from the patient depicted in Fig. 12-2. A thickened esophagus representing tumor *(arrow)* is seen at the level of the carina, with bulging of the membranous portion of the trachea *(T)*. Operative exploration revealed a T4 lesion despite negative bronchoscopy.

volvement on the extent of direct contact between the aorta and the tumor. If this extent of contact exceeds 90 degrees, aortic invasion is likely, but if less than 45 degrees, aortic invasion is uncommon (28). Pericardial invasion is also detected by loss of fat planes, with a sensitivity reported to be as high as 94% (27).

CT, unfortunately, is unreliable in the detection of lymph node metastases. Although CT can detect enlarged lymph

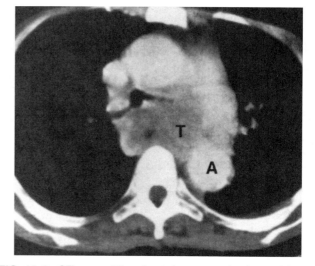

FIG. 12-4. CT scan of the chest demonstrating loss of the fat plane between a large esophageal tumor *(T)* and the descending thoracic aorta *(A)*. Operative exploration revealed a T4 lesion.

nodes, it cannot differentiate between reactive hyperplasia and malignancy. Conversely, the CT scan also cannot detect malignant tissue in normal-sized lymph nodes. Most studies report the sensitivity and specificity of CT scan for detecting metastatic lymph nodes to be approximately 40% and 90%, respectively (27).

Magnetic resonance imaging (MRI) has been compared to CT in the staging of esophageal cancer in several studies. It is generally agreed that MRI has no added benefit over CT for the detection of primary tumor invasion and metastatic spread of esophageal cancer (27). The added cost and limited availability of MRI actually make this imaging modality less desirable than CT.

Endoscopic Ultrasonography

In recent years, EUS has emerged as an important tool for the preoperative staging of several gastrointestinal malignancies, including esophageal cancer. High frequency ultrasound is utilized for these studies due to its high resolution. Although unlikely to determine the presence or absence of distant metastases, this modality is used frequently for assessing tumor penetration (T) and lymph node involvement (N) of esophageal cancer.

The great strength of EUS lies in its ability to visualize the esophageal wall in greater detail than any other imaging modality. Using this technique, the esophageal wall can be seen as a distinct five layer structure consisting of alternating light and dark bands. Each band corresponds to a histologic layer of the bowel wall. In a recent review of nearly 800 patients, EUS had an accuracy of 85% for predicting the depth of cancer invasion into the bowel wall (29) (Fig. 12-5). The least accurate stage to predict was T2, but even this stage could be predicted accurately in 80% of cases.

The detection of lymph node metastases, however, remains problematic. In the same series, the ability to accurately predict N0 disease was only 61% (29), indicating that specificity is a major problem with this technique. Although EUS can detect lymph nodes that appear abnormal (Fig. 12-6), it seems unable to determine if these abnormal nodes contain tumor. Transesophageal fine needle aspiration of suspicious nodes for cytology may play a role in improving the specificity of this modality.

The main technical limitation of EUS as a preoperative staging technique lies in the inability to pass the endoscope through the lesion in as many as 50% of cases (29). Thinner, nonoptical probes are currently being developed, and this problem may be overcome in the near future.

Although EUS is a useful technique for determining the depth of tumor invasion, its necessity in the preoperative workup of patients with esophageal cancer remains questionable. In the vast majority of cases the result of the EUS will not change the therapeutic strategy. Inoperability, as defined by tumor invasion into adjacent structures (T4), can be accurately detected with CT, as discussed previously, and since the standard of care is esophagectomy for patients with

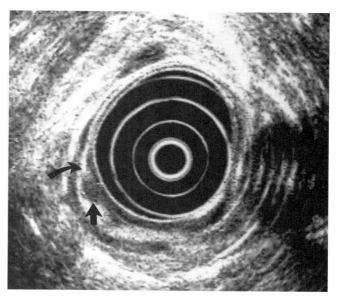

FIG. 12-5. Endoscopic ultrasonographic image of the distal esophagus in a patient with Barrett's metaplasia and some superficial ulceration. Biopsy revealed adenocarcinoma. A T1 lesion is seen via endosonography because the hypoechoic tumor *(straight arrow)* extends into the submucosa *(curved arrow),* but not into the muscularis propria.

T1, T2, and T3 lesions, it is not essential to assess the depth of wall penetration with EUS. Similarly, since lymph node involvement cannot be reliably assessed with EUS, therapeutic decisions cannot be based on it without histologic confirmation.

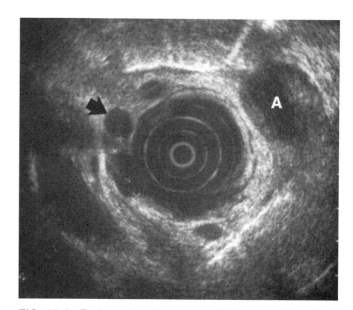

FIG. 12-6. Endoscopic ultrasonographic image of the distal esophagus in a patient with a T3 midesophageal squamous cell carcinoma, demonstrating enlarged paraesophageal lymph nodes *(arrow).* The aorta *(A)* is also visualized.

The clinical usefulness of EUS, therefore, is limited to the following. First, it is useful in assessing the response to neoadjuvant (induction) therapy in investigational protocols. Second, it can be used for selecting patients for therapeutic protocols that use the T stage as an inclusion criterion, and third, it can be used as a confirmatory tool when the CT scan suggests a T4 lesion prior to denying a patient a curative resection.

Bronchoscopy

Fiberoptic bronchoscopy is important in the staging of patients with tumors of the midesophagus. Findings range from simple bulging of the posterior membranous trachea and left mainstem bronchus to actual tumor invasion or fistula formation. Since newer generation CT scans can predict airway invasion with up to 97% accuracy, there is little role for routine preoperative bronchoscopy. However, in patients where the CT scan suggests tracheobronchial involvement, bronchoscopy is necessary prior to an attempt at resection to rule out airway invasion. If bulging of the posterior membranous trachea is the only bronchoscopic finding, operative assessment is frequently necessary.

Thoracoscopic Lymph Node Staging

Preoperative thoracoscopic and laparoscopic nodal staging, as advocated by Krasna (30), has been reported to be accurate for staging the lymph nodes in patients with esophageal cancer. In his series of 33 patients who underwent this type of preoperative staging followed by resection, this technique detected only one patient with metastatic lymph nodes, indicating that the added benefit of these procedures over nonsurgical techniques may be small. The role of thoracoscopic and laparoscopic lymph node staging for esophageal cancer has therefore yet to be determined.

Miscellaneous Studies

Positron emission tomography (PET) is an emerging modality that may be useful for noninvasively staging a variety of malignancies. PET relies on the abnormal glucose uptake by malignant cells to produce computer-generated images. When used in the preoperative staging of esophageal cancer, PET has been able to detect distant metastatic lesions which were unsuspected by CT scanning (31,32). With respect to nodal disease, preliminary data suggest that PET may be more sensitive than CT scanning, but still can miss metastatic nodes both adjacent and remote from the primary tumor (31,32).

Further metastatic workup prior to treatment for esophageal cancer is generally not indicated in the absence of clinical findings. For example, routine CT of the brain is a very low yield study since only approximately 1% of patients have brain metastases. Similarly, the yield of routine radionuclide bone scanning is also very low in the absence of bony symptoms and a normal serum alkaline phosphatase.

Any cervical or supraclavicular lymph nodes suspicious for metastatic disease should be biopsied prior to treatment, since a positive result will influence the therapeutic plan. Suspicious intraabdominal lymph nodes can be biopsied at the beginning of an attempt at resection and need not be biopsied at a separate sitting.

PATHOLOGIC STAGING

The American Joint Committee for Cancer Staging and End-Results Reporting classification for staging esophageal carcinoma is depicted in Table 12-4. The staging scheme follows the standard TNM system characteristic of most other types of cancer.

Although the T and visceral M classification for staging is generally agreed upon, the breakdown of the N descriptor has been the subject of debate. According to the AJCC system, N1 is applied to patients with positive regional lymph node metastases, and any positive nodes beyond the regional level are deemed M1. Currently, regional lymph nodes for an intrathoracic esophageal cancer include the mediastinal and perigastric lymph nodes, excluding the celiac axis nodes. Regional lymph nodes for a cervical esophageal lesion include the cervical and supraclavicular nodes. This breakdown is controversial, however, and some studies have attempted to clarify this issue by arbitrarily assigning specific lymph node groups as N1 depending on the location of the primary tumor (33).

Further confusing the lymph node issue are studies that report a change in survival based on the number of positive lymph nodes, not just the location. As an example, Skinner et al. (34) refer to less than five positive nodes as N1, while tumors with five or more positive nodes are deemed N2.

TABLE 12–4. *UICC staging system for esophageal cancer*

Stage	T	N	M
0	Tis	N0	M0
I	T1	N0	M0
IIA	T2–3	N0	M0
IIB	T1–2	N1	M0
IIIA	T3	N1	M0
	T4	Any N	M0
IV	Any T	Any N	M1
IVA	Any T	Any N	M1a
IVB	Any T	Any N	M1b

T descriptor: TX, primary tumor cannot be assessed; T0, no evidence of primary tumor; Tis, carcinoma *in situ;* T1, tumor invades lamina propria or submucosa; T2, tumor invades muscularis propria; T3, tumor invades adventitia; T4, tumor invades adjacent structures.

N descriptor: NX, regional lymph nodes cannot be assessed; N0, no regional lymph node metastases; N1, regional lymph node metastases.

M descriptor: MX, presence of distant metastases cannot be assessed; M0, no distant metastases; M1, distant metastases.

Adapted from Sobin and Wittekind (70).

TREATMENT

As mentioned previously, the treatment of esophageal carcinoma is stage dependent. Although cures for early disease have been reported following both surgical resection as well as radiation therapy (RT), esophagectomy is generally agreed to be the treatment of choice for curable lesions. Figure 12-7 displays an algorithm for the treatment of esophageal cancer.

Surgical resection

History

Czerny performed the first successful esophageal resection for cancer in a patient with carcinoma of the cervical esophagus in 1877. No attempt was made for reconstruction, and the patient survived for 1 year, being fed through a distal cervical esophagostomy. This was followed by the first transthoracic esophagectomy by Torek in a 67-year-old woman in 1913. In this case, esophagogastric continuity was restored via an extracorporeal rubber tube and the patient survived for 13 years. The first successful transhiatal esophagectomy was performed in 1931 by Turner, although this technique had been conceptualized by Denk 18 years earlier.

The first successful transthoracic esophagectomy with immediate reconstruction was reported by Oshawa in 1933, who operated on 19 patients using this technique. This was followed by Lewis in 1948 who described the initial mobilization of the stomach through a laparotomy, followed by right thoracotomy with esophagectomy, and immediate reconstruction via an intrathoracic esophagogastrostomy.

Types of Resections

The technique of esophagectomy varies widely between surgeons, institutions, and even countries, with each approach having its proponents and critics. With respect to the ap-proach, extent of resection and lymphadenectomy, all types of curative surgical techniques can be consolidated into three basic types of esophagectomy: Esophagectomy with thoracotomy (Ivor Lewis, left thoracotomy, left thoracoabdominal), esophagectomy without thoracotomy (transhiatal esophagectomy), and *en bloc* esophagectomy with radical lymphadenectomy.

Transthoracic Esophagectomy

Esophagectomy with thoracotomy, regardless of the type of incision, involves the dissection of the thoracic esophagus under direct vision. This is combined with a laparotomy if a right thoracotomy is performed, or if a left thoracotomy is

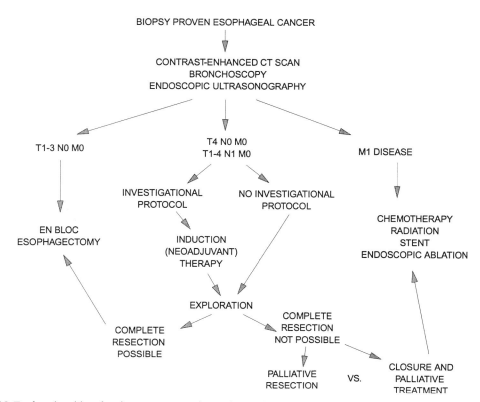

FIG. 12-7. An algorithm for the treatment of esophageal carcinoma. Bronchoscopy is only indicated for upper and middle third tumors. Preoperative noninvasive detection of nodal metastases is unreliable and must be confirmed by biopsy prior to clinical decision-making.

made, the left hemidiaphragm can be incised to expose the peritoneal cavity or the incision itself can be carried across the costal margin into the abdomen (thoracoabdominal). These approaches allow for the dissection of most intrathoracic and abdominal node-bearing areas. However, the degree of lymphadenectomy that is actually performed varies widely between surgeons.

A right thoracotomy is usually performed for lesions in the proximal two-thirds of the esophagus. The Ivor Lewis technique calls for the stomach mobilization and intraabdominal lymph node dissection to be carried out through a laparotomy prior to the thoracotomy. Once the stomach is mobilized and the hiatus dissected, the abdomen is closed and the patient is turned to the left lateral decubitus position. A right posterolateral thoracotomy through the fifth interspace is performed and the intrathoracic esophagus is dissected under direct vision. The azygous vein is divided, the mediastinal lymph nodes are dissected, and the mobilized stomach is brought up into the chest. A high intrathoracic anastomosis is then performed after resection of the thoracic esophagus and proximal stomach is performed. This can be done using either a hand sewn or stapled technique.

Alternatively, when approaching lesions through the right chest, it may be desirable to perform the thoracotomy initially, followed by the laparotomy. This is useful when the resectability of the primary tumor is in question, or when the surgeon wishes to create a cervical anastomosis. In this situation, the right thoracotomy is performed and the thoracic esophagus dissected with the patient in the left lateral decubitus position. The patient is then turned supine, a laparotomy made and the stomach mobilized. This is followed by a cervical incision and division of the cervical esophagus. The thoracic esophagus is then withdrawn into the abdomen for resection, and the stomach is transposed through the posterior mediastinum into the neck for the anastomosis.

Lesions of the distal third of the thoracic esophagus as well as the gastroesophageal junction are best approached through a left thoracotomy. A lateral thoracotomy through the sixth or seventh interspace is performed and the left hemidiaphragm is incised along its perimeter to expose the peritoneal cavity. The stomach is mobilized and the hiatal dissection is carried out. Exposure of the abdomen through this approach is usually sufficient such that it is rarely necessary to extend the thoracotomy anteriorly across the costal margin. Division of the costal margin is avoided whenever possible to decrease postoperative pain and pulmonary morbidity. Once the stomach is mobilized, the intrathoracic esophagus is dissected under direct vision up to the level of the aortic arch. An intrathoracic anastomosis can then be carried out below the level of the arch or, alternatively, the esophagus above the arch can be dissected bluntly up into the neck for a subsequent cervical anastomosis if desired. The diaphragm is then closed securely to prevent herniation of abdominal viscera into the chest.

When creating an intrathoracic anastomosis, two points must be considered. First, an adequate proximal margin must be obtained, which is usually considered to be 10 cm from the tumor. Second, the anastomosis should be placed as high as possible to lessen symptoms and sequelae of postoperative gastroesophageal reflux (34). This is easily accomplished on the right side by creating the anastomosis above the arch of the azygous vein. On the left side, creating a supraaortic anastomosis can be tedious and in such cases a cervical anastomosis is performed.

Transhiatal Esophagectomy

Transhiatal esophagectomy has enjoyed a revival of popularity over the past 20 years for two reasons. First, early series of transthoracic esophagectomy reported high rates of pulmonary complications, many of which were considered due to the thoracotomy incision alone. This led many surgeons searching for a less morbid way of resecting the esophagus. Second, advocates of the transhiatal approach view lymph node metastases as evidence of systemic spread. The implication of this thinking is that the presence of lymph node metastases signifies disease incurable by surgery alone. Indeed, the extent of resection for some malignant tumors (e.g., breast carcinoma) has decreased, with lymphadenectomy being performed simply for prognostic purposes. In addition, lymphadenectomy is thought not to improve survival in these instances as well. As a result, the concept of simple, palliative extirpation of the esophagus is thought by many to be sufficient therapy for carcinoma of this organ.

Transhiatal esophagectomy is performed through a laparotomy during which the replacement conduit is mobilized, the lymph nodes are dissected, and the thoracic esophagus is bluntly dissected free from the posterior mediastinum through the enlarged esophageal hiatus. A second incision is made in the neck and the blunt mobilization of the thoracic esophagus is continued through this incision as well. Once the entire esophagus is free, the cervical esophagus is transected and the specimen is retrieved through the posterior mediastinum into the abdomen. The proximal stomach is divided and the replacement conduit is placed up through the mediastinum into the neck. An anastomosis is then performed between the replacement conduit and the cervical esophagus.

Transhiatal esophagectomy differs from the transthoracic approaches in several ways other than simply the omission of the thoracotomy. First, the thoracic esophagus is dissected bluntly from the surrounding tissues usually under blind conditions. In some cases, the esophagus distal to the carina can be visualized with the aid of a widely opened hiatus and a lighted retractor; however, this is not a consistent occurrence, and the superior thoracic esophagus is never dissected under direct vision. Second, although access to intraabdominal lymph node bearing regions is similar to the previously described thoracic approaches, the extent of mediastinal lymphadenectomy that can be carried out via this approach is minimal. The implications of this minimalist approach in terms of long-term survival are controversial and will be addressed later in this chapter. However, the absence of a thorough lymphadenectomy can cause patients to be incorrectly staged, making survival data more difficult to interpret.

En Bloc Esophagectomy

First reported in 1963 by Logan (36) and subsequently by Skinner in 1983 (37), *en bloc* esophagectomy is an attempt to apply techniques of cancer surgery to carcinoma of the esophagus. In this operation the intrathoracic esophagus is resected along with the periesophageal tissues which include the pericardium, the thoracic duct, and both pleura. If the tumor is near the esophageal hiatus, a portion of the right crus is also taken in an *en bloc* fashion. This technique stems from the fact that the intrathoracic esophagus has no serosa, and the abutting tissues previously mentioned may be analogous to a serosal covering. The esophagectomy is combined with a radical lymphadenectomy consisting of dissection of the upper abdominal lymph node-bearing regions (left gastric, celiac, common hepatic, splenic, greater curvature, and paracardiac) as well as the intrathoracic regions (periesophageal, inferior pulmonary ligament, phrenic, and subcarinal).

In the *en bloc* technique, as with standard transthoracic resections, the location of the tumor in the esophagus dictates if a left or right-sided approach is used. If the tumor is in the upper or middle third, a right thoracotomy through the fifth interspace combined with a laparotomy is the best choice. If dealing with a tumor in the distal third or gastroesophageal junction, a left thoracotomy through the sixth interspace is used. Both techniques are followed with a cervical incision for the anastomosis.

During the thoracic portion of the dissection, the parietal pleura is opened posterior to the esophagus, which is then dissected off the aortic adventitia and anterior longitudinal ligament of the spine. This dissection is continued into the opposite hemithorax where this parietal pleura is opened as well. Anteriorly, the pericardium is opened and the dissection proceeds inside the pericardium to the opposite side, where the opposite parietal pleura is again incised. In this fashion, the esophagus is resected with the surrounding fat, lymph nodes, thoracic duct, pericardium, and parietal pleura. The thoracic duct is divided carefully at the aortic hiatus and again up near the aortic arch or azygous vein. If operating on the right side, the arch of the azygous vein is taken *en bloc* with the specimen as well. Above the level of the aortic or azygous arch, the esophagus is dissected bluntly up into the thoracic inlet. Attention is then turned to the esophageal hiatus which is opened widely. A cuff of the right crus is taken *en bloc* with the esophagus as well.

The abdominal portion of the *en bloc* esophagectomy includes the retroperitoneal dissection of all nodal and areolar tissue above the superior border of the pancreatic body and celiac axis. Splenectomy is not routinely performed. During both the thoracic and abdominal portions of this procedure, a systematic *en bloc* dissection of the lymph node-bearing areas in the mediastinum and superior portion of the abdomen is essential. The extent of lymphadenectomy will be discussed in further detail in the next section.

Extent of Lymphadenectomy

As previously mentioned, the spread of esophageal carcinoma occurs via lymphatic pathways and frequently involves both regional and distant lymph nodes. Two schools of thought have developed regarding the extent of lymphadenectomy that should be performed for esophageal cancer. The first opinion is one of minimal lymphadenectomy. Proponents of this approach suggest that esophageal cancer is a systemic disease at presentation and once lymph nodes are involved the possibility for cure with surgery alone is a chance occurrence. Therefore, the best resection is a palliative one, with the main goals being those of short operative time and minimal morbidity. Transhiatal esophagectomy, according to some advocates of this philosophy, best serves these goals. Although operative time is relatively short with this procedure, the issue of reduced morbidity and mortality is a controversial one and will be addressed later in this chapter.

The second school of thought concerning the extent of lymphadenectomy that should be performed during esophagectomy is one of complete lymph node dissection. Advocates of this approach argue that complete lymphadenectomy is the only way to correctly stage each patient, and subsequently the only way to obtain accurate survival data. In addition, several series of *en bloc* esophagectomy with radical lymphadenectomy report superior long-term survival when compared to series where patients underwent nonradical standard resections (Table 12-5).

Over the past 20 years an extension of this second school of thought has developed—the concept of the three-field lymph node dissection. While the traditional two-field radical lymphadenectomy includes both the upper abdominal and mediastinal node bearing regions, a three-field dissection includes both the deep cervical and recurrent laryngeal nerve lymph nodes. This approach has its roots in Japan, where preliminary series report that as many as 30% to 40% of patients with cancer of the thoracic esophagus undergoing esophagectomy with three-field lymphadenectomy will have cervical node metastases (38). This finding has been confirmed in a recent series reported on from the New York Hospital (22). Antagonists of this approach argue that the occult cervical lymph node metastases are simply just more evidence that esophageal cancer is a systemic disease at the time of diagnosis. However, studies from Japan report better survival and lower rates of locoregional recurrence following three-field lymphadenectomy compared to the two-field approach in patients with node-positive esophageal cancer (39). In addition, the added morbidity associated with the three-field dissection present in early reports has diminished with increasing experience with the technique (22). The survival advantage for three-field lymphadenectomy,

TABLE 12–5. *Operative mortality and survival following resection for carcinoma of the esophagus*

Reference (first author)	Year	No. of patients	Resection[a]	LN dissection[b]	Mortality[c]	Survival[d]
Orringer (64)	1993	417	THE	Nonradical	5%	27%
Mathisen (20)	1988	104	TTE	Nonradical	2.9%	15.4%
Lieberman (65)	1995	258	TTE, THE	Nonradical	5%	27%
Vigneswaran (66)	1993	131	THE	Nonradical	2.3%	20.8%
Lerut (67)	1992	54	EBE	Radical	7.4%	48.5%
		75	TTE	Nonradical	10.6%	41%
Skinner (68)	1987	31	EBE	Radical	9.7%	22%
		21	TTE	Nonradical	5%	0%
Hagen (69)	1993	30	EBE	Radical	10%	41%
		39	THE	Nonradical	12.8%	14%
Altorki (41)	1997	33	EBE	Radical	5.1%	34%[e]
		21	TTE, THE	Nonradical	6%	11%[e]

[a] THE, transhiatal esophagectomy; TTE, transthoracic esophagectomy; EBE, *en bloc* esophagectomy.
[b] Extent of lymph node dissection.
[c] Operative mortality rate.
[d] Five-year actuarial survival unless otherwise indicated.
[e] Four-year actuarial survival, only stage III lesions included in study.

however, has not been confirmed in the Western literature, further fueling this controversy.

Reconstruction

Following the performance of esophagectomy, regardless of the technique, continuity must be restored between the cervical esophagus and the remaining stomach. Issues that arise during this aspect of treatment include the selection of an appropriate esophageal replacement as well as the location for placement of the neoesophagus.

Choice of Conduit

The most popular organ used for esophageal replacement is the stomach. Advantages to its use in this setting are numerous: (a) the stomach has a rich blood supply, (b) only one anastomosis is needed, reducing operative time and the risk of anastomotic leaks, (c) the stomach reaches fairly easily to the cervical esophagus and pharynx, (d) no special preoperative preparation is needed.

Disadvantages are few and are mainly due to reflux postoperatively. Aspiration, esophagitis, and stricture have been reported to occur following esophagectomy when the stomach is used for reconstruction in a significant percentage of patients. Generally, the higher the anastomosis, the less severe the reflux.

The stomach can be fashioned into the neoesophagus in two ways. First, it can be left intact and transposed up to the neck or upper chest. This technique eliminates the chance of leak from a long gastric suture line that would be used to create a gastric tube. The intact stomach, however, is bulky and may produce respiratory embarrassment, especially if early delayed gastric emptying is present. Second, and most common, is the creation of a gastric tube. This is most commonly

created by resecting the majority of the lesser curvature with the esophagus and leaving the greater curvature gastric tube to survive on the blood supply from the right gastric and right gastroepiploic arteries. This tubularized replacement fits better in the mediastinum and is less likely to distend to the extent that the intact stomach might. Disadvantages of this approach include the presence of a long suture line and predisposition to reflux postoperatively, the latter of which is a concern whenever the stomach is used as the replacement conduit. Other types of gastric tubes include the reversed gastric tube, based on the left gastroepiploic artery and the nonreversed gastric tube, which is nourished from the right gastroepiploic artery (Fig. 12-8).

The next most common esophageal replacement is the colon. Advantages of colon interposition include the following: (a) relative ease in reaching to the neck, (b) residual peristalsis for propelling a food bolus, and (c) resistance to reflux due to the presence of mucus on the colonic epithelium. Disadvantages include added time to the procedure, the need for three anastomoses, and the need for preoperative bowel preparation. The left colon is more desirable than the right for several reasons. First, the size of the left colonic lumen is a closer match to the esophagus. Second, the right colon is bulky and may not reach to the neck, and third, the inconsistent presence of a marginal artery in the right colon may jeopardize a right colonic transposition. Contraindications to the use of a colon interposition are the presence of intrinsic colonic disease, mesenteric vascular disease, or a colonic motility disorder.

Other, less frequently used conduits include a pedicled loop of jejunum as well as a free jejunal graft. These techniques are not commonly utilized since a pedicled graft may not easily reach the neck due to the tethering anatomy of the mesenteric arcades. The need for five anastomoses (two microvascular) in the case of the free jejunal transfer may further prolong the operative procedure.

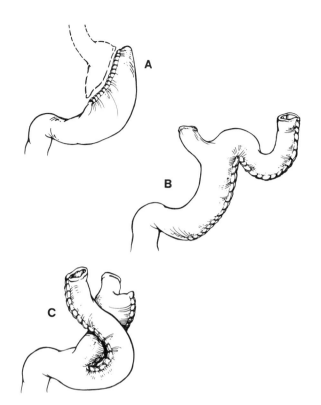

FIG. 12-8. Gastric tubes used for reconstruction following esophagectomy. **A:** Greater curve gastric tube, based on the right gastroepiploic artery. **B:** Reversed gastric tube based on the left gastroepiploic artery. **C:** Nonreversed gastric tube based on the right gastroepiploic artery.

Conduit Placement

Options for the location of the esophageal replacement include the posterior mediastinum, the intrapleural route, the substernal space, and a subcutaneous placement. The most commonly used route is the posterior mediastinum, the site of the native esophagus. The advantages of this location are the almost linear path of the graft as well as the decreased amount of length needed to reach the neck. Intrapleural placement is usually the next choice but can usually only be used if a transthoracic esophagectomy is performed. The retrosternal route is reported to be 25% longer than the posterior mediastinal route, and the food bolus must negotiate several rather abrupt turns prior to reaching the abdomen. Previous median sternotomy eliminates substernal placement of the conduit as an option. However, the retrosternal channel may be useful in cases when the posterior mediastinum is going to be irradiated in the postoperative period. Finally, the subcutaneous route is rarely used and is essentially a last resort if contraindications to the previously mentioned routes exist.

Operative Morbidity and Mortality

Acceptable operative mortality following esophagectomy used to be in the range of 20% to 30% as little as 20 years ago. With recent improvements in surgical technique, antibiotics and critical care, this figure is presently in the range of 5% to 10%, with many reports being even lower. Table 12-5 displays the operative mortality for recent series reported from major centers across the United States and Europe. In a recent literature review of 1,201 papers on the surgical treatment of esophageal carcinoma by Muller et al. (40), the overall hospital mortality rate was 13%. This figure was 18% when only the reports enlisting patients prior to 1960 were evaluated, but decreased to 11% if the evaluation was restricted to papers enrolling patients after 1980. This implies a learning curve phenomenon, and also reflects the previously mentioned advances in surgical care. No difference was seen in hospital mortality with respect to the type of resection performed, instead, the lowest hospital mortality rates were found in papers by surgeons having a personal experience with a large number of resections. This finding reiterates that esophageal resection has an appreciable learning curve.

Muller et al. (40) report an overall complication rate of 36% for 46,692 patients included in their review. Complication rates are difficult to interpret from one study to the next due to the lack of a consistent, objective definition of specific complications. In experienced hands, esophagectomy can be performed with very acceptable morbidity regardless of the approach. Specifically, the technique of *en bloc* esophagectomy with three-field lymphadenectomy and dissection of the recurrent laryngeal nodes can be performed with morbidity similar to the less radical, standard resections (41).

Traditionally, one of the most feared complications following esophagectomy is an anastomotic leak. Leaks tend to occur 5 to 10 days after the procedure and are generally caused by inadequate healing. Causes of inadequate healing include arterial or venous insufficiency, tension, gastric distension, technical errors, malnutrition, hypoxia, and hypotension (42). An anastomotic leak that occurs within the first 3 days postoperatively is more likely to be the result of a technically inadequate anastomosis or necrosis of the conduit, and generally reflects a more difficult problem (42).

In Muller's review, leakage rates were similar following gastric transposition whether the anastomosis was performed in a one layer, two layer, or stapled fashion (40). The overall incidence of clinically apparent leaks was 12%. If nonabsorbable suture was used, however, the leakage rate was 11% compared to 7% if absorbable suture was used, a statistically significant difference. It is generally accepted that cervical anastomoses leak at a higher rate than their intrathoracic counterparts, but the morbidity and mortality associated with a cervical leak is less than an intrathoracic one (42).

Pulmonary complications are commonplace following esophageal resection. In Muller's review (40), the incidence of postoperative pneumonia was similar whether the procedure was transthoracic (26%) or extrathoracic (21%). Atelectasis was found to be present more frequently after transthoracic resection when compared to the extrathoracic approach (23% versus 10%, respectively), but the definition of postoperative atelectasis traditionally is very subjective. One pulmonary complication that tends to be specific for *en bloc* esophagectomy with radical mediastinal lymphadenectomy is the relatively high incidence of bronchorrhea seen after this procedure (22). As a result, aggressive postoperative respiratory care is essential in these patients to prevent complications from this phenomenon.

Other major complications specific to esophagectomy include recurrent laryngeal nerve injury and chylothorax with wide ranges of incidence rates quoted in the literature. Initial reports listed the incidence of recurrent nerve injury after three-field lymph node dissection to be as high as 70% (39), but multiple recent series report this complication in only 6% or less of patients undergoing this procedure (22,41). The underlying theme is that operative experience is needed to keep these problems at a minimum, and that the type of resection does not matter as much as the expertise of the surgeon performing the resection.

Results

Long-term survival following esophagectomy for carcinoma is generally poor. This is mainly due to the high incidence of transmural invasion of the primary tumor and lymph node metastases. Table 12-5 lists the long-term survival reported in several major series from centers treating large numbers of patients with esophageal cancer. Also listed is the type of resection performed and the extent of lymphadenectomy. The first four studies represent series of patients who underwent standard, nonradical resections for esophageal carcinoma. The last four studies include groups of patients who underwent either standard, nonradical resections or *en bloc* esophagectomy with radical lymphadenectomy. None of the latter four studies are randomized trials; however, from the data shown, there is a suggestion that *en bloc* esophagectomy with radical lymph node dissection may yield better long-term survival when compared to less radical, standard resections. In Muller's review, *en bloc* resections showed a significantly better prognosis as well (40). However, no randomized trials exist to confirm this suspicion and it is unlikely that any will be performed because the patients undergoing the nonradical, standard resections always risk being understaged. We continue to perform *en bloc* esophagectomy with radical lymph node dissection because of the suggestion of a survival advantage, its comparable morbidity and mortality in experienced hands, and because it is the only way to accurately stage the patient.

Radiation Therapy

RT was first attempted for the treatment of esophageal carcinoma in 1907 when Guisez reported the use of endoesophageal brachytherapy less than 11 years after the discovery of radium.

Radiation Therapy as Primary Treatment

The results of RT administered with curative intent have in general been poor. Five-year survival rates have been in the range of 10% or less using this modality alone (43). It is difficult, however, to compare curative RT to surgical trials since many of the patients who receive curative RT are those denied an attempt at resection due to their poor state of health, or those with advanced tumors. The most frequent pattern of failure after curative RT has been local relapse, not systemic metastases (43). Future directions in the use of curative RT include the use of endoesophageal brachytherapy to boost external beam RT. Although some of these series show an improvement in survival when compared to historical controls, this difference may be attributable to patient selection (43).

Radiation Therapy as Adjuvant Treatment

Since a significant number of patients undergoing esophagectomy for carcinoma will experience locoregional failure, adjuvant RT makes intuitive sense. Several randomized trials explore the use of preoperative (44) and postoperative RT (45). Unfortunately, neither regimen has been shown to be of benefit in prolonging survival or decreasing the locoregional failure rate when compared to esophagectomy alone. Based on these data, adjuvant RT as a single agent cannot be considered the standard of care for patients with esophageal carcinoma.

Chemotherapy

Numerous studies have investigated various chemotherapeutic agents for the treatment of esophageal carcinoma, in both single-agent and multi-agent regimens. In total, over fifteen drugs have undergone enough evaluation to make preliminary statements about response rates. However, many limitations exist with the studies that report response rates for chemotherapeutic agents. These limitations include (a) the absence of uniform, objective response criteria, (b) small numbers of patients in each trial, necessitating pooling of patients from multiple trials, and (c) varying drug dosages and schedules. In addition, most trials deal mainly with squamous cell carcinoma, with very little data addressing adenocarcinoma of the esophagus. As a result of these trials, the most active single agents against esophageal carcinoma are cisplatin, 5-flourouracil (5-FU), vindesine, mitomycin, and paclitaxel. Multiagent chemotherapeutic regimens mainly contain variable combinations of these active single agents, the most common being the combination of cisplatin and 5-FU. Although response rates for combination chemotherapy exceed 50% in some series, none of the regimens developed thus far have induced complete remissions in a significant number of patients (46).

Chemoradiotherapy

Chemotherapy given concurrently with RT represents the most common way these two modalities are combined in the treatment of esophageal cancer. Again, the most frequently used chemotherapy regimen when combined with RT is cisplatin and 5-FU. In addition to being one of the most active combinations for esophageal cancer, both of these drugs may act as radiation sensitizers as well.

Multiple phase II trials for concurrent chemoradiotherapy exist which suggest an improvement in survival when compared to historical controls of RT alone (47). Several randomized, controlled trials of concurrent chemoradiotherapy versus RT alone substantiate this improvement in survival as well (48), but there has been no successfully completed phase III trial comparing concurrent chemoradiotherapy to surgical resection. In addition, both local and distant recurrence rates were noted to be decreased following concurrent chemotherapy and RT compared to RT alone. However, the local failure rate was still 34% in the phase III trial of chemoradiotherapy reported by Herskovic et al. (48). Unfortunately, toxicity for the combined modality regimens tends to be greater than that seen with RT alone (48).

Neoadjuvant (Induction) Therapy

Induction therapy for cancer is defined as a therapeutic intervention prior to an attempt at definitive local control. The rationale for induction therapy in the management of esophageal cancer is to hopefully reduce the incidence of micrometastases and to increase resectability of the primary tumor. Induction therapy for esophageal cancer has taken the form of preoperative chemotherapy or preoperative chemoradiotherapy.

Multiple phase II single arm studies of neoadjuvant chemotherapy exist. The most commonly used agents are cisplatin and 5-flourouracil, although cisplatin has been combined with other agents as well. Operative mortality seems to be comparable to surgery alone and the pathologic complete response rate has ranged from 3% to 10% (49). Although it has been concluded that induction chemotherapy does not adversely affect surgical outcome, an improvement in survival is suggested but cannot be consistently demonstrated.

Three small phase III randomized trials exist comparing induction chemotherapy followed by resection versus surgical resection alone. Two of these studies showed no improvement in overall survival for induction chemotherapy, but the subgroup of patients who responded to the chemotherapy did have a prolonged survival (50,51). The third study did not give response data, but the overall survival in the induction therapy group was no better than the patients who received surgery alone (52).

Induction chemoradiotherapy has again been studied in multiple phase II trials. Cisplatin based chemotherapy combined with at least 30 Gy of concurrent external beam RT have been the most tested regimens. In these trials, pathologic complete responses were seen in 20% to 25% of patients who received the induction therapy, with the 5-year survival in several series approaching 30% (52). Based on these encouraging results, a randomized, controlled trial of induction

chemoradiotherapy followed by surgery versus resection alone was recently reported (54). The induction therapy consisted of cisplatin and 5-FU with 40 Gy of concurrent external beam RT. The pathologic complete response rate was 25%, and the 3-year survival in the induction therapy group was 32%, compared to 6% in the surgery-alone group. Although a phase III trial, this study has been criticized because the 3-year survival in the surgery alone group was much lower than the historical 23% 5-year survival previously reported from that institution.

Palliative Measures

Since the vast majority of patients with esophageal cancer present with advanced, unresectable disease, palliation of symptoms plays a major role in the treatment of this disorder. The best technique to relieve dysphagia and restore the patient's ability to eat remains controversial and depends on the characteristics of both the individual patient and tumor.

Dilation

One of the simplest means of palliation for the patient with dysphagia is dilation of the tumor. Complication rates tend to be low (less than 10%), but the duration of its effect is short, usually lasting for only 2 to 4 weeks (55). As a result, dilation as the sole means of palliation is rarely used except when the patient's life expectancy is extremely short.

This technique, however, is commonly performed as a preparatory step for other palliative procedures. Prior to intubation with a plastic stent, the malignant stricture must be dilated. Similarly, tumors may need to be dilated prior to placement of brachytherapy catheters or before endoscopic laser therapy is instituted.

Surgery

Surgical palliation in the form of resection or bypass has a high rate of success in relieving dysphagia. However, mortality rates following these procedures in the clearly unresectable patient are high and approach 30% in some series (42). Given the short median survival of patients with unresectable esophageal cancer, and the abundance of other palliative approaches that are available, surgical resection or bypass in this patient population has generally fallen out of favor.

In the small group of patients where other attempts at palliation have been unsuccessful or contraindicated, surgical bypass may be indicated. The simplest method of bypass is performed by bringing the stomach up to the neck via the retrosternal route. This is carried out through a laparotomy and cervical incision, and usually utilizes some sort of gastric tube. The native esophagus can either be drained distally by a variety of techniques or vented by a red rubber catheter inserted into its proximal end and brought out through a separate stab wound in the neck.

Radiation Therapy

The main advantage of external beam RT as a palliative approach for the treatment of esophageal cancer is that it is truly noninvasive. In addition, RT tends to be a good technique for the relief of dysphagia, with success rates ranging from 50% to 70% (56). These rates, however, are typical for squamous cell carcinoma, with adenocarcinoma generally being much less sensitive to RT. Disadvantages include a comparably lengthy duration of treatment before relief is seen (4 to 6 weeks), as well as a significant complication rate (30%) (56). The untoward effects of external beam RT in the palliation of esophageal cancer include perforation, fistula formation, stricture formation, and esophagitis.

Endoluminal brachytherapy, either alone or in combination with external beam RT, has developed into a useful technique for palliating patients with esophageal cancer in recent years. Several series report success rates of 70% to 90% for the relief of dysphagia with complication rates similar to those reported for external beam RT alone (57). Another advantage of brachytherapy is the shorter duration of treatment when compared to external beam RT alone. Isotopes used include Cesium-137 and Iridium-192, which are administered in pellet form into the esophagus via catheters or a hollow bougie.

Laser and Photodynamic Therapy

The most commonly used endoscopic laser system utilized for palliation in patients with advanced esophageal carcinoma is the neodymium, yttrium-aluminum-garnet (Nd:YAG) laser. Advantages of the Nd:YAG laser include its ease of use, its ability to be used with flexible endoscopes, its excellent ability to coagulate, and its tissue penetration properties. Laser has a high success rate in restoring luminal patency, ranging from 90% to 100% in most series, although more than half of these patients will require repeat treatment prior to death (58). Luminal patency, however, does not always translate into restoration of a patient's ability to eat. As a result, the actual functional success rate for laser therapy in the palliation of esophageal carcinoma is approximately 70% to 80% (58).

The ideal tumor suitable for laser ablation is a short, noncircumferential, exophytic, nonangulating tumor in the distal esophagus. The technique favored by most clinicians is a retrograde approach, where the lesion is first dilated, followed by ablation of the distal portion of the tumor and working proximally. The advantage of this approach is the ability to treat the entire lesion in one or two sessions. In totally obstructing cases where the endoscope cannot be passed through the tumor, the antegrade approach is used. This technique allows for 1 to 2 cm of the tumor to be ablated at each session. Complications occur in 4% to 10% of patients in most series and mainly consist of perforation and bleeding (58).

Photodynamic therapy is an experimental therapy that entails giving an intravenous photosensitizer, such as porfimer sodium, which is selectively retained by the tumor due to a lymphatic defect which is not present in normal tissue. A laser (630 nm) is then applied to the tumor causing necrosis via the production of singlet oxygen, which damages the microvasculature of the tumor and renders it ischemic. Photodynamic therapy may be more effective than Nd:YAG laser for the ablation of upper third, circumferential lesions, especially those longer than 8 cm (59). However, 40% of patients require retreatment for subsequent tumor growth (59), and the complication rate has been significant in some series.

Esophageal Intubation

The placement of an esophageal prosthesis has been used for over 100 years in the palliation of esophageal carcinoma. Throughout the latter half of the 20th century, these prostheses have evolved into plastic tubes, 10 to 12 mm in internal diameter, with a funnel on the proximal end to prevent distal migration and a flange on the distal end to prevent proximal movement. These tubes are still a popular method for restoring the ability to eat worldwide in patients with obstructing esophageal cancers, with a success rate of more than 90% commonly reported (58). Situations particularly amenable to the use of endoesophageal prostheses include tracheoesophageal fistulas, long, tortuous malignant strictures, and failure of other palliative attempts.

Advantages of the plastic endoesophageal prostheses are immediate relief of dysphagia and their low cost. The main disadvantages are that the tumor must be dilatable prior to insertion of the stent and the inability to use this mode of palliation for tumors near the cricopharyngeus muscle. Complications are not uncommon and include perforation, tube migration, aspiration, hemorrhage, obstruction, and pressure necrosis (58).

Recently, a new type of endoesophageal prosthesis has emerged. These are the expandable metal stents, both covered and noncovered. These wire mesh stents can be placed over a guide wire and therefore do not require dilation prior to insertion, which reduces the risk of perforation. In addition, they are self-expanding and have a larger diameter than the plastic prostheses previously described. The covering, usually silicone, prevents ingrowth of tumor into the stent lumen and subsequent obstruction. Drawbacks include high cost as well as the inability to remove or reposition the stent after its placement. Preliminary reports suggest that this type of prosthesis has a very high success rate in terms of placement as well as a low complication rate when compared to their plastic counterparts (59).

Miscellaneous Palliative Measures

Other techniques currently in use for the palliation of advanced esophageal carcinoma include the use of electrocautery and direct injection of the tumor with chemicals which cause necrosis. However, these techniques require repeated administration and are less versatile than laser ablation. As a result, these techniques are not used with the same frequency as laser ablation and have not been as thoroughly investigated.

CONCLUSION

Carcinoma of the esophagus is a devastating disease, which usually presents in its advanced stages. Although squamous cell carcinoma is a frequent malignancy worldwide, it is uncommon in the United States. Instead, the incidence of adenocarcinoma is rising at a rapid rate, which is thought to be due to the increasing incidence of Barrett's esophagus. The treatment of esophageal cancer is stage related, and it is therefore essential to accurately stage the patient prior to the institution of therapy. Essential diagnostic and staging modalities include esophagoscopy with biopsy and contrast-enhanced CT scan of the chest and upper abdomen. EUS, although interesting, usually does not alter the treatment plan.

The standard treatment of esophageal cancer thought to be localized to the esophagus and regional lymph nodes is esophagectomy. Although several different techniques of esophagectomy are performed worldwide, several nonrandomized studies suggest that *en bloc* esophagectomy with radical lymphadenectomy may offer a survival advantage when compared to less radical, standard resections. In addition, the former technique is the only way to accurately stage the patient and can be performed with reasonable morbidity and mortality in experienced hands.

Chemotherapy and RT offer little as primary treatment modalities, but concurrent chemoradiotherapy may yield survival comparable with that of surgical resection. However, this has not yet been confirmed in a randomized, prospective setting. Some data suggest that induction chemotherapy or chemoradiotherapy followed by surgery may offer a survival advantage as well when compared to surgery alone, but again, further prospective, randomized trials are needed.

Since the majority of patients with esophageal cancer do not have limited disease at the time of presentation, palliative therapy plays an important role in the treatment of this disease. Choosing the best mode of palliation depends on the specific characteristics of both the patient and the tumor, but several different techniques can offer adequate palliation with minimal risk.

REFERENCES

1. Yang PC, Davis S. SEER report. Incidence of cancer of the esophagus in the U.S. by histologic type. *Cancer* 1988;61:612.
2. Marger RS, Marger D. Carcinoma of the esophagus and tylosis. A lethal genetic combination. *Cancer* 1993;72:17.
3. Wu YC, Ran SZ. Genetic etiology of oesophageal cancer: cytogenetic study of individuals in five cancer families in Linxian. *Acta Genet Sin* 1979;6:277.
4. Uchino S, Saito T, Inomata M, et al. Prognostic significance of the p53 mutation in esophageal cancer. *Jpn J Clin Oncol* 1996;26:287.
5. Brown LM, Silverman DT, Pottern LM, et al. Adenocarcinoma of the esophagus and esophagogastric junction in white men in the United States: alcohol, tobacco, and socioeconomic factors. *Cancer Causes Control* 1994;5:333.
6. Gray JR, Coldman AJ, MacDonald WC. Cigarette and alcohol use in patients with adenocarcinoma of the gastric cardia and lower esophagus. *Cancer* 1992;69:2227.
7. Hanaoka T, Tsugane S, Ando N, et al. Alcohol consumption and risk of esophageal cancer in Japan: a case-control study in seven hospitals. *Jpn J Clin Oncol* 1995;24:241.
8. Bradshaw E, Schonland M. Smoking, drinking, and oesophageal cancer in African males in Johannesburg, South Africa. *Br J Cancer* 1974;30:157.
9. Gabrial GN, Scrazer TF, Newberne PM. Zinc deficiency, alcohol, and a retinoid: association with esophageal cancer in rats. *J Natl Cancer Inst* 1982;68:785.
10. Li B, Taylor PR, Li JY, et al. Linxian nutrition intervention trials. Design, methods, participant characteristics, and compliance. *Ann Epidemiol* 1993;3:577.
11. Rogers MA, Vaughan TL, Davis S, Thomas DB. Consumption of nitrate, nitrite and nitrosodimethylamine and the risk of upper aerodigestive tract cancer. *Cancer Epidemiol Biomarkers Prev* 1995;4:29.
12. Zitsch RP, O'Brien CJ, Maddox WA. Pharyngoesophageal diverticulum complicated by squamous cell carcinoma. *Head Neck Surg* 1987;9:290.
13. Li H. Malignant Barrett's esophagus. *Eur J Cancer Prev* 1993;2:47.
14. Pera M, Trastek VF, Carpenter HA, et al. Influence of pancreatic and biliary reflux on the development of esophageal carcinoma. *Ann Thorac Surg* 1993;55:1386.
15. Burt M. Unusual malignancies. In: Pearson FG, Deslauriers J, Ginsberg RJ, Hiebert CA, McKneally MF, Urschel HC, eds. *Esophageal surgery.* New York: Churchill Livingstone, 1995:629.
16. Akiyama H, Tsurumaru M, Kawamura T, Ono Y. Principles of surgical treatment for carcinoma of the esophagus. Analysis of lymph node involvement. *Ann Surg* 1981;194:438.
17. Hamilton SR, Smith RRL, Cameron JL. Prevalence and characteristics of Barrett esophagus in patients with adenocarcinoma of the esophagus or esophagogastric junction. *Hum Pathol* 1988;19:942.
18. Akiyama H. *Surgery for cancer of the esophagus.* Baltimore: Williams & Wilkins, 1990.
19. Wong J. Esophageal resection for cancer: the rationale of current practice. *Am J Surg* 1987;153:18.
20. Mathisen DJ, Grillo HC, Wilkins EW, et al. Transthoracic esophagectomy: a safe approach to carcinoma of the esophagus. *Ann Thorac Surg* 1988;45:137.
21. Postlethwait RW. *Surgery of the esophagus.* 2nd ed. Norwalk, CT: Appleton-Century-Crofts, 1986:385.
22. Altorki NK, Skinner DB. Occult cervical nodal metastases in esophageal cancer: preliminary results of three-field lymphadenectomy. *J Thorac Cardiovasc Surg* 1997;113:540.
23. Quint LE, Hepburn LM, Francis IR, Whyte RI, Orringer MB. Incidence and distribution of distant metastases from newly diagnosed esophageal carcinoma. *Cancer* 1995;76:1120.
24. Korst RJ, Altorki NK. Extent of resection and lymphadenectomy for early Barrett's cancer. *Dis Esophagus* 1997;10:172.
25. Akiyama H, Kogure T, Itai Y. The esophageal axis and its relationship to the resectability of carcinoma of the esophagus. *Ann Surg* 1972;176:30.
26. Endo M, Takeshita K, Yoshida M. How can we diagnose the early stage of esophageal cancer? Endoscopic diagnosis. *Endoscopy* 1986;18:11.
27. Thompson WM, Halvorsen RA. Staging esophageal carcinoma. II. CT and MRI. *Semin Oncol* 1994;21:447.
28. Picus D, Balfe DM, Koehler RE, et al. Computed tomography in the staging of esophageal carcinoma. *Radiology* 1983;146:433.
29. Lightdale CJ. Staging esophageal carcinoma. I. Endoscopic ultrasonography. *Semin Oncol* 1994;21:438.
30. Krasna MJ. Thoracoscopic staging of esophageal staging. *Chest Surg Clin North Am* 1995;5:489–514.
31. Block MI, Patterson GA, Sundaresan RS, et al. Positron emission tomography improves preoperative staging of esophageal cancer. Presented at the 33rd annual meeting of the Society of Thoracic Surgeons, San Diego, February 3–5, 1997(abst).
32. Luketich JD, Schauer PR, Townsend DW, et al. The role of positron emission tomography in staging esophageal cancer. Presented at the 33rd annual meeting of the Society of Thoracic Surgeons, San Diego, February 3–5, 1997(abst).
33. Korst RJ, Venkatraman E, Bains MS, et al. A proposal for a new staging classification for esophageal cancer. Presented at the 23rd meeting of the Western Thoracic Surgical Association, Napa, June 1997(abst).

34. Skinner DB, Dowlatshahi KD, DeMeester TR. Potentially curable cancer of the esophagus. *Cancer* 1982;50:2571.

35. Pac M, Basoglu A, Kocak H, et al. Transhiatal versus transthoracic esophagectomy for esophageal cancer. *J Thorac Cardiovasc Surg* 1993;106:205.

36. Logan A. The surgical treatment of carcinoma of the esophagus and cardia. *J Thorac Cardiovasc Surg* 1963;46:150.

37. Skinner DB. *En bloc* resection for neoplasms of the esophagus and cardia. *J Thorac Cardiovasc Surg* 1983;85:59.

38. Kato H, Tachimori Y, Watanabe H, et al. Lymph node metastasis in thoracic esophageal carcinoma. *J Surg Oncol* 1991;48:106.

39. Fugita H, Kakegawa T, Yamana H, et al. Mortality and morbidity rates, postoperative course, quality of life, and prognosis after extended radical lymphadenectomy for esophageal cancer: comparison of three-field lymphadenectomy with two-field lymphadenectomy. *Ann Surg* 1995; 222:654.

40. Muller JM, Erasmi H, Stelzner M, Zieren U, Pichlmaier H. Surgical therapy of esophageal carcinoma. *Br J Surg* 1990;77:845.

41. Altorki N, Girardi L, Skinner D. *En bloc* esophagectomy improves survival for stage III esophageal cancer. Presented at the 77th meeting of the American Association for Thoracic Surgery, Washington, D.C., May 4–7, 1997(abst).

42. Urschel JD. Esophagogastrostomy anastomotic leaks complicating esophagectomy: a review. *Am J Surg* 1995;169:634.

43. Smalley SR, Gunderson LL, Reddy EK, Williamson S. Radiotherapy alone in esophageal carcinoma: current management and future directions of adjuvant, curative and palliative approaches. *Semin Oncol* 1994;21:467.

44. Launois B, Delarue D, Campion JP, et al. Preoperative radiotherapy for carcinoma of the esophagus. *Surg Gynecol Obstet* 1981;153:690.

45. Teniere P, Hay J, Fingerhut A, et al. Postoperative radiation therapy does not increase survival after curative resection for squamous cell carcinoma of the middle and lower esophagus as shown by a multicenter, controlled trial. *Surg Gynecol Obstet* 1991;173:123.

46. Ajani JA. Contributions of chemotherapy in the treatment of carcinoma of the esophagus: results and commmentary. *Semin Surg Oncol* 1994; 21:474.

47. John M, Flam MS, Agermowry P, et al. Radiotherapy alone and chemoradiation for nonmetastatic esophageal carcinoma. *Cancer* 1989; 63:2397.

48. Herskovic A, Martz K, Ali-Sarraf M, et al. Combined chemotherapy and radiotherapy compared with radiotherapy alone in patients with cancer of the esophagus. *N Engl J Med* 1992;326:1593.

49. Kelsen D. Chemotherapy for local regional and advanced esophageal cancer. In: Devita VT, Hellman S, Rosenberg SA, eds. *Cancer: principles and practice of oncology updates.* Philadelphia: JB Lippincott Co, 1988:1.

50. Roth JA, Pass HI, Flanagan MM, Graeber GM, Rosenberg JC, Steinberg S. Randomized clinical trial of preoperative and post-operative adjuvant chemotherapy with cisplatin, vindesine, and bleomycin for carcinoma of the oesophagus. *J Thorac Cardiovasc Surg* 1988;96:242.

51. Schlag P. Randomized study of preoperative chemotherapy in squamous cell cancer of the esophagus. CAO Esophageal Cancer Study Group (in German). *Chiurg* 1992;63:709.

52. Nygaard K, Hagen S, Hansen HS, et al. Preoperative radiotherapy prolongs survival in operable esophageal carcinoma: a randomized, multicenter study of preoperative radiotherapy and chemotherapy. The second Scandinavian trial in esophageal cancer. *World J Surg* 1992; 16:1104.

53. Forastiere AA, Oringer MB, Perez-Tamayo C, et al. Concurrent chemotherapy and radiation therapy followed by transhiatal esophagectomy for local-regional cancer of the esophagus. *J Clin Oncol* 1990; 8:119.

54. Walsh TN, Noonan N, Hollywood D, et al. A comparison of multimodal therapy and surgery for esophageal adenocarcinoma. *N Engl J Med* 1996; 335:462.

55. Lundell L, Leth R, Lind T, Lonroth H, Sjovall M, Olbe L. Palliative dilitation in carcinoma of the esophagus and esophagogastric junction. *Acta Chir Scand* 1989;155:179.

56. Caspers RJ, Welvaart K, Verkes RJ, Hermans JO, Leer JWH. The effect of radiotherapy on dysphagia and survival in patients with esophageal cancer. *Radiother Oncol* 1988;12:15.

57. Caspers RJL, Zwinderman AH, Griffioen G, et al. Combined external beam and low dose rate intraluminal radiotherapy in oesohageal cancer. *Radiother Oncol* 1993;27:7.

58. Reed CE, Endoscopic palliation of esophageal carcinoma. *Chest Surg Clin North Am* 1994;4:155.

59. Marcon NE. Photodynamic therapy and cancer of the esophagus [Review]. *Semin Oncol* 1994;21(6 Suppl 15):20.

60. Knyrim K, Wagner H-G, Bethge N, Keymling M, Vakil N. A controlled trial of an expansile metal stent for palliation of esophageal obstruction due to inoperable cancer. *N Engl J Med* 1993;329:1302.

61. Lu YK, Li YM, Gu YZ. Cancer of the esophagus and esophagogastric junction: analysis of results of 1,025 resections after 5 to 20 years. *Ann Thorac Surg* 1987;43:176.

62. Nishimaki T, Tanaka O, Suzuki T, Aizawa K, Hatakeyama K, Muto T. Patterns of lymphatic spread in esophageal cancer. *Cancer* 1994;74:4.

63. Fok M, Wong J. Squamous cell carcinoma. In: Pearson FG, Deslauriers J, Ginsberg RJ, Hiebert CA, McKneally MF, Urschel HC, eds. *Esophageal surgery.* New York: Churchill Livingstone, 1995:571.

64. Orringer MB, Marshall B, Stirling MC. Transhiatal esophagectomy for benign and malignant disease. *J Thorac Cardiovasc Surg* 1993; 105:265.

65. Lieberman MD, Shriver CD, Bleckner S, Burt M. Carcinoma of the esophagus. *J Thorac Cardiovasc Surg* 1995;109:130.

66. Vigneswaran WT, Trastek VF, Pairolero PC, Deschamps C, Daly RC, Allen MS. Transhiatal esophagectomy for carcinoma of the esophagus. *Ann Thorac Surg* 1993;56:838.

67. Lerut T, De Leyn P, Coosemans W, Van Raemdonck D, Scheys I, LeSaffre E. Surgical strategies in esophageal carcinoma with emphasis on radical lymphadenectomy. *Ann Surg* 1992;216:583.

68. Skinner DB, Little AG, Ferguson MK, Soriano A, Staszak VM. Selection of operation for esophageal cancer based on staging. *Ann Surg* 1986;204:391.

69. Hagen JA, Peters JH, DeMeester TR. Superiority of extended *en bloc* esophagogastrectomy for carcinoma of the lower esophagus and cardia. *J Thorac Cardiovasc Surg* 1993;106:850.

70. Sobin LH, Wittekind, C, eds. *TNM classification of malignant tumors.* 5th ed. New York: Wiley-Liss, 1997.

CHAPTER 13

Gastric Cancer

Mark S. Talamonti

Carcinoma of the stomach is one of the leading causes of cancer mortality worldwide. Despite evidence demonstrating a marked decline in the incidence of stomach cancer in the United States, management of patients with this malignancy continues to present multiple challenges for the gastrointestinal (GI) surgeon. Controversies exist regarding the extent of gastric resection and the role of extended lymph node dissections. Effective postoperative adjuvant therapies remain to be defined, and novel neoadjuvant approaches are currently considered investigational. In addition, the majority of gastric cancers in Western countries are detected at an advanced stage, and, thus, the surgeon is frequently faced with decisions regarding the role of surgical management in patients with likely incurable disease. This is reflected by the fact that the prognosis for stomach cancer in the United States remains extremely poor, with 5-year survival rates ranging between 5% and 15%. Even after potentially curative gastric resections, disease recurrence occurs in at least 80% of patients. The intent of this chapter is to review the biologic and pathologic characteristics of adenocarcinoma of the stomach. In addition, current strategies for diagnosis and staging will be discussed. Emphasis will be placed on relevant current data regarding surgical management of gastric cancer. Finally, recommendations regarding follow-up and monitoring for recurrence will be discussed.

EPIDEMIOLOGY OF GASTRIC CANCER

While the impact of gastric carcinoma is decreasing in the United States, worldwide this tumor continues to be a leading cause of cancer-related deaths. Only recently, with the increasing worldwide use of tobacco has lung cancer overtaken gastric cancer as the leading cause of cancer death overall. The incidence of this tumor is highest in Japan, South America, and Eastern Europe. The incidence of gastric cancer varies widely by country and population. In general, higher rates are seen among lower socioeconomic groups and in less well-developed nations, while gastric cancer is becoming increasingly uncommon in more industrialized nations. The factors that have led to these wide differences are incompletely understood. Dietary factors appear to have played a significant role.

As demonstrated by epidemiologic studies, there has been a significant decrease in incidence among migrants moving from high-incidence countries to low-incidence countries (1).

Most striking have been the changes in the incidence and distribution of gastric carcinoma in the United States over the past 60 years. Gastric carcinoma now ranks 14th in incidence among the major types of malignancy in this country. In the United States from 1930 to 1980, the incidence decreased from 38 to 10 per 100,000 for men and from 30 to 5 per 100,000 for women. In 1998, it is estimated that 22,600 new cases will occur and approximately 14,000 deaths will result from this cancer. Stomach cancer occurs infrequently before the age of 40 and its incidence peaks in the seventh decade. African-Americans, Hispanic-Americans, and Native Americans are two times more likely to develop gastric cancer than are Whites (2).

Despite the decrease in the incidence of the disease, the current 5-year survival rates have not shown a great deal of improvement over the past 30 years. The majority of patients with gastric carcinoma will present in advanced stages and ultimately succumb to their disease. In a 1995 study by the American College of Surgeons, 66% of patients with stomach cancer had locally advanced or metastatic disease at presentation. Resection rates ranged between 30% and 50%, and 5-year survival following potentially curative resection was related to stage at presentation. The survey of 16,992 patients by the American College of Surgeons found 5-year survival rates of 43% for stage I, 37% for stage II, 18% for stage III, and 20% for stage IV. As noted above, the principle reason for the failure to see dramatic improvements in survival rates, despite the significant decrease in incidence, is the fact that the majority of patients present with stage III or IV disease (3).

An extremely relevant change in the epidemiology of gastric carcinoma has to do with the distribution of the primary lesion within the stomach. In 1930, most cases of gastric carcinoma originated in the distal stomach. Since 1976, there has been a steady rise in the incidence of adenocarcinoma of the gastroesophageal junction and cardia. The reasons for this rapid increase in proximal malignancies remain unclear. In an earlier report from the American College of Surgeons, all lesions were grouped into one of three areas; the upper third was involved in 30.5%, the middle third in 13.9%, and the distal third in 26% of the patients. Ten percent involved the entire stomach and the site was unknown in 19% (4a). This is in contradistinction to the first quarter of this century, when two-thirds of gastric cancers were located in the antrum and prepyloric area and only 10% or fewer were in the cardia or gastroesophageal junction. In the United States, carcinoma of the cardia occurs mostly in Whites and shows a high male-to-female ratio. The simultaneous decrease in the incidence of distal gastric cancer and the marked increase in the numbers of proximal gastric cancers suggest that adenocarcinoma of the proximal stomach and gastroesophageal junction have a common pathogenesis that is different from distal gastric cancers. The surgical implications of such changes are important because in general the treatment of proximal gastric cancer is technically more difficult than the treatment of distal gastric cancer.

RISK FACTORS

There are a number of risk factors and predisposing diseases associated with the development of gastric cancer (Table 13-1). Diets rich in smoked or salted foods and low in fruits and vegetables and a decreased use of refrigeration have been linked to an increased incidence of gastric cancer. Highly salted or poorly preserved foods are associated with increased levels of nitrates and nitrites, which can combine to form potent N-nitroso compounds thought to be carcinogenic in gastric mucosa. The association of gastric cancer with lower socioeconomic status may be related to several dietary and environmental factors. The marked decline of gastric cancer in the United States over the past several decades has, in part, been attributed to improved refrigeration and the nationwide availability of fresh foods, including milk, vegetables, fruit juices, beef, and fish. This has been accompanied by a marked decline in the consumption of smoked, pickled, preserved, and spiced foods. Other possible environmental risk factors include cigarette smoking, alcohol abuse, and poor food storage. Occupational hazards include industrial exposure to certain carcinogens such as asbestosis, rubber production, and iron processing (5).

Precursor changes in the gastric mucosa associated with an increased risk of gastric carcinoma include the presence of chronic gastritis, both chronic atrophic and hypersecretory gastritis, adenomatous polyps, and chronic gastric ulcer. Patients with chronic atrophic gastritis and intestinal metaplasia are thought to be at increased risk for developing stomach cancer based on histologic studies demonstrating the presence of these changes in the mucosa surrounding intestinal-type gastric cancer. Theoretical models have been developed proposing chronic gastric mucosal injury as an initiating event leading to intestinal metaplasia and possible progression to dysplasia and ultimately invasive cancer (Fig. 13-1). In addition, investigators have demonstrated that the prevalence of atrophic gastritis and intestinal metaplasia is greatest in regions of the world that have the highest rates of gastric cancer (6).

Hyperplastic polyps are most common, accounting for 75% to 95% of gastric polyps. Hyperplastic polyps are associated with chronic gastritis and are usually asymptomatic. The hyperplastic polyp contains an overgrowth of histologically normal gastric epithelium and atypia is rare. Endoscopic biopsy to confirm the benign nature of these lesions is sufficient treatment. Adenomatous polyps are rare in the stomach and usually smaller than 2 cm. However, as seen with colon polyps the incidence of malignancy is associated with polyp size, number, and histology. Polyps larger than 2 cm in size have a 40% incidence of cancer within the polyp and surgical resection should be considered when the number of polyps exceeds the feasibility and safety of complete endoscopic removal, or when invasive carcinoma is present in the base of an incompletely removed polyp. New polyps develop in 25% to 33% of patients who have endoscopic removal of an adenomatous polyp. Thus, surveillance endoscopy is indicated in patients who have had adenomas resected (7).

Prior distal gastrectomy with vagotomy for benign gastric or duodenal ulcer disease has been proposed as a risk factor for subsequent malignancy in the gastric remnant. While retrospective reviews of the subject may have overstated the true risk, more recent prospective studies with long-term follow-up indicate that there is a 15- to 20-year latent period, after which the relative risk increases threefold to sixfold. Controversy exists regarding the role of endoscopic surveillance for patients having previously undergone distal gastrectomy for these reasons (8).

Genetic risk factors for gastric carcinoma include a family history of gastric cancer, blood type A, hypertrophic gastropathy (Menetrier's disease), and pernicious anemia.

The marked rise in the incidence of adenocarcinoma of the gastric cardia and distal esophagus appears to be strongly correlated with an increase in the incidence of Barrett's esophagus. Patients with hereditary, nonpolyposis colorectal cancer (Lynch syndrome) are also at increased risk for gastric cancer (5).

TABLE 13–1. *Risk factors for gastric cancer*

Precursor conditions
    Chronic atrophic gastritis and intestinal metaplasia
    Pernicious anemia
    Partial gastrectomy for benign disease
    Helicobacter pylori infection
    Menetrier's disease
    Gastric adenomatous polyps
    Barrett's esophagus

Genetic and environmental factors
    Family history of gastric cancer
    Blood type A
    Hereditary nonpolyposis colon cancer syndrome
    Low socioeconomic status
    Low consumption of fruits and vegetables
    Consumption of salted, smoked, or poorly preserved foods
    Cigarette smoking

Adapted from Fuchs and Mayer (5).

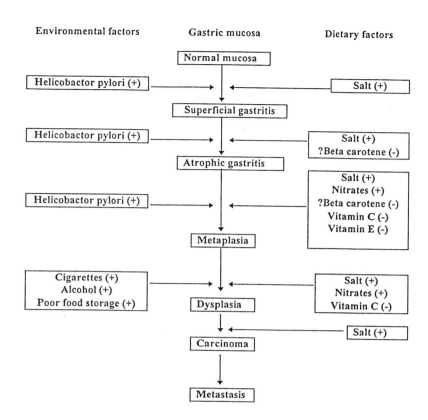

Environmental factors   Gastric mucosa   Dietary factors

FIG. 13-1. Environmental influences on gastric carcinogenesis, based on the Correa model. +, possible promoters; −, possible inhibitors. (Reprinted with permission from Wadstrom T. An update on *Helicobacter pylori. Curr Opin Gastroenterol* 1995; 11:69.)

Several studies have shown an increased incidence of gastric carcinoma in patients infected with *Helicobacter pylori (H. pylori)* (9–12). Persons infected with *H. pylori* had a three- to sixfold higher risk of gastric cancer than those without infection. These cancers mainly seem to be located in the distal stomach and restricted to an intestinal-type of cancer (to be discussed). This association appears to be independent of the association between *H. pylori* infection and gastric ulcer disease. The precise role of *H. pylori* infection and gastric carcinogenesis is not certain but appears to be related to the development of chronic atrophic gastritis. It is likely that *H. pylori* infection is one of a number of genetic or environmental cofactors required for the development of gastric carcinoma. Whether treatment of the *H. pylori* infection will decrease the risk of gastric carcinoma is currently unknown.

PATHOLOGY AND MOLECULAR BIOLOGY OF GASTRIC CANCER

Pathology

Adenocarcinoma accounts for over 95% of gastric malignancies. Lymphoma, carcinoid tumors, leiomyosarcoma, and squamous cell carcinoma make up the remaining 5%. Many pathologic classifications and descriptions for gastric cancer have been developed in an effort to predict prognosis at various stages and to help define optimal treatment protocols. The most widely used classification of gastric cancer was proposed in 1965 by Lauren (13) and divides stomach cancers into two basic types: intestinal and diffuse. This classification scheme based on tumor histology effectively characterizes two varieties of gastric adenocarcinomas that manifest distinctly different pathologic, epidemiologic, etiologic, and prognostic factors. The intestinal type is characterized by cohesive neoplastic cells forming gland-like tubular structures that are aligned by well-polarized columnar cells (Fig. 13-2). In general, the intestinal type of cancer is better circumscribed and more well differentiated than the diffuse type. The diffuse type of gastric cancer extends widely with no distinct margins and glandular structures are rarely present. Cell cohesion is absent and these tumors tend to be more infiltrative and poorly differentiated (Fig. 13-3). Individual cells can infiltrate and thicken the stomach wall without forming a discrete mass.

The intestinal type of gastric cancer is seen more frequently in geographic regions with a high incidence of gastric cancer. Intestinal tumors are found in anatomic regions of the stomach associated with chronic gastritis and intestinal metaplasia. These lesions tend to occur in the distal stomach and often have a prolonged precancerous phase. Intestinal type tumors are predominant in men and older patients and, in general, have a more favorable prognosis than the diffuse type of cancer. Decline in the incidence of gastric cancer, as noted above, appears to be largely due to a decrease in the incidence of intestinal type lesions. The diffuse type of gastric cancer is seen more frequently in populations considered at low risk for stomach cancer. Most proximal tumors of the fundus, cardia, and gastroesophageal junction are of the diffuse type and tend

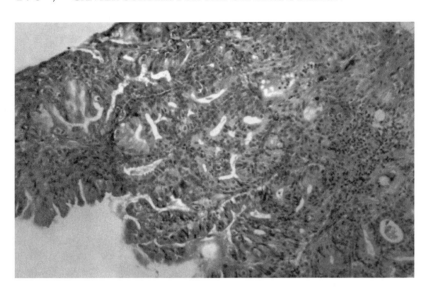

FIG. 13-2. Intestinal-type carcinoma demonstrating cohesive neoplastic cells forming gland-like tubular structures.

to be aggressively infiltrative at an early stage. Thus, this is frequently the most difficult type of tumor for the surgeon to achieve histologically negative margins of resection. Diffuse carcinomas are also seen more frequently in younger patients and, in general, have a worse clinical prognosis. The incidence of diffuse tumors is relatively constant among many countries and appears to be increasing overall.

A variant of the Lauren classification was proposed by Ming in 1977 (14). The primary emphasis in this classification is not the histologic glandular structures or differentiation of the tumors but rather their patterns of growth and spread. In the Ming classification, there are two main growth patterns. The expanding and infiltrative categories roughly correspond to the intestinal and diffuse types of the Lauren classification. The expanding type of tumors are most common and include tumors with fungating or polypoid appearance. These tumors more frequently have well-differentiated gland formation and cell cohesiveness, as described in the Lauren classification.

The infiltrative type of cancer, as described by Ming, is comparable to the diffuse lesion of Lauren. As noted, these tumors are made up of less cohesive cells that are seen to aggressively infiltrate all layers of the stomach wall. The expansile growth pattern accounts for 67% of gastric cancers, while the infiltrating growth pattern is seen in the remaining third of tumors. The reproducibility of this classification is based on the evaluation of only one parameter, regardless of cell type or histologic structure.

The pattern of spread of gastric cancer is related to tumor type. Favorable prognostic factors include a limited depth of invasion and an absence of lymph node metastases. Intestinal tumors that are expansive or exophytic and located in the antrum of the stomach, in general, have a more favorable outcome than diffuse lesions with a great deal of desmoplastic reaction located in the proximal stomach. The poorly differentiated infiltrative tumors typically elicit a dense desmoplastic reaction and spread commonly and early into the peritoneal

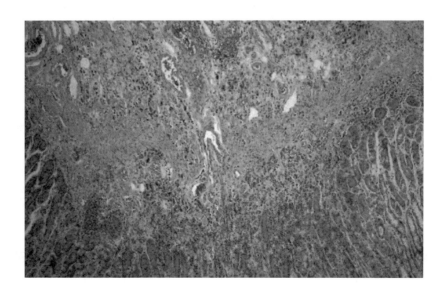

FIG. 13-3. Diffuse-type carcinoma with signet-ring cells demonstrating aggressive tissue invasion and lack of formed tubular elements.

cavity and lymph nodes. The well-differentiated intestinal type of tumors metastasize most commonly to the liver and lymph nodes and less commonly to the peritoneal cavity.

A less frequently used form of microscopic classification of gastric cancers was proposed by the World Health Organization (WHO) (15). This classification identifies cancers with distinctive growth patterns. Tumors are assigned a grade, based on the degree of differentiation and resemblance to metaplastic intestinal tissue. Thus, tumors are categorized as either well-differentiated, or moderately or poorly differentiated types. In addition, it further categorizes the histologic patterns of adenocarcinoma into four subtypes, based on growth patterns. Papillary tumors consist of slender or plump processes covered by cuboidal or columnar cells. Tubular carcinomas have well-defined glandular lumens. Mucinous tumors are also termed colloid cancers and contain abundant mucin secreted by the tumor cells. Finally, signet ring cells may be present, but they are not a predominant feature in these cancers. Signet ring carcinomas often produce marked desmoplastic reactions. The cells of this tumor type display little cohesion and, in general, correspond to the diffuse type of cancer or infiltrating lesions described above. As expected, these are associated with a worse clinical prognosis.

Gastric cancer classifications have also been proposed based on gross features of the tumor, and these descriptions remain very useful when discussing and characterizing endoscopic findings. In the United States, most cancers present at a more advanced stage and, thus, are grossly better described by the Borrmann classification (16). The type I lesion is a nodular polypoid lesion and is usually broad-based. The type II lesion is a fungating, circumscribed tumor and may have an ulceration on the dome. A type III lesion is an ulcerated tumor with a penetrating ulcer base. The base is infiltrated by neoplastic proliferation. Finally, the type IV lesion is a diffuse thickening of the stomach wall, usually without forming a discrete mass or becoming ulcerated. This type lesion corresponds to the appearance of linitis plastica. Five-year survival rates of 45%, 45%, 20%, and 6% are reported for types I to IV, respectively.

Mass screening programs in Japan established the concept of early gastric cancer. Early gastric cancer has been proposed as a unique form of gastric neoplasms. The distinction between early and advanced gastric carcinoma is based on the involvement of the muscularis propria. Early gastric carcinoma is limited to the mucosa and submucosa. It is thought to be highly curable with appropriate resection. The 5- and 10-year survival rates in Japan are greater than 90% and 80%, respectively. The incidence of early gastric cancer in the United States is only about 10%. In Japan, where annual screening by upper endoscopy is recommended for patients more than 50 years of age, early gastric cancer is found in up to 40% of patients (4a). The gross classification of early gastric carcinoma proposed by Japanese investigators has received wide acceptance (17) (Fig. 13-4). Despite differences in the endoscopic appearance of these early gastric cancers, the predominant prognostic factor that makes their behavior so favorable from a clinical point of view is the lack of invasion into the muscularis propria. This is reflected by the fact that only 10% of early gastric cancers will exhibit lymph node metastases. By the TNM classification, early gastric cancer would include all T1 tumors with any end stage of disease. The detection of early gastric cancer and its effective treatment continues to pose a problem for Western surgeons. In the American College of Surgeons series, stage I cancers accounted for approximately 18% of the cases and had a 5-year survival rate of 50% compared to 34% of early gastric cancer cases in a similar Japanese study with a survival rate of 95% (4a). There was essentially no difference in the percentage of stage I cancers diagnosed and treated in the ACS reports from 1982 and 1987. The identification of early gastric cancer in countries like the U.S. where the overall incidence is declining will remain a problem until cost-effective screening strategies can be defined and high-risk groups identified.

Molecular Biology

The molecular biology of stomach cancer as expected reflects the heterogeneity of its causes and subtypes. As studies in colorectal cancer begin to identify specific molecular changes that are correlated with patient survival, similar investigations into the role of oncogenes and tumor suppressor genes in the pathogenesis of gastric cancer are underway. Identification of the genetic and molecular variables among gastric cancers may lead to more directed therapeutic approaches and more accurate prediction of clinical outcome. As in studies of colorectal cancer, allelic deletions of the MCC (mutated in colon cancer),

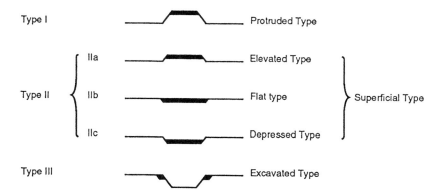

FIG. 13-4. Macroscopic classification of early gastric cancer. (Reprinted with permission from Nava HR, Arredondo MA. Diagnosis of gastric cancer: endoscopy, imaging and tumor markers. *Surg Oncol Clin North Am* 1993;2:371.)

APC (adenomatous polyposis coli), and p53 tumor suppressor genes have been reported in 33%, 34%, and 64% of gastric cancers, respectively (18). Unlike both colon and pancreatic cancers, gastric cancers rarely involve mutations in the ras oncogene. Abnormalities of several growth factors and receptors have also been identified in gastric cancer. Over expression of the receptor for epidermal growth factor has been noted in several studies and may be an independent prognostic factor. Although pathologic stage specifically related to presence or absence of lymph node metastases and depth of tumor invasion continues to be the strongest prognostic predictor of survival, molecular and biologic determinants such as flow cytometry measurements may soon be clinically relevant. Flow cytometry analysis of gastric tumors demonstrate that lesions with a large fraction of aneuploid cells tend to be more highly infiltrative and have a poorer prognosis. As our knowledge of the molecular pathogenesis of gastric carcinoma increases, molecular and biologic determinants will no doubt be added to pathologic staging in hopes of better predicting survival and determining treatment strategies.

CLINICAL MANIFESTATIONS

Most patients with gastric cancer are diagnosed with advanced stage disease, and this is reflected in the nonspecific symptoms that characterize early stages of this cancer. Early symptoms such as vague epigastric discomfort and indigestion are often ignored by the patient. In addition, these symptoms produced by gastric cancer are not specific and can also be caused by other benign upper GI disorders. It is not uncommon for patients with vague epigastric symptoms to be treated with a presumptive diagnosis of benign gastric ulcer disease for 2 to 6 months without diagnostic studies being performed. Anorexia, nausea, and weight loss are present in less than 50% of patients with early gastric cancer. As disease progression occurs these symptoms become more persistent and more pronounced. In the American College of Surgeons review, major symptoms included weight loss and abdominal pain in more than half the patients (4a). Nausea, anorexia, and dysphagia were noted in approximately one third of patients and melena in 20%. In some patients, symptoms may suggest the presence of a lesion in a specific location. Dysphagia is usually associated with tumors of the cardia or gastroesophageal junction. A complaint of early satiety is an infrequent symptom of gastric cancer, but it indicates a diffusely infiltrating tumor that has resulted in loss of distensibility of the gastric wall. Antral tumors may cause symptoms of gastric outlet obstruction. Massive upper GI bleeding is rare. Approximately 10% to 20% of patients will present with either hematemesis or melena (4a).

When the patient's only clinical symptoms consist of mild weight loss, vague epigastric pain, and occasional nausea and vomiting, the physical findings will usually be normal. The development of specific physical findings usually indicates extensive and incurable disease. The presence of an intraabdominal mass, hepatomegaly, or ascites is usually due to advanced intraabdominal disease. Other physical findings consistent with widespread metastatic disease include a palpable supraclavicular lymph node (Virchow's node) and a large ovarian mass (Krukenberg's tumor), or a large peritoneal implant in the pelvis (Blumer's shelf). Sister Mary Joseph's nodule, named after a nurse at the Mayo Clinic who discovered the phenomenon, is a visible and palpable secondary deposit at the umbilicus due to spread along the lymphatics in the falciform ligament.

Currently, there is no specific laboratory test or serum tumor marker specific for gastric cancer. Routine hematologic studies may disclose an iron deficiency anemia in these patients. Testing of the stools for occult blood may also be positive. The carcinoembryonic antigen level may be elevated in as many as 30% of patients with advanced tumors (17). It is insensitive as a means to detect or screen for early disease.

DIAGNOSIS AND SCREENING

Diagnosis

A barium contrast study is often the first diagnostic test performed to evaluate symptoms related to the upper GI tract. In Japan, the double contrast air barium study has been perfected and used for mass population screening (19,20). In the United States, primary care physicians will frequently obtain an upper GI contrast study when treating patients with persistent or refractory presumed peptic ulcer disease. The development and refinement of double-contrast radiographic techniques have improved the radiologist's ability to detect gastric cancer and to characterize gastric ulcers (21). The characteristics of a malignant gastric ulcer versus benign disease have now been well described (Table 13-2). Despite the improved sensitivity of barium contrast studies for screening and diagnosis, in most U.S. centers fiberoptic endoscopy is the study of choice because biopsy can be performed at the same procedure. Endoscopy and biopsy should be performed when an upper GI examination indicates the possible presence of a tumor or a presumed benign gastric ulcer has not completely healed within approximately 6 to 10 weeks of medical management. Fiberoptic endoscopy and biopsy have been reported to have a diagnostic accuracy of 95%. The accuracy of biopsy has been shown to be related to the number of biopsies taken (17,22). If up to 10 biopsies are taken from each lesion, the diagnostic accuracy approaches 100%. In addition to establishing the diagnosis of gastric cancer, endoscopic visualization of the esophagus, stomach, and duodenum can provide direct and useful surgical information about the extent of disease. The size, location, and morphology of the tumor, including the proximal and distal extent of disease, will be critically useful in planning the extent of surgical gastric resection.

Screening

The ability to diagnose gastric adenocarcinoma by radiography or endoscopy has prompted mass screening programs for populations at high risk. In Japan, annual screening has been recommended for persons 50 years of age or older. In

TABLE 13–2. *Benign versus malignant gastric ulcers: differential radiologic features*

Features	Benign	Malignant
Project beyond gastric wall	Yes	No
Convergence of folds	To edge of crater	Stop short of crater
Radiating folds	Smooth	Thickened, irregular, club-shaped
Ulcer shape	Linear, round, oval	Irregular
Position of ulcer mound	Central	Eccentric
Depth	Considerable depth	Shallow in relation to overall size
Ulcer collar	Smooth, symmetric	Eccentric
Margin	Smooth	Nodular, irregular
Peristalsis	Preserved	Diminished or absent
Healing	Complete in 8 weeks	Very rare
Multiplicity	10–30%	20%
Associated duodenal ulcer	50–60%	Uncommon
Location	Rarely in fundus or proximal greater curvature	Anywhere

Adapted from Gore et al. (21).

some Japanese studies, as many as 40% to 60% of newly diagnosed cancers are in an early stage. As noted previously, the 5-year survival rate for stage I cancer in Japan approaches 90%. When similar strict pathologic criteria are applied to early lesions diagnosed in the United States or other Western European countries, significantly improved 5-year survival rate results are demonstrated relative to later stages of disease (4a). However, with incidence rates approximately one-fifth of those observed in Japan, mass screening for gastric cancer cannot yet be economically justified in the United States. In the United States, the American Society of Gastrointestinal Endoscopy has recommended surveillance for patients with a history of gastric adenoma; adenomatous polyposis coli (including familial polyposis and Gardener's syndrome); and possibly for patients with Peutz-Jeghers syndrome and Menetrier's disease. In patients with adenomatous polyposis coli, gastroduodenoscopy with biopsy excision of polyps should be performed every 1 to 2 years. In patients with a prior history of a solitary adenoma, repeat endoscopy should be performed every 2 to 3 years to monitor for polyp recurrence (23).

PREOPERATIVE EVALUATION

Gastric cancer is usually diagnosed by upper GI endoscopy or barium studies. These techniques provide superb visualization of the mucosa but cannot determine the depth of mural invasion by tumor or the extent of metastatic involvement. By virtue of their cross-sectional imaging format and ability to demonstrate the extent of wall invasion, extraluminal tumor spread, lymph node, and distant metastases, CT scan and endoscopic ultrasound (EUS) have become the primary means of preoperative tumor staging.

Once the tissue diagnosis has been established, CT scan evaluation allows visualization of the stomach, perigastric area, and distant sites such as the liver, nodal basins, and peritoneum (24). Optimal luminal distention with barium, water, or gas is key to the evaluation of the gastric wall by CT scan. If not adequately distended, the normal stomach can appear pathologically thick. When properly distended, the normal

gastric wall is less than 5 mm on CT scan. The gastric wall near the gastroesophageal junction and cardia often appears thick due to axial images obliquely transversing the curved gastric wall. A wall thickness of over 1 cm is considered abnormal when the stomach is well distended. The CT scan findings of gastric cancer can vary and may include focal mural thickening with or without ulceration, a polypoid mass, or diffuse wall thickening with luminal narrowing as seen with linitis plastica. The use of helical CT scan techniques with i.v. contrast helps optimize identification of lymph node involvement and vascular encasement. Carcinomatosis with diffuse peritoneal seeding, malignant ascites, and adnexal and pelvic metastases are well depicted by CT scan. The reported accuracy of CT scan staging of gastric cancer has been quite variable. This is due no doubt in part to the continuing evolution of the technology. The major limitations of CT scan are categorizing the degree of gastric wall involvement and in identifying metastases in normal-sized lymph nodes. Understaging also occurs due to difficulty in identifying peritoneal carcinomatosis and small liver metastases. Reviews of more recent series examining state-of-the-art helical scanners suggest that serosal invasion can be detected with an accuracy of 70% to 80% (24). The overall accuracy of CT scan for evaluating lymph node disease is reported to be between 25% to 70% (24). The use of helical CT scan has increased the accuracy of staging and may be especially helpful in examining nodes not adjacent to the stomach. With helical CT scan, enlarged perigastric nodes can be distinguished from adjacent highly enhanced vessels during the early phase of scanning. A recent report using helical CT scan noted that 1% of nodes less than 5 mm, 45% of nodes 5 to 9 mm, and 72% of nodes over 9 mm were detected at CT scan. Metastatic involvement was not common in lymph nodes less than 15 mm, tumor was found in only 5% of nodes less than 5 mm, 21% of nodes 5 to 9 mm, and 23% of nodes 10 to 14 mm. Approximately 83% of the nodes larger than 14 mm contained cancer (25).

A new staging technique involves EUS. EUS uses a high-frequency (7.5 or 12 mHz) transducer at the end of an endoscope. It allows highly accurate staging of the depth of invasion of the primary tumor and is more accurate than CT scan for lymph node status in the perigastric region. The advantages of EUS lies in its ability to visualize routinely the gastric wall layers, the perigastric lymph nodes, and surrounding tissues. Most centers now consider EUS as a complimentary test to standard cross-sectional CT scan imaging (24). EUS is typically coupled with standard upper endoscopy during which tissue biopsies are performed. Normally, the diagnosis of carcinoma is made by endoscopic biopsy prior to EUS. EUS has difficulty in differentiating neoplastic involvement from benign inflammation and fibrosis. Lymphadenopathy is most frequently seen along the common hepatic artery, celiac axis, and hepatoduodenal ligament.

EUS has proven very accurate in demonstrating the depth of tumor invasion and lymph node involvement when compared with pathologic specimens (24,26,27). The overall accuracy for tumor staging is in the range of 80% to 90%. The reported diagnostic accuracy of EUS for determining nodal status is between 70% and 90%. A major problem in terms of diagnostic accuracy is the inability of EUS to detect non-enlarged nodes greater than 3 cm from the gastric wall. These are precisely the nodes in question when determining the role of extended lymph node dissection (to be discussed). EUS criteria for malignant involvement of lymph nodes do not rely solely on size but also consider the roundness, homogeneity, and hypoechogenicity of the lymph node, as well as its proximity to the tumor (26,27).

Accurate staging of gastric cancer is vital in designing appropriate patient treatment strategies. In addition to documenting the characteristics of the primary tumor such as depth of invasion and degree of differentiation, other important prognostic factors include the presence of distant metastases, lymph node metastases, and the ability to achieve complete surgical resection. EUS and CT scan are becoming increasingly accurate in terms of defining the extent of the primary tumor. When used in combination these studies provide important information regarding the extent of mural involvement, depth of tumor invasion, and possible contiguous organ invasion. This information is useful when planning the type of gastric resection and reconstruction to be performed. This is perhaps best illustrated by the treatment decisions required in patients with tumors of the proximal stomach. Submucosal infiltration of the distal stomach may go undetected on gross examination at laparotomy for a proximal gastric cancer. Resection of the distal esophagus and proximal stomach followed by esophagogastric anastomosis would fail to remove the true burden of residual disease, the distal stomach. If preoperative EUS or CT scan shows distal gastric involvement, then total gastrectomy with resection of the intra-abdominal esophagus and esophagojejunal anastomosis is more appropriate. Similarly, adenocarcinomas of the cardia, gastroesophageal junction, and distal esophagus are at risk for significant involvement of the more proximal esophagus that might be missed at surgery. Preoperative EUS and CT scan can help define the proximal extent of disease providing information crucial in planning the surgical approach.

STAGING AND PROGNOSIS

The pathologic stage of gastric cancer remains the most important determinant of the prognosis. In addition, accurate staging of gastric cancer is essential to assess the results of treatment protocols. Clinical trials confirm the importance of the depth at which the tumor has penetrated the stomach wall and the presence or absence of metastases to regional lymph nodes or distant organs in predicting disease-free and overall survival. The American Joint Committee on Cancer (AJCC) has incorporated these factors into a comprehensive TNM staging system (Table 13-3). The T category (tumor invasion)

TABLE 13–3. *Staging of cancer of the stomach*

Stage	T	N	M
0	Tis	N0	M0
IA	T1	N0	M0
IB	T1	N1	M0
IB	T2	N0	M0
II	T1	N2	M0
II	T2	N1	M0
II	T3	N0	M0
IIIA	T2	N2	M0
IIIA	T3	N1	M0
IIIA	T4	N0	M0
IIIB	T3	N2	M0
IV	T4	N1	M0
IV	T1	N3	M0
IV	T2	N3	M0
IV	T3	N3	M0
IV	T4	N2	M0
IV	T4	N3	M0
IV	Any T	Any N	M1

Primary Tumor (%): TX, primary tumor cannot be assessed; T0, no evidence of primary tumor; Tis, carcinoma *in situ* (intraepithelial tumor without invasion of the lamina propria); T1, tumor invades lamina propria or submucosa; T2, tumor invades the muscularis propria or the subserosa[a]; T3, tumor penetrates the serosa (visceral peritoneum) without invasion of adjacent structures[b,c]; T4, tumor invades adjacent structures[b,c].

Regional lymph nodes (N): NX, regional lymph node(s) cannot be assessed; N0, no regional lymph node metastasis; N1, metastasis in 1 to 6 regional lymph nodes; N2, metastasis in 7 to 15 regional lymph nodes; N3, metastasis in more than 15 regional lymph nodes.

Direct metastases (M): MX, presence of distant metastasis cannot be assessed; M0, no distant metastasis; M1, distant metastasis.

[a] A tumor may penetrate the muscularis propria with extension into the gastrocolic or gastrohepatic ligaments, or into the greater or lesser omentum without perforation of the visceral peritoneum covering these structures. In this case, the tumor is classified T2. If there is perforation of the visceral peritoneum covering the gastric ligaments or omenta, the tumor should be classified T3.

[b] The adjacent structures of the stomach include the spleen, transverse colon, liver, diaphragm, pancreas, abdominal wall, adrenal gland, kidney, small intestine, and retroperitoneum.

[c] Intramural extension to the duodenum or esophagus is classified by the depth of greatest invasion in any of these sites, including the stomach.

Adapted from American Joint Committee on Cancer (28).

includes T0 (no tumor); T1 (lamina propria or submucosal); T2 (muscularis or subserosa); T3 (extraserosal); and T4 (invasion of adjacent structures). The N category (regional lymph node involvement) includes N0 (no involvement); N1 (metastasis in 1 to 6 regional lymph nodes); N2 for metastasis in 7 to 15 regional lymph nodes; and N3 for metastasis in more than 15 regional lymph nodes. The M (metastases) category is defined as M0 for no distant metastasis and M1 for distant metastases. The TNM findings are then combined to determine the specific stage of disease (28). As noted in the report from the National Cancer Database of the American College of Surgeons Commission on Cancer and the American Cancer Society, the strongest correlation for survival was AJCC stage (Fig. 13-5). The 5-year survival rate for stage I was 43%, 37% for stage II, 18% for stage III, and 20% for stage IV (3). As noted previously in the United States, nearly 66% of patients present with either stage III or IV disease (4a).

The involvement of lymph nodes and the pattern of spread are particularly important for gastric cancers. There is considerable disparity between the published survival rates of patients with stomach cancer in Japanese and Western series. Although early diagnosis, a higher incidence of intestinal-type tumors, and the use of radical surgery in Japan may explain some of the differences, a major contributing factor may be differences in surgical and pathologic staging of gastric cancer in Japan. The anatomical classification of lymph nodes varies in the West and Japan and confuses the interpretation of the results of surgery.

The General Rules for Gastric Cancer Study in Surgery and Pathology, as published by the Japanese Research Society for Gastric Cancer, define the primary tumor stage based on the depth of invasion and the presence and extent of serosal invasion (29). Thus, unlike the AJCC system, which distinguishes the primary tumor based on depth of stomach wall layers involved with cancer, the Japanese system basically stratifies the primary tumor based on the presence or absence

of serosal involvement. The Japanese staging of lymph node involvement is also distinctly different than the AJCC system. The Japanese system describes four major nodal groups (N1 to N4) that encompass 16 separate locations of nodal tissue. Group 1 (N1) are nodes closest to the primary tumor and within the perigastric tissue along the greater and lesser curvatures, group 2 (N2) are nodes along major vessels from the celiac axis, group 3 (N3) are lymph nodes at the celiac axis, near the root of the superior mesenteric artery, in the hepato-duodenal ligament, and behind the pancreas. Group 4 (N4) are lymph nodes in the para-aortic tissue (Tables 13-4 and 13-5 and Fig. 13-6). The N3 and N4 designations would constitute distant metastatic disease (M1) in the AJCC system. It is important to note that the specific nodal tissue included in each nodal grouping varies depending on the anatomic location of the tumor. For example, a perigastric lymph node at the antrum is an N1 node for a distal stomach cancer while categorized as an N2 node for a carcinoma in the upper third of the stomach. Thus, the node stations in relation to the location of the primary tumor are used to define the stage of lymph node disease and ultimately are used to plan the surgical extent of nodal dissection. Adding to this confusion is the fact that the terminology used to describe different types of dissections has changed. Resections which remove the N1, N1 to N2, and N1 to N3 nodes used to be termed R1, R2, and R3, respectively, but are now termed D1, D2, and D3. The newer use of the terms R0 and R1 is a convention where R0 denotes a curative excision with no residual tumor in the patient and R1 indicates incomplete excision. In essence, the Japanese system of precise surgical dissection and pathologic staging of specific nodal basins, relative to the location of the primary tumor, is based on the assumption that there is an orderly spread of metastases from the primary tumor to regional lymph nodes and then to the next higher echelon of lymph nodes. Based on this assumption is the hypothesis that progressively more radical surgery encompassing progressively

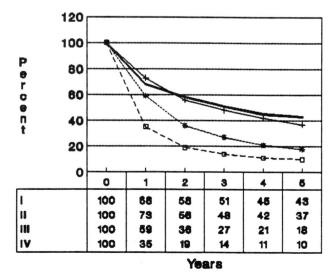
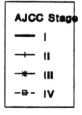

	0	1	2	3	4	5
I	100	68	58	51	45	43
II	100	73	56	48	42	37
III	100	59	36	27	21	18
IV	100	35	19	14	11	10

Years

FIG. 13-5. Relative 5-year gastric cancer survival rate by combined AJCC pathologic and clinical stage groups. (Reprinted with permission from Lawrence W Jr, Menck HR, Steele GD Jr, Winchester DP. The National Cancer Data Base report on gastric cancer. *Cancer* 1995;75:1734.)

TABLE 13–4. *Lymph node groupings according to site of tumor* [a]

Group	Location of primary tumor			
	Entire stomach	Lower third	Middle third	Upper third
N1	1–6	3–6	1, 3–6	1–4
N2	7–11	1, 7–9	2, 7–11	5–11
N3	12–14	2, 10–14	12–14	12–14

[a] 1–14 correspond to the lymph nodes described in Fig. 13-6.
Adapted from Behrns et al. (79).

higher echelons of lymph nodes will result in improved survival rates per stage of disease (30,31). Unfortunately, this has not been confirmed in Western series and this controversy will be discussed in a subsequent section.

Controversies regarding the role of extended lymph node dissections and the obvious differences between Western staging systems versus the Japanese staging systems cannot only be confusing for the practicing surgeon to interpret, but can raise the question about adequacy and completeness of staging and surgical treatment. Current recommendations regarding the role of extended lymphadenectomy and surgical resection will be discussed. At the present time, no distinct or obvious advantage to staging gastric cancer according to the Japanese rules has been demonstrated in Western patients. For the sake of uniformity and accuracy, it is thus recommended that until proven otherwise, the TNM staging system as advocated by the AJCC continue to be used for patients in the United States. Adherence to these recommendations and criteria has enabled the American College of Surgeons to es-

TABLE 13–5. *Japanese classification of regional gastric lymph nodes*

A. Perigastric lymph nodes (see corresponding drawing)
    1. Right pericardial
    2. Left pericardial
    3. Lesser curvature
    4. Greater curvature
    5. Suprapyloric
    6. Infrapyloric
B. Extraperigastric lymph nodes (see corresponding drawing)
    7. Left gastric artery
    8. Common hepatic artery
    9. Celiac artery
    10. Splenic hilus
    11. Splenic artery
    12. Hepatic pedicle
    13. Retropancreatic
    14. Mesenteric root
    15. Middle colic artery
    16. Para-aortic

Adapted from Kodama Y, Sugimachi K, Soejima K, et al. Evaluation of extensive lymph node dissection for carcinoma of the stomach. *World J Surg* 1981;5:242.

tablish the National Cancer Database. The establishment of this national database has allowed review of overall trends in treatment and outcome. In addition, while Western surgeons have examined the differences and discrepancies between the current TNM system and Japanese staging systems, our colleagues in pathology, medical oncology, and radiation oncology continue to use the TNM system as the basis and standard of care for all of their treatment decisions.

SURGICAL MANAGEMENT

Surgical resection is the only potentially curative modality for localized gastric cancer. The basic surgical approach for potentially curable gastric cancer has not essentially changed since the time of Billroth. Chances to maximize cure for patients with localized cancer are predicated upon a wide excision of the primary tumor with *en bloc* removal of the lymphatic drainage and any local or regional extension of disease. With the very limited effectiveness of radiotherapy and chemotherapy for stomach cancer, surgery still offers the best chance of cure for the patient with gastric carcinoma. Current surgical issues involve defining the extent of radicality and the adequacy of surgical resection. The main areas that are addressed are the extent of gastric resection, the adequacy of proximal and distal resection margins, the extent of lymph node dissection, and the role of splenectomy and adjacent organ resection for locally advanced cancer (32).

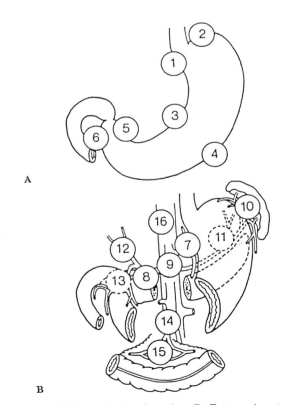

Fig. 13-6. A: Perigastric lymph nodes. **B:** Extraperigastric lymph nodes.

Extent of Gastric Resection

The appropriate extent of gastric resection for a given patient must take into account the location of the lesion and the known pattern of spread. Surgical strategy should provide the optimal cancer procedure with minimal morbidity. The most obvious and simplest solution to this problem would be to perform total gastrectomy upon any patient with a diagnosis of gastric carcinoma. However, the morbidity of this operation needs to be considered relative to the possibility that complete removal of the stomach may be excessive for patients with localized, distal gastric cancers (33). In addition, complete resection of the stomach may be inadequate therapy for a proximal tumor involving the cardia and gastroesophageal junction with significant esophageal extension. It becomes clear then that the selection of the most appropriate operation for gastric carcinoma is based on the location of the tumor and for this purpose the stomach is divided into thirds. The proximal third includes the gastroesophageal junction and cardia. The middle third consists of the body of the stomach and extends from the fundus to the incisura angularis of the lesser curvature. The distal third of the stomach includes

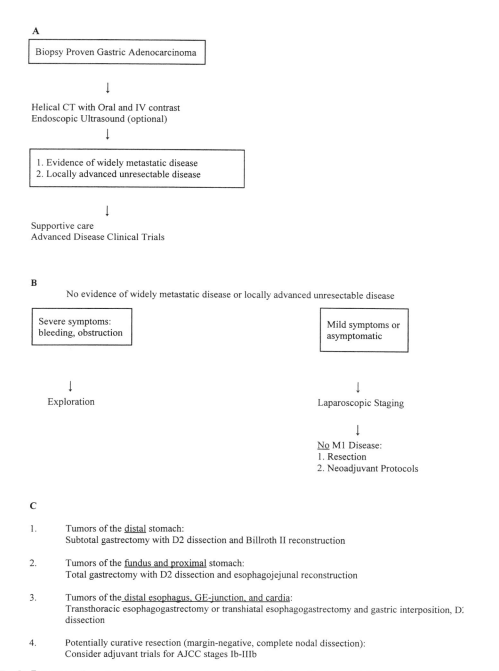

FIG. 13-7. A: Preoperative staging and management of metastatic disease. **B:** Management of localized gastric cancer. **C:** Types of surgical resections for localized gastric cancer.

the pyloric antrum and extends from the incisura angularis to the pylorus (34).

For patients with proximal lesions, the surgeon will have to make a choice between performing a transabdominal total gastrectomy with esophagojejunal anastomosis versus a combined transthoracic and transabdominal resection of the distal esophagus and proximal stomach with intrathoracic esophagogastric anastomosis (traditional Ivor-Lewis procedure) or transhiatal esophagectomy with cervical esophagogastric anastomosis. In general, if the tumor is limited to the proximal portion of the stomach with minimal extension past the GE junction, a total gastrectomy with intraabdominal esophagojejunal anastomosis is the procedure of choice. This can now be accomplished with acceptable morbidity and mortality (less than 5% in the Memorial Sloan-Kettering series) (34). The oncologic advantages of this operation is the assurance of achieving a completely negative histologic distal margin. It also facilitates complete perigastric lymph node removal relative to a proximal subtotal gastrectomy. Functionally, this procedure has the advantage of avoiding alkaline reflux gastritis associated with proximal subtotal gastrectomy. The most important point to stress, however, is the absolute necessity for obtaining negative histologic margins of resection (35). For tumors not involving the distal esophagus, GE junction, or cardia, a total gastrectomy with resection of the intraabdominal esophagus assures at least a 5- to 10-cm proximal margin and obviates the distal margin.

Cancer of the mid-stomach accounts for about 15% to 30% of all gastric cancers, and these lesions tend to remain asymptomatic until they are quite large and have metastasized to regional lymph nodes or distant sites. Whether to perform a total gastrectomy or an extended subtotal gastrectomy (75% to 85%) remains controversial. In general, however, most of these mid-body tumors are quite large and to achieve at least 5 cm of negative margins, a total gastrectomy is usually required. In addition, tumors of the fundus can metastasize to all of the perigastric lymph nodes so total gastrectomy is more likely to remove all of these lymph nodes. In comparative studies between high subtotal gastrectomy versus total gastrectomy, survival advantages have not clearly been defined (36). This is less likely due to the differences in the operation and more likely due to the fact that patients in the series who underwent either operation usually had stage III or IV disease. It is quite possible that in patients with earlier disease and potentially more curable disease, total gastrectomy would minimize the risk for marginal recurrence and would facilitate complete lymph node dissection. As noted, total gastrectomy with Roux-en-y reconstruction avoids the frequently debilitating complication of severe alkaline reflux gastritis.

About 35% of all gastric carcinomas occur in the distal third of the stomach. These lesions are usually diagnosed somewhat earlier than cancers in the more proximal two-thirds of the stomach because they can cause symptoms of pyloric obstruction even when relatively small. A distal subtotal gastrectomy with regional lymphadenectomy is the operation of choice for distal third gastric cancer (34). This requires resection of about 75% to 85% of the distal stomach including most of the lesser curvature where the margin of resection is often closest. At least 1 cm of the first portion of the duodenum should also be resected and a resection line 5 to 7 cm proximal to the tumor helps to insure adequate margins. Regardless of whether the tumor is located in the proximal mid-body or distal stomach, and regardless of the specific operation performed to achieve resection, intraoperative frozen section inspection of the proximal and distal resection margins is mandatory (35). As noted in the discussion of gastric carcinoma pathology, submucosal extension and diffuse submucosal infiltration is not uncommon with this malignancy. Intraoperative gross appearances can be deceiving and positive resection margins are uniformly associated with poor long-term survival and a high rate of local recurrence. Aside from the need for complete lymph node dissection, which will be discussed in the subsequent section, in addition to achieving wide margins of resection, removal of the greater and lesser omentum with perigastric lymph nodes is routinely performed for any gastric operation done for cancer. The Norwegian Stomach Cancer Trial prospectively studied the incidence of postoperative complications and mortality in more than 1,000 consecutive patients undergoing surgery for gastric cancer (37). The postoperative mortality rate among more than 760 patients undergoing resection was 8.3% and was highest in patients undergoing proximal resection (16%) and lower in those with total gastrectomy (8%), subtotal gastrectomy (10%), or distal resection (7%). Similar to the postoperative mortality, the complication rate was highest for proximal resections (52%), followed by total gastrectomy (38%), subtotal resection (28%), and distal resection (19%). Factors significantly related to the incidence of postoperative complications included advancing age, male sex, no antibiotic prophylaxis, and splenectomy (37).

A French cooperative prospectively randomized trial comparing total gastrectomy with subtotal gastrectomy has reported data on postoperative morbidity, mortality, and 5-year survival for carcinoma of the antrum (38). Analysis was performed for 169 patients with adenocarcinoma of the antrum operated upon with curative intent. The groups were well matched for the usual prognostic variables. The overall complication rate and postoperative mortality was 32% and 1.3%, respectively, for total gastrectomy and 34% and 3.2%, respectively, for subtotal gastrectomy. There was no difference in cumulative 5-year survival rates between groups (38). In conclusion, for more proximal lesions, total gastrectomy with esophagojejunal anastomosis probably provides better functional results, fewer complications, and lower operative mortality than proximal gastrectomy. For more distal tumors, high subtotal gastrectomy provides equivalent long-term survival and is associated with lower morbidity and mortality rates (39).

Extent of Lymphadenectomy

Perhaps no subject in gastric surgery has received as much attention as the role of extended lymphadenectomy for gastric carcinoma. As radical surgery for gastric cancer has become uniformly accepted in Japan, the operative mortality rate for extended dissections has declined and 5-year survival after curative resection has improved. The Japanese Research Society for Gastric Cancer defines a curative resection as one in which patients without peritoneal or hepatic involvement have a gastric resection with a lymph node dissection one level beyond that of pathological lymph node involvement (29). According to Maruyama (30), the 5-year survival rates of patients with metastases at node levels N0, N1, N2, N3, and N4 were 81.5%, 49.7%, 24%, 5.9%, and 1.9% respectively. The greater the total number of positive nodes, the higher the incidence of involved nodes at multiple levels. Five-year survival rates were inversely related to the number of nodal metastases.

In Japan, a rigorous effort has been made to codify the extent of the lymph node dissection according to the level of nodes dissected. The D1 gastric resection includes dissection of the N1 nodes, a D2 resection includes dissection of N1 and N2 nodes, and D3 dissection includes N1 to N3 nodes. In general, N1 represents the first echelon of draining nodes along the gastric and perigastric lymph node basin, and N2 includes the next echelon of extragastric nodes, primarily the celiac, hepatic, and splenic nodes, and selected nodes at other sites depending on the location of the primary tumor. For example, left periesophageal nodes would be N1 for proximal gastric carcinoma on the lesser curvature of the mid-stomach but would be considered N2 for carcinomas in the middle or distal third of the stomach. The N3 nodes include hepatoduodenal ligament nodes, although for distal gastric carcinomas hepatoduodenal ligament nodes would be N2. N4 nodes are the periaortic, pericaval, or mesenteric root lymph nodes. A retrospective review of data from 13 hospitals in Japan revealed an apparently steady improvement in survival, strongly supporting, at least in concept, the value of node dissection (31). Essential concepts underlying the adequacy of node dissection is to dissect the echelon of nodes that incorporate a level above the highest level of metastases, thus for positive N1 nodes a minimum of an N2 dissection is needed and positive N2 nodes would require an N3 dissection to adequately encompass them. Data from one Japanese study noting an improvement in 5-year survival rates after a D3 resection when compared with D2 resection (21.4% compared with 10%, respectively, for N2 nodes) support this position. Others Japanese studies have reported similar results with increased 5-year survival rates after a D2 or D3 resection compared with a D0 or D1 resection. In many of these Japanese reports, 5-year survival rates were significantly better than any Western series for both node negative and node positive patients. Node negative patients had a survival rate exceeding 75% and 5-year survival rates in node positive patients approached 50%.

Western surgeons have not uniformly embraced radical lymphadenectomy, arguing that an unequivocal survival advantage has yet to be demonstrated in Western series and that the increase in morbidity and cost has not been justified. Im-

portantly, some argue that any survival advantage of radical surgery is merely an artifact of more accurate pathologic staging, the so-called Will Rogers phenomenon (40). The stage migration of microscopic node positive patients into a higher TNM category would statistically improve survival in both the node negative and node positive groups. Because of these ongoing debates, several prospective Western series have examined this controversy.

There are now three randomized, controlled trials that have examined the problem of D1 versus D2 lymph node dissection in Western countries. A small trial consisting of 66 patients has been reported by Dent et al. (41) from Capetown in South Africa. With a median follow-up of 6.1 years, there has been no survival difference between the two groups and there has been no apparent difference in the site of recurrent disease between the D1 and D2 groups. The D2 group did, however, have a longer operation time, a greater requirement for blood transfusion, longer postoperative stay, and more reoperations for complications. However, this study was limited by the fact that the small number of patients entered in each group lacked statistical power.

In the Netherlands, a prospective randomized trial comparing D1 versus D2 dissections began in August of 1989 (42). Over 1,000 patients have been entered into this randomized trial. Bonenkamp (43) has pointed out several methodological problems in this type of study. An attempt at quality control was to be assured by having a Japanese instructor available to train the participating surgeons in the specific techniques of extended dissection. While long-term survival data from this study is not yet available, preliminary results reported by Bonenkamp (43) have shown a higher morbidity rate and even higher mortality rate in those patients receiving a more extended lymph node dissection. In addition, Bunt (44) has also published a report identifying several protocol violations in this study, which may blur the distinctions between whether patients actually had a more limited D1 dissection and the more aggressive D2 dissection. Clearly, it is unrealistic to assume that each patient will receive an exactly similar operation by a different surgeon. It is likely that there would be some overlap and some blurring of distinctions between the type of dissection relative to each patient and surgeon. This will be true in any type of prospective study examining surgical technique, and needs to be factored when interpreting the final survival outcomes. While the long-term survival data from this Netherlands study has yet to be reported, the data that have become available suggest that D2 patients had a higher operative mortality rate then the D1 patients (10% versus 4%) and had more complications (43% versus 25%) (42).

A similar study was undertaken in the United Kingdom (45). Approximately 400 patients were randomized between a standard, Western D1 lymph node dissection versus a D2 lymph node dissection that included distal pancreatectomy and splenectomy. Mature survival data from this study are also not yet available. However, preliminary results suggest an increased postoperative morbidity in the radical lymph node dissection group and increased mortality (6.5% versus 13%). This increased morbidity and mortality is thought to be largely accounted for by the distal pancreatectomy and splenectomy.

A nonrandomized but prospective study from Germany reported by Siewert (46) demonstrated a 5-year survival rate that was higher after a D2 resection when compared with the rate after a D1 resection. Among cases with stage II disease, the survival rates were 55% and 26%, respectively; for cases with stage III-A disease, the rates were 38.4% and 25.3%, respectively.

In the United States, several institutions have begun to examine their individual experiences with extended lymph node dissection for gastric cancer. At Memorial Sloan-Kettering Cancer Center, Smith et al. (47) reviewed the morbidity of radical lymphadenectomy in a prospective database of 185 potentially curative gastric resections. In 123 patients, at least two regional lymph node echelons were removed *en bloc* with the stomach, whereas 62 patients had less extended, or more traditional, dissections. The two groups were similar with regard to demographics and pathologic stage. Only postoperative abdominal drainage was found to be increased for radical resection. All other surgically related events occurred with no statistically significant difference between the two groups. They concluded that radical lymphadenectomy for gastric cancer could be performed as safely as lesser operations and should not be avoided because of the fear of complications. The relatively similar rates of postoperative complications in this series may be accountable by the fact that splenectomy and distal pancreatectomy were not routinely performed as originally described by the Japanese. Survival data were not reported in this preliminary report.

Volpe and Douglas (48) have recently reported the experience with extended lymph node dissection from the Roswell Park Cancer Center. They reviewed 101 patients who underwent potentially curative gastric resections. With a median follow-up of 33 months, the entire group had an estimated 5-year survival rate of 36% with a median survival of 33 months. The estimated 5-year survival rate for 46 patients who had an extended resection was 49% with a median survival of 50 months compared to 27% and 25.7 months, respectively, for 55 patients with a limited resection. Following extended resection, 74% of stage I patients survived 5 years, 75% of patients with stage II disease were alive at 5 years, as were 13% with stage IIIa and 30% with stage IIIb. Their data suggested that nearly one-third of patients who had metastases to lymph nodes in the N2 group and who had a methodical D2 lymphadenectomy survived 5 years.

Wanebo and others (49) have recently reexamined the data accumulated by the National Cancer Database of the American College of Surgeons. In the database of over 18,000 patients, approximately 3,800 were identified as having curative resection with more than 5 years follow-up. Based on a review of the operative reports and pathology reports, Wanabe et al. (49) defined three groups of patients. The first group were patients who were thought to have had by definition an N2

lymph node clearance which included dissection of the nodes along the celiac axis, hepatic artery, or splenic artery. The other two groups had patients who had a more limited lymph node dissection or who had no lymph nodes identified in the resection specimen. While clearly not a study designed to specifically address the role of extended lymph node dissection, this review of the National Cancer Database found no statistically significant difference in median survival time or overall survival rate between the groups that had a more limited lymph node dissection versus the group in which the surgical reports and pathology reports confirmed the presence of a more extended lymph node clearance.

Despite these ongoing debates, certain reasonable conclusions can be made from the series thus far reported. Without question, the presence of lymph node metastases is an independent predictor of poor survival. In addition, aggressive lymph node clearance improves local-regional control of disease and thus facilitates the ability of adjuvant treatments such as chemotherapy and radiation therapy to make an impact on the natural history of the disease. While the prospective randomized series performed in the West have yet to reach maturity, and thus survival benefits of extended dissection cannot yet be completely determined, there does appear to be an increased morbidity and mortality when distal pancreatectomy and splenectomy are included in the dissection. Whether extended lymph node dissection that spares the spleen and avoids pancreatectomy will provide a survival advantage compared to limited dissection of the first echelon of lymph nodes is unknown. Conversely, extended lymph node dissection to include the second echelon of lymph nodes (D2) without pancreatectomy or splenectomy probably adds little time, morbidity, or an increase in mortality to gastric resection. Thus, many surgeons have adopted a D2 dissection which includes a margin negative gastric resection, complete omentectomy, and extended lymphadenectomy which includes the first echelon (N1) lymph nodes and regional dissection of the N2 lymph nodes based on the location of the primary tumor.

Splenectomy and Extended Organ Resection

Prophylactic splenectomy during gastric resection for tumors not adjacent to or invading the spleen has not been demonstrated to improve outcome for similarly staged patients. Noguchi, in a review of surgery for gastric cancer in Japan, concluded that the evidence to support routine splenectomy with gastric resection in that country is not well established (50). The effect of splenectomy on morbidity and survival following curative gastrectomy for carcinoma was reviewed by Brady et al. (51) at Memorial Sloan-Kettering Cancer Center. In a retrospective analysis of 392 patients with potentially curative resection, significantly more complications occurred in patients undergoing splenectomy as part of extended gastric resections than in those who did not have the spleen removed (45% versus 21%). The splenectomy patients also had a higher percentage of infectious complications than the nonsplenectomy patients (75% versus 47%). No long-term survival benefit could be attributed to having splenectomy performed, and it was concluded that splenectomy increased the morbidity of potentially curative gastrectomy and should be avoided unless the spleen is close to or invaded by tumor. A more recent report from the American College of Surgeons specifically examined outcome related to stage and splenectomy. For any given stage of gastric cancer, a survival benefit could not be found which would have been directly attributable to splenectomy (4b).

The presence of locally advanced gastric carcinoma with direct invasion into adjacent organs is clearly a poor prognostic factor. Nevertheless, extended *en bloc* resections including the spleen, distal pancreas, and occasionally transverse colon have been reported. While it is difficult to demonstrate markedly improved 5-year survival rates in patients with locally advanced disease, significant palliation can be achieved with hopes of an extended survival. Consideration should be given to extended resection in the presence of locally advanced disease, in the absence of distant metastases, when it appears feasible to obtain negative margins of resection. *En bloc* resection which fails to remove all gross disease (debulking) is not indicated for adenocarcinoma of the stomach.

Laparoscopic Staging

To date, no randomized prospective trial has demonstrated an unequivocal survival advantage to either postoperative adjuvant chemotherapy or radiation therapy. A current Intergroup trial is examining the role of combined chemotherapy and radiation therapy following complete surgical resection and the results of this adjuvant trial are eagerly awaited. In addition, palliative resections for those in which there is incomplete removal of primary or nodal disease are uniformly associated with dismal long-term results. Because of the disappointing results of adjuvant therapy and the significant number of patients who undergo incomplete resections, neoadjuvant chemotherapy is being examined as a potential strategy to improve resectability and survival. Because of the poor prognosis associated with peritoneal carcinomatosis and the inefficacy of neoadjuvant chemotherapy in this situation, these patients should be excluded from trials of neoadjuvant chemotherapy. Failure to detect peritoneal or occult hepatic disease before treatment begins adversely biases response and resectability rates. The presence of peritoneal carcinomatosis can conclusively be excluded only by laparoscopy.

The ability of laparoscopy to detect nodal metastases, subclinical peritoneal disease, and occult hepatic metastases has been demonstrated in several different series. In one study by Watt et al. (52), laparoscopy had a diagnostic accuracy of 72% in assessing nodal involvement compared with 52% and 57% for ultrasonography and CT scan, respectively. Laparoscopy was also significantly more accurate than ultrasound and CT scan in detecting hepatic metastases with an accuracy of 96% compared with 83% and 85% for ultrasound

and CT scan, respectively. Not unexpectedly it was also the most accurate study for the detection of small peritoneal metastases. Possik reported results of staging laparoscopy in 360 patients with gastric cancer (53). Laparoscopy had a sensitivity of 83.3% in detecting peritoneal dissemination and 87.2% in detecting liver metastases as confirmed by laparoscopic biopsy or surgery. A more recent study by Bemelman suggests that the differences in diagnostic accuracy between laparoscopy and CT scan may be decreasing because of the remarkable advances in current CT scan technology (54). In only two of 56 patients was the planned laparotomy aborted because of findings at laparoscopy. In their study examining the role of staging laparoscopy in intraabdominal malignancy, Hemming et al. (55) noted potential areas of failure during laparoscopic exploration: nodes near the common bile duct and superior mesenteric artery and the lesser sac and superior pancreatic nodes. These areas can be addressed by dissection of the greater omentum, opening of the lesser sac, and careful inspection and sampling of the hiatus, posterior stomach, pancreas, and celiac axis. The most advantageous use of laparoscopy lies in detecting peritoneal and visceral metastases. Sendler (56) found peritoneal carcinomatosis in 23% of 111 patients during laparoscopy for pretreatment staging. The development of laparoscopic ultrasound probes has also increased the sensitivity for the detection of occult hepatic metastases by 10% to 20% (56).

Two recent series from M. D. Anderson and Memorial Sloan-Kettering confirmed the value of laparoscopy in the management of gastric cancer. Lowy et al. (57) from M. D. Anderson reported 71 patients who underwent preoperative CT and laparoscopy. Unsuspected peritoneal or hepatic metastases were found by laparoscopy in 20 patients (28%). The median survival for these patients was 5 months, and only one patient required reoperation for a palliative procedure. Similarly, Burke et al. (58) from Memorial Sloan-Kettering reviewed 111 patients in whom laparoscopic exploration was performed subsequent to a reportedly normal CT. Unsuspected metastatic disease was found in 37% with a sensitivity of 84% and a specificity of 100%. No patient whose initial operation was only laparoscopy required reoperation for palliation.

At Northwestern, a rather selective application of laparoscopy for patients with gastric cancer is currently in use. The location of the primary lesion and the patient's symptoms are important in determining the utility of laparoscopy versus the necessity of laparotomy. Surgical resection of a distal gastric lesion causing pyloric obstruction and vomiting or persistent bleeding appears to be warranted in the majority of patients. In patients with limited hepatic metastases, distal gastrectomy may provide reasonable palliation and allows the resumption of oral intake. Laparoscopy plays little role in these patients unless the preoperative EUS or CT scan demonstrate equivocal findings suggesting unresectability due to locally advanced disease.

Surgical palliation for more proximal cancers in patients with incurable disease is controversial. If EUS or CT scan suggest the presence of peritoneal or hepatic metastases or suspicious lymphadenopathy outside the field of resection but are not definitive, then laparoscopy is used to confirm this advanced disease before proceeding with a total gastrectomy. Patients with cancer of the cardia, gastroesophageal junction, or distal esophagus are currently enrolled in a randomized prospective trial of aggressive neoadjuvant chemoradiation. Accurate pretherapy evaluation of the liver, peritoneum, and nodal status is carried out with EUS, CT scan, and laparoscopy with laparoscopic ultrasound. A laparoscopic feeding jejunostomy tube is placed to help maintain the patient's nutritional status during the intensive chemotherapy. The preliminary experience with this approach has been quite favorable, and it is hoped that the long-term results will confirm the utility of this staging algorithm and the efficacy of the treatment protocol (Fig 13-7).

Treatment of Early Gastric Cancer

As noted in the section on pathology and screening, early gastric cancer is defined as gastric adenocarcinoma confined to the mucosa or submucosa irrespective of lymph node involvement. With the high incidence of early gastric cancer in Japan and the possibility of encountering this diagnosis in the United States, questions have arisen regarding surgical management of this early cancer. Questions exist regarding the extent of gastric resection and the role of lymph node dissection for patients with this lesion. Reports of early gastric cancer note that symptoms of this tumor mimic those of peptic ulcer disease and epigastric pain or dyspepsia in about two-thirds of these patients. Approximately 20% to 40% of patients will have anorexia, nausea, or vomiting, but weight loss is usually less than 10 lbs. However, the presence or absence of any specific symptom complex cannot differentiate early gastric cancer from late disease. The diagnosis, therefore, is essentially established by endoscopic biopsy which demonstrates carcinoma superficial to the muscularis propria.

Japanese series of early gastric cancer have identified specific characteristics of these early cancers that are predictors of lymph node metastasis. Mehara et al. (59) in Japan note that the 10-year survival rate for patients with early gastric cancer without nodal involvement ranges from 82% to 97% but falls to 57% to 87% with involved nodes. They stress the fact that tumors superficial to the muscularis propria with metastatic lymph nodes are still considered an early cancer. Nodal metastases in most series are found in approximately 7% to 10% of patients. Multivaried analysis by Maehara et al. demonstrated that independent risk factors for lymph node metastasis in early gastric cancer patients were large tumor size (greater than 2 cm), lymphatic vessel involvement, and invasion into the submucosal layer (59). Extended lymphadenectomy for patients with early gastric cancer has not proven beneficial if the lymph nodes resected are histologically negative. In patients with early gastric cancers that are large, have lymphatic vessel involvement or invasion into the submucosal layer, more aggressive lymph node dissection is probably warranted because of the increased risk of nodal metas-

tases. Experience with early gastric cancer at the Mayo Clinic and Memorial Sloan-Kettering emphasize the need for appropriate gastric resection and lymph node dissection (60,61). In the series from New York, the disease-free 5-year survival rate after gastrectomy was 76.4% and survival was not significantly correlated with sex, tumor site, macroscopic appearance of the tumor, extent of the gastric resection, or histopathologic type. Early gastric cancers more than 1.5 cm in diameter that invaded the submucosa or involved the regional lymph nodes resulted in significantly lower survival rates. In an early series from the Mayo Clinic, only 7.7% of the early gastric cancer patients had perigastric nodal metastases. The 10-year survival was 75% after subtotal gastrectomy and survival was correlated with the presence or absence of lymph node metastases.

In conclusion, in the United States, treatment of early gastric cancer should consist of subtotal gastrectomy with regional lymphadenectomy. Total gastrectomy should be limited to patients with multifocal or proximal early gastric cancer. The extent of lymph node dissection remains as controversial as with more advanced gastric carcinoma. Since the vast majority of patients with early gastric carcinoma will do extremely well even with limited lymph node dissection, an extended D2 dissection is difficult to justify. However, as noted by Lawrence and Shiu (61), recurrence after gastric resection is usually lethal and they recommend gastrectomy plus extended lymphadenectomy to achieve the highest possible cure rate. Adverse prognostic factors predicting an increased risk for nodal metastasis may be helpful in determining the extent of lymph node dissection.

Endoscopic treatment or nonoperative therapy of early gastric carcinoma has been described in series from Japan. Endoscopic resection or ablation of small protruded, well-differentiated early gastric cancer limited to the mucosa seems to be effective. Short-term survival in the series reported is thus far excellent and for poor risk patients and those refusing gastrectomy, endoscopic treatment may be appropriate.

**ADJUVANT CHEMOTHERAPY
FOR GASTRIC CANCER**

The majority of patients who present with gastric carcinoma and undergo potentially curative resection will still die from recurrent disease. Even patients without nodal metastases will have at least a 50% chance of dying within 5 years. As noted earlier, it is actually a very small percentage of patients in the United States who are diagnosed with early gastric cancer. Thus, the use of postoperative adjuvant therapy is reasonable in a disease in which subsequent local or distant failure is a likely probability. Few Western studies have shown any statistically significant survival benefit from adjuvant chemotherapy. Several Japanese series have demonstrated favorable results in limited subsets of patients. Over the past 20 years, several randomized controlled studies of surgery alone versus surgery plus adjuvant chemotherapy have been reported. There have been four main groups of chemotherapeutic agents used in these trials. Essentially, the chemotherapeutic agents that have been tested against gastric cancer include nitrosourea-containing protocols, mitomycin-C, 5-fluorouracil (5-FU), and adriamycin-based protocols either alone or in combination with 5-FU or mitomycin (39). Early studies examined the role of each of these different drugs as single agents for adjuvant treatment for gastric cancer.

Single agent 5-FU treatment has not prolonged life in patients undergoing potentially curative resection. In the United States, the Gastrointestinal Tumor Study Group (GITSG) reported a clinical benefit with 5-FU and methyl-CCNU treatment but the Veteran's Administration Surgical Oncology Group and the Eastern Cooperative Oncology Group reported no benefit over surgical treatment only (62). The regimens used in these three studies were identical, but there were differences in patient selection. The GITSG study treated only patients undergoing potentially curative surgery while the other two groups included patients with palliative resections. Other subsequent studies combining 5-FU with a second cytotoxic agent have shown no benefit.

Mitomycin-C is reported to prolong life in patients with advanced disease in several Japanese series. Two major Japanese trials failed to show significantly prolonged overall survival in groups treated with either surgery and postoperative mitomycin-C, or surgery alone. However, subgroup analysis suggested that stage II or III patients showed approximately a 10% to 20% improvement in 5-year survival rate (62). An early study from Spain demonstrated a prolonged improvement in survival in patients treated with mitomycin-C as an adjuvant treatment. After 10 years of follow-up, 16% of patients remained alive after surgery alone versus 52% of patients receiving mitomycin after resection. The best effective adjuvant treatment was seen in patients with T3N0M0 stage tumors. However, more recent trials involving mitomycin-C in the United States have not confirmed a significant benefit to this regimen. Japanese trials examining three drug combinations with mitomycin-C as the central drug and combined with 5-FU and cytosine arabinoside produced no overall significant improvement compared to single agent mitomycin-C (62).

In conclusion, Japanese series have suggested an improvement in overall survival when mitomycin-C is used as a single agent adjuvant therapy. At least one European study has confirmed this with at least a 5- to 10-year follow-up. Studies done in the United States have yet to show a convincing survival advantage for adjuvant mitomycin-C when used either alone or in combination with other agents.

More recently doxorubicin containing combination chemotherapy has been tested. Because of the activity of 5-FU and adriamycin in other solid tumors, this combination of drugs with mitomycin has undergone testing in several clinical trials. Coombs et al. (63) reported a trial examining postoperative 5-FU, doxorubicin, and mitomycin-C (FAM) versus surgery alone. With medium follow-up of more than 5 years, there was no difference in disease free survival or overall survival.

The Southwest Oncology Group recently evaluated FAM as adjuvant therapy for patients with resected stage I, II, or III gastric carcinoma (64). One hundred and ninety-three patients were entered in the study which was reported with a median follow-up of 9.5 years. The estimated 5-year disease free survival was approximately 30% in each group. Similarly, there was no statistically significant difference in overall survival between the two treatment groups. Interestingly, when all patients were reviewed, cases with a curative resection defined as having no evidence of residual disease in the abdomen and tumor-free margins of greater than 1 cm had a superior survival compared to cases not meeting this requirement. The overall 5-year survival rate for patients with a defined curative resection was 42% versus 15% in patients who had either inadequate or a questionably curative resection. The presence or absence of adjuvant treatment with FAM did not predict survival within these two groups.

In conclusion, no study has demonstrated a significant advantage to postoperative adjuvant 5-FU either alone or in combination. Similarly, adriamycin-based protocols (FAM) also seem to be ineffective as an adjuvant treatment. Japanese studies have demonstrated survival advantage to adjuvant mitomycin-C; this has not been generally confirmed in studies done in the United States. At the present time, no single agent chemotherapy protocol or combination drug regimen can be considered standard adjuvant care for gastric cancer. The most active agent in Japanese and European studies appears to be mitomycin-C.

ADJUVANT RADIOTHERAPY

The rationale for radiation therapy in the adjuvant setting is based on the patterns of failure after potentially curative surgery. As found with other GI malignancies, the incidence of locoregional failure increases with depth of penetration and the presence of lymph node metastases. As discussed earlier, the majority of patients will present with full thickness tumors penetrating the serosa of the stomach or with lymph node metastases present at the time of diagnosis. Two major randomized trials of postoperative radiation therapy with or without chemotherapy after potentially curative resections have been reported. In 1984, Moertel from the Mayo Clinic examined the role of postoperative radiation therapy (37.5 Gy) plus 5-FU versus surgery alone (65). Although there was a significant improvement in survival in the patients who were in the postoperative combined modality treatment group compared with surgery alone (23% versus 4%), this improvement may have been due to the 10 patients who were randomized to receive the postoperative combined modality therapy and refused. The 5-year survival of those 10 patients who refused the treatment was higher compared with the remaining 29 who were randomized to the treatment and accepted the treatment (30% versus 20%). However, locoregional failure was decreased in the patients who received postoperative combined modality therapy compared with those that were randomized to either surgery alone or refused the postoperative combined modality therapy (39% versus 54%).

The second trial involved the subset analysis of a randomized trial by Dent et al. (66). Limiting the analysis to 30 patients with locoregional disease that underwent a potentially curative resection, postoperative combined modality therapy had a negative impact on 2-year survival compared with surgery alone. Virtually all of the other randomized as well as nonrandomized trials of postoperative radiation therapy or combined modality therapy have included patients with residual disease.

Given the high incidence of locoregional failure as well as the moderate response rate with a combination of radiation plus 5-FU chemotherapy in the advanced gastric cancer setting, a phase III Intergroup trial has been activated that compares *en bloc* resection alone versus *en bloc* resection plus 45 Gy of radiation and 4 monthly cycles of 5-FU and leucovorin. This Intergroup trial is one of the few in which adequate doses 5-FU based chemotherapy are delivered. Until the results of the Intergroup trial are available, the use of postoperative radiation therapy in the adjuvant setting remains investigational. Standard treatment after a complete resection is observation alone. In the setting of locally unresectable or residual disease, postoperative radiation therapy and 5-FU based chemotherapy may decrease locoregional progression and improve survival (67).

An alternative method of delivering radiation therapy is intraoperative radiation. In this technique, patients receive a single dose of high-energy electrons delivered to the tumor bed at the time of gastrectomy. The theoretical advantage of this approach is the ability to deliver a more intensive dose of radiation to the tumor bed while excluding the surrounding normal tissues from the high-dose field. Two randomized phase III trials have examined this technique in an adjuvant setting. A limited randomized trial was reported from the National Cancer Institute (68). Patients with grossly resected stage III or IV disease were randomized to receive either 20 Gy intraoperative radiation or 50 Gy postoperative external beam radiation. The mean time to local failure was significantly improved in patients who received intraoperative radiation (21 versus 8 months). In addition, the postoperative complication rate was lower (40% versus 72%) and the median survival was higher (21 versus 10 months) in patients who received intraoperative radiation. None of these differences, however, reached statistical significance.

Takahashi and Abe randomized patients to surgery plus intraoperative radiation (28 to 35 Gy) versus surgery alone (69). There was improvement in survival with intraoperative radiation; however, it was limited to patients with stage III and IV disease. As noted, the more extensive surgical staging and possibly earlier presentation of gastric cancer in Japan make it difficult to compare this study with data from the United States. Limited data thus far suggests that intraoperative radiation may be beneficial in selected patients with gastric cancer. The optimal method by which to combine it with surgery and external beam radiation has yet to be determined.

The use of intraoperative radiation therapy for gastric cancer remains investigational.

INTRAPERITONEAL CHEMOTHERAPY

Because peritoneal or hepatic failure is so common, the use of postoperative intraperitoneal chemotherapy with hyperthermic perfusion has been studied by several centers in the United States and Japan (62). Early work done with intraperitoneal chemotherapy for colon cancer compared intraperitoneal 5-FU chemotherapy versus i.v. chemotherapy. These studies showed a change in the failure pattern with a marked decrease in peritoneal metastases using intraperitoneal chemotherapy when compared with i.v. treatment. There was no change in overall survival. Because of the even higher rate of peritoneal metastasis in gastric carcinoma, these observations have led to similar studies in stomach cancer (62).

Experience from Japan has shown that the combination of hyperthermia and mitomycin-C used in an adjuvant setting is technically feasible and safe. Patients who have undergone postoperative perfusion have not shown an increased incidence of postoperative complications. Intraperitoneal chemotherapy has also been examined in the adjuvant setting. Hamaze (70) used hyperthermic peritoneal perfusion for high-risk gastric cancer patients. Mitomycin-C was given in 42 patients with intraperitoneal treatment, whereas 40 patients underwent resection alone. The 5-year survival rate for patients receiving IP therapy was 64.3% versus 52.4% in the control group. This difference was not statistically significant. Peritoneal recurrence was found more frequently in the control group but again the difference was not statistically significant. Another phase III trial done by Hagiwara et al. (71) also examined intraperitoneal mitomycin-C after curative resection in high-risk patients. There was a highly significant survival difference in favor of the intraperitoneal treatment group at 2 years (68.6% versus 26.9%). Based on these studies, this technique is currently under investigation at several centers in the United States.

NEOADJUVANT THERAPY

Because of the disappointing results with adjuvant therapy and the significant number of patients who undergo incomplete resections, neoadjuvant chemotherapy is being examined as a potential strategy to improve resectability and survival (62). Ota (72) has summarized the advantages of preoperative chemotherapy. Initial treatment with systemic chemotherapy may reduce the size of the primary tumor and facilitate a complete margin negative resection. Therapy for occult, systemic disease is started early, before the patient has had time to recover from a major GI resection, and thus may be more biologically effective than postoperative therapy. In addition, early delivery of systemic chemotherapy allows one to assess the sensitivity of the tumor to the drugs used. If a primary tumor shows a measurable response, then the same antineoplastic agents are continued postoperatively. If there is tumor progression during chemotherapy, the initial drug combination is discontinued postoperatively and either a second chemotherapeutic regimen is used or no further treatment is given (72).

Fink et al. (73) recently reviewed the results of seven studies that examined response rates and resections after preoperative chemotherapy. Although the drug combinations varied between studies, complete or major clinical responses were seen in 24% to 63% of patients, but no complete pathological responses were seen in any of the resected specimens. In patients undergoing subsequent laparotomy, complete resections were done in 56% to 90% of patients without significant increases in morbidity or mortality relative to controls. Survival data were not available from all series; however, in one series the 2-year survival rate was 42%. Survival benefit was seen in those who had a major clinical response to chemotherapy and had subsequent complete tumor resection. Ajani (74) from M. D. Anderson has noted that because of the poor prognosis associated with peritoneal carcinomatosis and the inefficacy of neoadjuvant chemotherapy in this situation, these patients should be excluded from trials of neoadjuvant chemotherapy. Failure to detect peritoneal or occult hepatic disease before treatment begins adversely biases response and resectability rates. The presence of peritoneal carcinomatosis can be conclusively excluded only by laparoscopy. Thus, at the M. D. Anderson Cancer Center, patients entered on neoadjuvant trials of chemotherapy are routinely staged prior to treatment with laparoscopy. In a study from that institution, 48 patients who had gastric cancers that were potentially operable were treated preoperatively with three courses of etoposide, doxorubicin, and platinum (EAP) chemotherapy (74). Toxicity was substantial but generally manageable. The median duration of survival for all patients was 15.5 months. In a second study from the same institution, a similar protocol was used with cisplatin, 5-FU and etoposide. Seventy-two percent of patients had potentially curative resections. The median duration of survival was 15 months. Neoadjuvant chemotherapy given with or without postoperative intraperitoneal treatment is now being studied at several institutions. To date, no increase in operative morbidity or mortality has been reported. An aggressive strategy for high-risk gastric cancer combining neoadjuvant therapy using 5-FU, doxorubicin, and methyltrexate and postoperative intraperitoneal cisplatin and i.v. fluorouracil was recently reported from Memorial Sloan-Kettering (75). In this study, 56 patients were treated with preoperative FAMTX therapy. Eighty-nine percent of patients underwent surgical exploration and 61% had potentially curative resections. Comparison of the postoperative, pathologic tumor stage with the predicted tumor stage by preoperative EUS showed apparent down-staging in 51% of patients. Toxicity was acceptable and there was no increase in the rate of operative complications or mortality. Peritoneal failure was seen in 16% and was thought to be lower than expected.

PATTERNS OF RECURRENCE AND SURVELLIANCE RECOMMENDATIONS AFTER POTENTIALLY CURATIVE GASTRIC RESECTION

To develop effective adjuvant therapy following potentially curative gastric resections and to define cost-efficient means of monitoring for cancer recurrence, there must first be a thorough understanding of the patterns of disease failure. Despite complete resection of all gross disease with negative microscopic margins, disease recurrence is common. Carcinoma of the stomach can spread by local extension into adjacent structures and can develop lymphatic metastases, peritoneal metastases, and distant metastases. Patterns of locoregional failure and distant metastasis have been analyzed in clinical, reoperative, and autopsy series. While all of these studies have some limitations in terms of how patients were evaluated, with bias inherent in the mechanisms used to identify distant disease, certain patterns of locoregional failure and distant metastases become evident. Locoregional failures occur commonly within the region of the gastric bed and nearby lymph nodes. Clinical and reoperative evaluation suggest that locoregional recurrence in the gastric bed, anastomosis, or regional lymph nodes occurs in 20% to 50% of patients. Autopsy studies demonstrate locoregional failure ultimately in 50% to 70% of patients (39). Similarly, peritoneal seeding or distant metastases are seen in approximately 20% to 40% of patients at reoperation, but ultimately develop as a component of overall failure in 40% to 70% of patients (39). The most common sites of visceral metastasis are the liver followed by the lung. Predictably, patients at greatest risk for locoregional failure are those with locally advanced tumors penetrating through the serosa of the stomach and with advanced invasion into contiguous organs. In addition, patients with extensive lymph node metastases remain at risk for regional lymphatic recurrence. These data suggest the development of effective therapy for locoregional disease, in addition to extended resection, could be potentially beneficial in at least 20% to 40% of patients. The high rate of systemic metastases and peritoneal recurrence support investigational studies involving systemic neoadjuvant chemotherapy or postoperative intraperitoneal chemotherapy (39).

There are no currently accepted standards of care recommended for postoperative surveillance. This is based in part on the lack of effective treatment for recurrent or distant metastatic failure. Preliminary studies examining certain tumor markers such as CA19.9 and CEA suggest correlation with early disease recurrence. Currently, serial monitoring of tumor markers is probably not cost-efficient because there are few therapeutic options for recurrent gastric cancer. However, should effective therapies for recurrent disease develop, serial monitoring of gastric tumor specific markers for gastric cancer may become important. Similarly, no rigid recommendations can currently be made for periodic chest x-rays, CT scans, and routine blood studies. However, patients at high risk for both local recurrence and distant failure may be monitored selectively with frequent testing if considered eligible for investigational trials at the time that recurrent disease is detected.

GASTRIC LYMPHOMA

Lymphomas are the second most common gastric malignancy in the United States, comprising 2% to 9% of all malignancies in the stomach. The stomach is the most common site of extranodal lymphoma accounting for over one-half of all primary GI lymphomas. Most of these tumors are B-cell lymphomas of the non-Hodgkin's type. The clinical presentation of gastric lymphoma can be very similar to gastric adenocarcinoma and symptoms may include dyspepsia, pain, nausea, vomiting, perforation, or hematemesis. Diagnosis is best made with endoscopic biopsy. Staging studies should consist of a chest x-ray, CT scan of the abdomen, peripheral blood smear, or bone marrow aspirate and biopsy. Multiple staging systems exist for gastric lymphoma. Essentially for the general surgeon, the most important determination is whether the tumor involves the stomach and local perigastric lymph nodes (stages I and II), other intraabdominal nodes and organs (stage III), or disease exists outside the abdomen (stage IV). In general, patients with tumor involvement beyond regional lymph nodes such as the iliac or periaortic nodes are best treated with chemotherapy or a combination of chemotherapy and radiation. In addition, patients with tumor spread to other intraabdominal organs or disease outside of the abdomen are best treated with chemotherapy. The optimal treatment for early stage primary non-Hodgkin's gastric lymphoma is controversial. Several retrospective surgical studies show excellent long-term survival after gastric resection with or without radiation therapy. In a study by Talamonti et al. (76), patients undergoing complete surgical resection of early-stage gastric lymphoma had an 82% 5-year survival rate versus a 50% 5-year survival rate for patients treated with primary radiation therapy. In addition, other series have suggested an improved 5-year survival rate when surgery and radiation therapy are combined versus primary radiotherapy alone. What has complicated the issue of treatment for primary gastric lymphoma has been the impressive results of chemotherapy for more advanced stages of disease. In patients with stage III or IV primary gastric lymphoma, treatment primarily with chemotherapy has in general resulted in improved survivals compared to surgery alone or surgery with radiation therapy. In addition, the patient is spared the morbidity of gastric resection. However, controversy still exists regarding the role of primary chemotherapy versus surgical resection with or without radiation therapy for early stage disease. Thus, the necessity of obtaining accurate staging studies becomes quite clear. In general, patients with early stage disease (stage I or II) may be considered candidates for surgical resection. If the patient is elderly or a poor risk operative candidate, then consideration should be given to primary chemotherapy or primary radiation therapy. In general, most centers specializing in the treatment of lymphoma will treat patients with stage III or IV disease primarily with chemotherapy. Surgical resection is reserved for patients who develop complications of perforation or bleeding. In addition, radiotherapy and surgery should be considered for patients who have an incomplete response after aggressive primary chemotherapy is completed.

GASTRIC SARCOMA

The stomach is the most common site of GI soft tissue tumors. Most gastric smooth muscle tumors are benign. The vast majority of malignant gastric sarcomas are leiomyosarcomas. Most of these lesions are diagnosed by upper GI contrast studies which demonstrate extramucosal mass effects within the stomach wall. The clinical presentation may include weight loss, epigastric fullness, and upper GI bleeding. By the time the patient presents with symptoms, these tumors can frequently be very large and demonstrate invasion into contiguous organs. Endoscopy is frequently not helpful preoperatively because of the lack of mucosal erosion. Preoperative EUS may confirm the presence of a mass lesion arising from the deeper layers of the gastric wall. Series that have examined the results of surgical resection emphasize the need to obtain complete resection of the tumor with negative histologic margins and *en bloc* removal of any involved contiguous organs (77). Other prognostic factors in gastric leiomyosarcoma include histologic grade, size, and depth of the primary lesion. Formal gastric procedures such as total gastrectomy or high subtotal resection may not be required if 5 to 6 cm of normal gastric margin can be obtained. Involvement of the gastroesophageal junction or pylorus may necessitate formal resection. Overall survival following resection approaches 50% in patients with completely resected tumor. Adjuvant radiotherapy and chemotherapy have not been shown to improve results of complete *en bloc* resection alone.

GASTRIC CARCINOIDS

Gastric carcinoids account for less than 5% of all GI carcinoid tumors. Histologically, the tumors appear very similar to carcinoid tumors found in other locations within the GI tract. Most patients with gastric carcinoids are asymptomatic. Gastric carcinoids may be associated with pernicious anemia and almost all patients with gastric carcinoids have intestinal metaplasia with or without atrophic gastritis. When symptoms are present, they may be due to ulceration of the overlying mucosa. Endoscopic biopsy can establish the diagnosis, and preoperative EUS can determine the extent of stomach wall involvement. The prognosis is associated with the depth of penetration of the primary tumor and lymph node metastases may be present. Surgical resection with regional lymphadenectomy is recommended for most cases (78).

REFERENCES

1. Inamdar NV, Levin B. The epidemiology and causes of gastric cancer. *Surg Oncol Clin North Am* 1993;2:333.
2. Landis SL, Murray T, Bolden S, Wingo PA. Cancer statistics, 1998. *CA Cancer J Clin* 1998;48:6.
3. Lawrence W Jr, Menck HR, Steele GD Jr, Winchester DP. The National Cancer Data Base report on gastric cancer. *Cancer* 1995;75:1734.

4a. Wanebo HJ, Kennedy BJ, Chmiel J, Steele GD Jr, Winchester DP, Osteen R. Cancer of the stomach. A patient care study by the American College of Surgeons. *Ann Surg* 1993;218:583.

4b. Wanebo HJ, Kennedy BJ, Winchester DP, Stewart AK, Fremgen AM. Role of splenectomy in gastric cancer surgery: adverse effect of elective splenectomy on long-term survival. *J Am Coll Surg* 1997;185:177.

5. Fuchs CS, Mayer RJ. Gastric carcinoma [Review]. *N Engl J Med* 1995;333:32.

6. Wadstrom T. An update on *Helicobacter pylori. Curr Opin Gastroenterol* 1995;11:69.

7. Ginsberg GG, Al-Kawas FH, Fleischer DE, et al. Gastric polyps: relationship of size and histology to cancer risk. *Am J Gastrenterol* 1996;91:714.

8. Greene FL. Management of gastric remnant carcinoma based on the results of a 15-year endoscopic screening program. *Ann Surg* 1996;223:701.

9. Parsonnet J, Friedman GD, Vandersteen DP, et al. *Helicobacter pylori* infection and the risk of gastric carcinoma. *N Engl J Med* 1991;325:1127.

10. Forman D, Newell DG, Fullerton F, et al. Association between infection with *Helicobacter pylori* and risk of gastric cancer: evidence from a prospective investigation. *BMJ* 1991;302:1302.

11. Talley NJ, Zinsmeister AR, Weaver A, et al. Gastric adenocarcinoma and *Helicobacter pylori* infection. *J Natl Cancer Inst* 1991;83:1734.

12. Tatsuta M, Iishi H, Okuda S, Taniguchi H, Yokota Y. The association of *Helicobacter pylori* with differentiated-type early gastric cancer. *Cancer* 1993;72:1841.

13. Lauren P. The two histologically main types of gastric carcinoma: diffuse and the so-called intestinal-type carcinoma. *Acta Pathol Microbiol Scand* 1965;64:31.

14. Ming SC. Gastric carcinoma. A pathobiological classification. *Cancer* 1977;39:2475.

15. Watanabe H, Jass JR, Sobin LH. *Histologic typing of gastric and oesophageal tumors.* 2nd ed. Berlin: Springer-Verlag, 1990.

16. Brenes F, Correa P. Pathology of gastric cancer. *Surg Oncol Clin North Am* 1993;2:347.

17. Nava HR, Arredondo MA. Diagnosis of gastric cancer: endoscopy, imaging and tumor markers. *Surg Oncol Clin North Am* 1993;2:371.

18. Wright PA, Williams GT. Molecular biology and gastric carcinoma [Review]. *Gut* 1993;34:145.

19. Montesi A, Graziani L, Pesaresi A, et al. Radiologic diagnosis of early gastric cancer by routine double-contrast examination. *Gastrointest Radiol* 1982;7:205.

20. Oshima A, Hirata N, Ubukata T, et al. Evaluation of a mass screening program for stomach cancer with a case control design. *Int J Cancer* 1986;38:829.

21. Gore RM, Levine MS, Ghahremani GG, Miller FH. Gastric cancer. Radiologic diagnosis [Review]. *Radiol Clin North Am* 1997;35:311.

22. Graham DY, Schwartz JT, Cain GD, Gyorkey F. Prospective evaluation of biopsy numbers in the diagnosis of esophageal and gastric carcinoma. *Gastroenterology* 1982;82:228.

23. Parsonnet J, Axon AT. Principles of screening and surveillance. *Am J Gastroenterol* 1996;91:847.

24. Miller FH, Kochman ML, Talamonti MS, Gharemani GG, Gore RM. Gastric cancer. Radiologic staging [Review]. *Radiol Clin North Am* 1997;35:331.

25. Fukuya T, Honda H, Hayashi T, et al. Lymph-node metastases: efficacy of detection with helical CT in patients with gastric cancer. *Radiology* 1995;197:705.

26. Botet JF, Lightdale CJ, Zauber AG, et al. Preoperative staging of gastric cancer: comparison of endoscopic US and dynamic CT. *Radiology* 1991;181:426.

27. Caletti G, Ferrari A, Brocchi E, Barbara L. Accuracy of endoscopic ultrasonography in the diagnosis and staging of gastric cancer and lymphoma. *Surgery* 1993;113:14.

28. American Joint Committee on Cancer. Stomach. In: *AJCC cancer staging manual.* 5th ed. Philadelphia: JB Lippincott Co, 1997:71.

29. Kajitani T. The general rules for the gastric cancer study in surgery and pathology. Part I. Clinical classification. *Jpn J Surg* 1981;11:127.

30. Maruyama K, Gunven P, Okabayashi K, Sasako M, Kinoshita T. Lymph node metastases of gastric cancer. General pattern in 1931 patients. *Ann Surg* 1989;210:596.

31. Maruyama K, Okabayashi K, Kinoshita T. Progress in gastric cancer surgery in Japan and its limits of radicality. *World J Surg* 1987;11:418.

32. Mulholland MW. Gastric neoplasms. In: Greenfield LJ, Mulholland MW, Oldham KT, Zelenock GB, Lillemoe KD, eds. *Surgery: scientific principles and practice.* 2nd ed. Philadelphia: JB Lippincott Co, 1997:795.

33. Shiu MH, Moore E, Sanders M, et al. Influence of the extent of resection in survival after curative treatment of gastric carcinoma. A retrospective multivariate analysis. *Arch Surg* 1987;122:1347.

34. Smith JW, Brennan MF. Surgical treatment of gastric cancer. Proximal, mid, and distal stomach [Review]. *Surg Clin North Am* 1992;72:381.

35. Hallissey MT, Jewkes AJ, Dunn JA, Ward L, Fielding JW. Resection-line involvement in gastric cancer: a continuing problem. *Br J Surg* 1993;80:1418.

36. Shiu MH, Perrotti M, Brennan MF. Adenocarcinoma of the stomach: a multivariate analysis of clinical, pathologic and treatment factors. *Hepatogastroenterology* 1989;36:7.

37. Viste A, Haugstvedt T, Eide GE, Soreide O. Postoperative complications and mortality after surgery for gastric cancer. *Ann Surg* 1981;207:7.

38. Gouzi JL, Huguier M, Fagniez PL, et al. Total versus subtotal gastrectomy for adenocarcinoma of the gastric antrum. *Ann Surg* 1989;209:162.

39. Alexander RH, Kelsen DG, Tepper JC. Cancer of the stomach. In: DeVita VT, Hellman S, Rosenberg SA, eds. *Cancer: principles and practice of oncology.* 5th ed. Philadelphia: JB Lippincott Co, 1997:1021.

40. Cady B. Comments on the appropriateness of extended resection in gastric carcinoma. *Surg Oncol Clin North Am* 1993;2:459.

41. Dent DM, Madden MV, Price SK. Randomized comparison of R₁ and R₂ gastrectomy for gastric carcinoma. *Br J Surg* 1988;75:110.

42. Roder JD, Bonenkamp JJ, Craven J, et al. Lymphadenectomy for gastric cancer in clinical trials: update [Review]. *World J Surg* 1995;19:546.

43. Bonenkamp JJ, Songun I, Hermans J, et al. Randomised comparison of morbidity after D1 and D2 dissection for gastric cancer in 996 Dutch patients. *Lancet* 1995;345:745.

44. Bunt AM, Hermans J, Smit VT, van de Velde CJ, Fleuren GJ, Bruijin JA. Surgical/pathologic stage migration confounds compairsons of gastric cancer survival rates between Japan and Western countries. *J Clin Oncol* 1995;13:19.

45. Cuschieri A, Fayers P, Fielding J, et al. Postoperative morbidity and mortality after D1 and D2 resections for gastric cancer: preliminary results of the MRC randomised controlled surgical trial. *Lancet* 1996;347:995.

46. Siewert JR, Bottcher K, Roder JD, et al. Prognostic relevance of systematic lymph node dissection in gastric carcinoma. *Br J Surg* 1993;80:1015.

47. Smith JW, Shiu MH, Kelsey L, Brennan MF. Morbidity of radical lymphadenectomy in the curative resection of gastric carcinoma. *Arch Surg* 1991;126:1469.

48. Volpe CM, Koo J, Miloro SM, Driscoll DL, Nava HR, Douglass HO Jr. The effect of extended lymphadenectomy on survival in patients with gastric adenocarcinoma. *J Am Coll Surg* 1995;181:56.

49. Wanebo HJ, Kennedy BJ, Winchester DP, Fremgen A, Stewart AK. Gastric carcinoma: does lymph node dissection alter survival? *J Am Coll Surg* 1996;183:616.

50. Noguchi Y, Imada T, Matsumoto A, et al. Radical surgery for gastric cancer. A review of the Japanese experience. *Cancer* 1989;64:2053.

51. Brady MS, Rogatko A, Dent LL, Shiu MG. Effect of splenectomy on morbidity and survival following curative gastrectomy for carcinoma. *Arch Surg* 1991;216:359.

52. Watt I, Stewart I, Anderson D, et al. Laparoscopy, ultrasound and computed tomography in cancer of the esophagus and gastric cardia: a prospective comparison for detecting intra-abdominal metastases. *Br J Surg* 1989;76:1036.

53. Possik RA, Franco EL, Pires DR, et al. Sensitivity, specificity, and predictive value of laparoscopy for the staging of gastric cancer and for the detection of liver metastases. *Cancer* 1986;58:1.

54. Bemelman WA, van Delden OM, van Lanschot JJ, et al. Laparoscopy and laparoscopic ultrasonography in staging or carcinoma of the esophagus and gastric cardia. *J Am Coll Surg* 1995;181:421.

55. Hemming AW, Nagy AG, Scudamore CH, Edelmann K. Laparoscopic staging of intrabdominal malignancy. *Surg Endosc* 1995;9:325.

56. Sendler A, Dittler HJ, Feussner H, et al. Preoperative staging of gastric cancer as precondition for multimodal treatment [Review]. *World J Surg* 1995;19:501.

57. Lowy AM, Mansfield PF, Leach SD, Ajani J. Laparoscopic staging for gastric cancer. *Surgery* 1995;119:611.

58. Burke EC, Karpeh MS, Conlon KC, Brennan MF. Laparoscopy in the management of gastric adenocarcinoma [Review]. *Ann Surg* 1997;225:262.

59. Maehara Y, Orita H, Okuyama T, et al. Predictors of lymph node metastases in early gastric cancer. *Br J Surg* 1992;79:245.
60. Farley DR, Donohue JH. Early gastric cancer [Review]. *Surg Clin North Am* 1992;72:401.
61. Lawrence M, Shiu MH. Early gastric cancer. Twenty-eight–year experience. *Ann Surg* 1991;213:327.
62. Kelsen DP. Adjuvant and neoadjuvant therapy for gastric cancer [Review]. *Semin Oncol* 1996;23:379.
63. Coombes RC, Schein PS, Chilvers CE, et al. A randomized trial comparing adjuvant fluorouracil, doxorubicin, and mitomycin with no treatment in operable gastric cancer. *J Clin Oncol* 1990;8:1362.
64. Macdonald JS, Fleming TR, Peterson RF, et al. Adjuvant chemotherapy with 5-FU, adriamycin, and mitomycin-C (FAM) versus surgery alone for patients with locally advanced gastric adenocarcinoma: a Southwest Oncology Group Study. *Ann Surg Oncol* 1995;2:488.
65. Moertel CG, Childs DS, O'Fallon JR, et al. Combined 5-fluorouracil and radiation therapy as a surgical adjuvant for poor prognosis gastric cancer. *J Clin Oncol* 1984;2:1249.
66. Dent DM, Werner ID, Novis B, et al. Prospective randomized trial of combined oncologic therapy for gastric carcinoma. *Cancer* 1979;44:385.
67. Minsky BD. The role of radiation therapy in gastric cancer [Review]. *Semin Oncol* 1996;23:390.
68. Sindelar WF, Kinsella TJ. Randomized trial of resection and intraoperative radiotherapy in locally advanced gastric cancer [Abstract]. *Proc Am Soc Clin Oncol* 1987;6:91.
69. Takahashi T, Abe M. Intra-operative radiotherapy for carcinoma of the stomach. *Eur J Surg Oncol* 1986;12:247.
70. Kaibara N, Hamazoe R, Iitsuka Y, et al. Hyperthermic peritoneal perfusion combined with anticancer chemotherapy as prophylactic treatment of peritoneal recurrence of gastric cancer. *Hepatogastroenterology* 1989;36:75.
71. Hagiwara A, Takahashi T, Kojima O, et al. Prophylaxis with carbon-absorbed mitomycin against peritoneal recurrence of gastric cancer. *Lancet* 1992;339:629.
72. Ota DM, Ajani JA, Mansfield P. Preoperative chemotherapy for gastric carcinoma. *Surg Oncol Clin North Am* 1993;2:493.
73. Fink U, Stein HJ, Schuhmacher C, Wilke HJ. Neoadjuvant chemotherapy for gastric cancer: update [Review]. *World J Surg* 1995;19:509.
74. Ajani JA, Mansfield PF, Ota DM. Potentially resectable gastric carcinoma: current approaches to staging and preoperative therapy [Review]. *World J Surg* 1995;19:216.
75. Kelsen D, Karpeh M, Schwartz, G, et al. Neoadjuvant therapy of high-risk gastric cancer: a phase II trial of preoperative FAMTX and postoperative intraperitoneal fluorouracil-cisplatin plus intravenous fluorouracil. *J Clin Oncol* 1996;14:1818.
76. Talamonti MS, Dawes LG, Joehl RJ, Nahrwold DL. Gastrointestinal lymphomas. A case for primary surgical resection. *Arch Surg* 1990;125:972.
77. Ng EH, Pollock RE, Munsell MF, Atkinson EN, Romsdahl MM. Prognostic factors influencing survival in gastrointestinal leiomyosarcomas. *Ann Surg* 1992;215:68.
78. Gilligan CJ, Lawton GP, Tang LH, West BA, Modlin IM. Gastric carcinoid tumors: the biology and therapy of an enigmatic and controversial lesion [Review]. *Am J Gastrentrol* 1995;90:338.
79. Behrns KE, Dalton RR, van Heerden JA, et al. Extended lymph node dissection for gastric cancer. Is it of value? *Surg Clin North Am* 1992;72:433.
80. Kodama Y, Sugimachi K, Soejima K, et al. Evaluation of extensive lymph node dissection for carcinoma of the stomach. *World J Surg* 1981;5:242.

CHAPTER 14

Carcinoma of the Pancreas and Tumors of the Periampullary Region

Jeffrey A. Drebin and Steven M. Strasberg

Carcinoma of the exocrine pancreas is one of the most deadly malignancies, with an overall 5-year disease-free survival rate of under 3%. Most patients present with locally advanced or regionally disseminated disease, which precludes curative resection. Chemotherapy and radiation therapy are of modest palliative benefit, and typical survival is on the order of 4 to 6 months. Among those undergoing an attempted surgical resection, the 5-year disease-free survival is less than 30%. Furthermore, until recently, the operative morbidity and mortality of curative surgery for carcinoma of the pancreas, particularly the results of pancreaticoduodenectomy (Whipple procedure), were such that the benefit of such procedures for any patient were seriously questioned (1–3).

However, a number of factors justify a more aggressive approach to the treatment of patients with pancreatic cancer and other periampullary tumors. These include advances in our understanding of the pathophysiology of periampullary malignancies, improvements in surgical technique and the management of perioperative complications, and the development of novel agents and approaches to palliating patients with advanced disease. This chapter will review current approaches to the management of patients with pancreatic and periampullary tumors.

EPIDEMIOLOGY

Pancreatic carcinoma is a fairly common malignancy and a very common cause of cancer mortality. Carcinoma of the pancreas is responsible for approximately 28,000 deaths per year in the United States, ranking fifth behind carcinomas of the lung, colorectum, breast, and prostate as a cause of cancer deaths (4). Because of the relative rarity of breast cancer in men and the nonexistance of prostate cancer in women, pancreatic cancer is the fourth most common cause of cancer death in both men and in women. Other periampullary tumors, such as carcinomas of the distal bile duct, duodenum, and ampulla of Vater are decidedly less common, but are more often

resectable. Indeed, about one-third of resectable tumors of the periampullary region are of nonpancreatic origin.

The incidence of pancreatic carcinoma has increased three- to fourfold in the 20th century, but appears to have leveled off in recent decades. No doubt this, in part, reflects both improvements in the accuracy of diagnostic techniques as well as a genuine increase in incidence. Adenocarcinoma of the pancreas is more common in men than women (relative risk 1.5:1) and in blacks than in whites (relative risk 2:1). The risk of developing pancreatic cancer increases with age, and is most common in those in their 60s and 70s, though patients in their 40s and 50s are not uncommon; pancreatic cancer is rarely seen in patients under 30 years of age.

Environmental Risk Factors

Studies of environmental factors linked to the development of pancreatic carcinoma have identified a number of agents that may play a role in pancreatic carcinogenesis, as summarized in Table 14-1 (5–8). Cigarette smoking significantly increases the risk of this form of cancer, as it does for a variety of other tumors. Certain industrials solvents, particularly those used in metal refining, have been linked to the development of pancreatic cancer. Although alcohol consumption does not appear to be a risk factor for the development of pancreatic cancer, chronic pancreatitis almost certainly is (7). Consumption of coffee and other caffeinated beverages, which had been suggested to be a risk factors based on early studies, appears to be unrelated to the development of pancreatic cancer (6).

Perhaps the most controversial risk factor is diabetes. About 15% of patients with pancreatic cancer become diabetic in the 6 months preceding the diagnosis of their cancer. This most likely reflects local alterations in pancreatic function resulting from an occult tumor rather than rapid development of cancer following the onset of diabetes. However, among patients with long-standing diabetes there does appear to be an approximately twofold increased risk for the development of pancreatic cancer (8).

TABLE 14-1. *Risk factors for pancreatic cancer*

	Relative increase in risk
Proven risk factors	
Cigarette smoking	2–3-fold
Industrial chemical exposure	3–5-fold
Chronic pancreatitis	2–10-fold
Diabetes mellitus	2–3-fold
Unproven or disproven risk factors	
Coffee consumption	—
Alcohol consumption	—

Genetics and Molecular Biology

Though most cases of pancreatic cancer occur on a sporadic basis, families have been identified in which pancreatic cancer occurs with increased frequency. Analysis of such kindreds suggests that, in some cases, the predilection for pancreatic cancer is transmitted as an autosomal dominant characteristic with incomplete penetrance. A national registry of familial pancreatic cancer cases has been established at the Johns Hopkins Hospital.

Advances in our understanding of the contribution of oncogenes and tumor suppressor genes to the etiology of cancer have identified a number of genes that appear to play a role in the development of pancreatic carcinoma. Mutations involving the K-ras oncogene are seen in 80% to 90% of pancreatic cancers (9) and overexpression of the HER2/neu oncogene is seen in 50% to 60% of pancreatic cancers (10). These genetic events occur relatively early in the process of pancreatic carcinogenesis and have been identified in patients with premalignant lesions and *in situ* tumors. Cells containing K-ras mutations have been identified in pancreatic juice and stool of patients with pancreatic cancer (11), suggesting a possible approach to facilitate earlier diagnosis of pancreatic tumors.

Loss of the tumor suppressor genes p16 and p53 are seen in 80% and 70% of pancreatic cancers, respectively (12,13). Interestingly, patients with germ-line mutations of the p16 gene have a 20- to 40-fold increased risk of developing pancreatic cancer, suggesting that some of the familial cases of pancreatic cancer can be linked to this gene (14). As with other tumor susceptibility genes, the benefit of aggressive screening in at-risk populations remains unproven.

PATHOLOGY AND TUMOR BIOLOGY

Pancreatic carcinoma arises in the head of the pancreas approximately 75% of the time, with the remainder of lesions being distributed evenly in the body and tail of the gland. Although adenocarcinoma of the pancreas is the most common of the periampullary tumors, a variety of other pancreatic and nonpancreatic periampullary tumors have been described, as shown in Table 14-2. Many of these histologic tumor types are quite rare, but several are common enough to be seen outside of specialty centers, including cystic neoplasms of the

TABLE 14-2. *Histologic classification of pancreatic and periampullary tumors*

Benign tumors
  Serous cystadenoma
  Mature cystic teratoma
Tumors of indeterminate malignancy
  Mucinous tumors of the pancreas
  Intraductal tumors
  Solid and papillary tumors
  Neuroendocrine tumors
Malignant tumors
  Pancreatic origin
    Ductal adenocarcinoma
    Acinar cell carcinoma
    Adenosquamous carcinoma
    Anaplastic carcinoma
    Cystadenocarcinoma
    Pancreaticoblastoma
    Small cell carcinoma
  Nonpancreatic origin
    Ampullary carcinoma
    Bile duct carcinoma (cholangiocarcinoma)
    Duodenal carcinoma
    Lymphoma
    Sarcoma

Adapted from Bell (4).

pancreas and nonpancreatic tumors of the distal bile duct, duodenum, and ampulla.

Cystic neoplasms of the pancreas can be divided into benign tumors and malignant tumors (cystadenocarcinomas). Benign cystic tumors can be further divided on the basis of radiologic factors and by analysis of cyst fluid into lesions with little predilection to become malignant, termed serous cystadenomas, and those with a significant risk of malignant degeneration, termed mucinous cystadenomas. The frequent identification of cystadenocarcinoma in patients suspected of harboring a mucinous cystadenoma has led some to simply classify these lesions as mucinous tumors of the pancreas. A related but distinct lesion is mucinous ductal hyperplasia. This disorder is an abnormality of the pancreatic ductal epithelium in which the entire duct epithelium becomes dysplastic and may degenerate to overt malignancy. Cystadenocarcinomas of the pancreas are less biologically aggressive than pancreatic adenocarcinomas, with a high cure rate following complete resection. Since even serous cystadenomas can be locally invasive (Fig. 14-1), an aggressive approach to the removal of most serous cystadenomas as well as all mucinous tumors of the pancreas is justified.

Tumors of the distal bile duct, duodenum, and ampulla of Vater are much less common than pancreatic adenocarcinoma, but they comprise almost one-third of resectable periampullary lesions, as noted previously. Furthermore, these tumors tend to be biologically less aggressive than pancreatic carcinomas, with 5-year disease-free survival following resection ranging from 30% to 50% (15–17). It can be difficult, if not impossible, to distinguish these tumor types from routine carcinoma of the pancreas based on endoscopic, radio-

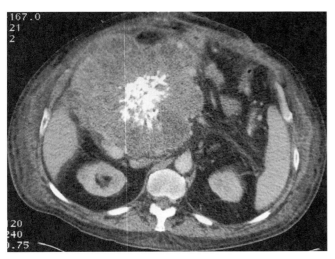

FIG. 14-1. Massive serous cystadenoma of the pancreas. The patient had undergone exploratory surgery 7 years previously, at which time his surgeon elected to leave the benign tumor *in situ* rather than proceeding with pancreaticoduodenectomy. The patient subsequently presented with biliary and duodenal obstruction from this lesion and went on to succumb to his disease.

TABLE 14-3. *Staging for pancreatic cancer*

Primary tumor (T)

TX	Primary tumor cannot be assessed
T0	No evidence of primary tumor
T1	Tumor limited to the pancreas
T1a	Tumor 2 cm or less in greatest dimension
T1b	Tumor more than 2 cm in greatest dimension
T2	Tumor extends directly to any of the following: duodenum, bile duct, or peripancreatic tissues
T3	Tumor extends directly to any of the following: stomach, spleen, colon, or adjacent large vessels

Lymph nodes (N)

NX	Regional lymph nodes cannot be assessed
N0	No regional lymph node metastasis
N1	Regional lymph node metastasis

Distant metastases (M)

MX	Presence of distant metastasis cannot be assessed
M0	No distant metastasis
M1	Distant metastasis

Stage grouping

I	T1, N0, M0
	T2, N0, M0
II	T3, N0, M0
III	Any T, N1, M0
IV	Any T, Any N, M1

logic or needle cytology criteria. Only histologic sectioning of a resected tumor mass can accurately classify the specific tumor type in some circumstances.

Pancreatic adenocarcinomas, bile duct carcinomas, duodenal carcinomas, and ampullary cancers tend to be aggressive tumors that disseminate early and tend to follow similar patterns of metastatic spread. Local invasion into adjacent structures is frequently seen, with encasement of the superior mesenteric/portal vein and the superior mesenteric artery, representing a common event which may preclude resection. Spread to regional lymphatics is common as is metastasis to the liver via the portal vein. Spread to peritoneal surfaces (carcinomatosis) is frequently seen in advanced disease, as are lung metastases. In contrast, mucinous tumors of the pancreas are less predictable in their biologic behavior, with some malignant tumors remaining indolent for months to years. They may be locally or regionally invasive without forming metastases. When mucinous tumors of the pancreas do disseminate they tend to form peritoneal implants but rarely develop liver or lung metastases.

The pathologic staging of pancreatic cancer and other periampullary tumors is based on the extent of tumor involvement of local and distant structures, as shown in Table 14-3. Stage I tumors are limited to the pancreas and immediate peripancreatic structures. Stage II tumors are regionally invasive. Stage III lesions are defined by positive lymph nodes. Stage IV lesions are defined by the presence of distant metastases. Patients with stage I, II, or III lesions are generally considered candidates for tumor resection, though this may be contraindicated in specific circumstances as discussed below. Patients with stage IV lesions are generally considered unresectable, though this view has recently been challenged (18,19).

PRESENTATION AND CLINICAL STAGING

Clinical Signs and Symptoms

Pancreatic cancer can be insidious in onset, and patients often have been vaguely unwell for several months prior to the development of the overt symptomatology that leads to the diagnosis of their illness. Common signs and symptoms of pancreatic cancer and other periampullary tumors are summarized in Table 14-4. Though painless jaundice is often thought of as the hallmark of a periampullary tumor, most patients in fact have mild to moderate abdominal pain. The presence of back pain is a particularly ominous symptom, reflecting retroperitoneal invasion by the growing tumor. The presence of weight loss is relatively common. It is worth noting that aggressive perioperative nutritional repletion has not been shown to be of definite benefit.

TABLE 14-4. *Signs and symptoms of pancreatic cancer*

Common signs and symptoms
  Jaundice
  Anorexia
  Weight loss
  Abdominal pain
Less common signs and symptoms
  Vomiting
  Palpable mass
  Palpable gallbladder (Courvoisier's sign)
  Back pain
  Splenomegaly
  Constipation
  Thrombophlebitis (Trousseau's sign)

Jaundice is related to the anatomic location of the primary tumor. It is common in tumors of the pancreatic head and in other periampullary tumors; it is quite rare in patients with primary tumors of the pancreatic tail. Liver function tests should be performed to distinguish obstructive jaundice from a primary hepatocellular process such as hepatitis. Patients with severe obstructive jaundice may have some degree of associated coagulopathy from hepatic dysfunction. Coagulation parameters should be tested in all jaundiced patients and those with coagulation abnormalites should receive preoperative vitamin K and/or perioperative fresh frozen plasma.

Radiologic Assessment

Patients suspected of having a pancreatic or other periampullary malignancy are generally evaluated by thin-cut contrast-enhanced computer tomagraphic (CT) scanning. This is of use in identifying the tumor mass as well as assessing the liver for metastasis. Vascular involvement of superior mesenteric vein, portal vein, and celiac and superior mesenteric arteries can also be determined by CT scanning (Fig. 14-2). Ultrasonography is useful in identifying the primary pancreatic mass but is less sensitive than CT and provides less information regarding local and regional dissemination. Magnetic resonance imaging has not proven superior to CT scanning for assessment of the primary tumor, metastatic disease or vascular encasement. Occasional patients with CT findings suggestive but not diagnostic of vascular encasement may benefit from preoperative visceral angiography, though improvements in CT methodology, particularly the use of dynamic contrast infusion and spiral techniques, have largely supplanted angiography.

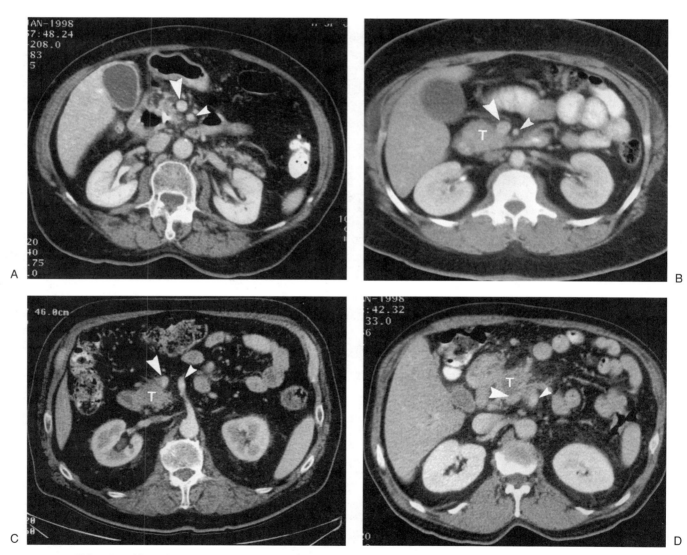

FIG. 14-2. Use of computed tomagraphy in assessment of superior mesenteric vein/portal vein and superior mesenteric artery involvement by tumor. **A:** No detectable tumor. **B:** Pancreatic tumor without evidence of vascular involvement. **C:** Pancreatic tumor invading the sidewall of the superior mesenteric vein, superior mesenteric artery free of disease. **D:** Pancreatic tumor encasing both superior mesenteric vein and artery. *Large arrow,* superior mesenteric vein; *small arrow,* superior mesenteric artery; *T,* tumor.

Patients with a periampullary or pancreatic mass on CT and no evidence of metastatic disease or vascular encasement require no further testing and can be taken to the operating room for surgical resection. At the time of definitive surgery, an initial laparoscopic staging of resectability may be performed, as discussed below. It is not necessary to obtain a tissue diagnosis preoperatively. Indeed, cytologic assessment of periampullary malignancies is notoriously inaccurate, rendering absence of malignant cells on percutaneous or endoscopic biopsy of little value in patient management. An additional concern with percutaneous techniques is the possibility of tumor dissemination as a result of the biopsy process, as has been suggested in some studies (20).

Endoscopic Retrograde Cholangiopancreatography

Patients with jaundice but no mass on CT are generally evaluated by endoscopic retrograde cholangiopancreatography (ERCP). This may reveal an irregular or tapering biliary stricture characteristic of an obstructing periampullary tumor (Fig. 14-3). Sometimes the biliary stricture is seen in conjunction with a pancreatic duct stricture—the double duct sign—which is highly suspicious for the presence of a malignancy (Fig. 14-3). Irregular strictures of the pancreatic duct may also be seen in patients with pancreatic carcinoma (Fig. 14-3). Such endoscopic findings, even in the absence of a pancreatic mass on CT scanning, justify proceeding to surgical resection. An aggressive surgical approach to patients with suspicious biliary strictures, particularly in those patients without a history of previous gallstone disease, will often result in removal of tumors at an early stage.

A question that dates back to Whipple's original report on pancreaticoduodenectomy is whether to decompress the bil-

iary tree prior to attempting to resect a periampullary tumor (21). Several randomized prospective trials have failed to show a benefit of preoperative biliary stenting by ERCP or percutaneous techniques (22–24). Furthermore, there is a significant incidence of complications in patients who undergo stenting prior to resection. Probably the critical factor in deciding whether to preoperatively decompress a jaundiced patient is the interval to surgery. If the patient can be operated upon in a few days to 1 week and is not symptomatic from jaundice it may be best to proceed directly to surgery; if there will be a delay of several weeks it may be best to stent the patient, both for comfort and to minimize the risk of cholangitis.

Tumor Markers

A number of tumor-associated antigens detectable in the serum of patients with pancreatic carcinoma have been described, the most useful being CA19-9 (25). CA19-9 is a mucin-associated carbohydrate antigen produced by normal pancreatic cells as well as pancreatic carcinoma cells. CA19-9 can be detected in serum and pancreatic juice. As with other tumor markers, the use of CA19-9 in the management of patients with pancreatic cancer is plagued by problems related to sensitivity and specificity. Small tumors often fail to produce enough CA19-9 to be detectable above the accepted serum threshold of 35 units/ml. Nonneoplastic disorders of the pancreas and biliary tract, particularly pancreatitis, are associated with elevations of CA19-9 which may reach several hundred units per milliliter. Patients with CA19-9 levels in the thousands almost definitely have pancreatic cancer but are generally quite symptomatic from their tumors and often unresectable. Thus there is little use for CA19-9 in screening asymptomatic populations. There may be a role for monitor-

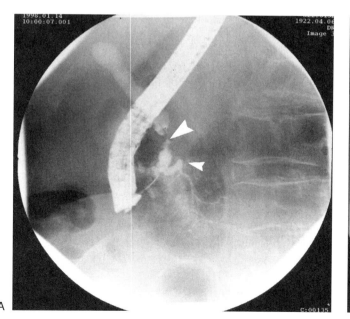
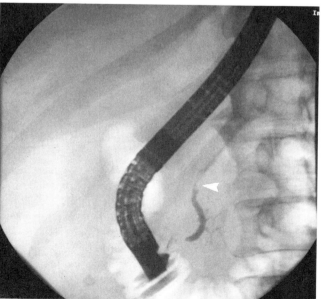

A   B

FIG. 14-3. ERCP findings in pancreatic cancer. **A:** Irregular distal bile duct stricture and pancreatic duct occlusion—the double duct sign. Same patient as Fig. 14-2A. **B:** Pancreatic duct stricture due to pancreatic malignancy. *Large arrow,* bile duct; *small arrow,* pancreatic duct.

ing CA19-9 in patients postoperatively following tumor resection, but in the absence of effective therapy for recurrent disease this is also of questionable value except in research protocols.

Analysis of tumor markers in pancreatic cyst aspirates may be of use in distinguishing pseudocysts from cystic neoplasms and in separating serous cystadenomas from mucinous tumors if radiologic criteria alone are inadequate. Interestingly, CA19-9 levels in cyst aspirates are of little use in separating these different lesions. However, it has been shown that analyzing the combination of amylase, carcinoembryonic antigen, CA-125, and tissue polypeptide antigen allows fairly accurate separation among the different cystic lesions of the pancreas (26,27). These studies are particularly useful in the elderly or medically frail patient in whom resection of a cystic lesion of the pancreas poses an unusually high risk. Such patients, in whom cyst fluid analysis suggests a low liklihood of malignancy, can be managed nonoperatively.

Laparoscopic Staging

Perhaps the most important recent advance in the preoperative staging of patients with pancreatic cancer and other periampullary tumors has been the development of laparoscopic staging procedures (20,28–30). Even with spiral CT scanning techniques suggesting resectability, there is a 20% to 30% incidence of either locally advanced disease or of small hepatic or peritoneal implants, undetected by radiologic imaging, which preclude resection. Given the improvements in biliary stenting, as discussed below, there may be no need for laparotomy in a patient with unresectable disease. Avoiding unnecessary laparotomy is an important goal of staging periampullary neoplasms.

Simple laparoscopy and biopsy allow the evaluation of visceral and peritoneal surfaces, and may reveal disease undetectable by other techniques. Patients may then avoid unnecessary open surgical procedures if adequate palliation of jaundice can be achieved with percutaneous or transhepatic biliary stent placement. Staging laparoscopy, with frozen section evaluation of biopsy specimens if necessary, can be carried out in 15 to 20 min and can be followed by formal laparotomy and tumor resection under the same anesthetic. Available data suggest that this technique alone can reduce the incidence of unresectable disease at laparotomy by one half (29).

Several more complex techniques may further enhance the utility of laparoscopic staging. Laparoscopic ultrasonography can reveal abnormalities beneath the visceral surfaces and, with the use of flow Doppler techniques, may identify vascular encasement or occlusion (28,29). Conlon et al. (30) have described a more thorough laparoscopic staging of periampullary tumors, including pathologic evaluation of celiac, periportal, and peripancreatic lymph nodes. Finally, the assessment of occult disease by cytologic assessment of peritoneal washings obtained at laparoscopy may further define patients with tumor dissemination who are unlikely to

benefit from extensive surgical resection (20). It is worth noting, however, that all of these techniques extend operative time and may require several days to obtain a definitive diagnosis in the case of lymph node biopsies or peritoneal cytology. Surgeons favoring these approaches often perform laparoscopic staging procedures and definitive resections under separate anesthetics, with a corresponding increase in cost and patient morbidity. The precise role of these more complex procedures will no doubt be determined in the coming years.

Endoscopic Ultrasonography

Another important advance in the staging of patients with periampullary tumors is the development of endoscopic ultrasonography (EUS) (31). EUS can assess tumor size, portal and mesenteric vascular involvement, and can obtain tissue samples from lesions located close to the stomach and duodenum. It has the advantage of not requiring a general anesthetic and can be performed outside an operating suite with mild sedation. EUS cannot evaluate lesions, such as peritoneal metastases, which are located at sites distant from the lumen of the gastrointestinal (GI) tract. Future studies will help define the precise role of laparoscopy and EUS in the staging of periampullary tumors.

Surgical Resection

Surgical resection remains the only demonstrated approach to curing pancreatic and periampullary malignancies. Most such tumors are resected by pancreaticoduodenectomy (Whipple procedure). This procedure was initially described as a two-stage operation (21), though it fairly rapidly evolved into a one-stage procedure (32). Although individual surgeons perform this procedure differently, in all cases the head of the pancreas, distal bile duct, and most of the duodenum and proximal jejunum are resected en bloc. In many cases, the entire duodenum, as well as the gastric antrum, are included with the resection specimen. Reconstruction involves the performance of pancreatic, biliary, and gastric or duodenal anastamoses to the remaining jejunum. A schematic drawing of a pancreaticoduodenectomy with distal gastrectomy (classic Whipple procedure) and reconstruction is shown in Fig. 14-4.

Pancreaticoduodenectomy is a demanding technical operation, requiring meticulous dissection around portal and mesenteric blood vessels and three distinct anastamoses; the morbidity and mortality associated with the Whipple procedure can be significant. Indeed, in the mid-1970s, it was seriously questioned whether patients with resectable pancreatic malignancies might be better managed with palliative bypass procedures (1–3). Over the past two decades, however, there has been a steady improvement in the results reported following pancreaticoduodenectomy with regards to morbidity and mortality, with a corresponding improvement in long-term survival of resected patients.

Standard Whipple

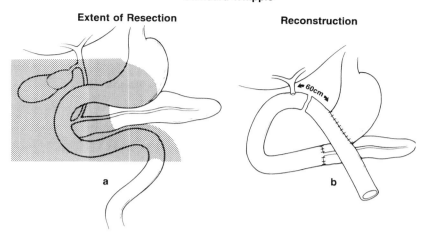

Extent of Resection

Reconstruction

a

b

FIG. 14-4. Classic Whipple procedure. **A:** Extent of resection. **B:** Method of reconstruction. (Reprinted, in adapted form, with permission from Strasberg SM, Drebin JA, Soper NJ. Evolution and current status of the Whipple procedure: an update for gastroenterologist. *Gastroenterology* 1997;113:983.)

Mortality

There has been a steep decline in the perioperative mortality rate of patients undergoing pancreaticoduodenectomy in recent years. Table 14-5 documents the results of case series of greater than one hundred operations in which the main indication for surgery was malignancy, published in the English language literature, since 1964. Similar trends are also seen in smaller case series published over this time. The median year of the case series is provided because this is more reflective of the era of the series than the date of publication.

During this time, 30-day postoperative mortality rates have declined from 20% to less than 5% in many institutions around the world. Near-zero mortality rates, which we define as less than 2%, are being reported with increasing frequency in case series numbering over 100 patients (44,46). These mortality rates are so low that many hundreds of cases would be required to determine precise mortality rates. Nonetheless, it is safe to make the general statement that extremely low mortality rates are now the norm for pancreaticoduodenectomies performed in specialized centers.

The reason for the precipitous decline in mortality rates is not completely understood. While it may, in part, reflect concentration of pancreaticoduodenectomy procedures at high volume centers (47,49), the improvement in mortality is no doubt multifactorial and parallels a general decline in operative mortality seen for other surgical procedures. Other contributing factors are improvements in intensive care, diagnostic and interventional radiology, and nutritional support. Prophylaxis and management of infection, venous thromboembolism, and GI hemorrhage have also improved greatly during this period. As a result, postoperative cardiopulmonary complications and GI hemorrhage, which used to be fairly common, have been sharply reduced. Other complications such as disruption of the pancreaticojejunal anastamosis, which were often fatal 30 years ago, now lead to death infrequently (50).

Morbidity

Though mortality rates have improved significantly, pancreaticoduodenectomy remains a procedure in which major morbidity is common. Complication rates are difficult to evaluate because there is no uniformly adopted method of reporting or even defining complications. Additionally, some series provide numbers of complications, whereas others report the number of patients with complications. Despite these limitations, it is apparent that some complications, such as pulmonary embolism, GI bleeding, pneumonia, and myocardial infarction, are much less common today than in the past.

Results for development of pancreatic fistula and biliary fistula in large series are shown in Table 14-5. Leakage at the pancreaticojejunal anastamosis is still a major complication of this procedure. There does not appear to have been much improvement in the incidence of this complication over the years, though individual case series have occasionally shown markedly lower pancreatic fistula rates (51). At the present time the pancreaticoenteric anastamosis continues to be the weak point of the operation, leakage being most common when the pancreatic duct is small and the gland very soft. However, in the current era, leakage at the pancreaticojejunostomy generally leads to an increased length of hospital stay but rarely to reoperation or death (50).

A number of studies have looked at the utility of somatostatin analogues, such as octreotide, in preventing the development of pancreatic fistula. Though somatostatin analogues have proven effective in European studies in patients undergoing a range of pancreatic surgical procedures (52,53), these studies did not show a significant benefit in the subset of patients undergoing pancreaticoduodenectomy. Furthermore, a randomized trial of octreotide in patients undergoing Whipple resections in the United States has failed to demonstrate any benefit from the prophylactic use of this agent to prevent pancreatic fistula (54). Octreotide is expensive and, when administered subcutaneously, uncomfortable for patients; we

TABLE 14-5. *Morbidity and mortality of pancreaticoduodenectomy in case series of over 100 operations*[a]

Reference	Median year of series[b]	Duration of series (years)	No. of patients	Mortality rate (%)			Complication rate (%)	
				Single surgeon	Single institution	Multiple institutions	Pancreatic fistulae	Biliary fistulae
Monge et al. (34)	1951	22	239		19		13	5
Warren et al. (35)	1957	30	348		16		8	7
Smith (36)	1959	26	224	7			8	
Herter et al. (37)	1959	28	102		15		9	4
Nakase et al. (38)	1962	26	822			21	14	4
Warren et al. (35)	1966	9	139		10		7	21
Yeo et al. (39)[b]	1982	24	201		5			
Andersen et al. (40)	1983	15	117		8		16	5
Tsao et al. (41)	1986	13	101		2		15	5
Nitecki et al. (42)	1986	10	186		3			
Geer and Brennan (43)	1987	7	146		5		2	2
Trede et al. (44)	1987	4	118	0			8	3
Swope et al. (45)	1989	4	299			8		
Cameron et al. (46)[b,c]	1989	3	145		0		19	6
Gordon et al. (47)[b,d]	1990	5	271		2			
		5	230			14		
Fernandez del Castillo et al. (48)	1992	3	142	0			7	4

[a] Adapted from Strasberg et al. (33).

[b] These data are from the same institution and there is case overlap in the series.

[c] These series by definition have zero mortality as they are reported as consecutive cases without a mortality. The other case series in this table are presented as series collected over defined time periods. The series by Trede et al. (44) was a single surgeon series (personal communication from the author).

[d] The two sets of data in this one report compare results in a tertiary care center with results in the remaining hospitals in that state.

do not routinely use it in the management of patients undergoing pancreaticoduodenectomy. Other technical aspects of the pancreaticojejunal anastamosis are discussed below.

The rate of biliary fistula has declined moderately over time (Table 14-5). Improvements in biliary fistula rates most likely reflect improved understanding of the blood supply of the bile duct. The bile duct normally receives blood via longitudinal arteries that run from the liver distally, and from the pancreas proximally. Pancreaticoduodenectomy eliminates this latter source, leaving the bile duct dependent on flow from the liver. Dividing the bile duct above the cystic duct insertion, that is, in the common hepatic duct rather than the common bile duct, provides better blood supply to facilitate healing of the biliary-enteric anastamosis.

Probably the most common postoperative complication seen in patients undergoing pancreaticoduodenectomy is delayed gastric emptying. Though not well understood, it is thought that disruption of enterogastric signaling following duodenectomy is responsible for the gastric motility problems so frequently seen. Though perhaps more common in patients undergoing pyloric preservation (55), delayed emptying is also seen in patients undergoing classic Whipple resection with hemigastrectomy (56). Delayed gastric emptying is seen in over 20% of patients and may range in severity from mild nausea and inability to eat, to persistant vomiting requiring nasogastric suction for days to weeks postoperatively. Problems with gastric emptying are rarely life threatening but can significantly prolong postoperative hospitalization. A randomized prospective trial of erythromycin demonstrated modest but statistically significant benefits in improving gastric emptying after pancreaticoduodenctomy, presumably through the effects of erythromycin on motilin receptors (56). Based on these results, we routinely administer intravenous erythromycin in the postoperative period.

Outcome

With improvements in perioperative morbidity and mortality, there has also been some improvement in 5-year survival rates for patients undergoing pancreaticoduodenectomy for pancreatic cancer. Five-year survival rates following Whipple resection for ampullary, bile duct, and duodenal malignancies have always been reasonable, ranging from 30% to 50% in most series, while resection of a mucinous tumor of the pancreas results in 5-year survival rates of over 75%. By contrast, the long-term survival of patients with pancreatic adenocarcinoma has generally been extremely poor. A recent review of the world literature dating back over the past 50 years suggests that the overall 5-year survival of patients following attempted curative resection for adenocarcinoma of the pancreas is on the order of 4% (57). Furthermore, some of these patients recurred beyond 5 years, suggesting that they in fact had not been cured by resection of their tumors.

Several large case series from high-volume centers suggest that better long-term results are now being obtained, with up to 20% of resected patients with documented pancreatic ade-

nocarcinoma surviving 5 years (39,44). In patients with negative resection margins, small tumors, and no evidence of lymph node metastases, the results may be even better, with over 40% of such patients expected to survive 5 years. It is important to note, however, that these survival curves are based on actuarial rather than actual survival, and not all recent series have noted such results (58). Those who believe that results have improved point to improvements in diagnosis, surgical technique, and the use of adjuvant chemotherapy and radiation therapy as possible contributing factors. These encouraging results will no doubt be confirmed or refuted with the accumulation of additional patients and prolonged follow-up.

Steps in Performing Pancreaticoduodenectomy

Though there are a variety of approaches to this procedure, the general method developed by Cameron is widely used and is described here (59). The upper abdomen is exposed via either an upper midline or bilateral subcostal incision. On entering the abdomen, a thorough examination of serosal surfaces is made to exclude metastatic disease and any suspicious lesions are examined by frozen section biopsy. The duodenum is Kocherized and the head of the pancreas is mobilized off the vena cava and aorta; posterior invasion of these structures by tumors of the periampullary region is quite uncommon. The superior mesenteric artery is palpated. If tumor extends around or to the left of the superior mesenteric artery, the tumor is generally considered unresectable.

If the tumor appears resectable, the Kocher manuever is carefully extended to the third duodenum, and the superior mesenteric vein is identified in the pancreaticoduodenal groove. The anterior surface of the superior mesenteric vein is exposed, and dissection up to and beneath the pancreatic neck is carried out. Small branches are carefully divided between ligatures; even small branches may produce impressive bleeding if evulsed or casually divided with the cautery. By staying flush on the anterior surface of the superior mesenteric vein, it is usually possible to develop a plane beneath the pancreatic neck. Dense tumor encasement in this region may be reason to consider the lesion unresectable, though more limited superior mesenteric vein or portal vein involvement may be successfully managed with segmental vein resection, as discussed below.

Attention is then turned to the perihilar dissection. The undersurface of the porta is palpated for an aberrant hepatic artery, most commonly a right hepatic artery arising from the superior mesenteric artery. If such an artery is identified, it must be carefully preserved in subsequent dissection; if involved by tumor, it may be resected with the tumor specimen *en bloc*, but arterial reconstruction must be carried out in order to insure that the biliary blood supply is adequate for anastamotic healing. The gallbladder is taken down and the common hepatic duct is mobilized. The common duct may be retracted laterally using a vessel loop or more conveniently divided at this stage of the procedure. In the event the tumor proves unresectable, a palliative end-to-side hepaticojejunostomy can be constructed using the cut end of the duct.

The common hepatic artery is identified and is mobilized proximally, revealing the gastroduodenal artery. Tumor involvement of the hepatic artery or celiac trunk is generally considered to be unresectable, though tumor involvement of the gastroduodenal artery near its origin can generally be mobilized with an adequate margin. Rarely, in patients with atherosclerotic disease of the celiac artery, the arterial supply to the liver occurs via retrograde flow through the gastroduodenal artery into the hepatic artery. In such cases, ligating the gastroduodenal artery will reduce or eliminate hepatic arterial inflow, with resulting risks to biliary anastamotic healing as noted above. In order to insure that flow in the gastroduodenal artery is occurring in an antegrade fashion, the gastroduodenal artery is occluded with a small vascular clamp and persistance of flow in the hepatic artery is verified. The gastroduodenal artery is then ligated proximally and distally, with an additional suture ligature on the proximal side, and divided. The portal vein is then readily exposed, lying posterior and medial to the bile duct and posterior and lateral to the hepatic artery.

The anterior surface of the portal vein is dissected inferiorly, with dissection carried beneath the pancreatic neck. Again, dense tumor involvement in this region may make the tumor unresectable, though with current preoperative staging methods this is uncommon. Working from the portal vein down and from the superior mesenteric vein up, the neck of the pancreas is fully mobilized off the underlying venous structures. Successful completion of this mobilization generally means the tumor can be resected, though involvement with the posterior or lateral wall of the portal vein, or at the root of the superior mesenteric artery, may still compromise the surgical margin.

The stomach (for a classic Whipple) or the postpyloric duodenum (for a pylorus preserving Whipple, as discussed below) is divided, and the distal segment is mobilized back to the right of the pancreatic neck. The pancreatic neck is then divided using the cautery or a scalpel. Bleeding from longitudinal pancreatic arteries may be managed with suture ligatures if necessary. Following division of the pancreatic neck, a margin is sent for frozen section; if involved by tumor the pancreas can be further mobilized distally and an additional segment of the body of the pancreas resected.

The portal/superior mesenteric vein is then completely mobilized off the underlying uncinate process of the pancreas. All branches are carefully divided between ligatures. This mobilization, though tedious, is critical; fully resecting the uncinate without compromising the superior mesenteric artery is greatly facilitated by fully mobilizing the portal vein. The bile duct is then divided, if this was not done previously.

Dissection of connective tissue and lymphatics posterolateral to the portal vein is then carried from the top down. At the superior edge of the uncinate, this dissection is carried medially to the root of the superior mesenteric artery. Subsequent division of the uncinate flush on the superior mesen-

teric artery is facilitated by medial retraction of the mobilized portal/superior mesenteric vein. There are numerous small vascular branches in the uncinate, all of which must be divided between ligatures or suture ligated. Even with appropriate preoperative staging, the uncinate margin may be close or microscopically involved by tumor, and the technique of division directly on the superior mesenteric artery is a useful method to maximize this margin.

The jejunum is next divided approximately 20 cm distal to the ligament of Treitz. The mesentery of the proximal jejunum is then divided between ligatures and the connective tissue at the ligament of Treitz is mobilized. The proximal jejunum and distal duodenum are then reflected under the superior mesenteric artery and vein, leaving only a few small duodenal attachments holding the specimen in place. These are divided between ligatures and the specimen is removed.

Reconstruction is performed using the retained jejunal segment. This is brought through a defect in the transverse mesocolon to the right of the middle colic vessels. The pancreaticojejunostomy anastamosis is performed initially to the most proximal segment of remaining jejunum. This can be done using either an intussuscepting technique or a duct-to-mucosa technique, as discussed below. The common hepatic duct is then anastamosed end-to-side to the jejunum, using a single layer of absorbable sutures. Finally, a gastrojejunostomy is performed 60 cm distal to the biliary anastamosis. We perform a two-layered, hand sewn anastamosis for the gastrojejunostomy, though a stapled anastamosis can also be satisfactory. The jejunal loop is tacked to the defect in the mesocolon with interrupted sutures and the defect at the ligament of Treitz is closed with a running suture in order to avoid internal hernias at these sites. Closed suction drains are placed adjacent to the biliary and pancreatic anastamoses and brought out through separate stab incisions. The abdomen is then copiously irrigated and closed.

Technical Aspects of Pancreaticoduodenectomy

Variations in pancreaticoduodenectomy technique between experienced surgeons are the rule, and several other approaches can be reviewed in surgical atlases and texts (60–62). However, there are certain strategic aspects to the successful performance of this operation that are worth emphasizing. Probably first and foremost is that this is not an operation that should be carried out by surgeons who do pancreatic surgery on an infrequent basis. Studies from multiple centers have demonstrated a strong relationship between surgical volume and outcome in patients undergoing pancreaticoduodenectomy (47,49). The statewide mortality rates in Maryland and New York show remarkably similar findings, with mortality three- to fivefold higher in patients undergoing surgery at low-volume centers, defined as doing fewer than five cases per year, compared with centers doing 20 or more cases per year. A significant fraction of pancreaticoduodenectomies are still performed in low-volume centers (63), which may account for the higher morbidity and mortality reported in national surveys as opposed to reported rates at high-volume centers. Other specific technical issues are discussed below.

Total Pancreatectomy

The oldest controversy regarding resection of tumors in the periampullary region was between a classic Whipple-type pancreaticoduodenectomy with preservation of the pancreatic body and tail and a total pancreatectomy. Advocates of total pancreatectomy claimed that the more extensive resection offered the opportunity to resect extensive or multifocal disease, and more thoroughly removed potentially involved peripancreatic nodes (64,65). In addition, by completely removing the pancreas it was not necessary to perform a pancreaticoenteric anastamosis, eliminating the risk of a postoperative pancreatic fistula.

Patients undergoing total pancreatectomy did uniformly develop diabetes, which was frequently quite brittle and difficult to control. Furthermore, it has been shown that pancreatic carcinomas are rarely multifocal (66) and that a total pancreatectomy per se does not remove a significantly greater number of the lymph nodes to which periampullary tumors are likely to metastasize (67). Improvement in our ability to manage pancreatic anastamotic leaks has changed this once dreaded complication into one which is rarely a cause of mortality (50,68). Finally, analysis of a number of studies of partial and total pancreatectomy for periampullary tumors failed to show a benefit for total pancreatectomy, and suggested an equivalent or inferior outcome when compared to a Whipple-type pancreaticoduodenectomy. Thus total pancreatectomy has been largely discredited as an operation for periampullary tumors except for the relatively rare cases in which direct tumor extension into the body and tail of the pancreas, or extensive mucinous ductal hyperplasia, make a total pancreatectomy the only way to completely excise the primary neoplasm.

Regional Pancreatectomy

Based on careful study of the patterns of local and lymphatic metastases in pancreatic carcinoma, Fortner's group (69) at the Memorial Sloan-Kettering Cancer Center championed a more extensive operation for periampullary tumors, which they termed "regional pancreatctomy." This operation removed not only the pancreatic mass (with either a total or subtotal pancreatectomy) but also included resection and reconstruction of the superior mesenteric vein-portal vein confluence and an extensive *en bloc* regional lymph node dissection (70). In some patients, resection and reconstruction of the superior mesenteric artery or hepatic artery was performed as well.

Fortner (70) recently summarized his experience with this procedure in 56 patients, which demonstrated a near universal occurrence of major morbidity and a 30-day surgical mortality of over 5%. In addition, it appears that several other patients survived over 30 days but succumbed to surgical complications after a continuous postoperative hospitalization in excess of 30 days. Long-term survival in patients undergoing this procedure was closely related to tumor size, with an estimated 33% 5-year survival in patients with tumors less than 2.5 cm in diameter and a 12% survival in patients with tumors 2.5 to 5.0 cm in size; no patients with larger tumors survived 5 years. The survival figures obtained with regional pancreatectomy are not significantly better than those reported with the standard Whipple-type pancreaticoduodenectomy (39), while the morbidity and mortality are clearly greater.

Sindelar et al. (71) at the National Cancer Institute also found the regional pancreatectomy to be associated with a significantly greater morbidity and mortality than standard pancreaticoduodenectomy. Furthermore, they analyzed the sites of tumor recurrence in patients undergoing regional pancreatectomy and found that the majority of patients developed both local–regional recurrence as well as evidence of distant metastases (72). Thus the more radical operation was not successful in providing better local control or survival when compared with pancreaticoduodenectomy.

Although few surgeons now perform the regional pancreatectomy as originally conceived by Fortner, two of its principles, namely portal vein resection and extensive regional lymph node resection, are being carried out elsewhere and may have a role in selected patients. These will be discussed individually below.

Portal Vein Resection

Among the many factors complicating resection of periampullary tumors is the close proximity of major vessels in the porta hepatis, particularly the portal vein. In a number of studies, tumor involvement of the portal vein has been associated with a poor outcome (73,74). This may reflect a difference in the biology of such tumors, with tumors which are more aggressive and destined to do poorly being more likely to invade the portal vein. By contrast, it is also possible that portal vein invasion is simply a consequence of where the tumor anatomically arises, and that if it can be adequately resected with negative margins such patients may do as well as patients undergoing resection who do not have portal vein involvement. Though somewhat controversial, the current data favor the latter conclusion.

The first reports of superior mesenteric vein-portal vein resection for periampullary tumors date to the 1950s. However, it is only recently that large series of patients undergoing portal vein resection have been reported (75,76). Results from both M. D. Anderson and Memorial-Sloan-Kettering suggest that patients undergoing *en bloc* resection of the portal vein have a morbidity and mortality comparable to patients undergoing a standard pancreaticoduodenectomy. Analysis of resected specimens from patients whose tumors had invaded the portal vein suggest that they are no more likely to have positive lymph nodes or to be aneuploid than with tumors which did not invade the portal vein (75). Thus, vein invasion does not appear to reflect a difference in tumor biology and most likely is the unfortunate result of tumor anatomy.

While the recent data are not yet mature with regard to survival in patients undergoing portal vein resection, preliminary analysis of these studies suggest that patients undergoing portal vein resection and reconstruction who have negative surgical margins do no worse than patients in which the portal vein is uninvolved (74–76). It seems reasonable to conclude that in patients with tumors involving the portal vein, which are otherwise resectable with negative margins, *en bloc* resection of the portal vein is warranted.

From a technical standpoint, resection of the portal (or superior mesenteric) vein can be relatively simple or quite complex. Involvement of a small segment of the side wall of the vein can be locally resected followed by primary venorrhaphy. Longer or more circumferential involvement generally requires segmental vein resection. Reconstruction can often be carried out with primary anastamosis if the resected segment is less than 2 to 3 cm and the anastamosis can be performed without undue tension. Resection of longer segments generally requires interposition grafting using autologous vein. Either the saphenous vein, internal iliac vein, or the internal jugular vein can be used in reconstruction of the portal/superior mesenteric vein, and can generally be harvested unilaterally without significant morbidity.

It is important to note that there are still situations in which portal/superior mesenteric vein involvement can be an indication of unresectability. Circumferential involvement (encasement) of the portal or superior mesenteric veins, and particularly occlusion of the portal vein with resulting mesenteric venous hypertension, render resection exceedingly difficult, if not impossible, in most circumstances. Tumors that encase the portal vein often invade or encase the superior mesenteric artery as well. We do not perform pancreaticoduodenectomy in patients whose preoperative staging demonstrates encasement of the portal or superior mesenteric veins, a position taken at other high volume centers as well (75,76).

Extended Lymphadenectomy

Periampullary malignancies frequently metastasize to lymph nodes beyond the limits of a standard pancreaticoduodenectomy (67). In an effort to eradicate regional nodal disease prior to the development of distant metastases, a number of groups have championed the performance of an extended lymphadenectomy in addition to the standard pancreaticoduodenectomy (77,78). This procedure involves the wide resection of lymphatic tissue from the celiac axis to the iliac bifurcation, including resection of nodal tissues between the portal vein and the superior mesenteric artery; resection of the portal vein-superior mesenteric vein confluence is often included and renders this portion of the case simpler from a technical point of view.

The Japanese have aggressively adopted this technique, and a number of series demonstrate favorable results compared with historical controls or concurrent patient populations that received a standard pancreaticoduodenectomy (78). However, other series have not shown such a difference (79). In analyzing the results of multiple series of patients undergoing pancreaticoduodenectomy with extended lymph node dissection, it was concluded that the perioperative morbidity and mortality, as well as 5-year survival results, were not different than the results of the standard Whipple type pancreaticoduodenectomy (80). In part this no doubt reflects the fact that, as in other malignancies, lymph node metastases reflect a more advanced stage of disease in which systemic spread beyond the boundaries of possible resection has occured. A prospective randomized trial of extended lymphadenectomy is clearly needed in order to determine whether this procedure is of benefit to patients with periampullary malignancies.

Pylorus Preservation

Longmire and Traverso introduced the pylorus-preserving pancreaticoduodenectomy in an effort to minimize complications of the procedure related to the hemigastrectomy, specifically dumping, marginal ulceration, and bile reflux gastritis (81). The pylorus preserving Whipple procedure preserves the entire stomach and pylorus, as well as the proximal 3 to 6 cm of duodenum, which is anastamosed to the jejunum to restore GI continuity. While this portion of duodenum is occasionly invaded by tumor, in many cases it can be preserved without apparent compromise of the tumor margin. Studies have confirmed preservation of pyloric function with resulting decreases in dumping and enterogastric reflux (82).

Surgeons critical of pylorus preservation raise a number of pursuasive arguments, however. The incidence of marginal ulceration is quite low in the era of H-2 receptor blockers and proton pump inhibitors. Furthermore, delayed gastric emptying, which can occur after either pylorus preserving or classic Whipple resection, is thought to be more common after pylorus preservation, though this view is not universally held (55,56). Finally, the adequacy of pylorus preservation as a cancer operation has never been been formally demonstrated in a randomized study. It must be noted, however, that available data from case series do not suggest a markedly different 5-year survival among patients with periampullary tumors undergoing either type of pancreaticoduodenectomy (39,41). Given the marginal benefits and potential drawbacks of pylorus preservation, we rarely perform this procedure for patients undergoing pancreaticoduodenctomy for malignant disease though this procedure is commonly performed at other high volume centers (39).

Pancreaticojejunostomy

As mentioned above, leakage at the pancreaticoenteric anastamosis remains a significant source of morbidity. Furthermore, this complication was reported in one large series to double the average postoperative hospital stay, from 2 to 4 weeks (83). Different types of pancreaticojejunostomies have been performed in an effort to minimize leakage from this anastamosis; most are variations on one of two very different techniques, as shown in Fig. 14-5. The first approach, the so called intussuscepting or dunking anastamosis, is performed by mobilizing the body of the pancreas 3 to 4 cm off the underlying splenic vein and then invaginating the cut end of the pancreas into the open end of the jejunal limb, which is sutured around the pancreas. This anastamosis is not dependent on the size of the pancreatic duct, though it may be technically difficult in certain circumstances, particularly when the pancreas is quite thick. A variation of this technique is to intussuscept the pancreas into the stomach (83).

The alternative approach, the duct-to-mucosa anastamosis, is performed by anastamosing the cut edges of the pancreatic duct to the intestinal mucosa via a small defect in the jejunum, using fine absorbable sutures. A reinforcing layer of sutures between the pancreatic capsule and the jejunal serosa are commonly placed in order to take tension off of the anastamosis. This anastamosis is satisfying from a physiologic viewpoint, but may be technically quite difficult in the presence of a nondilated pancreatic duct or a soft pancreas. Pancreatic fistula rates in series reported using either the duct-to-

mucosa technique or the intussuscepting technique appear to be equivalent, and both are widely performed. A number of factors undoubtedly play a role in the success of pancreaticoenteric anastamoses; it is our belief that delicate handling of the pancreas and careful atraumatic placement of sutures may be as important as the specific type of anastamosis constructed.

Laparoscopic Pancreaticoduodenectomy

The Whipple procedure has not escaped the wave of enthusiasm for attempting every open surgical procedure via minimally invasive techniques. Only small series reporting laparoscopic pancreaticoduodenectomy have thus far been presented. One of the largest experiences was reported by Gagner and Pomp (84). They attempted eight laparoscopic Whipple resections, of which four required conversion to an open procedure and four were completed laparoscopically (84). The mean operating time in patients successfully resected via the laparoscope was in excess of 9 h, and the average postoperative hospital stay was 31 days. These are significantly longer than representative results for open procedures, which commonly take about 6 h and require a postoperative hospitalization of 10 to 14 days. Thus it is difficult to make the case at present that a minimally invasive approach to pancreaticoduodenectomy is associated with improved patient outcome. Furthermore, the adequacy of laparoscopic Whipple resection as a cancer operation is unknown.

Distal Pancreatectomy

Patients with adenocarcinoma of the pancreas involving the body or tail of the pancreas are generally not symptomatic until their tumors have reached an advanced stage and thus are rarely resectable at the time of diagnosis. Furthermore, the long-term outcome following attempted surgical resection of more distal pancreatic adenocarcinomas is poor (85,86). Probably the one subset of patients most likely to benefit from distal pancreatectomy are those with mucinous tumors of the pancreas, previously termed cystadenomas and cystadenocarcinomas. These tumors have a high cure rate following surgical resection and thus warrent aggressive surgical measures regardless of their size or anatomic location.

Distal pancreatectomy is a less daunting technical undertaking than pancreaticoduodenectomy, involving *en bloc* resection of the spleen and pancreatic tail. As with the Whipple procedure, it is critical to achieve an adequate resection margin, in this case the proximal pancreatic margin, and the pancreas should be widely mobilized from the retroperitoneum to ensure removal of adjacent lymphatic tissue. The stump of the pancreas can be transected with a stapler or oversewn, and a peripancreatic closed suction drain should be left in place. In experienced hands pancreatic tail leaks are uncommon.

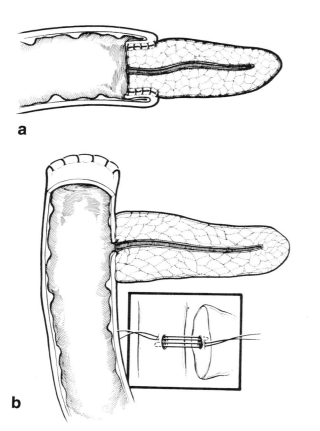

a

b

FIG. 14-5. Techniques of pancreaticojejunostomy. **A:** Intussuscepting anastamosis. **B:** Duct-to-mucosa anastamosis. (Reprinted, in adapted form, with permission from Strasberg SM, Drebin JA, Soper NJ. Evolution and current status of the Whipple procedure: an update for gastroenterologist. *Gastroenterology* 1997;113:983.)

ADJUVANT AND NEOADJUVANT THERAPY

Adjuvant Therapy

The modest success of surgical resection in producing long-term cures of patients with pancreatic and other periampullary tumors has led to a number of studies using chemotherapy and radiation therapy to diminish local and systemic recurrence following surgery. The classic study of adjuvant therapy for pancreatic carcinoma was performed by the Gastrointestinal Tumor Study Group (GITSG). This study prospectively randomized patients undergoing resection with curative intent to either no additional therapy or to combined bolus 5-fluorouracil and external beam radiation therapy. Despite small numbers of patients in each arm of the study, a significant difference in outcome was observed between the two groups, with treated patients surviving 20 months, versus 11 months for untreated controls (87). The GITSG subsequently completed a confirmatory trial in a larger patient population (88). Case series from several institutions, although nonrandomized, also support a beneficial role for adjuvant chemotherapy and radiation therapy in patients undergoing resection of pancreatic carcinomas (39,89,90).

Neoadjuvant Chemotherapy and Radiation Therapy

Recently, several groups have reported results from studies of preoperative neoadjuvant therapy in patients with periampullary tumors (91,92). Such therapy is theoretically attractive from several perspectives. Shrinking of the primary tumor mass may make technical aspects of surgical resection easier. Data from animal experiments suggest that such therapy may reduce the incidence of tumor dissemination at the time of surgery. Furthermore, up to one-third of eligible patients may fail to receive postoperative adjuvant therapy in a timely fashion due to the development of postoperative complications.

Against these advantages must be weighed several disadvantages, however. Significant tumor shrinkage has been rarely seen in neoadjuvant trials. More common is the development of local or distant disease progression, precluding curative resection, which has been noted with disturbing frequency. Furthermore, the effects of preoperative radiation and chemotherapy on surgical healing and complications such as biliary and pancreatic fistulae have not been established. It is our belief that postoperative adjuvant fluorouracil and external beam radiation therapy should be considered standard therapy, and should be offered to all patients except for those participating in clinical trials. Given the limited benefit of such therapy, enrollment in clinical trials of novel adjuvant and neoadjuvant regimans should be encouraged.

MANAGEMENT OF ADVANCED DISEASE

Modern approaches to surgical management of pancreatic carcinoma and other tumors of the periampullary region and the use of adjuvant therapy have made pancreatic resection safer and more effective. Such therapy has resulted in significant extension of survival for many patients. However, long-term eradication of disease is still the exception among patients with pancreatic carcinoma undergoing attempted curative resection. Furthermore, only 5% to 10% of patients with pancreatic carcinoma present at an early enough stage to be eligible for resection. Thus, the vast majority of patients with pancreatic cancer either present with advanced disease or develop it in the setting of tumor recurrence. For physicians involved in the palliative management of patients with advanced pancreatic cancer there are a number of important issues to be addressed.

Palliation of Pain

Advanced pancreatic cancer can be extremely painful, and most patients experience moderate or severe pain in the course of their illness. Pancreatic malignancies commonly invade neural and perineural tissues. Invasion of neural structures in the retroperitoneum by the growing pancreatic tumor mass is associated with a steady unrelenting pain which can be psychologically devastating. There are a number of important aspects to the management of such patients, including the use of long-acting analgesics in appropriate doses, and consideration for celiac plexus ablation. While the use of long-acting oral or topical narcotic preparations should be well understood by all physicians who care for patients with advanced cancer, the use of celiac plexus blockade is less often appreciated.

Probably the best study of celiac plexus ablation was performed by Lillemoe et al. (93). They randomized patients with unresectable disease, who were undergoing laparotomy for palliative biliary and gastric bypass, to receive injections of either 50% alcohol or saline into the celiac ganglia bilaterally. The study was carried out in a double-blind, prospective fashion, and outcomes of interest included pain, narcotic usage, and survival among treated patients. This study convincingly demonstrated that patients undergoing chemical splanchnicectomy had significant relief of pain and required less narcotic usage than patients receiving saline. The benefit of such therapy appeared to last for 4 to 6 months. Interestingly, in the subset of patients with moderate to severe pain at the time of treatment there was a statistically significant survival advantage among those treated with alcohol injection. While celiac plexus block can be easily and safely performed at the time of a palliative surgical bypass procedure, it can also be performed percutaneously, with or without CT guidance, in patients who have no other indication for laparotomy.

Palliation of Jaundice

Most patients with tumors of the periampullary region present with jaundice. While pancreaticoduodenectomy is an effective method of relieving jaundice, most patients present with disease too extensive for attempted curative surgical resection. There are multiple approaches to the management of jaundice in such patients, including endoscopic and percutaneous biliary stent placement, and surgical biliary bypass. There have been several trials comparing surgical with nonsurgical approaches to biliary tract obstruction (94). In general these trials have demonstrated a lower initial morbidity among those undergoing nonoperative stenting. However, the stent occlusion rates were significantly higher than the failure rates of surgical biliary bypass, resulting in more frequent bouts of cholangitis and the need for multiple procedures over time in patients managed nonoperatively.

The greater long-term morbidity among stented patients was felt to be approximately equivalent to the greater short-term morbidity among patients undergoing surgical bypass, leading to the conclusion that the treatments were approximately equivalent. It has been suggested that patients with a relatively short life expectancy due to extensive disease, and those with increased operative risk due to other medical problems, might be best managed with biliary stenting. By contrast, patients thought to have less extensive disease and to be reasonable operative candidates might benefit more from surgical biliary bypass (94).

The recent development of expandable wall stents has, in our view, changed this treatment algorithm. Wall stents can be placed endoscopically or percutaneously, but unlike older stent technology, wall stents have a sigificantly longer time to stent failure. In one recent study it was demonstrated that the stent occlusion rate among patients receiving wall stents was less than 30% at 10 months (95). Since the median survival of patients with advanced pancreatic cancer ranges from 4 to 8 months and rarely exceeds 1 year, most patients receiving a wall stent will be adequately palliated for life. The rare patients who outlive the functional life of a wall stent can generally be restented by endoscopic or percutaneous techniques. It is, therefore, our practice to spare patients with unresectable pancreatic and periampullary tumors the morbidity and mortality of surgical biliary bypass in favor of wall stent placement.

It is worth noting, however, there are still times when surgical biliary bypass is preferred. The most common is when a patient undergoing laparotomy for attempted curative resection is found to have unresectable disease. In such cases it is our practice to perform surgical gastric and biliary bypass as well as an intraoperative chemical splanchnicectomy. Another group of periampullary tumor patients who benefit from surgical biliary bypass are those with duodenal obstruction at the time of diagnosis. Such patients generally require laparotomy for creation of a gastrojejunostomy, and should have a surgical biliary bypass under the same anesthetic. The precise type of biliary bypass created is largely a choice of the operating surgeon. While choledochojejunostomy to a defunctionalized jejunal loop is our preferred approach to surgical biliary bypass, cholecystojejunostomy is an acceptable alternative except in cases in which the tumor is encroaching on the cystic duct.

Palliation of Gastric Outlet Obstruction

Approximately 15% of patients with periampullary tumors have symptoms of gastric outlet obstruction at the time of diagnosis, and another 20% to 30% of patients will develop symptomatic duodenal obstruction in the course of their disease. Surgical gastrojejunostomy is the preferred approach to palliating such patients. When carcinomatosis involving the small bowel is also present, it is our practice to place a gastrostomy tube along with performing surgical bypass of the gastric and/or intestinal obstruction. Patients with carcinomatosis almost invariably reobstruct in a matter of weeks and the presence of a gastrostomy tube can greatly facilitate terminal care by avoiding the need for nasogastric suction in most patients.

Chemotherapy and Radiation Therapy in Advanced Disease

Advanced pancreatic carcinomas and other tumors of the periampullary region respond fairly poorly to chemotherapy and radiation therapy. While aggressive combination therapy has been suggested to provide a modest extension of survival in several case series (96), there are few data from randomized prospective trials favoring its general use.

Recently gemcitabine, a new chemotherapeutic agent, has been approved for use in the palliative management of patients with advanced pancreatic cancer. In prospective randomized trials, treatment with gemcitabine has been shown to produce a higher tumor response rate and a statistically significant prolongation of survival compared to treatment with 5-fluorouracil (97). Furthermore, using criteria of clinical benefit such as analgesic consumption, maintenance of weight, and performance status, gemcitabine also appears to be beneficial. It is important to emphasize that these benefits were modest, with median survivals of 5 months and 1-year survival of 18%; clearly better agents are still needed. A number of new chemotherapeutic and biologic agents with activity against pancreatic cancer are entering clinical trials and eligible patients should be encouraged to enroll in such trials.

CONCLUSION

Malignancies of the pancreas and periampullary region remain a difficult clinical problem and a major source of cancer mortality. However, improvements in operative technique and perioperative management now allow pancreaticoduodenectomy to be performed with minimal mortality and reasonable, though still significant, morbidity. Adjuvant chemotherapy and radiation therapy appear to improve survival after resection, and long-term survival is being achieved by a significant fraction of resected patients. Unfortunately, most patients present with locally or systemically disseminated disease, precluding curative resection. For such patients, improvements in preoperative staging and palliative management avoid unnecessary exploratory surgery and offer the hope of improving the quality, if not the duration, of survival.

REFERENCES

1. Shapiro TM. Adenocarcinoma of the pancreas: a statistical analysis of bypass vs. Whipple resection in good risk patients. *Ann Surg* 1975; 182:715.
2. Crile G. The advantages of bypass operations over radical pancreato-duodenectomy in the treatment of pancreatic carcinoma. *Surg Gynecol Obstet* 1970;130:1049.
3. Hertzberg J. Pancreatico-duodenal resection and by-pass operation in patients with carcinoma of the head of the pancreas, ampulla, and distal end of the common duct. *Acta Chir Scand* 1974;140:523.
4. Bell RH Jr. Neoplasms of the exocrine pancreas. In: Bell RH Jr, Rikkers LF, Mulholland MW, eds. *Digestive tract surgery: a text and atlas.* Philadelphia: Lippincott–Raven Publishers, 1996:849.
5. Fuchs CS, Colditz GA, Stampfer MJ, et al. A prospective study of cigarette smoking and the risk of pancreatic cancer. *Arch Intern Med* 1996; 156:2255.
6. Ahlgren JD. Epidemiology and risk factors in pancreatic cancer. *Semin Oncol* 1996;23:241.
7. Lowenfels AB, Maisonneuve P, Cavallini G, et al. Pancreatitis and the risk of pancreatic cancer. International Pancreatitis Study Group. *N Engl J Med* 1993;328:1433.
8. Gullo L, Pezzilli R, Morselli-Labate AM. Diabetes and the risk of pancreatic cancer. Italian Pancreatic Cancer Study Group. *N Engl J Med* 1994;331:81.
9. Almoguera C, Shibata D, Forrester K, Martin J, Arnheim N, Perucho M. Most human carcinomas of the exocrine pancreas contain mutant c-K-ras genes. *Cell* 1988;53:549.
10. Day JD, Digiuseppe JA, Yeo C, et al. Immunohistochemical evaluation of HER-2/neu expression in pancreatic adenocarcinoma and pancreatic intraepithelial neoplasms. *Hum Pathol* 1996;27:119.
11. Abbruzzese JL, Evans DB, Raijman I, et al. Detection of mutated c-Ki-ras in the bile of patients with pancreatic cancer. *Anticancer Res* 1997; 17:795.
12. Caldas C, Hahn SA, da Costa LT, et al. Frequent somatic mutations and homozyygous deletions of the p16 (MTS1) gene in pancreatic adenocarcinoma. *Nat Genet* 1994;8:27.
13. Redston MS, Caldas C, Seymour AB, et al. p53 mutations in pancreatic carcinoma and evidence of common involvement of homocopolymer tracts in DNA microdeletions. *Cancer Res* 1994;54:3025.
14. Goldstein AM, Fraser MC, Struewing JP, et al. Increased risk of pancreatic cancer in melonama-prone kindreds with p16INK4 mutations. *N Engl J Med* 1995;333:970.
15. Fong Y, Blumgart LH, Lin E, Fortner JG, Brennan MF. Outcome of treatment for distal bile duct cancer. *Br J Surg* 1996;83:1712.
16. Rose DM, Hochwald SN, Klimstra DS, Brennan MF. Primary duodenal adenocarcinoma: a ten-year experience with 79 patients. *J Am Coll Surg* 1996;183:89.
17. Talamini MA, Moesinger RC, Pitt HA, et al. Adenocarcinoma of the ampulla of Vater. A 28-year experience. *Ann Surg* 1997;225:590.
18. Lillemoe KD, Cameron JL, Yeo CJ, et al. Pancreaticoduodenectomy; does it have a role in the palliation of pancreatic cancer? *Ann Surg* 1996;223:718.
19. Howard JM. Pancreaticoduodenectomy (Whipple resection) with resection of hepatic metastases for carcinoma of the exocrine pancreas. *Arch Surg* 1997;132:1049.
20. Warshaw AL. Implications of peritoneal cytology for staging of early pancreatic cancer. *Am J Surg* 1991;161:26.
21. Whipple AO, Parsons WB, Mullins CR. Treatment of carcinoma of the ampulla of Vater. *Ann Surg* 1935;102:763.
22. Pitt HA, Gomes AS, Lois JF, et al. Does preoperative percutaneous biliary drainage reduces operative risk or increase hospital cost? *Ann Surg* 1985;201:545.
23. Lygridakis NJ, van der Heyde MN, Lubbers NJ. An evaluation of preoperative biliary drainage in the surgical management of pancreatic head carcinoma. *Acta Chir Scand* 1987;153:665.
24. Lai EC, Mok FP, Fan ST, et al. Preoperative endoscopic drainage for malignant obstructive jaundice. *Br J Surg* 1994;81:1195.
25. Safi F, Roscher R, Beger HG. The clinical relevance of the tumor marker CA 19-9 in the diagnosing and monitoring of pancreatic carcinoma. *Bull Cancer* 1990;77:83.
26. Lewandrowski KB, Southern JF, Pins MR, Compton CC, Warshaw AL. Cyst fluid analysis in the differential diagnosis of pancreatic cysts: a comparison of pseudocysts, serous cystadenomas, mucinous cystic neoplasms and mucinous cystadenocarcinoma. *Ann Surg* 1993;217:41.
27. Yang JM, Southern JF, Warshaw AL, Lewandrowski KG. Proliferation tissue polypeptide antigen distinguishes malignant mucinous cystadenocarcinomas from benign cystic tumors and pseudocysts. *Am J Surg* 1996;171:126.
28. John TG, Greig JD, Carter DC, Garden OJ. Carcinoma of the pancreatic head and periampullary region: tumor staging with laparoscopy and laparoscopic ultrasound. *Ann Surg* 1995;221:165.
29. Callery MP, Strasberg SM, Doherty GM, Soper NJ, Norton JA. Staging laparoscopy with laparoscopic ultrasonography: optimizing resectability in hepatobiliary and pancreatic malignancy. *J Am Coll Surg* 1997; 185:33.
30. Conlon KC, Dougherty E, Klimstra DS, Coit DG, Turnbull AD, Brennan MF. The value of minimal access surgery in the staging of patients with potentially resectable peripancreatic malignancy. *Ann Surg* 1996; 223:134.
31. Palazzo L, Roseau G, Gayet B, et al. Results of a prospective study with comparison to ultrasonography and CT scan. *Endoscopy* 1993;25:143.
32. Trimble IR, Parsons JW, Sherman CP. A one-stage operation for the cure of carcinoma of the ampulla of Vater and head of the pancreas. *Surg Gynecol Obstet* 1941;73:711.
33. Strasberg SM, Drebin JA, Soper NJ. Evolution and current status of the Whipple procedure: an update for gastroenterologist. *Gastroenterology* 1997;113:983.
34. Monge JJ, Judd ES, Gage RP. Radical pancreatoduodenectomy: a 22-year experience with the complications, mortality rate, and survival rate. *Ann Surg* 1964;160:711.
35. Warren KW, Choe DS, Plaza J, Relihan M. Results of radical resection for periampullary cancer. *Ann Surg* 1975;181:534.
36. Smith R. Progress in the surgical treatment of pancreatic disease. *Am J Surg* 1973;125:143.
37. Herter FP, Cooperman AM, Ahlborn TN, et al. Surgical experience with pancreatic and periampullary cancer. *Ann Surg* 1982;195:274.
38. Nakase A, Matsumoto Y, Uchida K, Honjo I. Surgical treatment of cancer of the pancreas and the periampullary region: cumulative results in 57 institutions in Japan. *Ann Surg* 1977;185:52.
39. Yeo CJ, Cameron JL, Lillemoe KD, et al. Pancreaticoduodenectomy for cancer of the head of the pancreas. 201 patients. *Ann Surg* 1995; 221:721.
40. Andersen HB, Baden H, Brahe NE, Burcharth F. Pancreaticoduodenectomy for periampullary adenocarcinoma. *J Am Coll Surg* 1994;179:545.
41. Tsao JI, Rossi RL, Lowell JA, Pylorus-preserving pancreatoduodenectomy. Is it an adequate cancer operation? *Arch Surg* 1994;129:405.
42. Nitecki SS, Sarr MG, Colby TV, van Heerden JA. Long-term survival after resection for ductal adenocarcinoma of the pancreas. Is it really improving? *Ann Surg* 1995;221:59.
43. Geer RJ, Brennan MF. Prognostic indicators for survival after resection of pancreatic adenocarcinoma. *Am J Surg* 1993;165:68.
44. Trede M, Schwall G, Saeger HD. Survival after pancreatoduodenectomy. 118 consecutive resections without an operative mortality. *Ann Surg* 1990;21:447.
45. Swope TJ, Wade TP, Neuberger TJ, Virgo KS, Johnson FE. A reappraisal of total pancreatectomy for pancreatic cancer: results from U.S. Veterans Affairs hospitals, 1987–1991. *Am J Surg* 1991;168:582.
46. Cameron JL, Pitt HA, Yeo CJ, Lillemoe KD, Kaufman HS, Coleman J. One hundred and forty-five consecutive pancreaticoduodenectomies without mortality. *Ann Surg* 1993;217:430.
47. Gordon TA, Burleyson GP, Tielsch JM, Cameron JL. The effects of regionalization on cost and outcome for one general high-risk surgical procedure. *Ann Surg* 1995;221:43.
48. Fernandez del Castillo C, Rattner DW, Warshaw AL. Standards for pancreatic resection in the 1990s. *Arch Surg* 1995;130:295.
49. Lieberman MD, Kilburn H, Lindsey M, Brennan MF. Relation of perioperative deaths to hospital volume among patients undergoing pancreatic resection for malignancy. *Ann Surg* 1995;222:638.
50. Cullen JJ, Sarr MG, Ilstrup DM. Pancreatic anastomotic leak after pancreaticoduodenectomy: incidence, significance and management. *Am J Surg* 1994;168:295.
51. Howard JM. Pancreatojejunostomy: leakage is a preventable complication of the Whipple resection. *J Am Coll Surg* 1997;184:454.
52. Montorsi M, Zago M, Mosca F, et al. Efficacy of octreotide in the prevention of pancreatic fistula after elective pancreatis resections: a prospective, controlled, randomized clinical trial. *Surgery* 1995;117:26.
53. Buchler M, Freiss H, Klempa I, Hermanek P, Sulkowski U. Role of octreotide in the prevention of postoperative complications following pancreatic resection. *Am J Surg* 1992;163:125.

54. Lowy AM, Lee JE, Davidson BJ, Pisters PW, Evans DB. The role of octreotide in the prevention of pancreatic fistula after pancreaticoduodenectomy for periampullary malignancy: a prospective standardized trial. *Gastroenterology* 1996;110:1401.

55. Warshaw AL, Torchiana DL. Delayed gastric emptying after pylorus preserving pancreaticoduodenectomy. *Surg Gynecol Obstet* 1985;160:1.

56. Yeo CJ, Barry MK, Sauter PK, et al. Erythromycin accelerates gastric emptying after pancreaticoduodenectomy. *Ann Surg* 1993;218:229.

57. Gudjonsson G. Carcinoma of the pancreas: critical analysis of costs, results of resections, and the need for standardized reporting. *J Am Coll Surg* 1995;181:483.

58. Nitecki SS, Sarr MG, Colby TV, van Heerden JA. Long-term survival after resection for ductal adenocarcinoma of the pancreas. Is it really improving? *Ann Surg* 1995;221:59.

59. Cameron JL. *Atlas of surgery*. Toronto: B. C. Decker, 1990.

60. Evans DB, Lee JE, Pisters PW. Pancreaticoduodenectomy (Whipple operation) and total pancreatectomy for cancer. In: Nyhus LM, Baker RJ, Fischer JE, eds. *Mastery of surgery*. 3rd ed. Boston: Little, Brown and Company, 1996:1233.

61. Ashley SW, Brennan MF, Reber HA. Surgery for tumors of the pancreas. In: Bland, KI, Karakousis CP, Copeland EM, eds. *Atlas of surgical oncology*. Philadelphia: WB Saunders, 1994:473.

62. Pappas TN. Pancreaticoduodenectomy: Whipple procedure. In: Sabiston DC Jr, ed. *Atlas of general surgery*. Philadelphia: WB Saunders, 1994:579.

63. Janes RH, Niederhuber JE, Chmiel JS, et al. National patterns of care for pancreatic cancer. Results of a survey by the Commission on Cancer. *Ann Surg* 1996;223:261.

64. VanHeerden JA, McIlrath DC, Ilstrup DM, et al. Total pancreatectomy for ductal adenocarcinoma of the pancreas: an update. *World J Surg* 1988;12:658.

65. Brooks JR, Brooks DC, Levine JD. Total pancreatectomy for ductal cell carcinoma of the pancreas. *Ann Surg* 1989;209:405.

66. Kloppel G, Lohse T, Bosslet K, et al. Ductal adenocarcinoma of the head of the pancreas: incidence of tumor involvement beyond the Whipple resection line. *Pancreas* 1987;2:170.

67. Cubilla AL, Fortner J, Fitzgerald PJ. Lymph node involvement in carcinoma of the pancreas area. *Cancer* 1978;41:880.

68. Yeo CJ, Cameron JL, Maher MM, et al. A prospective randomized trial of pancreaticogastrostomy versus pancreaticojejunostomy after pancreaticoduodenectomy. *Ann Surg* 1995;222:580.

69. Fortner JG. Regional pancreatectomy for cancer of the pancreas, ampulla, and other related sites. *Ann Surg* 1984;199:418.

70. Fortner JG, Klimstra DS, Senie RT, et al. Tumor size is the primary prognosticator for pancreatic cancer after regional pancreatectomy. *Ann Surg* 1996;223:147.

71. Sindelar WF. Clinical experience with regional pancreatectomy for adenocarcinoma of the pancreas. *Arch Surg* 1989;124:127.

72. Johnstone PA, Sindelar WF. Patterns of disease recurrence following definitive therapy of adenocarcinoma of the pancreas using surgery and adjuvant radiotherapy: correlations of a clinical trial. *Int J Radiat Oncol Biol Phys* 1993;27:831.

73. Cameron JL, Crist DW, Sitzmann JV, et al. Factors influencing survival after pancreaticoduodenectomy for pancreatic cancer. *Am J Surg* 1991;161:120.

74. Furukawa H, Kosuge T, Makai K, et al. Helical computed tomography in the diagnosis of portal vein invasion by pancreatic head carcinoma. *Arch Surg* 1998;133:61.

75. Fuhrman GM, Leach SD, Staley CA, et al. Rationale for *en bloc* vein resection in the treatment of pancreatic adenocarcinoma adherent to the superior mesenteric-portal vein confluence. *Ann Surg* 1996;223:154.

76. Harrison LE, Klimstra DS, Brennan MF. Isolated portal vein involvement in pancreatic adenocarcinoma. A contraindication for resection? *Ann Surg* 1996;224:342.

77. McFadden DW, Reber HA. Cancer of the pancreas: radical resection—supporting view. *Adv Surg* 1994;27:257.

78. Ishikawa O, Ohhigashi H, Sasaki Y, et al. Practical usefulness of lymphatic and connective tissue clearance for carcinoma of the head of the pancreas. *Ann Surg* 1988;208:215.

79. Satake K, Nishiwaki H, Yokomatsu H, et al. Surgical curability and prognosis for standard versus extended resection for T1 carcinoma of the pancreas. *Surg Gynecol Obstet* 1992;175:259.

80. Yeo CJ, Cameron JL. Arguments against radical (extended) resection for adenocarcinoma of the pancreas. *Adv Surg* 1994;27:273.

81. Traverso LW, Longmire WP. Preservation of the pylorus in pancreaticoduodenectomy. *Surg Gynecol Obstet* 1978;146:959.

82. Williamson RC, Bliouras N, Cooper MJ, et al. Gastric emptying and enterogastric reflux after conservative and conventional pancreaticoduodenectomy. *Surgery* 1993;114:82.

83. Yeo CJ, Cameron JL, Maher MM, et al. A prospective randomized trial of pancreaticogastrostomy versus pancreaticojejunostomy after pancreaticoduodenectomy. *Ann Surg* 1995;222:580.

84. Gagner M, Pomp A. Laparoscopic pancreatic resection: is it worthwhile? *Gastroenterology* 1996;110:A1387(abst).

85. Brennan MF, Moccia RD, Klimstra D. Management of adenocarcinoma of the body and tail of the pancreas. *Ann Surg* 1996;223:506.

86. Nordback IH, Hruban RH, Boitnott JK, Pitt HA, Cameron JL. Carcinoma of the body and tail of the pancreas. *Am J Surg* 1992;164:26.

87. Kalser MH, Ellenberg SS. Pancreatic cancer: adjuvant combined radiation and chemotherapy following curative resection. *Arch Surg* 1985;120:899.

88. Anonymous. Further evidence of effective adjuvant combined radiation and chemotherapy following curative resection of pancreatic cancer. *Cancer* 1987;59:2006.

89. Foo ML, Gunderson LL, Nagorney DM, et al. Patterns of failure in grossly resected pancreatic ductal adenocarcinoma treated with adjuvant irradiation—5-fluorouracil. *Int J Radiat Oncol Biol Phys* 1993;26:483.

90. Jessup JM, Posner M, Huberman M. Influence of multimodality therapy on the management of pancreas carcinoma. *Semin Surg Oncol* 1993;9:27.

91. Spitz FR, Abbruzzese JL, Lee JE, et al. Preoperative and postoperative chemoradiation strategies in patients treated with pancreaticoduodenectomy for adenocarcinoma of the pancreas. *J Clin Oncol* 1997;15:928.

92. Hoffman JP, Lipsitz S, Pisansky T, Weese JL, Solin L, Benson AB III. Phase II trial of preoperative radiation therapy and chemotherapy for patients with localized, resectable adenocarcinoma of the pancreas: an Eastern Cooperative Oncology Group study. *J Clin Oncol* 1997;16:317.

93. Lillemoe KD, Cameron JL, Kaufman HS, Yeo CIJ, Pitt HA, Sauter PK. Chemical splanchnicectomy in patients with unresectable pancreatic cancer: a prospective randomized trial. *Ann Surg* 1993;217:447.

94. Lillemoe KD, Pitt HA. Palliation: surgical and otherwise [Review]. *Cancer* 1996;78[Suppl 3]:605.

95. Neuhaus H, Hagenmuller F, Griebel M, Classen M. Percutaneous cholangioscopic or transpapillary insertion of self-expanding biliary metal stents. *Gastrointest Endosc* 1991;37:31.

96. Blackstock AW, Cox AD, Tepper JE. Treatment of pancreatic cancer: current limitations, future possibilities. *Oncology* [Review] 1996;10:301.

97. Burris HA III, Moore MJ, Anderson J, et al. Improvements in survival and clinical benefit with gemcitabine as first-line therapy for patients with advanced pancreas cancer: a randomized trial [comment in: *J Clin Oncol* 1998;16:803]. *J Clin Oncol* 1997;15:2304.

CHAPTER 15

Primary Hepatic and Biliary Malignancy

Richard Schulick and Yuman Fong

The liver represents a common site for cancer. Any cell type of the liver and biliary tract may give rise to malignancy. Tumors arising from the hepatocyte are by far the most common, and hepatocellular carcinoma (HCC) is responsible for more than 1 million deaths a year. Other cells associated with the liver, such as biliary epithelium, can give rise to primary malignancies, including cholangiocarcinoma and gallbladder carcinoma. Surgery remains the most effective form of therapy for primary hepatic and biliary malignancies, and radical resection represents the only curative option. Resection of hepatic or biliary neoplasms, however, often requires radical procedures and complex biliary reconstructions that have only recently become safe in routine practice. In addition, many other surgical procedures are effective palliation for these cancers, including ablative therapies for nonresectable HCC, or biliary bypasses for nonresectable biliary tumors. The three most common primary hepatic and biliary malignancies are HCC, cholangiocarcinoma, and gallbladder carcinoma. The current chapter reviews the epidemiology, diagnosis, and therapy of these malignancies as well as the long-term outcome of treatment. The data supporting effectiveness of each modality for each disease will be emphasized. For technical details of surgical procedures, the reader is referred to standard surgical texts for liver surgery (1).

HEPATOCELLULAR CARCINOMA

Epidemiology

HCC represents one of the most common solid tumors in the world. This results from an association of this malignancy with cirrhosis of the liver. Any cause of liver injury and cirrhosis predisposes the patient to development of HCC, including chemical injury from ethanol or other environmental agents, and metabolic disease involving the liver such as porphyria cutanea tarda, hemochromatosis, a_1-antitrypsin deficiency, and Wilson's disease. By far, the most important association is to cirrhosis resulting from chronic viral hepatitis (2). In areas with a high incidence of viral hepatitis such as sub-Saharan Africa and Southeast Asia, the incidence of

HCC is as high as 30 to 60 per 100,000. In the United States, it is estimated that the incidence is less than 2 per 100,000 (3). Because this cancer is responsible for more than 1 million deaths annually around the world, it is a major public health problem. The incidence of HCC is significantly higher in men than in women with the male/female ratio approaching 8:1. The incidence tends to increase and then level off with age. In addition, it seems that hepatic adenomas may be a premalignant lesion that may lead to the development of HCC.

Diagnosis

Patients with HCC have remarkably few symptoms until a very advanced stage. Patients may present with malaise, anorexia, abdominal pain, abdominal fullness, and weight loss. Patients should be questioned as to a history of hepatitis, ethanol abuse, or family history of metabolic diseases such as hemochromatosis or a_1-antitrypsin deficiency. Most patients with HCC have underlying liver dysfunction from cirrhosis. Therefore, routine liver function tests are a poor screening test for the presence of HCC. Serum alpha-fetoprotein (AFP) level is a relatively sensitive test for the presence of HCC. An AFP level of more than 500 ng/mL in a patient with a liver mass is diagnostic of HCC. All patients with suspected HCC should also have hepatitis serologies tested, including hepatitis B surface antigen, and anti–hepatitis C antibody.

Radiologic assessment of HCC is very important in making the diagnosis and then deciding which of the many modalities of treatment to use. On ultrasound, a lesion typically will have a thin halo, lateral shadows, and posterior echo enhancement. Ultrasound is the most common imaging study used to screen patients with cirrhosis and is often the first imaging study used to examine the liver in a patient suspected of have an HCC. This has resulted mainly from the wide availability of ultrasound. Ultrasound is in fact a poor test for characterizing liver lesions in patients with cirrhosis, where regenerating nodules can be mistaken for tumor. Dynamic computed tomography (CT) is more useful. In the early phase, the tumor is hyperdense, but in the late phase the tumor becomes hypodense. Angiographic appearance is even more diagnostic, with HCC characteristically hypervascular (Fig. 15-1A). The drawback of angiography is clearly the invasive nature of the study and the cost. Consequently, angiography is more often used for therapy in embolizing these lesions than for making a diagnosis (Fig. 15-1B). Magnetic resonance imaging (MRI) is becoming the imaging modality of choice for evaluation of HCC. On MRI, HCC appears to be low in intensity on T1-weighted images, and intermediate in intensity on T2-weighted images. MRI can also be useful in distinguishing HCC from benign lesions such as hemangiomas and regenerating nodules. HCC also has a great propensity for extension into and along major vasculature. MRI is therefore particularly useful in the assessment of HCC because of the superior ability of MR to image portal veins and hepatic veins. On CT or MRI, three general growth patterns of HCC can be appreciated. The tumor may demonstrate an "invading" growth pattern, invading all structures in its path (Fig. 15-2A). Alternatively, the tumor may push structures such as major blood vessels ahead of it, in a "pushing" pattern (Fig. 15-2B). Lastly, the tumor may grow largely removed from the liver, "hanging" from the organ of origin by only a small stalk (Fig. 15-2C). Pushing and hanging lesions are much easier to resect than the invading variety, and therefore have better prognosis.

In patients without chronic liver disease and without elevated serum AFP levels, fine-needle aspiration may be useful to differentiate focal nodular hyperplasia or hepatic adenoma from HCC. This can be particularly helpful if radiologic imaging is not characteristic and if the risks of surgical resection are high for the patient.

Therapy

Resection

Partial Hepatectomy

Surgical excision represents the only potentially curative therapy for HCC. Resectability for hepatomas, as for any hepatic tumor, depends on (a) the patient's general medical condition, (b) the malignant disease isolated to the liver, and (c) anatomic resectability. The results of surgical resection are influenced greatly by the preoperative liver functional status. Cirrhosis adversely influences surgical outcome in many ways, including response to anesthesia. Cirrhosis also poses additional technical challenges for the surgeon in that the parenchyma is hard, making retraction and isolation of intraparenchymal vessels difficult. This makes hemorrhage a particular concern during resection of HCC. Patients with cirrhosis are also likely to have thrombocytopenia from hypersplenism, further exacerbating the potential for hemorrhage. Finally, cirrhosis is associated with decreased regenerative capacity, increasing the risk of liver failure after partial resections. For these reasons, hepatic resection for patients with cirrhosis carries a significantly higher operative risk than those for noncirrhotic patients.

The adverse influence of cirrhosis on surgical outcome is well documented by clinical data. Table 15-1 illustrates clinical data for liver resection in patients without cirrhosis. It is clear that in noncirrhotic patients partial hepatic resection can be performed with less than a 5% operative mortality and is associated with a 5-year survival in excess of 30% (4–8). For noncirrhotic patients with resectable HCC, therefore, surgical resection represents the treatment of choice. For cirrhotic

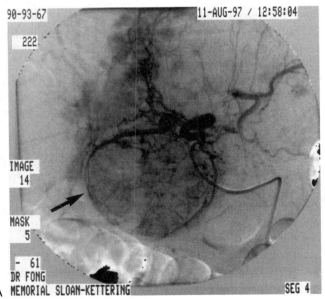 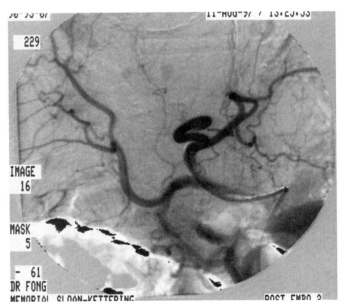

FIG. 15-1. A: Angiography of hepatocellular carcinoma (*arrow*) demonstrating a lesion with rich vascularity. **B:** The same lesion on angiography after transcutaneous arterial embolization. Note that the tumor vascularity is no longer noticeable.

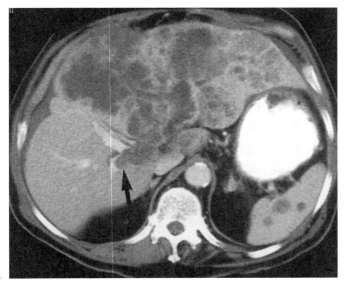

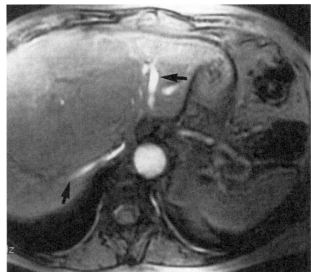

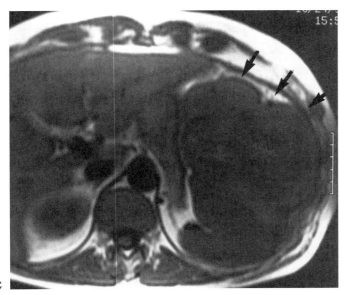

FIG. 15-2. **A:** "Invading" type of HCC demonstrated by CT. Note that this lesion has diffusely infiltrated the entire left lobe of the liver. It has also occluded the left, and main, portal vein, and a tongue of tumor can be noted within the right posterior portal vein (*arrow*). **B:** "Pushing" type of HCC demonstrated by MRI. Note that this tumor, which occupies the central portion of the liver, has pushed the left portal vein and right portal vein ahead of it without invading these vessels (*arrows*). This type of tumor is often encapsulated. **C:** "Hanging" type of HCC. MRI demonstrating a left upper quadrant mass (*arrows*) that appears distinct from the left liver. In fact, this is a 12-cm HCC attached only by a narrow stalk to the left lateral segment.

patients, however, the operative mortality is over 10% even at the centers with the best results (Table 15-2). Nevertheless, cirrhotic patients who survive the operation have a 5-year survival of approximately 30% (4–10).

Patient selection for surgery depends first and foremost on hepatic function. Over the years, many complex methods of evaluating liver function have been tested to assist in patient selection. Assessment by Childs' classification remains the most useful and most widely used. Few surgeons are willing to perform hepatic resection for patients with Childs C liver status. Even for patients with cirrhosis classified as Childs B, operative mortality is reported to be as high as 30%. There-

TABLE 15–1. *Results of hepatic resection for hepatocellular carcinoma in the noncirrhotic patient*

Institution	n	Operative mortality	Survival		
			1-year	3-year	5-year
Shanghai Second Military College (4)	55	2%	NR	NR	NR
Keio University (5)	39	3%	85	45	30
Chang Gung Mem Hospital (6)	65	2%	59	40	32
Shimane University (7)	52	6%	87	66	55
Memorial Sloan-Kettering Cancer Center (8)	70	1%	80	60	40

NR, not reported.

TABLE 15–2. *Results of hepatic resection for hepatocellular carcinoma in cirrhotic patients*

Institution	n	Operative mortality	Survival 1-year	3-year	5-year
Japan survey (9)	153	30%	30	15	12
Tokyo University (93)	72	19%	75	35	15
Shanghai Second Military College (4)	126	12%	NR	NR	NR
Kyushu University (10)	50	12%	79	62	30
Keio University (5)	119	13%	85	60	45
Chang Gung Memorial Hospital (6)	55	7%	52	41	33
Shimane University (7)	177	12%	77	43	21
Memorial Sloan-Kettering Cancer Center (8)	30	14%	80	60	40

NR, not reported.

fore, most surgeons will only consider resection for patients with Childs A liver function reserve.

Multiple lesions do not preclude surgical resection (7,8), since 5-year survival can still be expected to be between 24% (8) and 28% (7). Presentation with intraductal tumor and obstructive jaundice does not preclude long-term survival after surgical resection (5). Therefore, it is very important in a patient who presents with HCC and jaundice to distinguish biliary obstruction from hepatic insufficiency as the cause for the jaundice. HCC has a great propensity for vascular extension, and presence of tumor thrombus within the main portal vein or vena cava (Figs. 15-2, 15-3) is an ominous sign, and should be regarded as a contraindication to resection (5,11). This is the reason that patients being considered for resection should have preoperative evaluation of portal veins and hepatic veins by either doppler ultrasound or MRI (Fig. 15-3), since even small tumors may have significant extension of tumor intravascularly. Liver resections accompanied by portal venous tumor thrombectomies are unlikely to yield long-term survival.

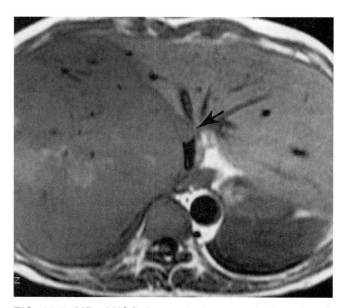

FIG. 15-3. MR of HCC demonstrating vascular invasion. A tongue of tumor can be seen within the vena cava (*arrow*).

Total Hepatectomy and Transplantation

From a theoretical standpoint, total hepatectomy and liver transplantation is an attractive option for the patient with cirrhosis and cancer. This treatment modality allows tumor excision as well as replacement of dysfunctional liver parenchyma. In practice, many obstacles exist to limit the usefulness of transplantation. The greatest obstacle is availability of organs for transplant. There are 3,000 to 4,000 livers available for transplant in this country yearly. In countries in the Far East, where there are greater social obstacles for organ donation, livers are in even greater shortage. A thorough cost-effectiveness analysis needs to be performed to justify use of these precious organs for patients with malignancies rather than for patients with benign disease. The costs associated with the transplantation procedure is also a major obstacle. Though perioperative morbidity and mortality is declining, in most centers, mortality is still substantial. Table 15-3 summarizes some of the published data to date. It is clear that operative mortality can be as high as 20% and 1-year survival as low as 42% (12). In patients with liver dysfunction in either the Childs B or C categories, however, total hepatectomy with liver transplantation represents the only potentially curative option.

Long-term results of HCC treated by transplantation are also related to extent of original liver involvement. As expected, the best results are recorded in patients who had small HCC discovered incidentally during transplantation performed for liver insufficiency (13). Patients with tumors smaller than 5 cm had a mean survival of 55 months, whereas those with tumors larger than 5 cm had a mean survival of only 24 months (14). For patients with severe liver dysfunction, total hepatectomy and transplantation is a better option than partial hepatectomy. For patients without cirrhosis or with Childs A classification cirrhosis, partial hepatectomy should be considered first. Total hepatectomy with transplantation may be necessary in this group if removal of tumor requires extensive resection of nonneoplastic liver.

Arterial Interruption

Hepatic arterial ligation was at one time the treatment of choice for HCC when lesions were found unresectable at the time of surgery and is mentioned mainly for historic interest.

TABLE 15–3. *Results of total hepatectomy with orthotopic transplantation for hepatocellular carcinoma*

Institution	n	Operative mortality	Survival		
			1-year	3-year	5-year
University of Pittsburgh (14)	80	13	64	45	45
King's College (12)	50	23	42	NR	NR
Medizinische Hochschule Hannover (94)	87	24	55	30	20
Massachusetts General Hospital (13)	24	17	71	42	NR
University of Pittsburgh (95)	105	NR	66	39	36
UCLA (21)	44	17	71	42	NR
Hopital Paul Brousse (11)	60	5%	75	49	NR
Mount Sinai Hospital (96)	57	0	72	57	NR

NR, not reported.

The operative mortality from such a procedure is as high as 13% in some series (15). The high mortality rate results from the high risk of liver hypoperfusion with arterial ligation in a population with portal hypertension. Percutaneous selective tumor embolization (Fig. 15-1B) is a much safer method for treating liver tumors when vascular interruption is desired and has largely replaced surgical arterial ligation.

Cryosurgery

Cryoablation is becoming an increasingly popular method for treating HCC. In this modality, vacuum-sealed probes that are cooled by liquid nitrogen or argon are introduced into tumors. Freezing is then performed under ultrasound guidance until the ice ball is more than 2 cm beyond the tumor margin. The tumor is then thawed and frozen again to improve tumor kill. It has great theoretical advantage in the treatment of tumors in cirrhotic patients in that very little nonmalignant parenchyma is damaged. The major disadvantage is the need for general anesthesia and laparotomy. Tumors near major vasculature are also difficult to freeze because of the risks of bleeding and because warm blood circulating in the vessels make complete freezing impossible. A number of series have been published clearly demonstrating safety of such an ablative approach in experienced hands (16,17). At present, however, this treatment must still be regarded as experimental. Comparative studies to nonsurgical ablative methods such as ethanol injection (18–20) or embolization are sorely needed. In our practice, we are prepared to perform cryoablation whenever an operation is performed to attempt resection. If a patient is found unresectable at the time of surgery, and the patient has already incurred the risks of anesthesia and laparotomy, we will proceed with cryoablation if it is technically feasible. We will also perform cryoablation for patients with clearly unresectable cancers who fail nonsurgical forms of ablative therapy.

Ethanol Injection

Percutaneous ethanol injection is highly effective treatment for small HCC (18–20). In this technique, absolute alcohol is injected into liver tumors percutaneously under CT or ultra-sound guidance. Most investigators will only inject tumors less than 4 cm in size and usually less than 4 in number. This method has the advantage of being nonoperative. There are indications that for the smallest lesions this method may be curative. Comparative trials of this modality to surgery in the treatment of small HCC is needed.

Chemotherapy/Intraarterial Infusion Chemotherapy

Systemic chemotherapy has had little success in the treatment for HCC. Chemotherapeutic regimens tested in this disease have included ones based on 5-FU, doxirubicin, cis-platinum, methyl-CCNU, or mitomycin (21). The response rate is uniformly less than 15%, with median survival for systemic chemotherapy reported at 3 months. Investigators have also examined the role for hepatic arterial chemotherapy for HCC (22,23). The drug regimens examined are usually based on either doxyrubicin or mitomycin-C. In one recent series, intraarterial FUDR, mitomycin, and subcutaneous alpha-interferon were administered to patients with HCC (24), and a response in six of the 10 highly selected patients was noted. Although these are encouraging results, the high risks of general anesthesia and laparotomy in patients with advanced liver dysfunction, as well as the risks of chemotherapy in patients who have liver dysfunction and thrombocytopenia, are likely to limit the feasibility of intraarterial chemotherapy to a very small group of patients with HCC.

Follow-Up

Follow-up after treatment for HCC is extremely important for a number of reasons. Recurrent disease can occur in up to two-thirds of patients after potentially curative resection. Metachronous second primaries can occur in the cirrhotic patient population where the field defect due to liver injury can predispose patients to new cancers. Recurrent or new cancers can be treated effectively if discovered early. Other medical problems associated with chronic hepatitis, ethanol abuse, metabolic disorders, and cirrhosis also demand close medical follow-up. Furthermore, patient reassurance if no recurrence is found, and the audit of therapeutic results, are additional reasons for follow-up.

Patterns of Recurrence

Recurrence rate after resection of HCC has been reported to be 20% to 80% (25–27) at 5 years, and the liver is the site of recurrence in up to 91% of these patients (28). Other common sites of metastases include lung, adrenals, other intra-abdominal spread, and bones (29).

Incidence of New Primary

It is clear that cirrhosis from any cause can lead to malignant transformation of the hepatocyte. Sixty percent to 80% of patients presenting with HCC have cirrhosis from associated liver parenchymal disease, most often due to chronic viral hepatitis from either hepatitis B or hepatitis C. The risk for development of HCC in the setting of hepatitis B–related cirrhosis is approximately 0.5%/year (2), while development of HCC in the setting of hepatitis C may occur in as many as 5% of cirrhotic patients per year (30). The possibility of developing second neoplasms demand that long-term follow-up be continued, even after the possibility of recurrence is remote.

Associated Medical Conditions

Follow-up must also aim to prevent and treat complications of associated parenchymal disease. Patients may need counseling for alcoholism. Patients with hemochromatosis should be treated for iron overload. Most importantly, patients should be treated for complications of portal hypertension. It is estimated that up to one-quarter of patients who die after diagnosis of liver cancer succumb to gastrointestinal bleeding from portal hypertension (29). Patients with cirrhosis should be assessed for worsening liver failure and portal hypertension.

Outcome of Treatment of Recurrence

A major reason for follow-up of patients with HCC is that reresection may be potentially curative for recurrences, with 5-year survival between 20% and 82% (26–28,31–40) (Table 15-4). One study comparing repeat liver resections with first time resections found no difference in blood loss, operation time, and incidence of complications (37). Therefore, in patients found to have both adequate liver reserve and technically resectable tumors, repeat hepatic resection is the therapy of choice.

Many ablative techniques have also been used for the treatment of recurrent HCC, including cryoablation, embolization, percutaneous ethanol injection (PEI). In selected cases of recurrent HCC of less than 3 cm treated by PEI, recurrent disease treated with PEI had a 5-year survival rate of 47% (41). Transcatheter arterial embolization (TAE) has also been considered a useful therapy for both recurrent and unresectable HCC.

Recommended Follow-Up

The routine follow-up of a patient after resection of HCC should include an office visit 2 to 3 weeks after hospital discharge. Liver function tests as well as tumor markers are assessed. For classical HCC, the tumor marker is AFP (42), while for the fibrolamellar variant of HCC it will be neurotenin or other markers (43,44) which have been found to be elevated in the preresectional blood test. A return of tumor markers to normal postoperatively will prompt the routine follow-up.

The routine follow-up consists of office visits every 3 months with history, examination, and measurement of liver function tests and tumor markers. History elicited from patients during follow-up should inquire for symptoms of worsening portal hypertension or liver failure. The patients should be questioned for symptoms of biliary obstruction including itching, and changes in stool or urine color. New right upper quadrant pain or bone pain should prompt investigation by appropriate radiological examinations. Physical examination should seek new masses, worsening ascites, and jaundice.

Patients will also be followed by an abdominal CT every 6 months. A chest x-ray is also obtained yearly. The reason

TABLE 15–4. *Results of repeat resection for HCC*

Author	Date	n	Reresection no.	Five-year survival
Nagasue (31)	1990	161	20	27%
Lin (32)	1991	188	90	24%
Matsuda (33)	1992	100	16	51%
Zhou (27)	1993	392	65	42%
Wu (34)	1993	NR	72	36%
Kakazu (35)	1993	268	18	82%
Imaoka (28)	1993	275	15	77%
Nakajima (36)	1993	149	14	92%
Shimada (37)	1994	NR	33	40%
Suenaga (38)	1994	134	18	37%
Lo (26)	1994	277	12	26%
Bismuth (39)	1995	222	14	NR
Kawasaki (40)	1995	112	21	NR

n, number of patients undergoing primary resection; reresection no., number of patients undergoing reresection; NR, not reported.

for the diligent follow-up for abdominal and particularly liver follow-up is that these are the most common sites of recurrence and recurrences in the liver can still be treated with potential cure and good palliation. Outcome of treatment for pulmonary or bony recurrence is never curative and much more dismal. Therefore, follow-up at these sites are undertaken with less diligence.

Five years after resection, office visits are reduced to every 6 months. After the first 5 years, potential for recurrence (26) or new metachronous tumors still exist. Complications resulting from cirrhosis and portal hypertension may also arise.

CHOLANGIOCARCINOMA

Epidemiology

Cholangiocarcinomas are a rare cancer that arises from the biliary epithelium, and occurs in less than 4,500 patients in the United States each year (45). Cholangiocarcinoma has a relatively even distribution between men and women with a male/female ratio of 1.3:1. The incidence of bile duct cancer is most frequent between 50 and 70 years of age, with the average between 60 and 65 years of age. A little more than half of cholangiocarcinomas occur in the upper third of the common bile duct, in the area of the hepatic hilus. These are commonly referred to as hilar cholangiocarcinomas and will be the focus of the discussion in this chapter. More distal lesions are usually treated as for adenocarcinoma of the head of the pancreas and are discussed in another chapter. Hilar cholangiocarcinoma is a surgical disease as resection is the most effective treatment option and the only curative option.

Diagnosis

A vast majority of patients with cholangiocarcinoma present with painless jaundice, though mild right upper quadrant pain, pruritus, anorexia, malaise, and weight loss may also be reported. A few patients will have the cancer discovered upon diligent workup for otherwise asymptomatic elevations of alkaline phosphatase and gamma glutamyl transferase.

Abdominal ultrasound is the most reasonable first test. It is noninvasive and can establish the level of biliary obstruction while ruling out cholelithiasis or choledocholithiasis as causes of biliary obstruction. CT scans are also usually performed. The findings to be noted on these imaging tests include a dilated intrahepatic biliary tree with a normal collapsed gallbladder and nondilated extrahepatic biliary tree. The scans should be scrutinized for patency of portal veins. In addition, signs of hepatic lobar atrophy should be sought since this is associated with a high incidence of ipsilateral portal vein involvement by tumor. In most centers, angiography and percutaneous cholangiography are used to evaluate the extent of vascular and biliary involvement, respectively. Endoscopic retrograde cholangiopancreatography (ERCP) has little role to play in high biliary obstruction since opacification of the entire biliary tree is difficult and infectious complications are

frequent. The role of magnetic resonance cholangiopancreatography (MRCP) is currently under investigation and offers the potential of evaluating parenchymal, vascular, biliary, and nodal involvement with a single noninvasive examination (46). It is difficult to obtain pathologic confirmation of cholangiocarcinoma except in very advanced cases. For the majority of cases, patients are offered surgical therapy based on clinical suspicion and radiographic appearance.

Therapy

Untreated, the majority of patients with bile duct cancers die within 1 year of diagnosis (47,48). Surgical excision is the treatment of choice, with no other therapy offering potential of cure. The immediate causes of death are most commonly hepatic failure or cholangitis related to tumor growth and inadequate drainage of the biliary tree (49,50). The objectives of management of cholangiocarcinomas must include not only complete removal of tumor, but also biliary drainage. It has become clear over the last three decades that curative treatment of tumors involving the upper third of the bile duct very much depends on aggressive excision that often requires a major liver resection. Until as recently as one decade ago, treatment of hilar cholangiocarcinomas was associated with as high as a 30% mortality (51–55). Recent results have indicate a major improvement in safety of these operations such that resections of hilar tumors can be accomplished, even when liver resections are required, with a mortality of less than 10% (52,54,56,57).

Partial Hepatectomy

The goals of surgical management for cholangiocarcinomas are both eradication of tumor and establishment of adequate biliary drainage. Complete surgical excision accomplishes both these goals and is the treatment of choice for cholangiocarcinoma since no other therapy offers the potential for cure. The tumors of the hepatic ducts and the biliary confluence are particularly difficult to treat because symptoms often appear late in the course of disease when the lesion has already involved adjacent structures including the portal vein or adjacent hepatic parenchyma. Complete resection, therefore, requires not only biliary resection but also major liver resection and often major vascular and biliary reconstruction. It is not surprising, therefore, that until recently, the surgical therapy for proximal biliary malignancies consisted mainly of biliary-enteric bypass as palliation for jaundice and cholangitis. The therapeutic approach to cholangiocarcinomas was largely nihilistic due to lack of familiarity with the disease, difficulties in delineating the extent of disease, and the technical challenge of resecting such lesions (58–60).

It is only recently that an aggressive resectional approach has been adopted for this disease (52,56,57,61,62). Improvements in sonography, CT, MRI, and angiography have greatly facilitated preoperative diagnoses and staging of cholangiocarcinoma. This has allowed improved patient selection and surgical planning. Combined with improvements in surgical techniques and perioperative care, the mortality and morbidity of surgical resections have been reduced to acceptable levels. The results of the major studies on resection of high bile duct cancer are summarized in Table 15-5. Mortality of early series was as high as 33% (63). Over the last decade, surgical approaches have become increasingly aggressive, as demonstrated by the increasing number of hepatic resections which have been performed for bile duct cancers (51–55). The operative mortality in experienced centers has dropped to acceptable levels (52,54,56,57), close to 0% for local resection and less than 10% when concomitant hepatic resection is necessary. Median survival is approximately 24 months (52,54,57), which compares very favorably with median survivals of 6 to 12 months for patient receiving only palliative bypasses. In addition, surgical resection not only provides improved survival but also improved quality of survival (64).

The greatest risk factors for recurrence are margin positive resection (65), node positive tumor (66), and vascular involvement by tumor.

Adjuvant Therapy

To date, no chemotherapeutic regimen has consistently shown activity with cholangiocarcinoma (50). Although chemotherapy based on 5-fluorouracil is often offered to patients with nonresectable disease, the likelihood of response is less than 10%. There is certainly no proven role for adjuvant chemotherapy in the treatment of cholangiocarcinoma.

In nonresectable cases of cholangiocarcinoma, many investigators have examined the use of external beam radiation therapy (61,67–71). To date, no study has clearly demonstrated efficacy for this modality. Anecdotal reports of long-term survivors after external beam radiotherapy show that some individuals may benefit from such treatment, but this must be weighed against the potential complications such as duodenal or bile duct stenosis, and duodenitis. The most encouraging results reported involve use of intraoperative (69,72) or interstitial radiation (70,73). Our current practice is to use combined interstitial radiation and external beam radiation in nonresectable cases after palliative bypass. In resected cases adjuvant radiotherapy is not justified.

Follow-Up of Patients After Resection of Cholangiocarcinoma

The most likely site of recurrence after resection of a hilar cholangiocarcinoma is locally within the bile duct, regional lymph nodes, or liver. If recurrence occurs, further therapy is only palliative. Surgical reexcision is usually impossible because of the delicate anatomic area within which hilar cholangiocarcinomas occur, and the radical procedures that are required for resection of the primary tumor the first time. Chemotherapy or radiotherapy has not been demonstrated to be effective in the treatment of recurrent cholangiocarcinomas. Therapy is therefore directed at palliation of symptoms.

Follow-up is therefore directed at diagnosis of symptomatic recurrences to direct palliative therapy, or directed at diagnosis of benign complications of surgical treatment such as biliary strictures or peptic ulcer disease. Patients with a Roux-en-Y biliary reconstruction have a higher chance of developing peptic ulcer disease. The main symptoms of recurrence that demand palliation are pruritus or cholangitis associated with jaundice. For biliary drainage to relieve jaundice or cholangitis, either surgical drainage (74) or drainage by percutaneous transhepatic cholangiogram (PTC) can be effective (75). Endoscopic drainage has little role in the relief of jaundice in a patient who has had a Roux-en-Y biliary re-

TABLE 15–5. *Results of therapy of hilar cholangiocarcinoma*

Author	n	Resectability (%)	Hepatic resection (%)	Mortality (%)	Survival (months) Mean	Median
Longmire (60)	34	18	6	10	—	—
Fortner (97)	26	34	31	33	14	—
Launois (63)	18	61	33	18	17	—
Akwari (98)	38	11	0	0	33	—
Tompkins (99)	45	47	0	23	—	10
Cameron (61)	27	37	0	0	18	—
Beazley (62)	61	26	20	19	17	—
Blumgart (64)	94	19	13	11	17	—
Alexander (100)	83	9	7	0	—	21
Iwasaki (101)	46	22	20	0	—	25
Iida (102)	41	56	56	4	—	8
Cameron (56)	96	55	8	2	—	18
Hadjis (55)	131	21	12	7	25	—
Altaee (51)	70	21	19	—	—	—
Baer (52)	48	44	23	4	34	—
Nagorney (57)	79	15	10	5	—	—

n, total number of patients reported; mortality, perioperative mortality for curative resections; survival, survival of patients resected with curative intent.

construction. Stenting, however, is associated with a high rate of recurrent cholangitis and jaundice, and therefore, in patients with limited local recurrence, hepaticojejunostomy may be more effective palliation. However, in patients with very advanced disease and limited life span, PTC may be chosen to avoid operative intervention. For limited recurrences, intraluminal brachytherapy (74) or external beam radiotherapy (76) may also improve palliation and even survival. In these cases, we favor adequate biliary drainage combined with brachytherapy and external beam radiation.

Current Recommendations for Follow-Up

The routine follow-up of a patient after resection of cholangiocarcinoma will include an office visit 2 to 3 weeks after hospital discharge. Physical examination and liver function tests will be performed to assess for postoperative recovery and complications.

Further routine follow-up consists of office visits every 3 months with history, examination, and measurement of liver function tests. Though a rising alkaline phosphatase is a good indicator of evolving biliary obstruction, patients recovering from liver resection and biliary obstruction may have persistent elevations of alkaline phosphatase. Furthermore, it is estimated that as high as 10% of all patients with biliary surgical reconstruction may eventually present with a benign anastomotic stricture. Use of tumor markers are not recommended, although a fair percentage of biliary malignancies will express CEA and other tumor markers such as CA 19-9. The reason these markers are not useful clinically is due to their high cost, and the low likelihood of effective tumor therapy if recurrence occurs. It is palliation of clinical symptoms that is the main goal in treatment of recurrences. If a patient presents with jaundice, itching or sepsis, a workup is performed to determine cause and extent of disease, and appropriate palliative therapy.

The use of routine imaging studies to follow cholangiocarcinoma after resection is even more questionable. These tests are even more expensive than tumor markers. An asymptomatic finding on these imaging studies is unlikely to prompt clinical intervention and is sure to prompt anxiety. Except as a tool to audit outcomes of clinical trials in this disease, we see no clear reason to routinely obtain imaging studies on patients after resection. When patients become symptomatic with jaundice, then an abdominal sonogram should be obtained. This allows for assessment of intrahepatic ductal dilatation as well as portal vein patency. Need for further imaging with CT or direct cholangiography will usually be dictated by the sonographic findings.

GALLBLADDER CARCINOMA

Epidemiology

Gallbladder cancer is also a rare malignancy, with approximately 6,000 to 7,000 new cases diagnosed nationally each year. It is a malignancy with a dismal outlook due to its in-

sidious onset, propensity for metastases, and rapid disease progression. This tumor occurs more frequently in women (female to male ratio = 3 : 1) and peak incidence is in the seventh decade (77). It is associated with cholelithiasis, and importantly is found incidentally in 1% of all gallbladders removed for gallstones.

Diagnosis

In patients with symptoms, abdominal pain consistent with biliary colic or acute cholecystitis is the most common symptom. The majority of patients are found to have gallbladder cancer during workup or treatment of cholelithiasis or choledocholithiasis. Some patients present with jaundice, hepatomegaly, palpable mass, or ascites.

Ultrasound examination may identify a mass within or replacing the gallbladder. CT scan may identify a gallbladder mass and may also reveal invasion into the liver parenchyma. Angiography may be necessary to assess extent of vascular involvement, and in patients who are jaundiced direct cholangiography is often useful to delineate extent of biliary involvement. As with cholangiocarcinoma, MRCP is a single noninvasive imaging modality that may allow complete assessment of biliary, vascular, liver parenchymal, and nodal involvement (46). The limited availability of MRCP, and variability of quality of this examination, however, limit its use to experienced centers, and multiple imaging modalities are still necessary in most centers for assessment of gallbladder cancer (Fig. 15-4).

Therapy

Cholecystectomy With or Without Partial Hepatectomy

Gallbladder cancer is a fast growing tumor that, if not completely excised, rapidly leads to the death of the patient. In a collected review of 5,836 patients with gallbladder cancer, Piehler (78) found that the overall mean survival was 2 to 5 months, while the 5-year survival was 4%. The 5-year survival of the patients subjected to resection with curative intent was 16.7%, while among the 2,115 patients who were unresectable, there was a single 5-year survivor (78). Surgical resection represents the treatment of choice and the only potentially curative therapy available. No effective alternative options exists. Response to chemotherapy of any type is consistently less than 10%, and data on the use of radiotherapy is far from convincing.

There is little doubt that results of treatment as well as scope of operation necessary is related to depth of penetration of the tumor (Table 15-6). For tumors restricted to the mucosa of the gallbladder (T1), there is near universal agreement that simple cholecystectomy is adequate (79–82). The extent of surgical resection for deeper penetration than T1 is controversial, with recommendations ranging from simple cholecystectomy to radical excision that includes hepatectomy. For advanced local disease, some groups have even

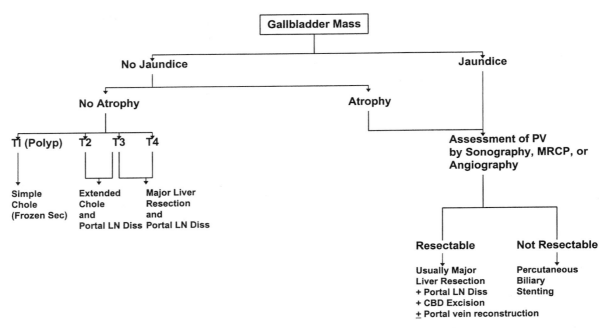

FIG. 15-4. Gallbladder cancer suspected on CT/sonography.

advocated radical resections including hepatectomy and pancreatectomy. To understand the rationale for the resections recommended by advocates of an aggressive approach, one has to examine the pattern of local spread of gallbladder cancer. This tumor routinely spreads by direct extension to the adjacent liver bed, and adjacent organs such as duodenum or stomach. Lymphatic spread of gallbladder cancer often involves nodes in the porta hepatis, in the parapancreatic region, in the celiac region, and in the aortal-caval nodal basins. For tumors with penetration through the submucosa but not yet through the serosa (T2), or tumors that involve the serosa but less than 2 cm into the liver (T3), radical cholecystectomy involving resection of the gallbladder bed as well as portal lymph nodes have been advocated. Proponents of this aggressive approach advocate the liver resection on the basis that it is often hard to distinguish T2 from T3 tumors at the time of surgery, and resection of the liver allows the best chance for tumor clearance. Portal node dissection is justified by the significant numbers of patients with T2 or T3 tumor with nodal metastasis. For patients with T2 tumors, data

would support such an aggressive approach. For patients with T2 tumor undergoing simple cholecystectomy, the 5-year survival is reported to be 24% to 40% (82,83), while those undergoing radical resection are reported to have a 5-year survival of 88% to 100% (82,84,85). For T4 (tumors with a greater than 2-cm extension into liver or with invasion of other adjacent organs) lesions many clinicians are nihilistic, discouraged by the high likelihood of intraperitoneal and hematogenous spread, and the significant morbidity of the radical procedures that may be necessary for excision of local disease. Recent series, however, also support a very aggressive approach at resection of these large tumors, particularly if no indications of nodal involvement is found (Table 15-7). With aggressive resection, long-term survival can be achieved for stage II or IV patients (80–82,85–87) (Fig. 15-5).

As indicated in the previous sections, even extended hepatic resections can now be performed safely in major centers. Whereas radical resections of the type described here at one time were associated with operative mortality of greater than 30%, in most recent reports, the operative risk is now

TABLE 15-6. *Results of surgical therapy for gallbladder cancer*

Institution	T1 or T2 lesions		T3 or T4 lesions	
	Cholecystectomy	Radical	Cholecystectomy	Radical
University of Virginia, 1982 (103)	33%	—	3%	13%
Tohoku University, 1987 (79)	57%	100%	0%	23%
Hamamatsu University, 1989 (86)	—	100%	—	15%
Mayo Clinic, 1990 (80)	—	—	0%	29%
Nigata University, 1992 (82)	—	72%	—	37%

TABLE 15-7. *Results of radical resections for gallbladder cancer*

Institution	Year	Mortality	Resected (n)	Stage III–IV	Five-year survival
Hamamatsu University (26)	1989	0	15	87%	25%
Mayo Clinic (80)	1990	2%	42	40%	33%
Japan Multicenter (81)	1991	5%	1686	50%	51%
Niigat University (82)	1992	0	40	53%	65%
Kyushu University (87)	1994	0	32	75%	53%
MSKCC (85)	1996	0	23	78%	51%

uniformly less than 5% (80–82,85–87) (Table 15-7). Medical criteria for patient selection are as for any liver resection (see above section on HCC).

Any noncirrhotic patient found to have a mass in the gallbladder fossa and found to have no endoscopic evidence of cancer in the colon should be suspected of having gallbladder cancer. Any mid-bile duct obstruction not due to gallstones should be suspected of being gallbladder cancer. Ultrasonography and/or computer assisted tomography should be performed to assess the depth of penetration through the gallbladder wall, liver involvement, and any signs of additional intraabdominal spread. Surgical exploration should be performed for all patients with no contraindications for excision of tumor. If a T1 tumor is suspected, a complete cholecystectomy and biopsy of regional nodes should be performed after thorough examination of the abdominal cavity for any signs of tumor dissemination. The pathology and depth of penetration should be confirmed by frozen section, and the procedure terminated if a T1 tumor is confirmed. For T2 or T3 lesions, a radical cholecystectomy should be performed consisting of wide excision of the gallbladder along with excision of the gallbladder bed. The common bile duct and common hepatic duct should be excised along with all associated lymphatic tissues and the confluence of the bile duct. Reconstruction is then performed by hepaticojejunostomy, connecting the right and left hepatic ducts to a loop of jejunum. For T4 lesions, a more radical excision of the liver, such as a extended right hepatectomy, usually needs to be performed.

Incidentally/Laparoscopically Discovered Gallbladder Cancer

Gallbladder cancer is often discovered during pathologic examination after cholecystectomy for presumed benign gallstone disease. There is good evidence that patients with depth of penetration of gallbladder cancer of T2 or greater and no signs of distant disease should be evaluated for and offered a radical resection to eradicate all disease (88). Since the popularization of laparoscopic cholecystectomy in this decade, increasing numbers of gallbladder cancer are now found incidentally during laparoscopic procedures. There is also mounting evidence that such tumors should be treated with a radical second operation (89–92). Patients presenting with gallbladder cancers after a recent simple cholecystectomy pose additional technical challenges. Because of the recent surgery, there is often severe inflammation in the right upper quadrant that hinders distinction of tumor from inflamed tissues. Determination of ductal or nodal involvement by tumor is always difficult at the time of reoperation. Indeed, during a second operation for incidentally discovered gallbladder cancer, an extended right hepatectomy along with excision of the extrahepatic biliary tree and periductal lymphatic tissues is almost

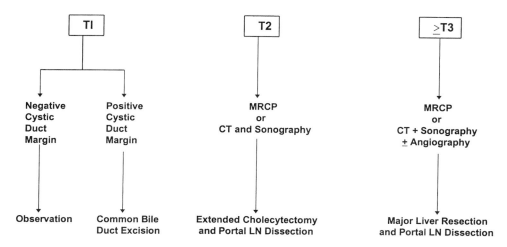

FIG. 15-5. Gallbladder cancers presenting for therapy after cholecystectomy.

always necessary. This resection allows adequate excision of the lymphatic tissues at the confluence of the bile ducts, greater confidence of negative ductal margins, and permits biliary reconstruction to only one side of the liver. The disadvantage is that a large portion of normal liver parenchyma is sacrificed, and consequently transient postoperative liver dysfunction is not unusual. In patients who presents after laparoscopic excision of a cancerous gallbladder, surgical therapy should include excision of laparoscopic port-sites.

When a patient presents with T1 gallbladder cancer discovered pathologically after simple cholecystectomy, the pathology is reviewed to determine if the entire gallbladder has been removed and if the cystic duct margin is clear of tumor. If the cystic duct margin is positive, a local bile duct excision is offered to the patient. If all margins are negative, no further therapy is warranted. If patient has a tumor proven to be T2 or greater, a radical second operation is offered after a thorough extent of disease work-up, if there are no medical contraindications.

Follow-Up After Resection for Gallbladder Cancer

The most common site of recurrence after resection of gallbladder cancer is intraabdominal, specifically in the liver or in the celiac or retropancreatic nodal basins. Jaundice is not an uncommon sign. Recurrence may also present as carcinomatosis. If recurrent disease is found after resection, prognosis is exceedingly poor. Death is likely to be due to biliary sepsis or liver failure.

Since gallbladder cancer is usually treated by a very radical surgical resection and a complex reconstruction, diagnosis of local recurrent disease is extremely difficult and excision of such a recurrence even more so. The exception is T1 gallbladder cancer previously treated with a simple cholecystectomy. A local recurrence in these patients may be treatable with a more radical resection. For most tumors, however, local recurrence is usually found in the context of other intraabdominal spread. Therefore, treatment of recurrence has little potential for cure. No study has proven efficacy for chemotherapy or radiation in the treatment of recurrent tumor. Any decision to offer unproven therapy to patient with recurrent disease must be considered in the context of the limited life spans of patients with recurrent gallbladder cancer.

The main goal of follow-up after resection of gallbladder cancer is to provide palliation for symptomatic recurrences. The main symptoms associated with recurrence requiring palliation are pruritus or cholangitis associated with jaundice or bowel obstruction associated with carcinomatosis. The other goals of follow-up are to detect benign complications of surgical treatment (biliary stricture, ulcer disease, etc.), to provide patient reassurance, and to audit results of treatment. When jaundice, pruritus or cholangitis is found, a nonsurgical palliative approach is usually favored. Because of the fast growth of tumor and rapid demise of the patients, the hospitalization and recovery time from a surgical bypass is usually not justified. Patients with recurrent gallbladder cancer and symptomatic jaundice is usually treated by PTC.

Current Recommendations

The routine follow-up of a patient after resection of gallbladder cancer will include an office visit 2 to 3 weeks after hospital discharge. Physical examination and liver function tests will be performed to assess for postoperative recovery and complications. Further routine follow-up consists of office visits every 3 months with examination and measurement of liver function tests. Although CEA is often expressed by gallbladder cancer and serum CEA levels have been advocated as a tool in diagnosis of this malignancy, use of this tumor marker in follow-up is not recommended. We also do not favor using complex imaging studies to assess for recurrence. Because it is unlikely that an asymptomatic recurrence will be treated, the financial cost of measuring tumor markers or imaging studies is not justified. When patients become symptomatic with jaundice, then an abdominal sonogram should be obtained. This allows for assessment of intrahepatic ductal dilatation as well as portal vein patency. Need for further imaging with CT or direct cholangiography will usually be dictated by the sonographic findings.

REFERENCES

1. Blumgart LH. Liver resection—liver and biliary tumours. In: Blumgart LH, ed. *Surgery of the liver and biliary tract*. New York: Churchill Livingstone, 1988:1251.
2. Beasley RP. Hepatitis B virus. The major etiology of hepatocellular carcinoma [Review]. *Cancer* 1988;61:1942.
3. Okuda K. Epidemiology of primary liver cancer. In: Tobe T, Kameda H, Okudaira M, Ohto M, Endo Y, Mito M, et al. *Primary liver cancer in Japan*. New York: Springer-Verlag, 1992:3.
4. Wu MC, Chen H, Zhang XH, Yao XP, Yang JM. Primary hepatic carcinoma resection over 18 years. *Chin Med J (Engl)* 1980;93:723–728.
5. Tsuzuki T, Sugoika A, Ueda M, et al. Hepatic resection for hepatocellular carcinoma. *Surgery* 1990;107:511.
6. Chen MF, Hwang TL, Jeng LB, Jan YY, Wang CS, Chou FF. Hepatic resection in 120 patients with hepatocellular carcinoma. *Arch Surg* 1989;124:1025.
7. Nagasue N, Kohno H, Chang YC, et al. Liver resection for hepatocellular carcinoma. *Ann Surg* 1993;217:375.
8. Vauthey JN, Klimstra D, Franceschi D, et al. Factors affecting long-term outcome after hepatic resection for hepatocellular carcinoma. *Am J Surg* 1995;169:28.
9. Okuda K, The Liver Study Group of Japan. Primary liver cancer in Japan. *Cancer* 1980;1:19.
10. Kanematsu T, Takenaka K, Matsumata T, Furuta T, Sugimachi K, Inokuchi K. Limited hepatic resection effective for selected cirrhotic patients with primary liver cancer. *Ann Surg* 1984;199:51.
11. Bismuth H, Chiche L, Adam R, Castaing D, Diamond T, Dennison A. Liver resection versus transplantation for hepatocellular carcinoma in cirrhotic patients. *Ann Surg* 1993;218:145.
12. O'Grady JG, Polson RJ, Rolles K, Calne RY, Williams R. Liver transplantation for malignant disease. *Ann Surg* 1988;207:373.
13. Haug CE, Jenkins RL, Rohrer RJ, et al. Liver transplantation for primary hepatic cancer. *Transplantation* 1992;53:376.
14. Yokoyama I, Todo S, Iwatsuki S, Starzl TE. Liver transplantation in the treatment of primary liver cancer. *Hepatogastroenterology* 1990; 37:188.
15. Mokka RE, Larmi TK, Huttunen R, Kairaluoma MI. Evaluation of the ligation of the hepatic artery and regional arterial chemotherapy in the treatment of primary and secondary cancer of the liver. *Ann Chir Gynaecol Fenn* 1975;64:347.
16. Zhou XD. [Improved cryosurgery for primary liver cancer] [Chinese]. *Chung-Hua Chung Liu Tsa Chih [Chin J Oncol]* 1992;14:61.
17. Tang ZY, Yu YQ, Zhou XD, et al. Cytoreduction and sequential resection: a hope for unresectable primary liver cancer. *J Surg Oncol* 1991;47:27.

18. Livraghi T, Bolondi L, Lazzaroni S, et al. Percutaneous ethanol injection in the treatment of hepatocellular carcinoma in cirrhosis. A study on 207 patients. *Cancer* 1992;69:925.

19. Shiina S, Tagawa K, Unuma T, et al. Percutaneous ethanol injection therapy for hepatocellular carcinoma. A histopathologic study. *Cancer* 1991;68:1524.

20. Sironi S, Livraghi T, DelMaschio A. Small hepatocellular carcinoma treated with percutaneous ethanol injection: MR imaging findings. *Radiology* 1991;180:333.

21. Farmer DG, Rosove MH, Shaked A, Busuttil RW. Treatment of hepatocellular carcinoma [Review]. *Ann Surg* 1994;219:236.

22. Ramming KP. The effectiveness of hepatic artery infusion in treatment of primary hepatobiliary tumors. *Semin Oncol* 1983;10:199.

23. Nakamura K, Takashima S, Takada K, et al. Clinical evaluation of intermittent arterial infusion chemotherapy with an implanted reservoir for hepatocellular carcinoma. *Cancer Chemother Pharmacol* 1992; 31[Suppl]:S93.

24. Atiq OT, Kemeny N, Niedzwieki D, Botet J. Treatment of unresectable primary liver cancer with intrahepatic fluorodeoxyuridine and mitomycin c through an implantable pump. *Cancer* 1992;69:920.

25. Mizutani J, Hiraoka T, Yamashita R, Miyauchi Y. Promotion of hepatic metastases by liver resection in the rat. *Br J Cancer* 1992;65:794.

26. Lo CM, Lai EC, Fan ST, Choi TK, Wong J. Resection for extrahepatic recurrence of hepatocellular carcinoma. *Br J Surg* 1994;81:1019.

27. Zhou XD, Yu YQ, Tang ZY, et al. Surgical treatment of recurrent hepatocellular carcinoma. *Hepatogastroenterology* 1993;40:333.

28. Imaoka S, Sasaki Y, Masutani S, et al. Palliative surgical treatment for recurrent and non-resectable hepatocellular carcinoma. *Hepatogastroenterology* 1993;40:342.

29. Okuda K, Ohtsuki T, Obata H, et al. Natural history of hepatocellular carcinoma and prognosis in relation to treatment. *Cancer* 1985;56:918.

30. Di Bisceglie AM. Hepatitis C and hepatocellular carcinoma [Review]. *Semin Liver Dis* 1995;15:64.

31. Nagasue N, Uchida M, Makino Y, et al. Incidence and factors associated with intrahepatic recurrence following reseciton of hepatocellular carcinoma. *Gastroenterology* 1993;105:488.

32. Lin ZY. [Recurrence and treatment of primary liver cancer after radical hepatectomy] [Chinese]. *Chung-Hua Wai Ko Tsa Chih [Chin J Surg]* 1991;29:93.

33. Matsuda Y, Ito T, Oguchi Y, Nakajima K, Izukura T. Rationale of surgical management for recurrent hepatocellular carcinoma. *Ann Surg* 1993;217:28.

34. Wu MC, Chen H, Yan YQ. Rehepatectomy of primary liver cancer. *Semin Surg Oncol* 1993;9:323.

35. Kakazu T, Makuuchi M, Kawasaki S, et al. Repeat hepatic resection for recurrent hepatocellular carcinoma. *Hepatogastroenterology* 1993; 40:337.

36. Nakajima Y, Ohmura T, Kimura J, et al. Role of surgical treatment for recurrent hepatocellular carcinoma after hepatic resection. *World J Surg* 1993;17:792.

37. Shimada M, Matsumata T, Taketomi A, Yamamoto K, Itasaka H, Sugimachi K. Repeat hepatectomy for recurrent hepatocellular carcinoma. *Surgery* 1984;115:703.

38. Suenaga M, Sugiura H, Kokuba Y, Uehara S, Kurumiya T. Repeated hepatic resection for recurrent hepatocellular carcinoma in eighteen cases. *Surgery* 1994;115:452.

39. Bismuth H, Chiche L, Castaing D. Surgical treatment of hepatocellular carcinomas in noncirrhotic liver: experience with 68 liver resections. *World J Surg* 1995;19:35.

40. Kawasaki S, Makuuchi M, Miyagawa S, et al. Results of hepatic resection for hepatocellular carcinoma. *World J Surg* 1995;19:31.

41. Tanikawa K, Majima Y. Percutaneous ethanol injection therapy for recurrent hepatocellular carcinoma. *Hepatogastroenterology* 1993; 40:324.

42. Belghiti J, Di Carlo I, Ferreira LL, Bezeaud A, Sauvanet A, Fekete F. [Prognostic value of pre- and postoperative alpha fetoprotein in the follow-up of patients with surgically-treated hepatocellular carcinoma] [Italian]. *Minerva Chir* 1993;48:25.

43. Warnes TW, Smith A. Tumour markers in management and diagnosis [Review]. *Bailleres Clin Gastroenterol* 1987;1:63.

44. Sheppard KJ, Bradbury DA, Davies JM, Ryrie DR. High serum vitamin B12 binding capacity as a marker of the fibrolamellar variant of hepatocellular carcinoma [Letter]. *BMJ* 1983;286(6358):57.

45. Longmire WP Jr. Tumours of the extrahepatic biliary radicals. *Curr Probl Cancer* 1976;1:1.

46. Soto JA, Barish MA, Yucel EK, Siegenberg D, Ferrucci JT, Chuttani R. Magnetic resonance cholangiography: comparison with endoscopic retrograde cholangiopancreatography. *Gastroenterology* 1996;110:589.

47. Kuwayti K, Baggenstoss AH, Stauffer MH, Priestly JI. Carcinoma of the major intrahepatic and extrahepatic bile ducts exclusive of the papilla of Vater. *Surg Gynecol Obstet* 1957;104:357.

48. Okuda K, Kubo Y, Okazaki N, et al. Clinical aspects of intrahepatic bile duct carcinoma including hilar carcinoma: a study of 57 autopsy proven cases [Review]. *Cancer* 1977;39:232.

49. Sako S, Seitzinger GL, Garside E. Carcinoma of the extrahepatic ducts. Review of the literature and report of six cases. *Surgery* 1957;41:416.

50. Ottow RT, August DA, Sugarbaker PH. Treatment of proximal biliary tract carcinoma: an overview of techniques and results [Review]. *Surgery* 1985;97:251.

51. Altaee MY, Johnson PJ, Farrant JM, Williams R. Etiologic and clinical characteristics of peripheral and hilar cholangiocarcinoma. *Cancer* 1991;68:2051.

52. Baer HU, Stain SC, Dennison AR, Eggers B, Blumgart LH. Improvements in survival by aggressive resections of hilar cholangiocarcinoma. *Ann Surg* 1993;217:20.

53. Bengmark S, Ekberg H, Evander A, Klofver-Stahl B, Tranberg KG. Major liver resection for hilar cholangiocarcinoma. *Ann Surg* 1988;207:120.

54. Bismuth H, Nakache R, Diamond T. Management strategies in resection for hilar cholangiocarcinoma. *Ann Surg* 1992;215:31.

55. Hadjis NS, Blenkharn JI, Alexander N, Benjamin IS, Blumgart LH. Outcome of radical surgery in hilar cholangiocarcinoma. *Surgery* 1990;107:597.

56. Cameron JL, Pitt HA, Zinner MJ, Kaufman SL, Coleman J. Management of proximal cholangiocarcinomas by surgical resection and radiotherapy. *Am J Surg* 1990;159:91.

57. Nagorney DM, Donohue JH, Farnell MB, Schleck CD, Ilstrup DM. Outcomes after curative resections of cholangiocarcinoma. *Arch Surg* 1993;128:871.

58. Altermeier WA, Gall EA, Zinninger MM, Hoxworth PI. Sclerosing carcinoma of the major intrahepatic bile ducts. *Arch Surg* 1957;75:450.

59. Klatskin G. Adenocarcinoma of the hepatic duct at its bifurcation within the prota hepatis. *Am J Med* 1965;38:241.

60. Longmire WP, McArthur MS, Bastounis EA, Hiatt J. Carcinoma of the extrahepatic biliary tract. *Ann Surg* 1973;178:333.

61. Cameron JL, Broe P, Zuidema GD. Proximal bile duct tumors: surgical management with silastic transhepatic biliary stents. *Ann Surg* 1982;196:412.

62. Beazley RM, Hadjis N, Benjamin IS, Blumgart LH. Clinicopathological aspects of high bile duct cancer. Experience with resection and bypass surgical treatment. *Ann Surg* 1984;199:623.

63. Launois B, Campion J, Brissot P, Gosselin M. Carcinoma of the hepatic hilus. Surgical management and the case for resection. *Ann Surg* 1978;190:151.

64. Blumgart LH, Hadjis NS, Benjamin IS, Beazley R. Surgical approaches to cholangiocarcinoma at confluence of hepatic ducts. *Lancet* 1984;1:66.

65. Yeo CJ, Pitt HA, Cameron JL. Cholangiocarcinoma [Review]. *Surg Clin North Am* 1990;70:1429.

66. Reding R, Buard JL, Lebeau G, Launois B. Surgical management of 552 carcinomas of the extrahepatic bile ducts (gallbladder and periampullary tumors excluded). Results of the French Surgical Association Survey. *Ann Surg* 1991;213:236.

67. Terblanche J, Louw JH. U tube drainage in the palliative therapy of carcinoma of the main hepatic duct system. *Surg Clin North Am* 1973; 53:1245.

68. Longmire WP Jr. The diverse causes of biliary obstruction and their remedies. *Curr Probl Surg* 1977;14:1.

69. Iwasaki Y, Ohto M, Todoroki T, Okamura T, Nishimura A, Sato H. Treatment of carcinoma of the biliary system. *Surg Gynecol Obstet* 1977;144:219.

70. Fletcher MS, Brinkley D, Dawson JL, Nummerley H, Wheeler PG, Williams R. Treatment of high bile duct carcinoma by internal radiotherapy with iridium-192 wire. *Lancet* 1981;2:172.

71. Kopelson G, Gunderson LL. Primary and adjuvant radiation therapy in gallbladder and extrahepatic biliary tract carcinoma. *J Clin Gastroenterol* 1983;5:43.

72. Todoroki T, Iwasaki Y, Okamura T, et al. Intrahepatic radiotherapy for advanced carcinoma of the biliary system. *Cancer* 1980;46:2179.

73. Ikeda H, Kuroda C, Uchida H, et al. [Intramural irradiation with Iridium 192 wires for extrahepatic bile duct carcinoma. A preliminary report] [Japan]. *Nippon Igaku Hoshasen Gakkai Zasshi [Nippon Acta Radiol]* 1979;39:1356.

74. Kuvshinoff BW, Armstrong JG, Fong Y, et al. Palliation of irresectable hilar cholangiocarcinoma with biliary drainage and radiotherapy. *Br J Surg* 1995;82:1522.

75. Polydorou AA, Cairns SR, Dowsett JF, et al. Palliation of proximal malignant biliary obstruction by endoscopic endoprosthesis insertion. *Gut* 1991;32:685.

76. Shiina T, Mikuriya S, Uno T, et al. Radiotherapy of cholangiocarcinoma: the roles for primary and adjuvant therapies. *Cancer Chemother Pharmacol* 1992;31[Suppl]:S115.

77. Diehl AK. Epidemiology of gallbladder cancer: a synthesis of recent data. *J Natl Cancer Inst* 1980;65:1209.

78. Piehler JM, Crichlow RW. Primary carcinoma of the gallbladder [Review]. *Surg Gynecol Obstet* 1978;147:929.

79. Ouchi K, Owada Y, Matsuno S, Sato T. Prognostic factors in the surgical treatment of gallbladder carcinoma. *Surgery* 1987;101:731.

80. Donohue JH, Nagorney DM, Grant CS, Tsushima K, Ilstrup DM, Adson MA. Carcinoma of the gallbladder. Does radical resection improve outcome? *Arch Surg* 1990;125:237.

81. Ogura Y, Mizumoto R, Isaji S, Kusuda T, Matsuda S, Tabata M. Radical operations for carcinoma of the gallbladder: present status in Japan. *World J Surg* 1991;15:337.

82. Shirai Y, Yoshida K, Tsukada K, Muto T, Watanabe H. Radical surgery for gallbladder carcinoma. Long-term results. *Ann Surg* 1992;216:565.

83. Yamaguchi K, Tsuneyoshi M. Subclinical gallbladder carcinoma. *Am J Surg* 1992;163:382.

84. Matsumoto Y, Fujii H, Aoyama H, Yamamoto M, Sugahara K, Suda K. Surgical treatment of primary carcinoma of the gallbladder based on the histologic analysis of 48 surgical specimens. *Am J Surg* 1992;163:239.

85. Bartlett DL, Fong Y, Fortner JG, Brennan MF, Blumgart LH. Long-term results after resection for gallbladder cancer. Implications for staging and management [Review]. *Ann Surg* 1996;224:639.

86. Nakamura S, Sakaguchi S, Suzuki S, Muro H. Aggressive surgery for carcinoma of the gallbladder. *Surgery* 1989;106:467.

87. Chijiiwa K, Tanaka M. Carcinoma of the gallbladder: an appraisal of surgical resection. *Surgery* 1994;115:751.

88. Shirai Y, Yoshida K, Tsukada K, Muto T. Inapparent carcinoma of the gallbladder—an appraisal of a radical second operation after simple cholecystectomy. *Cancer* 1988;62:1422.

89. Drouard F, Delamarre J, Capron J. Cutaneous seeding of gallbladder cancer after laparoscopic cholecystectomy [Letter]. *N Engl J Med* 1991;325:1316.

90. Pezet D, Fondrinier E, Rotman N, et al. Parietal seeding of carcinoma of the gallbladder after laparoscopic cholecystectomy. *Br J Surg* 1992;79:230.

91. Clair DG, Lautz DB, Brooks DC. Rapid development of umbilical metastases after laparoscopic cholecystectomy for unsuspected gallbladder carcinoma. *Surgery* 1993;113:355.

92. Fong Y, Brennan MF, Turnbull A, Coit DG, Blumgart LH. Gallbladder cancers discovered during laparoscopic surgery: potential for iatrogenic tumor dissemination. *Arch Surg* 1993;128:1054.

93. Nagao T, Inoue S, Goto S, et al. Hepatic resection for hepatocellular carcinoma: clinical features and long-term prognosis. *Ann Surg* 1987;205:33.

94. Pichlmayr R, Weimann A, Steinhoff G, Ringe B. Liver transplantation for hepatocellular carcinoma: clinical results and future aspects [Review]. *Cancer Chemother Pharmacol* 1992;31[Suppl]:S157.

95. Iwatsuki S, Starzl TE, Sheahan DG, et al. Hepatic resection versus transplantation for hepatocellular carcinoma. *Ann Surg* 1991;214:222.

96. Schwartz ME, Sung M, Mor E, et al. A multidisciplinary approach to hepatocellular carcinoma in patients with cirrhosis. *J Am Coll Surg* 1995;180:596.

97. Fortner JG, Kallum BO, Kim DK. Surgical management of carcinoma of the junction of the main hepatic ducts. *Ann Surg* 1976;184:68.

98. Akwari OE, Kelly KA. Surgical treatment of adenocarcinoma. Location: junction of the right, left, and common hepatic ducts. *Arch Surg* 1979;114:22.

99. Tompkins RK, Thomas D, Wile A, Longmire WP. Prognostic factors in bile duct carcinoma: analysis of 96 cases. *Ann Surg* 1981;194:447.

100. Alexander F, Rossi RL, O'Bryan M, Khettry U, Braasch JW, Watkins E Jr. Biliary carcinoma. A review of 109 cases. *Am J Surg* 1984;147:503.

101. Iwasaki Y, Okamura T, Ozaki A, et al. Surgical treatment for carcinoma at the confluence of the major hepatic ducts. *Surg Gynecol Obstet* 1986;162:457.

102. Iida S, Tsuzuki T, Ogata Y, Yoneyama K, Iri H, Watanabe K. The long-term survival of patients with carcinoma of the main hepatic duct junction. *Cancer* 1987;60:1612.

103. Wanebo HJ, Castle WN, Fechner RE. Is carcinoma of the gallbladder a curable lesion? *Ann Surg* 1982;196:624.

CHAPTER 16

Colon Cancer

Susan Galandiuk and Todd J. Waltrip

In 1997, an estimated 94,100 new cases of colon cancer were diagnosed in the United States and 46,600 people have died of colon cancer. Nationwide, cancer of the colon and rectum is second only to lung cancer, in both cancer incidence and deaths (1). The highest incidence of colon cancer occurs in patients over 50 years old and peaks in the 7th decade; this includes hereditary cancers, which present earlier. Five-year survival rates in the United States are just over 50% for all stages of colon cancer (Table 16-1).

RISK FACTORS

Many factors, environmental and genetic, have been variably linked to colon cancer (Table 16-2). The high incidence of colon cancer in the Western world has been attributed to diets that are relatively low in fiber and/or high in fat. This theory is supported by the observation that people who migrate to Western countries from an area with low rates of colon cancer apparently "lose" this protective diet factor. Smoking, which also increases the risk of developing colon cancer, becomes most significant after 20 to 35 years, emphasizing the need for preventive measures that discourage teenagers and young adults from smoking (2). Both estrogen replacement therapy and aspirin reduce the risk of colon cancer (3,4).

It is suspected that most, if not all, colon cancers arise in polyps. A corresponding increased risk of colon cancer exists in patients with a personal or family history of colorectal polyps. Patients with a family history of colon cancer have two to four times the normal risk of developing colon cancer. Patients with a personal history of colon cancer are at a higher risk not only of developing recurrent disease, but also of developing metachronous colon cancer. Inflammatory bowel disease also is associated with an increased colon cancer risk, with the risk associated with ulcerative colitis being much higher than that with Crohn's disease.

Genetic syndromes that have been linked to colon cancer include hereditary nonpolyposis colon cancer (HNPCC) and familial adenomatous polyposis (FAP) syndromes. Patients with a history of colon cancer in several family members or with a known family history of FAP should have genetic counseling to evaluate the need for genetic testing for both FAP and HNPCC (5). HNPCC is an autosomal dominant trait that is usually associated with right-sided colon cancers, often occurring at a younger age than in the general population. The two forms of this disease are referred to as Lynch I and Lynch II syndromes. The former is associated only with colon cancer, while the latter includes tumors of the stomach, duodenum, uterus, ovary, and/or pancreas, in addition to colon cancer (6). HNPCC results from mutations in the DNA mismatch repair genes *MSH2, MLH1, PMS1,* and *PMS2.* Carriers of one or more of these defects have approximately a 90% lifetime risk of developing some type of cancer (7).

FAP is an autosomal dominant trait characterized by multiple adenomatous colon polyps that are typically tubular adenomas. The disease is often, although not exclusively, associated with mutations in the adenomatous polyposis coli *(APC)* gene. FAP carries a 100% lifetime risk of developing colon cancer and can only be prevented by timely colectomy (5). In a variant known as Gardner's syndrome, patients may also develop duodenal villous adenomas, desmoid tumors, osteomas, and epidermoid cysts.

Genes linked to cancers are categorized as either tumor suppressor genes or oncogenes. Oncogenes, when activated from their protooncogene form, "actively" alter cell structure or function. Suppressor genes, on the other hand, are usually present in normal cells. Alterations in cell structure or function occur when these genes are inactivated by mutations. Oncogenes include *K-ras, s-arc, trk,* and *c-myc.* Tumor suppressor genes involved in colon cancer include *p53, APC,* and *DCC* (deleted in colon cancer). *P53* is the most commonly mutated gene in human cancers. It is frequently mutated in left-sided colon cancers, but rarely in right-sided or transverse colon lesions. The *DCC* gene is frequently deleted in sporadic colon cancer (8).

Gene mutations associated with cancer can be further divided as either predictive or prognostic. Predictive mutations are germ line mutations, meaning they are present in all cells of the body. For colon cancer, these mutations include *APC, MLH1,* and *MSH2.* Tests for mutations in these genes can be used to predict future colon cancer risk. Prognostic mutations,

TABLE 16–1. *Stage-dependent 5-year survival rates after curative resection of colon cancer*

Stage	Stage grouping			Five-year survival rate	Duke's stage
	T	N	M		
0	Tis	N0	M0	—	—
I	T1	N0	M0	70–100%	A
	T2	N0	M0	—	A
II	T3	N0	M0	63–90%	B
	T4	N0	M0	—	B
III	Any T	N1	M0	33–76%	C
	Any T	N2, N3	M0	—	C
IV	Any T	Any T	M1	0–19%	—

Adapted from Link et al. (1).

on the other hand, are present only within a tumor. For colon cancer, they include *p53, K-ras,* and *DCC*.

The widespread availability of polymerase chain reaction techniques allows detection of some of the common mutations in many of these genes. Tests are commercially available for *APC, MLH1, MSH2, p53, K-ras,* and *DCC*. An extension of these genetic tests is the detection of *K-ras* mutations in DNA shed in patients' stools. While detecting only one specific mutation, this test holds promise for future tests that might aid in screening or determining prognosis for cancers (9).

SCREENING OF ASYMPTOMATIC PATIENTS

The goal of screening is the detection of earlier stage cancers, with more favorable cure rates. A recent consensus statement by eight medical societies, including the American Cancer Society and the American Gastroenterological Association, recommended that screening begin at age 50 for patients without risk factors, and at age 40 for patients with a family history of either colon cancer or adenomatous polyps (5). Screening should include one of the following:

- Annual fecal occult blood testing
- Flexible sigmoidoscopy every 5 years
- Air-contrast barium enema every 5 to 10 years
- Colonoscopy every 10 years

The most effective screening procedure, in terms of both cost and effectiveness, has been difficult to define.

TABLE 16–2. *Risk and protective factors for colon cancer*

Risk factors	Protective factors
Diet high in fat or low in fiber	Diet high in fiber or low in fat
Smoking	Aspirin
Personal or family history of colon polyps	Estrogen replacement therapy
Inflammatory bowel disease	
Alcohol, in excess	
Family history of sporadic colon cancer	
Hereditary cancer syndromes	

Fecal occult blood testing requires that the patient make six slides: three consecutive stools each smeared onto two slides. The sensitivity of this test is highest when the slides are rehydrated. The mortality rate from colon cancer was reduced by up to 33% when this was used as the sole screening test. However, the cost is substantial, patient compliance is often poor, and there are a significant number of false-positive results that mandate further evaluation (10,11).

Colonoscopy is the most sensitive endoscopic modality, with 95% sensitivity, compared to rigid and flexible sigmoidoscopy, with 30% and 50% sensitivity, respectively (12). A 90% reduction in the risk of colon cancer has been reported with one-time screening colonoscopy in the 6th decade, provided that all polyps are removed at that time (13).

Air-contrast barium enema has an 83% sensitivity (12). It costs less than colonoscopy but can miss up to 30% of cancers identified at colonoscopy (14).

PREOPERATIVE ASSESSMENT

Carcinoembryonic antigen (CEA) is a glycoprotein produced by colon cancer cells as well as by certain normal cells. Despite a high sensitivity, serum CEA levels are not as good as screening tests since their specificity is less than 50% (15). CEA is least sensitive in detecting Duke's A and B colon cancers. It is most frequently elevated in patients with hepatic metastases and least frequently elevated in patients with local recurrence. There is no conclusive evidence that serum CEA level monitoring provides a survival advantage (16). Serum CEA levels should, however, be obtained preoperatively as a baseline value, in order to facilitate postoperative follow-up. Of the available serum liver function tests, lactate dehydrogenase has both a sensitivity and specificity between 85% and 95%, and is therefore a good predictor of hepatic metastases (15).

Synchronous colon cancers occur in 3% to 8% of patients, and to exclude these lesions, the entire colon must be evaluated preoperatively with either colonoscopy or barium enema (17). Patients with incomplete obstruction should have a colonoscopy instead of a barium enema in order to avoid postoperative complications associated with barium, including inspissation and impaction. Women should have a gynecologic examination to exclude simultaneous gynecologic pathology, such as ovarian metastases, which would alter operative management.

Routine preoperative computerized tomography (CT) scanning is controversial, as it rarely alters operative management. A promising new technique, endoscopic ultrasound, is invaluable in the staging of rectal cancer, but it is used less frequently with colon cancer, since local invasion will not likely alter the decision to operate. Endoscopic ultrasound may become increasingly important in the preoperative evaluation when laparoscopic resection is planned. Endoscopic ultrasound can determine the depth of colon cancer invasion with 83% specificity and can also detect lymph node metastases with sensitivity and specificity of 68% and 70%, respectively (18).

TREATMENT

Traditional Surgical Approach

Margins

The goal of surgery is resection of the tumor-bearing portion of the colon, with tumor-free margins of resection, and resection of the lymphovascular pedicle (19). The optimal margin of resection has been controversial, ranging anywhere from 2 to 10 cm, depending on the tumor stage. Currently, a 10-cm proximal margin and a 2-cm distal margin are common practice (19,20). A comparison of segmental colon resection versus formal left hemicolectomy showed no difference in patient survival up to 12 years postoperatively (21,22).

Vascular Ligation

The "no touch" technique of colon resection refers to ligation of the lymphovascular pedicle prior to colon mobilization. An early nonrandomized, retrospective report on this technique showed slightly improved survival at 5 years compared to conventional resection (23). A recent multicenter, randomized study (24) demonstrated no significant difference in survival at 5 years when comparing "no touch" and conventional techniques.

Obstructing Lesions

The treatment of obstructing lesions has evolved. It was recognized nearly 20 years ago that fecal diversion did not reduce the high mortality of emergency right hemicolectomy (25). While it is now widely accepted that obstructing right colon lesions are amenable to resection and primary anastamosis, obstructing left colon lesions generally have been treated with resection and fecal diversion. Recently, obstructing lesions of the left colon without perforation have been safely resected with immediate reconstruction, often following antegrade, on-table colon lavage (26,27). Perforation with generalized peritonitis is best treated with resection and diversion. Perforated colon cancer has the highest mortality of any type of colon perforation. The tumors themselves may be of advanced size, but may also be smaller with perforation of the proximal colon. A relative immunocompromised state in cancer patients may worsen both the septic and malignant disease (28).

On-Table Lavage

To safely perform on-table colon lavage, it is important that the hepatic and splenic flexures of the colon are free to move, and it is often necessary to mobilize both flexures. A Foley catheter is inserted into the cecum through the stump of the appendix or through the terminal ileum or cecum (if the patient has previously had an appendectomy). Corrugated anesthesia tubing is sterilized and inserted into the distal colon. Umbilical tape is used to secure the tubing into the colon. The free end of the tubing is draped over the side of the operating table and placed into a large plastic bag. The colon is then irrigated with warm isotonic saline until clear. Patients who are medically unfit or unstable at the time of surgery should not undergo on-table lavage, as the procedure does add significant time to the operation (26,27).

Tumor Adhesion

Adhesion of a carcinoma to an adjacent organ or tissue associated with cancer should be considered malignant, and not be divided. The adhesions should be resected en bloc with the specimen, as division of such adhesions is associated with an increased rate of local recurrence.

Local Invasion of Tumor

Many tumors that invade adjacent structures can be resected en bloc. If there is extensive invasion into the abdominal wall, it is often helpful to place metallic clips at the margins of the resection to aid in postoperative radiation therapy, if it is planned. Large defects in the abdominal wall left after resection can be repaired with flap reconstruction. Operations that involve extensive resection and reconstruction are best performed using a multidisciplinary team approach. Figures 16-1 and 16-2 summarize the treatment options for most presentations of colon cancer.

Young Patients

A unique group of patients with colon cancer are those less than 40 years of age. Traditionally, this group was thought to have a much worse prognosis than the typical patient over 50 years old. Recent studies, however, have shown that young patients with colon cancer have similar stage-related survival. Their apparent poorer prognosis is likely due to the fact that they present with more advanced cancers (29).

Oophorectomy

Prophylactic oophorectomy at the time of colon resection is controversial. The incidence of synchronous metastases to the ovaries ranges from 2% to 8%. Various nonrandomized studies have offered a variety of treatment recommendations, but there is no consensus on the role of prophylactic oophorectomy (19). It is wise preoperatively to discuss with patients (especially women in their reproductive years) the possibility that their ovaries may be removed. If there is any gross abnormality, oophorectomy should be performed (Fig. 16-3).

Radioimmunoguided Surgery

An intraoperative technique that has shown promise is radioimmunoguided surgery (RIGS), which permits intraoperative detection of occult cancer that might otherwise be missed. The patient receives an injection of a radiolabeled murine

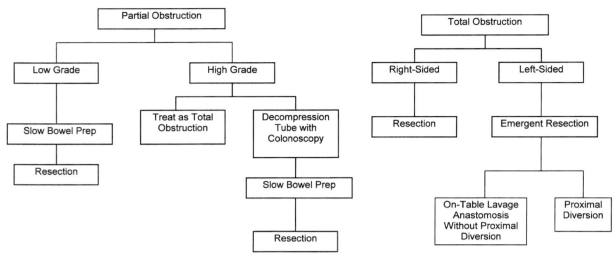

FIG. 16-1. Algorithm for treatment of obstructing colon cancer.

monoclonal antibody to colon cancer about 3 weeks preoperatively, and a hand-held gamma detection probe is used at the time of laparotomy to assess the extent of disease. This technique was found to be more sensitive than either clinical or pathologic examination in detecting regional spread of the cancer (30).

Laparoscopic Colon Resection

With the expanding spectrum of laparoscopic procedures, it was only a matter of time before colon resections were performed using laparoscopy. There are many differences between open and laparoscopic colon resections (Table 16-3). It can be difficult to localize smaller tumors using the laparoscope, and there have been several reports of the wrong segment of colon being resected laparoscopically. For this reason, great care must be taken in preoperative localization beyond simple visualization at the time of colonoscopy. If the lesion is small, consideration may be given to colonoscopic India ink injection adjacent to the tumor to facilitate intraoperative identification. The surgeon is limited by the inability to palpate organs, but this limitation is somewhat offset by lap-

aroscopic ultrasound probes, which allow excellent visualization of the liver. The sensitivity and specificity of ultrasonography is actually higher than that of manual palpation of the liver (22). Currently, a laparoscopic probe is being developed for RIGS.

In a comparison of open versus laparoscopic colon resections in pigs (31), the laparoscopic procedure took twice as long. Gastric function, however, returned more quickly in the laparoscopic resection group. The clinical significance of an earlier return of gastric function is difficult to interpret, since the return of bowel function was identical in both groups. Pfeifer and associates (32) compared open and laparoscopic colon resections and found no significant difference in either length of hospital stay or total cost, and patients reported no difference in either perceived pain or their satisfaction with cosmesis.

A unique problem that has been reported with laparoscopic colon cancer resections is port site recurrence. Approximately

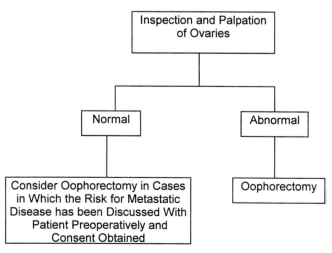

FIG. 16-2. Treatment algorithm for perforated colon cancer.

FIG. 16-3. Algorithm for oophorectomy in patients with colon cancer.

35 such port site recurrences were reported over a 2-year period in two studies, with an incidence as high as 21% (33,34). This is a significant problem that often requires extensive abdominal wall resection and reconstruction, frequently combined with radiation and chemotherapy.

Perioperative Care

There has been significant concern that blood transfusions during and after colon resections lead to poorer survival. This issue is controversial, with the overwhelming majority of literature over the past 15 years supporting a poorer prognosis in patients who receive blood transfusions. Recent reports have refuted this association (35,36).

Traditionally, following colon resection, nasogastric tubes are removed only when bowel function has returned. Many studies have examined the role of nasogastric tubes and early postoperative feeding in open colon resections. In two studies, nasogastric tubes were removed immediately postoperatively, a clear liquid diet begun the night of surgery, and a regular diet started the following day. In both reports, diets were generally well-tolerated, with only a slightly higher incidence of nausea and vomiting in patients on early feeding regimens (37,38). These reports emphasize that there are many different ways to manage patients postoperatively. The availability of newer, prokinetic agents may greatly affect perioperative care of such patients. There are ongoing clinical trials to investigate such agents (39).

Adjuvant Chemotherapy

In the United States, adjuvant chemotherapy is a relatively new modality that has had a positive impact on colon cancer patient survival. The goal of adjuvant therapy is to extend survival and reduce recurrence by eliminating occult disease and micrometastases (40). The most frequently used combination of agents is 5-fluorouracil (5-FU) with levamisole, though recently, folinic acid (leucovorin) has also been used with 5-FU. 5-FU is an antimetabolite that interferes with DNA synthesis. Serum CEA levels can be falsely elevated in patients who are receiving 5-FU. Levamisole increases the antitumor activity of the immune system. Folinic acid is a water soluble vitamin that "rescues" some cells from the toxic effects of 5-FU.

Postoperative adjuvant chemotherapy has been shown to decrease mortality rates for patients with stage III disease by 20% to 30% (41,42). Its use in stage II disease, except in study protocols, should be limited to T4 tumors or tumors with adverse prognostic characteristics (1). Adjuvant chemotherapy is usually begun 3 to 5 weeks postoperatively and continued for several months to a year, depending on the specific protocol.

In addition to adjuvant chemotherapy, adjuvant immunotherapy is being investigated. Trials with agents such as BCG (Bacillus Calmette-Guerin) vaccine are being conducted, with some preliminary studies showing promise (43). Ongoing trials are also evaluating the use of monoclonal antibodies that bind CEA and induce antitumor immunity (44).

Recurrent Disease

The goal of postoperative surveillance is the early detection of potentially resectable disease, since resection of such recurrences is the only real chance for cure. The most common factors leading to identification of recurrent disease are symptoms and elevated serum CEA levels (45). The most common symptom of recurrent disease is pain; other symptoms include intestinal obstruction, abdominal mass, gastrointestinal bleeding, anorexia, and weight loss. Many nonspecific symptoms can also herald recurrence (46). If the entire colon is evaluated preoperatively, follow-up colonoscopy is recommended after 1 to 3 years. If normal, colonoscopy can then be performed every 5 years. Patients whose entire colon is not evaluated preoperatively, should have colonoscopy 1 year after resection. If normal, subsequent colonoscopy can be performed every 5 years (5).

Preoperative elevation in CEA levels is a good predictor of the likelihood of tumor recurrence. The CEA is much less expensive than routine radiologic examination for detecting asymptomatic, recurrent disease (47). DNA ploidy and grade of anaplasia have been found to be anywhere from weak to good indicators of the risk of recurrence (48,49). CA195, CA19-9, and other markers are not useful in predicting recurrence (48).

One study (16) examined over 1,000 colon cancer patients who were followed postoperatively. One group had CEA levels monitored, while levels were not measured in the second group. Only 2.3% of patients were potentially cured as a result of CEA monitoring. A comparable 2% of patients without CEA monitoring were also cured of recurrent disease. Such results have led to questioning the often intensive and expensive postoperative monitoring that benefits an extremely small number of patients (45,50).

Intraluminal recurrence is uncommon and is often a subtle manifestation of a large extraluminal recurrence that cannot be identified endoscopically until it grows into the lumen. The recurrence at the suture line often manifests later than the extraluminal recurrence (46). Endoscopic ultrasound may be useful in evaluating such recurrences.

In addition to standard examinations such as CT scan, barium enema, and colonoscopy, immunoscintigraphy has shown some promise as a means of localizing recurrent disease. Immunoscintigraphy consists of intravenous injection of a radio-labelled, tumor-specific monoclonal antibody, which allows visualization with nuclear medicine cameras (51). It may be helpful in the difficult scenario of an elevated serum CEA without any recurrence detected using conventional diagnostic modalities (52).

Another diagnostic modality being investigated is positron emission tomography (PET). One study has shown it to have greater than 90% sensitivity in detecting both hepatic metastases and recurrent cancer at other sites. This was superior to CT scans, which had a sensitivity between 55% and 70% (53).

In many studies, resection of local recurrence has not resulted in cure, but survival has been prolonged by resection either alone or combined with intraoperative radiation (46,54).

Surgery for Metastatic Disease

Fifty percent of patients with colon cancer will develop metastatic disease, 60% of which will be liver metastases (55). Hepatic metastases occur in a somewhat predictable pattern. Right-sided colon cancers more frequently involve the right lobe of the liver, while left-sided colon cancers metastasize equally to both lobes of the liver (56). Resection of hepatic metastases is typically performed when there are three or fewer metastases in the liver, without evidence of extrahepatic disease. Patients with higher CEA levels prior to hepatic resection have a better survival rate following resection (57). In a review of 74 patients undergoing hepatic resection for metastatic disease, the mortality rate was 7%, and survival rates were 24% at 5 years and 12% at 10 years. There were significant correlations between survival and (a) the number of metastases, (b) unilobular versus bilobular disease, and (c) the extent of resection performed (58). While hepatic resection has a significant mortality rate in itself, substantial survival can be achieved, and surgery offers the only chance of cure (Table 16-4).

Hepatic resection for metastatic colorectal cancer has traditionally been delayed. A repeat CT scan is done several months after the colon resection to determine the extent of disease, and hepatic resection is performed, if the disease fits criteria for resection. The delay is to allow the level of tumor aggressiveness to become apparent, since there can be micrometastases in the liver at the time of colon resection that might not become apparent for some time. On the other hand, some surgeons perform resection of small, peripheral liver metastases at the time of colon resection.

Cryosurgery, a newer treatment option for liver metastases, is potentially curative for patients with otherwise unresectable disease that is confined to the liver. It involves rapid freezing with liquid nitrogen, followed by a slow thaw. Cryosurgery can be used in patients with multiple, bilobular, and even centrally located lesions. Survival rates following cryosurgery are reported to be similar to those of hepatic resection (55).

Resection of metastatic disease in the lung can also prolong survival, and in some cases, result in cure. In one review of pulmonary metastases, the chest x-ray was abnormal in over 90% of patients, and serum CEA levels were elevated in nearly 50% of patients. Resection of these metastases, both solitary and multiple, is effective in improving survival rates, with a 5-year survival rate of 40% in one series (59).

Resection of extensive peritoneal seeding has been combined with hyperthermic, intraperitoneal chemotherapy, resulting in complications in over a third of patients. This treatment remains experimental (60).

Medical Treatment of Metastatic Disease

Since the late 1950s, 5-FU has been the most effective agent for metastatic colon cancer. As a single agent, however, its response rate is only 11%. When 5-FU was combined with either leucovorin or folinic acid, there was improvement in response rates. For disease resistant to these agents, second-line treatments such as irinotecan (CPT-11), oxaliplatin, and even monoclonal antibodies are being developed (61,62). CPT-11 arrests DNA replication by binding the enzyme topoisomerase I (63).

Hepatic artery infusion chemotherapy for unresectable liver metastases, while making good intuitive sense, has not resulted in much improvement in survival compared to systemic chemotherapy (64–66), and has been aborted in many patients because of a high rate of peptic ulcer disease and hepatotoxicity (65). For these reasons, this treatment is not recommended outside of investigational protocols.

GENE THERAPY

The most promising treatment of the future is gene therapy, which has already been performed in its crudest form as bone marrow transplants. While successful in vitro transfer of genes in colon cancer patients cannot yet be done, there are many possible strategies (Table 16-5) (67). Ideally, gene ther-

TABLE 16–4. *Survival after hepatic resection for colorectal metastases*

Study, year	No. of patients	Five-year survival rates (%)	Operative mortality rates (%)
Hughes, 1989	800	32	NA
Foster, 1981	231	23	6
Scheele, 1990	219	39	5.5
Adson, 1984	141	25	4
van Ooijen, 1992	118	21	7.6
Savage, 1992	104	18	NA
Iwatsuki, 1989	86	38	0
Nordlinger, 1987	80	25	5

Adapted from McMasters and Edwards (55).

TABLE 16–5. *Approaches to gene therapy in cancer*

Increase tumor immunogenicity
Increase immune system function against tumor
Block oncogene activity
Insert normal-functioning suppressor gene

Adapted from Schmidt-Wolf and Schmidt-Wolf (67).

apy would eliminate defective genes and replace them with normal genes. Genes are transferred into cells by genetically engineered viruses, liposomes, or binding molecules. Retroviruses have been used most commonly (68).

CONCLUSION

Colon cancer is a common problem, but little progress has been made in treatment in the past several decades. The greatest opportunities for further advances seem to lie in prevention, early detection with surgical resection, and gene therapy. Given the enormous financial resources used to treat patients with advanced colon cancer, a more widespread institution of screening programs could be administered, which would enable surgeons to cure many more patients with early stage colon cancer. Early treatment of such cancers would likely be less expensive overall. The deterrents to early detection of colon cancer are a combination of physician and public awareness, financial allocation, and patient compliance. Screening guidelines must not only be utilized by well-informed surgeons and gastroenterologists, but more importantly, by primary care physicians who have frequent contact with their patients.

REFERENCES

1. Link KH, Staib L, Kreuser E, Begar HG. Adjuvant treatment of colon and rectal cancer: impact of chemotherapy, radiotherapy, and immunotherapy on routine postsurgical patient management. *Recent Results Cancer Res* 1996;142:311.
2. Giovannucci E, Rimm EB, Stampfer MJ, et al. A prospective study of cigarette smoking and risk of colorectal adenoma and colorectal cancer in U.S. men. *J Natl Cancer Inst* 1994;86:183.
3. Thun M, Namboodiri M, Heath C. Aspirin use and reduced risk of fatal colon cancer. *N Engl J Med* 1991;325:23.
4. Calle EE, Miracle-McMahill HL, Thun MJ, Heath CW. Estrogen replacement therapy and risk of fatal colon cancer in a prospective cohort of postmenopausal women. *J Natl Cancer Inst* 1995;87:517.
5. Winawer SJ, Fletcher RH, Miller L, et al. Colorectal cancer screening: clinical guidelines and rationale. *Gastroenterology* 1997;112:594.
6. Lynch HT, Smyrk T, Watson P, et al. Hereditary colon cancer. *Semin Oncol* 1991;18:337.
7. Vasen HF, Wijnen JT, Menko FH, et al. Cancer risk in families with hereditary nonpolyposis colorectal cancer diagnosed by mutation analysis. *Gastroenterology* 1996;110:1020.
8. Tsiotou AG, Krespis EN, Sakorafas GH, Krespi AE. The genetic basis of colorectal cancer—clinical implications. *Eur J Surg Oncol* 1995;21:96.
9. Villa E, Dugani A, Rebecchi AM, et al. Identification of subjects at risk for colorectal carcinoma through a test based on *K-ras* determination in the stool. *Gastroenterology* 1996;110:1346.
10. Mandel JS, Bond JH, Church TR, et al. Reducing mortality from colorectal cancer by screening for fecal occult blood. *N Engl J Med* 1993;328:1365.
11. Smith LE. The fecal occult blood testing controversy. *Dis Colon Rectum* 1993;36:799.
12. Rex DK, Rahmani EY, Haseman JH, Lemmel GT, Kaster S, Buckley JS. Relative sensitivity of colonoscopy and barium enema for detection of colorectal cancer in clinical practice. *Gastroenterology* 1997;112:117.
13. Lieberman D. Cost-effectiveness of colon cancer screening. *Gastroenterology* 1995;86:1789.
14. Rex DK, Mark D, Clarke B, Lappas JC, Lehman G. Flexible sigmoidoscopy plus air-contrast barium enema versus colonoscopy for evaluation of symptomatic patients without evidence of bleeding. *Gastrointest Endosc* 1995;42:132.
15. Fischer KS, Zamboni WA, Ross DS. The efficacy of preoperative computed tomography in patients with colorectal carcinoma. *Am Surg* 1990;56:339.
16. Moertel CG, Fleming TR, Macdonald JS, Haller DG, Laurie JA, Tangen C. An evaluation of the carcinoembryonic antigen test for monitoring patients with resected colon cancer. *JAMA* 1993;270:943.
17. Evers BM, Mullins RJ, Matthews TH, Broghamer WL, Polk HC Jr. Multiple adenocarcinomas of the colon and rectum: an analysis of incidences and current trends. *Dis Colon Rectum* 1988;31:518.
18. Cho E, Nakajima M, Yasuda K, Ashihara T, Kawai K. Endoscopic ultrasonography in the diagnosis of colorectal cancer invasion. *Gastrointest Endosc* 1993;39:521.
19. Nogueras JJ, Jagelman DG. Colorectal cancer: principles of surgical resection. *Surg Clin North Am* 1993;73:103.
20. McGinnis LS. Surgical treatment options for colorectal cancer. *Cancer* 1994;74:2147.
21. Rouffet F, Hay JM, Vacher B, et al. Curative resection for left colonic carcinoma: hemicolectomy vs. segmental colectomy. *Dis Colon Rectum* 1994;37:651.
22. Ota D. Laparoscopic colon resection for cancer. *Adv Surg* 1996;29:141.
23. Turnbull RB, Kyle K, Watson FR, Spratt J. Cancer of the colon: the influence of the "no-touch isolation" technique on survival rates. *Ann Surg* 1967;166:420.
24. Wiggers T, Jeekel J, Arends JW, et al. No-touch isolation technique in colon cancer: a controlled prospective trial. *Br J Surg* 1988;75:409.
25. Garrison RN, Shively EH, Baker C, Steele M, Trunkey D, Polk HC Jr. Evaluation of management of the emergency right hemicolectomy. *J Trauma* 1979;19:734.
26. McGregor JR, O'Dwyer JO. The surgical management of obstruction and perforation of the left colon. *Surg Gynecol Obstet* 1993;177:203.
27. Biondo S, Jaurrieta E, Jorba R, et al. Intraoperative colonic lavage and primary anastomosis in peritonitis and obstruction. *Br J Surg* 1997;84:222.
28. Kriwanek S, Armbruster C, Dittrich K, Beckerhinn P. Perforated colorectal cancer. *Dis Colon Rectum* 1996;39:1409.
29. Lee PY, Fletcher WS, Sullivan ES, Vetto JT. Colorectal cancer in young patients: characteristics and outcome. *Am Surg* 1994;60:607.
30. Cote RJ, Houchens DP, Hitchcock CL, et al. Intraoperative detection of occult colon cancer micrometastases using 125 I-radiolabeled monoclonal antibody CC49. *Cancer* 1996;77:613.
31. Bessler M, Whelan RL, Halverson A, Allendorf JDF, Nowygrod R, Treat MR. Controlled trial of laparoscopic-assisted vs. open colon resection in a porcine model. *Surg Endosc* 1996;10:732.
32. Pfeifer J, Wexner SD, Reissman P, et al. Laparoscopic vs. open colon surgery. *Surg Endosc* 1995;9:1322.
33. Johnstone P, Rohde DC, Swartz SE, Fetter JE, Wexner SD. Port site recurrences after laparoscopic and thoracoscopic procedures in malignancy. *J Clin Oncol* 1996;14:1950.
34. Wexner SD, Cohen SM, Ulrich A, Reissman P. Laparoscopic colorectal surgery—are we being honest with our patients? *Dis Colon Rectum* 1995;38:724.
35. Busch OR, Hop WC, Hoynck van Papendrecht MA, Marquet RL, Jeekel J. Blood transfusions and prognosis in colorectal cancer. *N Engl J Med* 1993;328:1372.
36. Vente JP, Wiggers T, Weidema WF, Jeekel J, Obertop H. Peri-operative blood transfusions in colorectal cancer. *Eur J Surg Oncol* 1989;15:371.
37. Binderow SR, Cohen SM, Wexner SD, Nogueras JJ. Must early postoperative oral intake be limited to laparoscopy. *Dis Colon Rectum* 1994;37:584.
38. Reissman P, Teoh TA, Cohen SM, Weiss EG, Nogueras JJ, Wexner SD. Is early oral feeding safe after elective colorectal surgery? *Ann Surg* 1995;222:73.
39. Ritchie J. Mass peristalsis in the human colon after contact with oxyphenisatin. *Gut* 1970;11:91.
40. Francini G, Petrioli R, Lorenzini L, et al. Folinic acid and 5-fluorouracil as adjuvant chemotherapy in colon cancer. *Gastroenterology* 1994;106:899.
41. Moertel CG, Fleming TR, Macdonald JS, et al. Flourouracil plus levamisole as effective adjuvant therapy after resection of stage III colon carcinoma: a final report. *Ann Intern Med* 1995;122:321.
42. Haller DG. An overview of adjuvant therapy for colorectal cancer. *Eur J Cancer* 1995;31:1255.
43. Hoover HC Jr, Brandhorst JS, Peters LC, et al. Adjuvant active specific immunotherapy for human colorectal cancer. *J Clin Oncol* 1993;11:390.
44. Pervin S, Chakraborty M, Bhattacharya-Chatterjee M, Zeytin H, Foon KA, Chatterjee SK. Induction of antitumor immunity by an anti-idiotype antibody mimicking carcinoembryonic antigen. *Cancer Res* 1997;57:728.

45. Ohlsson B, Breland U, Ekberg H, Graffner H, Tranberg KG. Follow-up after curative surgery for colorectal carcinoma. *Dis Colon Rectum* 1995;38:620.

46. Gwin JL, Hoffman JP, Eisenberg BL. Surgical management of non-hepatic intra-abdominal recurrence of carcinoma of the colon. *Dis Colon Rectum* 1993;36:540.

47. McCall JL, Black RB, Rich CA, et al. The value of serum carcino-embryonic antigen in predicting recurrent disease following curative resection of colorectal cancer. *Dis Colon Rectum* 1994;37:875.

48. Fielding LP, Pettigrew N. College of American Pathologists Conference XXVI on clinical relevance of prognostic markers in solid tumors: report of the colorectal cancer working group. *Arch Pathol Lab Med* 1995;119:1115.

49. Galandiuk S, Wieand HS, Moertel CG, et al. Patterns of recurrence after curative resection of carcinoma of the colon and rectum. *Surg Gynecol Obstet* 1992;174:27.

50. Makela JT, Laitinen SO, Kairaluoma MI. Five-year follow-up after radical surgery for colorectal cancer. *Arch Surg* 1995;130:1062.

51. Corman ML, Galandiuk S, Block GE, et al. Immunoscintigraphy with ^{111}In-Satumomab pendetide in patients with colorectal adenocarcinoma: performance and impact on clinical management. *Dis Colon Rectum* 1994;37:129.

52. Galandiuk S. Immunoscintigraphy in the surgical management of colorectal cancer. *J Nucl Med* 1993;34:541.

53. Ogunbiyi O, Flanagan F, Dehdashti F, et al. Staging of recurrent and metastatic colorectal cancer: comparison of positron emission tomography and CT. Presented at Annual Cancer Symposium of Society for Surgical Oncology, Chicago, March 20–23, 1997.

54. Polk HC Jr, Spratt JS. Recurrent cancer of the colon. *Surg Clin North Am* 1983;63:151.

55. McMasters KM, Edwards MJ. Liver cryosurgery: a potentially curative treatment option for patients with unresectable disease. *J Ky Med Assoc* 1996;94:222.

56. Shirai Y, Wakai T, Ohtani T, Sakai Y, Tsukada K, Hatakeyama K. Colorectal carcinoma metastases to the liver: does primary tumor location affect its lobar distribution? *Cancer* 1996;77:2213.

57. Wang JY, Chiang JM, Jeng LB, Changchien CR, Chen JS, Hsu KC. Resection of liver metastases from colorectal cancer: are there any truly significant clinical prognosticators? *Dis Colon Rectum* 1996;39:847.

58. Wanebo, HJ, Chu QD, Vezeridis MP, Soderberg C. Patient selection for hepatic resection of colorectal metastases. *Arch Surg* 1996;131:322.

59. McCormack PM, Burt ME, Bains MS, Martini N, Rusch VW, Ginsberg RJ. Lung resection for colorectal metastases: 10-year results. *Arch Surg* 1992;127:1403.

60. Jacquet P, Stephens AD, Averbach AM, et al. Analysis of morbidity and mortality in 60 patients with peritoneal carcinomatosis treated by cytoreductive surgery and heated intraoperative intraperitoneal chemotherapy. *Cancer* 1996;77:2622.

61. Bleiberg H. Role of chemotherapy for advanced colorectal. cancer: new opportunities. *Semin Oncol* 1996;23:42.

62. Kemeny N. Colorectal cancer—an undertreated disease. *Anticancer Drugs* 1996;7:623.

63. Rivory LP. Irinotecan (CPT-11): a brief overview. *Clin Exp Pharmacol Physiol* 1996;23:1000.

64. Vauthey JN, Marsh R, Cendan JC, Chu NM, Copeland EM. Arterial therapy of hepatic colorectal metastases. *Br J Surg* 1996;83:447.

65. Ogata Y, Shirouzu K, Akagi Y, Hiraki M, Isomoto H. Hepatic arterial chemotherapy for liver metastases from colorectal cancer. *Kurume Med J* 1996;43:41.

66. Sutanto-Ward E, Arisawa Y, Tremiterra S, Sigurdson ER. Regional chemotherapy for colorectal hepatic metastases: evidence for improved survival with new drug combinations. *Ann Surg Oncol* 1996;3:36.

67. Schmidt-Wolf GD, Schmidt-Wolf IG. Cancer and gene therapy. *Ann Hematol* 1996;73:207.

68. Mastrangelo MJ, Berd D, Nathan FE, Lattime EC. Gene therapy for human cancer: an essay for clinicians. *Semin Oncol* 1996;23:4.

CHAPTER 17

Rectal Cancer

Joseph P. Muldoon

Rectal cancer will be diagnosed in approximately 36,000 people in the United States in 1998 (1). This is a serious health concern in North America and Europe, especially since cure rates are only 50% after resection. Although histologically similar to colon cancer, rectal cancer is best considered separately because of several factors: (a) the rectum is located within the tight confines of the pelvis and below the peritoneal reflection, (b) it is surgically accessible through the abdomen or the perineum because of the distal location, and (c) there is a higher propensity for local recurrence, with devastating implications on the patient's quality of life.

The surgeon's approach to rectal cancer continues to evolve. New technologies have allowed for better preoperative staging and better surgical decision making. The approach to mid and distal rectal cancers is becoming more controversial, with emphasis on sphincter preservation, in appropriate circumstances. The place for preoperative versus postoperative adjuvant therapies is a debated topic.

PRESENTATION

Rectal bleeding is the most common initial symptom bringing the patient with rectal cancer to medical attention. This bleeding is usually red in color, sometimes coating the stool, usually occurs with or shortly after bowel movements, and is of small to moderate amounts. The patients may also note progressive decrease in stool caliber, feeling of incomplete evacuation of stool, and/or anal mucous seepage. Pelvic or coccygeal pain, tenesmus, obstruction, and weight loss are symptoms seen in advanced disease. Often times, patients are referred to the surgeon with a diagnosis of rectal cancer, but not infrequently the referral is for treatment of bleeding hemorrhoids, reaffirming the importance of digital rectal and proctoscopic/sigmoidoscopic examinations of these patients.

EVALUATION

Physical examination begins with a general examination to evaluate for concurrent illnesses and to look for evidence of metastatic disease such as jaundice, lymphadenopathy, hepa-

tomegaly, or ascites. A thorough evaluation of the anorectum should be performed. Digital examination is especially helpful in low cancers for estimating distance from the anal verge, mobility, anterior or posterior location, and texture of the tumor. When performed by an experienced examiner, depth of rectal wall penetration can be accurately assessed in 75% to 80% of the cases (2). Anoscopy allows evaluation of the anal canal, exposing very low tumors abutting the anal canal. Proctoscopy can visualize the tumor and facilitate biopsy, and is an accurate method for measuring the distance of the cancer from the dentate line as well as the percentage of wall circumference involved by the tumor.

Because synchronous colon cancer is reported in up to 6% of patients with colorectal cancer, all of these patients require full evaluation of the colon by colonoscopy or barium enema if possible. Patients with obstructing or near obstructing lesions sometimes cannot be evaluated with these tests initially.

Blood tests important in the evaluation include complete blood count, serum electrolytes, and liver function tests, including serum bilirubin, alkaline phosphatase, AST, and ALT. Serum carcinoembrionic antigen levels should be drawn preoperatively. All patients should undergo a chest x-ray to rule out pulmonary metastases.

Other tests used in the preoperative evaluation of rectal cancer include computed tomography (CT) scan, magnetic resonance imaging (MRI), and transrectal ultrasound (TRUS).

Computed Tomography

CT of the abdomen and pelvis should be performed on all patients with rectal cancer, preoperatively, looking for evidence of metastatic disease and to evaluate the extent of local disease. It is considered accurate in the diagnosis of liver metastases, especially those greater than 1.5 cm. Studies by Williams et al. (3) demonstrated 97% accuracy, when assessed at laparotomy, for hepatic metastases greater than 1.5 cm. This accuracy drops off significantly, however, when the lesions are less than 1.5 cm. New helical CT scanners allow for biphasic and triphasic intravenous contrast evaluations of the liver. Evaluation of the liver is performed during the arterial contrast and venous contrast phases, optimizing the sensitivity of the test. If suspicious hepatic lesions are identified, biopsy can also be performed with CT guidance to confirm the diagnosis in appropriate cases.

The accuracy of CT scan for evaluation of local disease, including depth of rectal wall penetration (T stage) and presence of lymph node metastases, is not as good (33% to 83%). Shank et al. (4) prospectively evaluated the accuracy of preoperative locoregional staging. When separate radiologists staged the tumors by CT scan alone, interobserver agreement was only 37%. Indeed when the same observer studied the same subject twice at different times, the agreement between readings was only 51%. Overall agreement with Duke's stage was only 33%. The inability to accurately diagnose lymph node metastases has been demonstrated in several studies (5,6). Patients considered for sphincter-preserving operations, especially local resection, should undergo further testing, including endorectal ultrasound.

Endorectal Ultrasound

To assess the extent of local disease, endorectal ultrasound is the most accurate and cost effective modality. Using a 7.5- to 10-MHz transducer, excellent visualization of the layers of the rectal wall can be obtained. Depth of rectal wall penetration can accurately be predicted in 85% to 90% of patients when the test is performed by an experienced operator (7). Evaluation of lymph nodes is less impressive, but is superior to CT and MRI. Hildebrant et al. (8) demonstrated accuracy in diagnosing lymph node metastases in 72% versus lymph node inflammation with specificity of 83%. Because there is often difficulty in interpretation, conservative judgment of lymph node disease is appropriate (9).

Proper technique and operator experience are the keys to reliable preoperative staging. Use of a proctoscope for precise placement of the probe is recommended. It should be noted that this modality is much less accurate in determining rectal wall penetration if the patient has undergone radiation therapy.

Magnetic Resonance Imaging

MRI with the use of endorectal surface coil is being examined as a modality for preoperative evaluation of local disease. It appears that this method is accurate in estimating rectal wall penetration. Limitations in its ability to diagnose lymph node metastases make it no better, at this time, than CT. Availability of this test and expense make endorectal ultrasound a more viable option for now.

MANAGEMENT

The optimal management of patients with rectal cancer requires a team approach, which includes surgeon, radiation oncologist, and medical oncologist. After an appropriate preoperative work-up, the treatment plan best suited to the indi-

vidual patient can be implemented. Surgery remains the mainstay in the treatment of rectal cancer and in early cancers may be all that is needed. The primary goal of curing the patient is closely followed by attempts at sphincter preservation. The use of adjuvant therapies, including radiation and chemotherapy, is often essential in achieving these goals, but the timing of these therapies is often physician and patient dependent.

OPERATIVE MANAGEMENT

The location and stage of the tumor determine the operative management of rectal cancer. For ease of discussion the rectum will be divided into thirds. The rectum 12 to 16 cm from the anal verge is the upper third; 7 to 12 cm is the middle third; and less than 7 cm from the anal verge represents the distal third of the rectum. Rectal cancer involving the upper third of the rectum, or the rectum above the peritoneal reflection, is best treated by anterior resection in the majority of cases. Polyps containing early carcinomas or superficial cancers can sometimes be removed locally using transanal endoscopic microsurgery or endoscopic snaring. Cancers of the mid and distal rectum are more controversial and the operative choices in this area require more detailed discussion. In this discussion we will emphasize sphincter-preserving operations (Fig. 17-1).

Operative Procedures

Abdominoperineal Resection

Abdominoperineal resection (APR) has long been considered the gold standard for treatment of rectal cancers below 8 cm. This idea is being challenged by many surgeons who are demonstrating that sphincter preservation can be achieved on tumors less than 8 cm from the anal verge with equal oncologic efficacy (10,11). Abdominoperineal resection remains an important operation in selected patients with rectal cancers. Patients with rectal cancers involving the levator muscles or sphincter muscles have an absolute indication for APR, unless they are medically unable to undergo the operation. Patients with low bulky tumors, cancers within 8 cm of the anal verge in patients with poor sphincter function, and patients with low tumors and are bed ridden, are usually best treated by APR as opposed to sphincter-preserving operations. Preoperative marking of the stoma site should be performed in all these patients to ensure optimization of patient comfort and accessibility.

Low Anterior Resection With Sphincter Preservation

Low anterior resection (LAR) has replaced abdominoperineal resection as the primary surgical approach to rectal cancer. To justify using sphincter-preserving operations for low rectal cancers, it had to be proven that the oncologic principles of the operation were not compromised, that the procedures could be performed safely, and that functional results were preferable to patients when compared to APR.

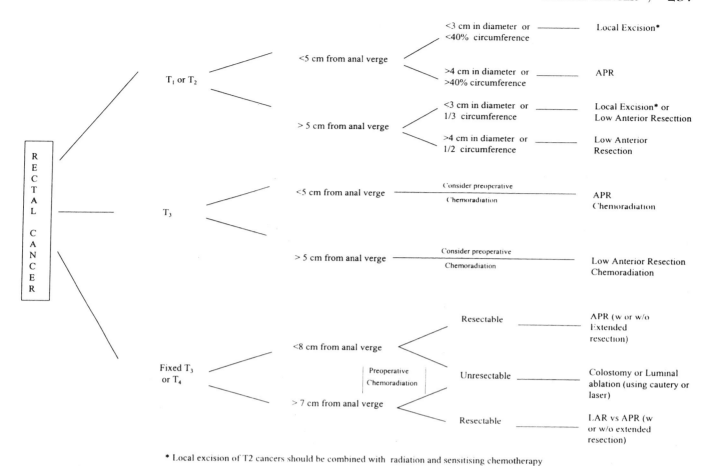

FIG. 17-1. Algorithm of the treatment of rectal cancer.

The goal of resection is removal of all local disease. Better understanding of the routes of tumor spread in rectal cancer has guided present recommendations for resection margins. Two main routes of spread are defined: (a) to the lymph nodes, proximally, which travel with the arterial supply, and (b) laterally, into the mesorectum and perirectal soft tissues. The techniques of pelvic dissection for the removal of rectal cancer are discussed elsewhere in this volume. An emphasis on adequate resection margins, including total mesorectal excision, without coning down on the rectum, will remove the likelihood of leaving tumor bearing mesorectal tissue behind. Autonomic nerve preservation is an important part of the technique because this significantly decreases the incidence of bladder and sexual dysfunction postoperatively. Using these techniques, oncologic principles of resection can be maintained using LAR.

After a thorough exploration of the abdomen and pelvis, the proximal extent of resection is determined. Most commonly, the bowel is divided at the distal descending or proximal sigmoid colon. The sigmoid colon can be used if the luminal diameter is adequate and there is not excessive muscular hypertrophy or diverticuli. The arterial supply is divided just distal to the left colic artery because prospective trials have not demonstrated benefit from high ligation of the infe-

rior mesenteric artery (12). The splenic flexure must always be mobilized to establish adequate length for a tension-free anastamosis. When length is still not adequate, the left colic artery and inferior mesenteric vein can be divided to gain additional length. The distal extent of the resection should include a minimum of 2 cm of normal rectum (preferably 3 to 4 cm) beyond the tumor. Williams et al demonstrated that intramural tumor spread rarely extends beyond 1 cm distally (13). Therefore, selected patients with cancers as low as 5 cm from the anal verge may be treated with LAR.

The use of stapling devices has greatly facilitated the creation of low anastamoses. Using a double stapling technique, anastamoses at the level of the levator muscles can safely be performed. A limitation on the use of stapling devices for low anastamoses is the patient with the deep and narrow pelvis. Intraoperative maneuvers, including the application of pressure on the perineum from below and the use of stapling devices with roticulating heads, minimizes this problem. Using these techniques, the distal line of transection can be placed within 2 cm of the dentate line. If preferred, the surgeon can perform a mucosal stripping of the residual distal colonic mucosa from a perineal approach and proceed with a colonic pull-through and handsewn anastamosis.

When a very low anterior anastamosis or coloanal anastamosis is performed, one should consider a diverting ileostomy or transverse colostomy. This will protect against a postoperative leak and can be taken down 6 to 12 weeks after surgery when the anastamosis is well healed. This is especially pertinent in patients who have received preoperative radiation. Because transverse loop colostomies are difficult to manage and bulky, a diverting loop ileostomy is recommended.

Patient Selection for Performing Sphincter-Preserving Resections

The distance of the tumor from the anal verge is the single most important determining factor in the selection of patients for these procedures. Tumors 6 cm or more from the anal verge can almost always be resected with restoration of intestinal continuity. Using present techniques, mobile tumors located 5 cm from the verge can be resected with sphincter preservation. Gross invasion of the anal sphincter complex or levator muscles precludes the performance of LAR.

Bulky tumors and those tumors with circumferential involvement may make attempts at sphincter preservation difficult and ill advised. The decision again is often reliant on the distance of the tumor from the anal verge. Body habitus may effect the ability to perform LAR. Obese patients, those with a narrow pelvis, and patients with an enlarged prostate may pose a significant technical challenge. Patients with poor sphincter function preoperatively are poor candidates for these procedures. Patients who are bed ridden may be better served by APR with end colostomy. Because of the 6–12 mo period of adaptation and initial functional results, patients with short life expectancies may be better served with a colostomy.

Functional Results of LAR with Coloanal Anastamosis

Although these sphincter-preserving techniques are possible in the majority of patients with rectal cancers, the functional outcomes of these procedures is often initially less than ideal. Stool frequency and incontinence to varying degrees result in significant morbidity and patient frustration. Several authors have demonstrated that functional outcome worsens as the anastamosis is performed more distally, with anastamoses within 6 cm of the anal verge having demonstrably poorer function (14). The reason for the worsened functional results is the decreased capacity of the neorectum and reduced resting anal pressures seen after these operations. Functional results are worst during the first year after surgery, with gradual improvement over the initial 9 months. This improvement is secondary to increasing capacity of the neorectum over time.

The functional results of these low anastamoses appear to be improved by the construction of a colonic J pouch. The J pouch is constructed using a GIA stapler to create a 5- to 10-cm pouch. This is then either anastamosed above the anal sphincters using an EEA stapler or handsewn from below after pulling the pouch through the anal canal. Follow-up studies are still forthcoming on this technique, but there appear to be better continence scores in those patients with colonic J pouches when compared to straight coloanal anastamoses (15).

The length of the J pouch may have an effect on long term functional results. Parc et al. (16) reported a series of 24 patients who underwent very low anastamoses with construction of 12-cm J pouches. One quarter of these patients had difficulty with incomplete evacuation and spontaneous defecation thereby becoming reliant on suppositories and enemas to induce defecation. Because of this experience, Parc has reduced the size of the pouches to 6 cm. Hida et al. (17) compared patients in whom a 5-cm versus a 10-cm pouch had been constructed. They found that the 5-cm J pouch provided adequate reservoir function without compromising evacuation.

Evaluation of the patient's anal sphincter function preoperatively is important if low anastamosis is considered. This can usually be assessed by digital examination, though those patients with a borderline exam and mild incontinence symptoms should undergo anal manometry. Those with poor sphincter function are best treated by APR and end colostomy.

Overall, patient satisfaction is high after sphincter-preserving operations for rectal cancer. Despite an often initially difficult adjustment period, functional results improve over a period of months. There is variability of stool frequency, but most patients have three or less bowel movements per day. Minor soiling and gas incontinence occur in 10% to 40% of patients, and some patients require protective pads. Most patients gladly accept these results when offered the alternative of APR.

Local Excision for Rectal Cancer

Some cancers involving the lower rectum are amenable to local excision via a variety of approaches. Initial investigation of this possibility was done by Morson et al. (18) and has recently been studied prospectively by Bleday and Ota (19,20). This modality is reserved for a select group, comprising approximately 5% to 15% of patients with rectal cancer. Good results are dependent on accurate patient selection. Several factors, including T stage, presence of lymph node metastases, tumor size, and histological characteristics of the tumor, must be considered (Table 17-1).

Patients with T_1 rectal cancers that are completely excised with adequate margins require no further treatment. Those undergoing local resection for T_2 lesions should be offered radiation with chemotherapy, while patients found to have T_3 tumors on pathologic examination should be urged to undergo a formal resection (low anterior with/without coloanal anastamosis, or abdominoperineal resection). These recommendations are founded on pathology studies reporting the incidence of lymph node metastases in up to 20% of patients with T_2 tumors. Local failure rates reported by Minsky after local resection and radiation averaged 3% (T_1), 10% (T_2), and 24% (T_3) (21). In Bleday's study, recurrence was associated with positive margins following resection, and lymphatic invasion (19). Forty-eight patients were studied (21 T_1, 21 T_2, and five T_3) with an overall recurrence rate of 8%.

TABLE 17–1. *Characteristics of rectal cancers amenable to local excision*

Characteristics	Yes	No
T stage	T_1 and T_2[a]	T_3 and T_4
Lymph node status	N0	Evidence of hypoechoic LN's on TRUS
Size	<3 cm or <40% rectal circumference	>3 cm or 40% of circumference
Gross examination	Mobile, not ulcerated	Fixed, ulcerated
Histology	Well and moderately differentiated	Poorly differentiated, >60% mucinous histology, lymphatic or angioinvasion
Location	Proximal extent <8 cm for anal verge	
Patient characteristics	Poor health risk; patient refuses abdominal surgery or colostomy	

[a]Local resection of T_2 cancers should be combined with radiation and/or chemotherapy.

Local Excision

The techniques used for local excision of rectal tumors include transanal, transsphincteric, and transcoccygeal approaches. The approach used is dependent upon tumor location, presence of anal stricture, and physician preference. All patients should undergo a full mechanical and antibiotic bowel preparation, and we administer intravenous antibiotics (cefoxitin) before surgery. These procedures can be performed under general or regional anesthesia depending upon patient and physician preference. Positioning of the patient is dependent upon tumor location. The lithotomy position is preferred for posterior tumors, while the prone jackknife position is used for anterior tumors and patients undergoing resection using the transcoccygeal approach.

The transanal approach is the approach used in the majority of patients. With adequate anesthesia and the available anal retractors, most tumors of the lower rectum can be resected transanally. Using this approach also minimizes the likelihood of complications such as fistula and incontinence which are more commonly seen with the transcoccygeal and transsphincteric approaches.

After the anus is manually dilated, anal retractors are placed to expose the tumor. The margins of resection are scored with the electrocautery. Margins should include 1 cm or more of normal rectum around the tumor. Stay sutures are placed proximally above the lesion. The lesion is then removed with the full thickness of rectal wall, exposing perirectal fat. Hemostasis is secured with electrocautery, the specimen is oriented and margins can be sent for frozen section to assess adequacy of margins. The rectal wall is then reapproximated transversely using interrupted absorbable sutures. All patients should be proctoscoped after completion of the case to ensure adequate luminal diameter.

Posterior approaches were commonly used procedures, but with improved anal retractors, new technologies, and the safety of transabdominal surgeries, these approaches are falling from favor. The transcoccygeal approach as described by Kraske is performed through a posterior approach and involves removal of the coccyx and a posterior proctotomy. This approach allows for excellent exposure, especially for anterior tumors (22). The postoperative complications of this approach make it less appealing than the transanal approach. Posterior fecal fistula and wound infections occur with a reported incidence of 2% to 29%, and significant postoperative pain syndromes are reported (23).

The transsphincteric or York-Mason approach requires complete transection of the anal sphincter complex for exposure (24). Like the transcoccygeal approach the exposure is excellent, but the risk of incontinence postoperatively makes this approach less attractive then transanal excision.

Transendoscopic Microsurgery

Transendoscopic microsurgery (TEM) is a form of minimal access surgery, performed through a transanal route, utilizing specialized instruments and stereoscopic optics. It follows the same principles and indications as the more traditional transanal surgery described above. The benefit of this technology is that it expands the boundaries of the traditional procedures to the level of the rectosigmoid region. The principles of local resection should be the same as the more conventional techniques previously mentioned and therefore provide equivalent results. Special training in these techniques and the expense of the instruments, coupled with the relative small percentage of rectal cancers amenable to local resection, make this technology beneficial to only a few surgeons within a practicing community.

Fulgaration and Local Destruction

In select cases, local destruction of rectal cancers is warranted. Patients with short life expectancy or inability to survive a major resection because of severe cardiac or pulmonary disease may be candidates. Most commonly, electrofulgaration is used, but the same results can be obtained with lasers. To be effective, full-thickness destruction of the tumor must be effected.

ADJUVANT THERAPIES

Radiation

Radiation therapy is an important adjuvant therapy in the treatment of rectal cancer. Potential benefits of adjuvant radiation include improved locoregional control; and improved resectability of large bulky tumors and those fixed to adjacent structures, possibly providing negative margins during a curative resection. Although controversial, it may improve long-term survival.

Selection of patients who will benefit from adjuvant radiation include patients with advanced T stage T_3 or T_4, which carry a 20% and 50% recurrence rate, respectively, when treated with surgery alone and patients with lymph node metastases (20% local recurrence rate when treated with surgery alone).

The timing of adjuvant radiation therapy is dependent on patient and physician biases. Most studies have demonstrated improvement in local control with either preoperative or postoperative treatment. Preoperative treatment improves the resectability of some tumors and may decrease the presence of viable cells at the time of resection. When postoperative treatment is chosen, one is assured of treating only those patients who are at high risk of recurrence. The advantages and disadvantages of preoperative versus postoperative radiation for rectal cancer are listed in Table 17-2. An important limitation lies in our ability to accurately stage rectal cancer preoperatively. TRUS is probably the best modality available for establishing the extent of local disease and should be used when considering preoperative radiation in patients who are suspected to have T_2 versus T_3 disease. Evaluation for the presence of lymph node metastases is difficult using present technologies often times proving inaccurate. A conservative approach to patients in whom the findings are equivocal is warranted.

Standard radiation therapy regimens call for 45 to 50 Gy over 5 weeks pre- or postoperatively. These regimens include 5-FU to potentiate the radiation effects. When properly performed, this therapy is well tolerated with low long-term morbidity. The Swedish study group has published data on high dose radiation (25 Gy) delivered in five fractions over 1 week preoperatively followed by surgery (25). They demonstrated significant improvement in local recurrence and overall survival in patients receiving preoperative radiation versus patients undergoing surgery alone. There were no increases in postoperative mortality in these patients (26,27).

Radiation alone has been advocated as treatment for selected, favorable, invasive rectal cancers. Kodner et al. (28) utilized a combination of external beam and endocavitary radiation, and reported local control rates of 93% for ideal lesions. The definition of ideal lesions is similar to those amenable to local excision: T_1 or T_2 lesions that are less than 3 cm in size, with favorable histology. The protocol utilized 4,500 cGy external beam, followed by 6,000 cGy of endocavitary radiation. Local failures in these patients were successfully treated by salvage APR.

Chemotherapy

Chemotherapy has two roles in the treatment of rectal cancer: (a) to eradicate distant micrometastases and (b) to potentiate the effects of radiation therapy on local disease. Indications for the use of adjuvant chemotherapy in rectal cancer include patients with stage II or stage III disease. In a trial that compared radiation alone, 5-FU plus MeCCNU, radiation and 5-FU plus MeCCNU, or surgery alone, there was a significant improvement in overall survival in the group that re-

---

TABLE 17–2. *Advantages and disadvantages of preoperative versus postoperative radiation*

Advantages
  Postoperative
    Accurate tumor staging
    Will not overtreat (<T3N0) patients or patients with disseminated disease found at surgery
    Offers patients immediate surgery
  Preoperative
    Accurate delivery of the maximum dose to the tumor at risk
    Reduced dose requirements in smaller nonadvanced lesions (lower cost/shorter course)
    Complete removal of all irradiated tissue except the distal postanastamotic bowel
    Less likelihood of small bowel fixation and radiation induced injury to the small bowel
    Less likelihood of compromised margins if tumor shrinkage occurs?
    Increased resectability
    Better locoregional control
    Possibly improved survival if given with preoperative chemotherapy
Disadvantages
  Postoperative
    Potentially compromised margins for large bulky tumors fixed to surrounding structures
    Irradiated bowel is left behind
    Decreased fecal reservoir due to radiation fibrosis of the neorectum after sphincter-sparing operations
    Difficulty in screening the small bowel from radiation
    Inability to accurately deliver the radiation to the tumor bed after surgery
  Preoperative
    Delay in surgical therapy (10 weeks for 4,500 cGy or 5 days for 2,000 cGy)
    Potential overtreatment for early or disseminated tumors
    Need for more extensive surgery to remove all radiated bowel proximally
      (removal of sigmoid colon and splenic flexure mobilisation)
    Patient fear of tumor spread during therapy

ceived radiation plus chemotherapy versus those patients receiving surgery alone ($p = 0.01$) (29). The NCCTG demonstrated improvement in 5-year disease-free survival as well as improved local and distant failure rates in patients who received radiation and chemotherapy versus those receiving radiation alone (30). Subsequent evaluation has revealed that MeCCNU does not improve outcome but does significantly increase treatment related toxicity as well as potentially increasing the risk of treatment related leukemias (31). This agent is therefore no longer used in the treatment of rectal cancer. Other agents are being investigated in combination with 5-FU. Leukovorin and 5-FU combinations are most commonly used in the United States at this time. Ongoing studies are investigating the use of 5-FU with radiation versus the addition of leukovorin and/or levamisole to 5-FU and radiation. Further questions to be answered include the method of 5-FU administration, bolus versus continuous infusion, and the timing of the therapy.

The role of preoperative chemoradiation therapy is being explored because of potential benefits, including tumor downstaging and increased resectability rates. Minsky et al. (21) demonstrated improved resectability rates and tumor downstaging with preoperative treatment using 5-FU and leukovorin with radiation. Improvement in local control and 20% complete response rates have been reported by Landry et al. (32). Active trials investigating preoperative chemoradiation include NSABP R-03, the Intergroup 0147, the EORTC study, and the Swedish study group all of which are comparing preoperative chemoradiation with preop radiotherapy alone. Patient accrual has been very poor in the U.S. studies, and there is question as to whether they will be completed. As mentioned previously, patient compliance improves with preoperative therapy and small bowel radiation injury appears to be decreased. Good randomized controlled studies are needed to determine the effect on survival and local recurrence.

Newer anticancer agents are being investigated in the treatment of colon and rectal cancer. Irinotecan (CPT-11) and tomudex are two agents that have shown effective antitumor activity against rectal cancer. These agents as well as others will continue to be investigated in the treatment of rectal cancer. Patients with stage IV disease have not been shown to have a survival benefit from systemic intravenous chemotherapy. Open protocols are available using new combinations and newer agents for patients with stage IV disease.

POSTOPERATIVE MONITORING/SURVEILLANCE

All patients treated for rectal cancer should undergo postoperative surveillance. The selection of follow-up tests and the timing of these tests are controversial. Guidelines for what might be considered an aggressive follow-up protocol are presented in Table 17-3. Digital rectal exam and proctoscopy are probably the best way to diagnose local recurrence in these patients. The aggressive screening with follow-up CEA, CT scans, and blood studies may lead to earlier diagnosis of recurrence but rarely leads to cure for these patients. Therefore, follow-up programs can be individualized depending upon patient and physician preference.

RECURRENT RECTAL CANCER AND METASTATIC DISEASE

Recurrent rectal cancer falls into three groups: (a) patients with local recurrence, (b) patients with metastatic disease, and (c) those with both. Reports of local recurrence rates range from 3% to 30%, representing a significant problem for these patients. With the addition of chemoradiation to the treatment regimen the incidence of local recurrence has decreased but has not been cured. Patients with local recurrence have a 5-year survival rate of 4%, and their final months are often unpleasant because of pain caused by the recurrence. Factors associated with an increased risk for recurrence include (a) Dukes stage (A 9.1%, B 16.7%, C 40.8% after APR, 1962) (33), (b) location of tumor (distal one-third more than upper and middle one-third) (34), (c) presence or absence of venous, lymphatic, or perineural invasion (35), (d) presence of obstruction or perforation (36), and (e) degree of tumor differentiation, ploidy and predominance of mucinous cancer (37). Adequate resection and adjuvant chemoradiation in appropriate cases help to minimize the likelihood of local recurrence and aggressive follow-up will help identify those patients in whom salvage surgery can be performed. In patients with unresectable local recurrence, radiation can

TABLE 17–3. *Monitoring/surveillance protocol for follow-up of patients with rectal cancer*

1. Physical exam including digital rectal exam every 3 months for 2 years, then every 6 months to 5 years.
2. CBC + blood chemistries every 3 months for 2 years, then every 6 months to 5 years.
3. If CEA was elevated at diagnosis or within 1 week of resection, repeat CEA every 6 months for 2 years, then annually for 5 years.
4. Chest x-ray every 12 months for 5 years if stage B2 or C, or every 6 months for 10 cycles if resected liver or abdominal metastases, or every 3 months for 20 cycles if resected lung metastases.
5. Abdominal CT every 6 months for four cycles, then every 12 months for 3 years if resected liver or abdominal metastases, or every 6 months for four cycles, then every 12 months for 3 years if resected rectal tumor.
6. Chest CT every 6 months for four cycles if resected lung metastases.
7. Proctoscopy should be performed every 6 months after resection for the first 3 years, then yearly to 5 years. Colonoscopy in 1 years and every 3 years if negative for multiple synchronous polyps or if patient has new polyp on surveillance colonoscopy.

be helpful if not previously used, but chemotherapy has not been shown to provide significant improvements in survival. Pain control is a major issue in these patients, and pain service consultation should be sought in these cases.

Metastatic recurrence can be isolated, coupled with local recurrence, or diffuse. Those patients with isolated hepatic metastases may be candidates for resection, regional infusional chemotherapy, or systemic chemotherapy. Patients with widely metastatic disease are probably best treated with chemotherapy on protocol or when symptomatic.

REFERENCES

1. Landis S, Murray T, Bolden S, Wingo PA. Cancer statistics, 1998. *CA Cancer J Clin* 1998;48:6.
2. Nicholls RJ, York Mason A, Morson BC, et al. The clinical staging of rectal cancer. *Br J Surg* 1982;69:404.
3. Williams NS, Durdey P, Quirk P. Pre-operative staging of rectal neoplasm and its impact on clinical management. *Br J Surg* 1985;72:868.
4. Shank B, Dershaw DD, Caravelli J, et al. A prospective study of the accuracy of preoperative computed tomographic staging of patients with biopsy-proven rectal carcinoma. *Dis Colon Rectum* 1990;33:285.
5. Freenz PC, Marks WM, Ryan JA, et al. Colorectal carcinoma evaluation with CT: preoperative staging and detection of postoperative recurrence. *Radiology* 1986;158:347.
6. Kramann B, Hildebrant U. Computed tomography versus endosonography in the staging of rectal carcinoma: a comparative study. *Int J Colon Dis* 1986;1:216.
7. Deen K, Madoff R, Belemonte C, et al. Preoperative staging of rectal neoplasms with endorectal ultrasonography. *Semin Colon Rectal Surg* 1995;6:78.
8. Hildebrant U, Klein T, Feifel G, et al. Endosonography of pararectal lymph nodes: in vitro and in vivo evaluation. *Dis Colon Rectum* 1990;33:863.
9. Orrom WJ, Wong WD, Rothenberger DA, et al. Endorectal ultrasound in the preoperative staging of rectal tumors: a learning experience. *Dis Colon Rectum* 1990;33:654.
10. Heald RJ, Ryall RD. Recurrence and survival after total mesorectal excision for rectal cancer. *Lancet* 1986;1:1479.
11. Lasson AL, Ekelund GR, Lindstrom CG. Recurrence risks after stapled anastamosis for rectal carcinoma. *Acta Chir Scan* 1984;150:85.
12. Corder AP, Karanjia ND, Williams JD, Heald RJ. Flush aortic tie versus selective preservation of the ascending left colic artery in low anterior resection for rectal carcinoma. *Br J Surg* 1992;79:680.
13. Williams NS, Dixon MF, Johnston D. Reappraisal of the 5 centimetre rule of distal excision for carcinoma of the rectum: a study of distal intramural spread and of patients' survival. *Br J Surg* 1983;70:150.
14. Lewis WG, Martin IG, Williamson ME, et al. Why do some patients experience poor functional results after resection of the rectum for carcinoma? *Dis Colon Rectum* 1995;38:259.
15. Ho YH, Tan M, Seow-Choen F. Prospective randomized controlled study of clinical function and anorectal physiology after low anterior resection: comparison of a straight and colonic J pouch anastamosis. *Br J Surg* 1996;83:978.
16. Parc R, Tiret E, Frileux P, et al. Resection and colo-anal anastomosis with colonic reservoir for rectal carcinoma. *Br J Surg* 1986;73:139.
17. Hida J, Yasutomi M, Fujimoto K, et al. Functional outcome after low anterior resection for rectal cancer using the colonic J pouch: prospective randomized study for determination of optimum pouch size. *Dis Colon Rectum* 1996;39:986.
18. Morson BC, Bussey HJ, Samoorian S. Policy of local excision for early cancer of the colorectum. *Gut* 1977;18:1045.
19. Bleday R, Breen E, Jessup JM, et al. Prospective evaluation of local excision for small rectal cancers. *Dis Colon Rectum* 1997;40:388.
20. Ota DM, Skibber J, Rich TA. M. D. Anderson Cancer Center experience with local excision and multimodality therapy for rectal cancer. *Surg Oncol Clin North Am* 1992;1:147.
21. Minskey B, Cohen A, Enker W, et al. Preoperative 5-fluorouracil, low dose leukovorin, and concurrent radiation therapy for rectal cancer. *Cancer* 1994;73:273.
22. Kraske P. [Zur Exstirpation hochsitzender Mastdarmkrebse] [German]. *Verh Dtsch Ges Chir* 1885;14:464.
23. McCready DR, Ota DM, Rich TA, et al. Prospective phase I trial of conservative management of low rectal lesions. *Arch Surg* 1989;124:67.
24. Mason AY. Trans-sphincteric surgery of the rectum. *Prog Surg* 1974; 13:66.
25. Pahlman L, Glimelius B. Pre- or postoperative radiotherapy in rectal and rectosigmoid carcinoma: report from a randomized multicenter trial. *Ann Surg* 1990;211:187.
26. Improved survival with preoperative radiotherapy in resectable rectal cancer. Swedish Rectal Cancer Trial. *N Engl J Med* 1997;336:980. [For erratum, see *N Engl J Med* 1997;336:1539.]
27. Minsky BD. Adjuvant therapy for rectal cancer a good first step [Editorial]. *N Engl J Med* 1997;336:1016.
28. Kodner IJ, Gilley MT, Shemesh EI, et al. Radiation therapy as definitive treatment for selected invasive rectal cancer. *Surgery* 1993;114:850.
29. Prolongation of disease-free interval in surgically treated rectal carcinoma. Gastrointestinal Tumor Study Group. *N Engl J Med* 1985;312:1465.
30. Krook JE, Moertel CG, Gunderson LL, et al. Effective surgical adjuvant therapy for high-risk rectal carcinoma. *N Engl J Med* 1991;324:709.
31. O'Connell MJ, Martenson JA, Weiand HS, et al. Improving adjuvant therapy for rectal cancer by combining protracted infusion fluorouracil with radiation therapy after curative surgery. *N Engl J Med* 1994;331:502.
32. Landry JC, Koritz M, Wood WC, et al. Preoperative irradiation and fluorouracil chemotherapy for advanced rectosigmoid carcinoma: phase I–II study. *Radiology* 1993;188:423.
33. Gilbertsen VA. The results of the surgical treatment of cancer of the rectum. *Surg Gynecl Obstet* 1962;114:313.
34. Morson BC, Vaughan EG, Bussey HJ. Pelvic recurrence after excision of the rectum for carcinoma. *BMJ* 1963;2:13.
35. Michelassi F, Block GE, Vannucci L, et al. A 5- to 21-year follow-up and analysis of 250 patients with rectal adenocarcinoma. *Ann Surg* 1988;208:379.
36. Phillips RK, Hittinger R, Blesovsky L, et al. Local recurrence following curative surgery for large bowel cancer. II. The rectum and rectosigmoid. *Br J Surg* 1984;71:17.
37. DeCosse JJ, Wong RJ, Quan SH, Friedman NB, Sternberg SS. Conservative treatment of distal rectal cancer by local excision. *Cancer* 1989;63:219.

CHAPTER 18

Neoplasms of the Anus

Wayne DeVos

The anus is an anatomic structure that is often neglected or even ignored by both patient and physician. However, the tissues that compose the anus, like any other area of the body, are susceptible to neoplastic changes that may threaten not only its integrity but also the life of the patient. Unfortunately, perhaps more than any other organ, the anus is considered to be private and embarrassing to discuss, much less be examined. Thus, malignancies of the anus, rationalized as hemorrhoids, or simply ignored, or worse, misdiagnosed, may go untreated for months or even years. For this reason, improved physician awareness and patient education are critical in the management of anal neoplasms.

Anal precancerous and cancerous lesions are rare, accounting for only 2% to 4% of all anorectal neoplasms. In the general population, the incidence of squamous cell carcinoma of the anus, the most common of the anal malignancies, is only approximately one in 100,000 patients. All lesions of the anus are reachable by the examiner's index finger, and while symptoms and signs overlap considerably, a reasonable index of suspicion is all that is required to help patient and doctor differentiate the common benign mass from the rare malignancy. When caught early, with appropriate care the patient can expect colostomy-free survival rates approaching 100%.

Although significant advances in the medical treatment of anal cancer have made radical primary surgical therapy of historic interest only, the surgeon remains an important member of the medical team caring for a patient with an anal malignancy for several reasons: first, benign anal disease is often referred to the surgeon for definitive care, and the ability to differentiate benign from malignant disease is critical at that juncture. Second, at the time of diagnosis, and in follow-up surveillance, an examination under anesthesia with or without biopsies often will be required, and are best completed by a surgeon. Third, while primary squamous cell carcinoma of the anal canal is now with rare exception treated with combined modality therapy, a small subset of patients will be candidates for local surgical therapy. Also, surgical resection, local or radical, is often the most appropriate alternative for many of the other anal malignancies. Fourth, whether sur-

gical or combined modality therapy is chosen as the initial treatment, a significant risk of recurrence is the rule for most anal tumors. Repeat resection or more radical surgical treatment must be strongly considered when recurrence is discovered, and therefore the surgeon must be available, often for many years, following definitive primary treatment of an anal cancer.

The anal canal and surrounding tissue is histologically complex, and thus can degenerate into many pathologically different premalignant and malignant lesions. At the level of the anorectal ring, the mucosa is composed of columnar epithelium. Proceeding distally, this merges with the cuboidal epithelium of the transitional zone at the level of the dentate line and extending 1 to 2 cm proximally. This tissue has variable histologic characteristics, and can have the appearance of urothelium (hence, transitional zone). Distal to the dentate line the lining of the anal canal is composed of modified, non-keratinizing squamous epithelium which lacks dermal elements such as hair and glands. Finally, at the level of the anal verge, the modified epithelium gives way to normal keratinizing squamous epithelium.

Classically, importance has been attached to the careful determination of the pathological boundaries of the anal canal and anal margin, primarily secondary to the reported differential behavior of squamous cell cancer depending on whether it originated in the anal margin (relatively less aggressive) or the anal canal (relatively more aggressive with poorer prognosis and requirement for more intensive therapy). Unfortunately, in spite of this potential importance, much confusion still exists regarding the true boundaries of these areas.

Little controversy exists regarding the surgical anal canal, which corresponds to the limits of the internal sphincter, extending from the anorectal ring to the intersphincteric groove (Fig. 18-1). With respect to the pathological anal canal, published reports are generally in agreement regarding its proximal extent, placing it at the proximal limit of the internal sphincter, at the level of the anorectal ring. However, the distal extent of the pathologic anal canal, and therefore the beginning of the anal margin, has been placed

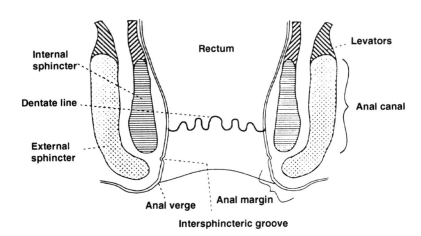

FIG. 18-1. Anatomy of the anal canal and anal margin. (Reprinted with permission from Beck DE, Wexner SD, eds. *Fundamentals of anorectal surgery.* New York: McGraw-Hill, 1992:233.)

at the dentate line (1), at the level of the intersphincteric groove (2) or at the level of the anal verge (3). This is potentially an important distinction since the lining of the anus between the dentate line and the anal verge is unlike either the transitional or columnar epithelium proximally, or the squamous epithelium distally. The question thus becomes: should neoplasms of the modified squamous epithelium of the distal surgical anal canal be included with those of the squamous epithelium beyond the anal verge, or with the transitional epithelium of the anal canal proximal to the dentate line?

In reality, the controversy is of importance more for academic reasons than for purposes of treatment. Certainly, when comparing treatment regimens, protocols and results, correct identification of the anatomical and histological origin of the tumor is critical. In practice, however, treatment of cancer of the anus is most often predicated not on the tissue of origin, but on the relationship of the tumor to the anal sphincter (for purposes of local resectability), and the dentate line (for identification of potential lymph node drainage basins). Thus, invasive neoplasms of the surgical anal canal between the anorectal ring and the intersphincteric groove, regardless of their histology, are generally not candidates for wide local excision secondary to almost certain resultant compromise of the sphincter muscle and consequent embarrassment of fecal continence. Small tumors of the skin distal to the intersphincteric groove, however, are often candidates for local treatment, with melanoma the only exception. While it is certainly true that lymphatic drainage of the surgical anal canal proximal and distal to the dentate line differ, this is less important today given the excellent results with combined modality therapy (Figs. 18-2, 18-3).

Therefore, since the relationship of the neoplasm to the internal sphincter is most often the critical factor in the determination of treatment, division of the anal canal from the anal margin at the intersphincteric groove seems most clinically relevant. Tumors of the anal canal are therefore those that arise from the transitional epithelium above the dentate line, the ductal epithelium of the anal glands, or the modified squamous epithelium of the distal anal canal beyond the dentate line, and include squamous cell carcinoma, epidermoid carcinoma (squamous, basaloid, cloacogenic, or transitional), and adenocarcinoma. If wide local excision of any of these tumors would lead to compromise of sphincter function, then chemoradiation therapy or, if necessary, abdominoperineal resection must be considered. Neoplasms of the anal margin beyond the intersphincteric groove may originate from the modified epithelium of the distal surgical anal canal or the keritinized epithelium of the perianal skin, and include squamous cell carcinoma, basal cell carcinoma, melanoma, and the precancerous lesions Paget's disease and Bowen's disease. As these tumors are more removed from the sphincteric muscle, they may be candidates for wide local excision with or without adjuvant therapy.

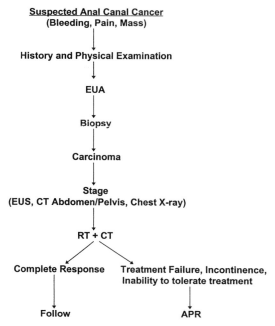

FIG. 18-2. Suspected anal canal cancer.

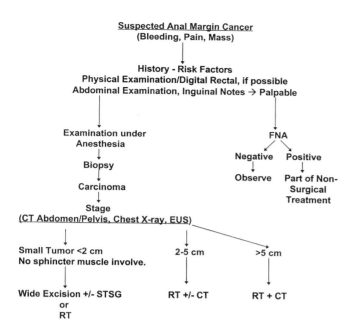

Suspected Anal Margin Cancer
(Bleeding, Pain, Mass)

History - Risk Factors
Physical Examination/Digital Rectal, if possible
Abdominal Examination, Inguinal Notes → Palpable

Examination under Anesthesia → Biopsy → Carcinoma → Stage (CT Abdomen/Pelvis, Chest X-ray, EUS)

FNA → Negative → Observe / Positive → Part of Non-Surgical Treatment

Small Tumor <2 cm No sphincter muscle involve. → Wide Excision +/- STSG or RT

2-5 cm → RT +/- CT

>5 cm → RT + CT

FIG. 18-3. Suspected anal margin cancer.

EPIDERMOID CANCER OF THE ANAL CANAL

Histology

The anal canal, situated between the anorectal ring and the intersphincteric groove, is composed of the transitional zone proximal to the dentate line and modified squamous epithelium distal to the dentate line (Fig. 18-1). Squamous cell carcinoma arising in the distal anal canal is generally nonkeratinizing and of a homogeneous histology. Squamous cell carcinoma arising at and proximal to the dentate line in the transitional zone can demonstrate multiple histologically distinct patterns, and, depending on the most prominent features, has been termed squamous, transitional, cloacogenic, basaloid, or mucoepidermoid carcinoma. Although distinguishing features have been found with regards to risk factors and prevalence, ultimately the different subtypes exhibit the same behavior and response to therapy; therefore, they are generally considered as a single, epidermoid neoplastic group, heterogeneous in histology, but homogeneous in behavior.

Squamous cell carcinoma of the distal anal canal behaves similarly to that of the proximal anal canal, though some significant differences exist with respect to lymphatic drainage and association with the sphincteric muscle at early stages. Whereas the lymphatic drainage of the anal canal distal to the dentate line generally involves the inguinal lymph node changes, the lymphatic drainage of the anal canal proximal to the dentate line involves the perirectal and pelvic lymph node complexes. Nonetheless, when a neoplasm of either area involves the dentate line, lymphatic drainage to either the inguinal region or perirectal and pelvic region can occur. As described earlier, in some reports neoplasms of the distal surgical anal canal have been grouped together with those of the

anal margin beyond the anal verge, which has led to confusion in the comparison of therapy and outcome.

Risk Factors

Premalignant Lesions

Bowen's Disease

Bowen's disease is characterized by the confinement of squamous cell carcinomatous changes to the epithelium. Only approximately 100 cases have been described in the literature (2). The diagnosis is often made after a long period of symptoms, which include itching, pruritis, burning, and bleeding. On examination, the appearance of Bowen's disease is typically that of a raised, scaly, brown red plaque in the perianal tissues, though it can also have the appearance of a raw, broad-based poorly healing sore. For this reason, critical to the early diagnosis of Bowen's disease is a high index of suspicion for any lesion which does not demonstrate healing following appropriate treatment. Diagnosis is based on the microscopic evaluation of tissue from punch biopsies, which can be obtained in the office under local anesthesia (Fig. 18-4).

The clinical course of Bowen's disease is generally benign: both progression to invasive cancer and association with other malignancies are rare. Nonetheless, while the small number of reported cases has precluded establishment of any definitive protocol, wide local excision with negative intraoperative margins is generally felt to be the most appropriate treatment. Given the propensity of Bowen's disease to spread locally, mapping of the anoderm should be completed at the time of the wide local excision. This involves the submission to frozen section of 3 mm punch biopsies taken from all four quadrants at the level of the dentate line, the anal verge, and

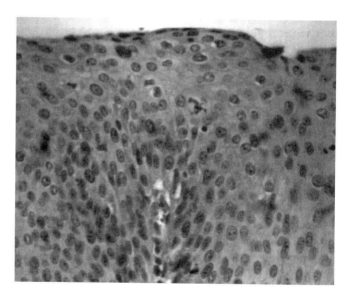

FIG. 18-4. Perianal Bowen's disease. (Reprinted with permission from Beck DE, Wexner SD, eds. *Fundamentals of anorectal surgery.* St. Louis: McGraw-Hill, 1992:233.)

approximately 3 cm from the anal verge, as described by Beck and Fazio (4) (Fig. 18-5).

Though most series are small, prognosis is generally good with a low percentage of recurrence. If invasive cancer is found associated with the Bowen's disease, treatment is based on the characteristics of the invasive cancer. Long-term surveillance following successful excision is important and any suspicious lesion should be biopsied.

Buschke-Lowenstein Tumors

Also called giant condyloma or verrucous condyloma, Buschke-Lowenstein tumors (BLK) is a slowly growing, exophytic, cauliflower-like lesion which is locally infiltrative and carries little metastatic potential (5). Differentiation from anal condyloma is generally possible secondary to the appearance of a central umbilical support in benign warts. Differentiation from invasive carcinoma is generally possible on microscopic analysis and therefore careful analysis of the surgical specimen is important to rule out focal points of invasive cancer, which may be present in up to 50% of BLK tumors (5). Recurrence is

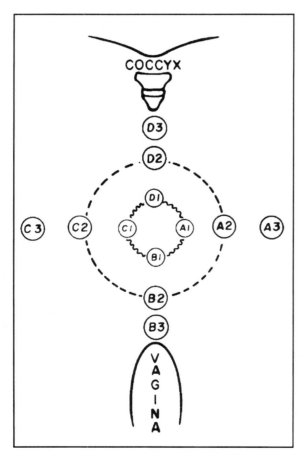

FIG. 18-5. Anal mapping for biopsies in Bowen's disease and Paget's disease. *1,* dentate line; *2,* anal verge; *3,* perineum 3 cm from anal verge. (Reprinted with permission from Beck DE, Wexner SD, eds. *Fundamentals of anorectal surgery.* St. Louis: McGraw-Hill, 1992:233.)

common, and therefore wide local excision with negative margins is critical. Careful postoperative surveillance should be carried out for up to 10 years, with frequent examinations and biopsy of any suspicious new lesions.

Anal Intraepithelial Neoplasia

Also called carcinoma *in situ* or dysplasia, anal intraepithelial neoplasia (AIN) has recently become increasingly important secondary to its increased observation in immune compromised patients and its possible premalignant behavior. AIN has similar characteristics to cervical intraepithelial neoplasia (CIN), both with respect to histologic appearance as well as to the association of these lesions with human papilloma virus. However, unlike CIN, which is a proven precursor lesion to invasive carcinoma of the cervix, the role of AIN in the development of anal carcinoma has not yet been established. However, the association of human papilloma virus with AIN has been well established (6–8). HPV 6 and 11 have been found to be associated with condyloma acuminata and low grade dysplasia (AIN I and II), while high grade dysplasia (AIN III) has been found in association with HPV 16, as well as in association with early invasive carcinoma (9). While it appears unlikely that low grade AIN progresses to high grade AIN, association of AIN III with HPV 16 and with local invasive cancer suggests that it may be a premalignant lesion. While currently the appropriate management of AIN has not been established, a reasonable approach to AIN III when found either alone or with association with anal warts would be ablation either by simple excision, fulguration or application of cytotoxic creams such as 5-fluorouracil (5-FU) (9).

Environmental and Social Risk Factors

Tobacco

Cigarette smoking has been linked in epidemiological studies to an increased risk of anal carcinoma (10–12). In Daling's report in 1992, 60% of patients with anal carcinoma were smokers versus 25% of the control group (10). Relative risk increased with increased number of pack years, while the cessation of smoking was associated with a decreased risk of developing anal carcinoma. The mechanism of increased risk has been hypothesized as either through an effect on the immune system or through a mechanism of synergy with human papilloma virus.

Benign Anorectal Disease

Most surgeons who care for patients with benign diseases of the anus have been asked the question will hemorrhoids lead to cancer? Several large population based studies have addressed this question. In two of the largest, risk for anal cancer was actually found to decrease with increasing duration of the benign anal disease (including hemorrhoids, fissures, anorectal abscesses, and fistula-in-ano), suggesting no link

(13,14). Other studies have suggested a slightly increased risk of developing invasive cancer in patients with chronic benign anal disease (11). While it is possible that patients with benign anorectal disease are at increased risk for anal cancer, whether an increased risk for such a rare phenomenon as anal cancer will change the management of such common benign diseases as hemorrhoids, fistula-in-ano, and fissure-in-ano is unclear. Nevertheless, awareness of the possible association with elevated risk of her cancer underlines the important of a high index of suspicion for any benign disease which does not respond appropriately to standard management (15).

Sexual Behavior

Multiple studies have demonstrated an increased relative risk of anal cancer with the practice of anal receptive intercourse. This is true both for the male gay population as well as for the female heterosexual population (12,14,16). Several risk factors related to sexual promiscuity and venereal disease have also been identified that are associated with an increased risk of anal cancer. These include infection with human papilloma virus (8,16–18), anal warts (11), heterosexual promiscuity (14), and infection with human immunodeficiency virus (HIV) (19–21).

Immune Suppression

Immune suppression associated with kidney transplants has been found to increase significantly the risk of human papilloma virus and anal cancer (22). This risk has been estimated to be approximately 100 fold. A link between anal cancer and anal Crohn's disease has only recently been suggested (23). The possible mechanisms include immune suppression secondary to chronic disease, immune suppression with medical treatment of the Crohn's disease, and/or chronic inflammatory process of the anus. Nonetheless, there have been only a few case reports, and the extremely low incidence of anal cancer in Crohn's disease patients makes relative risk establishment difficult. Nonetheless, as with other benign chronic diseases of the anus, a high index of suspicion should be maintained for any chronic inflammatory process in any immune-compromised patient which changes after a long period of stability, as this may indicate neoplastic degeneration.

Presentation

Anal canal cancer occurs in the United States and the United Kingdom with a frequency of 0.5 to 1 per 100,000. Average age at presentation is in the sixth to seventh decade, with a female/male ratio of approximately 2:1. Recent studies in Sweden, Denmark, and the United States have demonstrated an increase in the incidence of anal cancer over the past 20 years, with a most substantial increase in two patient groups (24–26). In both the Swedish and Danish study, the increase in women was the most substantial. In the United States SEER-based study (24), over the time period studied, when compared with the general population risk for developing anal cancer, there was a significantly greater increase in risk of developing anal cancer in women and in never-married white men in the San Francisco Bay area. A significant increase in the percentage of women who smoke and the probability that white men who have never married overlap significantly with the population of homosexual males are two possible reasons for the significant increase seen in these two subgroups.

Anal carcinoma is frequently diagnosed late. In his 1987 review, Jensen et al. (27) found that 55% of patients with anal carcinoma were initially incorrectly diagnosed, with an average resulting delay of correct diagnosis in that group of 15 months, compared with 6 months of symptoms prior to diagnosis in patients correctly identified as having anal cancer. The most common symptoms include bleeding, pain, and mass effect at the anus (28–30). Interestingly, in one study approximately 25% of patients were completely asymptomatic at diagnosis (30). The most common physical findings include a mass in the majority of patients (9) (Figs. 18-6, 18-7); additionally, the digital rectal examination is often painful. Ten percent to 20% of patients will present with synchronous inguinal lymphadenopathy, though on biopsy only approximately half of these will demonstrate metastatic cancer (31,32).

Evaluation

All patients suspected of harboring anal carcinoma should undergo a complete history and physical, with special attention paid to historical risk factors, inguinal lymphadenopathy,

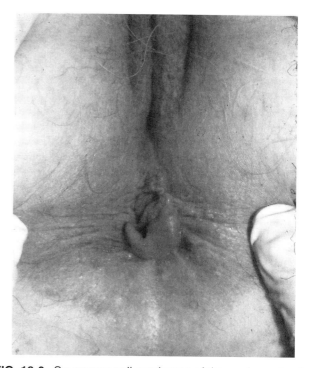

FIG. 18-6. Squamous cell carcinoma of the anal canal, relatively hidden at the time of presentation.

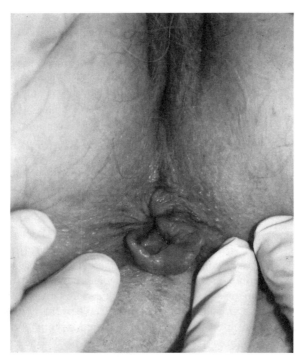

FIG. 18-7. Same tumor as in Fig. 18-6, during examination under anesthesia.

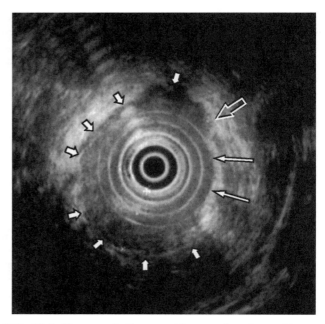

FIG. 18-8. Transanal ultrasound image of anal canal tumor. The tumor is 2.1 cm at its greatest depth of invasion, but does not extend into the perianal fat. It was therefore staged as a T2 lesion both with the AJCC and the ultrasound staging systems. *Small arrows,* outline of the tumor; *large arrow,* normal internal sphincter; *narrow arrow,* external sphincter.

abdominal masses, and digital rectal examination if possible. If an examination cannot be completed successfully in the office, progression to the operating room is appropriate to complete the examination. Biopsies of the anal mass can also be done at that time. Careful characterization of the mass, its size, distance from the anal verge and its relationship to the anus is critical in planning therapy. Finally, palpable inguinal lymph nodes should be examined by fine-needle aspiration (FNA) to rule out metastatic disease.

Further diagnostic tests include computerized tomography of the abdomen and pelvis for the evaluation of hepatic and retroperitoneal metastases, and chest x-ray to rule out the presence of pulmonary metastases. Recent experience with the application of endoluminal ultrasound (EUS) has shown that important information regarding tumor size, relationship to the sphincter muscle, and association of perirectal lymph nodes can be obtained with good accuracy for depth of invasion and moderate accuracy for presence of metastatic lymph

nodes (33,34) (Fig. 18-8). This information has become particularly useful given the difficulty of estimating the exact size of the tumor based only on clinical examination. EUS is also being shown to be useful for postoperative surveillance (35).

While no one staging method has been universally adopted, the AJCC recommendations are generally used (35) (Table 18-1). Unfortunately, this staging system is limited by its lack of information regarding association of the tumor to the sphincteric musculature and perianal and perirectal fatty tissue. An alternate tumor staging method is that based on ultrasound image (36) (Table 18-1). Since staging is important for comparison and prognosis, ultrasound staging, which allows more accurate estimation of depth of invasion with respect to the sphincter musculature, may be more useful. Certainly, as nonsurgical methods of treatment are refined, any method of evaluation that significantly improved staging accuracy will be useful.

TABLE 18–1. *Comparison of TNM staging system using ultrasound versus the American Joint Commission on Cancer (AJCC) criteria for tumor (T) staging*

T stage	AJCC stage (35)	Ultrasonic stage (36)
T1	Tumor 2 cm or less in greatest dimension	Tumor confined to mucosa
T2	Tumor more than 2 cm but not more than 5 cm in greatest dimension	Tumor invading sphincter muscle
T3	Tumor more than 5 cm in greatest diameter	Tumor invading perianal or perirectal fat
T4	Tumor of any size invades adjacent organ(s), e.g., vagina, urethra, bladder (involvement of the sphincter muscle[s] alone is not classified as T4)	Tumor invading adjacent organ (e.g., prostate, vagina)

Treatment

As recently as the mid 1970s, radical surgery was felt to be the most appropriate approach to anal cancer, with the best chance of long-term survival (28–31,37). While radiation treatment had been attempted following World War I, methods of application were relatively toxic, and a successful operation with the placement of a colostomy was felt to result in better long-term cure and/or palliation than radiation with its attendant toxicity (38).

In their review of the surgical treatment of anal cancer, Beck and Wexner (2) found a 5-year survival rate in all U.S. series of 27% to 71%, with an average of 55%. Recurrence was frequent: in Clark's study, recurrence following wide local excision was 78%, and recurrence following abdominal perineal resection was approximately 60% (37). This dismal local control rate was echoed in other series.

Refinement in radiation delivery encouraged several clinicians to reattempt management of anal cancer nonsurgically (39–42). With improved techniques of delivery, and the use of interstitial radiation, several authors were able to demonstrate similar or better 5-year survival when compared historically to abdominal perineal resection, but most significantly, this survival was largely without permanent colostomies. In Beck and Wexner's review (2) of all published reports of using radiation therapy only, they found 5-year survival to be reported between 46% and 92%, with an average of 68%. Recurrent disease remained a significant problem, however, with local recurrence averaging 26% and distant recurrence averaging approximately 17%.

In 1974, Nigro (43), at Wayne State University published a report describing his experience with three patients with bulky anal cancers, for which he used a combination of neoadjuvant chemotherapy and radiation therapy in an attempt to improve the odds of subsequent radical resection. He reasoned that, given the high rate of mortality following surgical treatment of anal cancer, the propensity of anal cancer to metastasize, and the limited ability to resect the locally aggressive tumor given the anatomical constraints of the pelvis, the use of multimodality therapy would be useful to shrink the tumor and improve clearance at the time of surgery. As support for this reasoning, he cited recent success with combined modality therapy in the treatment of squamous cell carcinoma of the stomach. He also reasoned that the use of adjuvant chemotherapy would allow a decreased dose of radiation therapy and thereby decrease toxicity. The regimen he applied involved radiation given in divided doses, coupled with the infusion of 5-FU and mitomycin C (Table 18-2). This was to be followed by abdominal perineal resection 6 to 8 weeks following completion of the therapy.

Nigro (43) was able to complete abdominal perineal resection in his first two patients and discovered no residual tumor in either specimen. His third patient refused surgery following completion of therapy and remained disease free. In 1984, Nigro (44) reported on 104 patients with anal cancer whom he had treated with the same regimen of combined modality

TABLE 18–2. *Nigro protocol for combined modality therapy for squamous cell cancer of the anal canal*

External beam radiation
3,000 cGy delivered to the pelvis in 15 fractions of 200 cGy each on days 1–15
Systemic chemotherapy
5-Fluorouracil, 1,000 mg/m^2/24 h continuously on days 1–4 and repeated on days 28–31
Mitomycin C 15 mg/m^2 i.v. bolus on day 1

Data from ref. 43.

therapy. While the early patients all underwent abdominal perineal resection, the majority of the group underwent only excision of the scar. In this study, Dr. Nigro demonstrated excellent initial complete response, and improved disease- and colostomy-free survival when compared historically with abdominal perineal resection alone.

Multiple reports followed demonstrating significant improvement in local control, decreased distant recurrence, and significant improvement in disease-free survival with a modest improvement in overall survival (45–52). Five-year survival was generally between 70% to 87%. However, some series showed less impressive 5-year survival rates (52), and the inherent weakness found in retrospective, uncontrolled series reports became the basis for the establishment of several prospective randomized trials in the late 1980s. In the past 2 years, three of these trials have matured. One of these trials addressed the benefit of mitomycin C, which is felt to be responsible for the majority of the toxicity of the chemotherapeutic regimen (53); the other two trials, one based in Europe (54) and one based in the United Kingdom (55), addressed the effect of the addition of chemotherapy to radiation on local recurrence and colostomy-free survival and long-term survival.

In the United States Intergroup trial, the effect of mitomycin C was evaluated by randomizing 310 patients to receive either 45 Gy of radiation and 5-FU only, or 45 Gy of radiation and 5-FU combined with mitomycin C (53). Biopsy was completed approximately 2 months posttreatment, and if positive, follow-up chemoradiation was completed using a 9-Gy boost of radiation and a combination of 5-FU and Cisplatin. Analysis at 4 years demonstrated a significant improvement in colostomy-free survival, a significant improvement in complete response, and significant decrease in local recurrence. No significant difference was observed in long-term survival (65% at 5 years for the entire group).

In 1996, the results of the UKCCR Anal Cancer Trial Working Party were published (55). In this trial, 585 patients were randomized to receive either 45 Gy of radiotherapy alone or in combination with 5-FU and mitomycin C. After a median follow-up of 42 months, 59% of radiotherapy patients had local failure versus 36% of combined modality therapy, giving a 46% reduction in the risk of local failure when combined modality therapy was used. While the risk of disease-specific death was reduced in the combined modality therapy arm, at 3 years follow-up there was no apparent overall survival advantage (58% for radiotherapy alone, 65% for combined modality therapy).

In 1997, Bartelink and associates published the results of the European Organization for Research and Treatment of Cancer (EORTC) phase III trial comparing isolated radiotherapy versus concomitant radiotherapy and chemotherapy in the treatment of anal cancer (54). 110 patients were randomized to receive either 45 Gy of radiation, followed by a boost of 15 to 20 Gy in the case of partial or complete response, respectively; or, in the combined modality therapy arm, 5-FU and mitomycin C were given concomitantly with the radiation therapy. With a follow-up of 5 years, locoregional control rate was improved by 18% and colostomy-free survival was improved by 32% in the group receiving combined modality therapy. No significant difference was found with respect to side effects, and the ultimate survival rate remained similar in both treatment arms (58% in the entire group).

The main points which can be derived from these prospective randomized trials are as follows: (a) chemotherapy combined with radiation therapy is well tolerated without a significant increase in morbidity to the patients; (b) the addition of chemotherapy to radiation therapy improves local disease control, reduces local recurrence, reduces the odds of requiring a colostomy, and improves disease-specific survival; (c) although mitomycin C is responsible for a significant portion of the toxicity when used in combination with 5-FU and radiation, it is also responsible for a significant portion of the benefit derived from addition of chemotherapy to radiation; and (d) the addition of adjuvant chemotherapy to radiation does not improve overall survival significantly. This last observation may seem surprising, particularly given the significantly improved local control and disease-specific survival. That the numbers of patients treated in the trials was not large enough to show more than a trend may explain this lack of improved overall survival; also, these results may reflect the outcomes to be expected from a large, multi-institutional study rather than a single institutional report. Also, it is possible that some other, not as yet recognized factor increases non–disease-related mortality in the chemotherapy arm.

Therefore, with the maturation of these trials, a solid basis of data has been provided on which clinical decisions can be made in the treatment of anal cancer. Clearly, the majority of patients presenting with squamous cell carcinoma of the anus regardless of histological subtype will be appropriate candidates for combined modality therapy. At this time, if clinical examination 6 to 8 weeks following completion of therapy shows no evidence of residual tumor, biopsy is no longer recommended. Follow-up is then recommended with examinations every 3 months for at least 2 years, and abdominal pelvic and CAT scan 1 year following treatment. Any suspicious new growth in the anal region or in the lymph node drainage basins should be biopsied to rule out metachronous cancer.

Abdominal perineal resection is currently recommended only for patients who have intractable incontinence to stool following therapy, and to patients who fail primary therapy and either will not tolerate or fail salvage therapy (see below).

Recent evidence regarding the use of EUS suggests that the addition of periodic examinations posttreatment with ultrasound will assist in the earlier discovery of recurrent cancer. The procedure can be performed with a minimum of morbidity, and can be completed every 3 to 4 months in the first 2 years. Experience is still small with this technique, but early results suggest that ultrasound can improve early detection of anal cancer recurrence (34,35). Hopefully, with increased experience at major centers which handle significant numbers of patients with anal cancer, long-term follow-up with ultrasound will help determine its utility.

Special Considerations

Treatment of Local Recurrence

In spite of excellent results with combined modality therapy in the maintenance of colostomy-free survival and decreased local recurrence, the problem with local recurrence is still substantial. Salvage combined modality therapy using 5-FU and mitomycin C has demonstrated disappointing results, with only 19% surviving 5 years in a survey of the Veteran's Administration Hospitals by Longo et al. (56) in 1994. This has been echoed by others. Unfortunately, only somewhat better survival is offered by completing abdominal perineal resection at the time of recurrence, with 5-year survival rates at 40% to 60% (41,57). While no specific trials have matured, recent evidence suggests the replacement of mitomycin C with cisplatin significantly improved salvage rate for recurrent anal cancer (53). In that phase III Intergroup trial, 5-FU and cisplatin were used with boost radiation in patients who had failed initial therapy at two months. With this regimen, a 50% complete response rate was obtained in the patients with recurrence. Cisplatin in the place of mitomycin C has been shown to have excellent response rates in early phase II trials for primary cancers (58,59). Currently, an RTOG phase III trial is being designed to investigate the use of cisplatin instead of mitomycin C as primary therapy for anal carcinoma. Hopefully, future trials will also address the use of cisplatin in the treatment of recurrent or persistent anal cancer.

Synchronous Inguinal Lymphadenopathy

Biopsy proven synchronous inguinal lymph node involvement is present in 10% to 20% of patients with cancer and is a poor prognostic indicator (54). Given its morbidity, bilateral inguinal lymph node dissection in the absence of proven metastases is not advised. However, even in the face of biopsy proven cancer in the inguinal nodes, lymph node dissection is currently felt not to be necessary in the face of appropriate inguinal lymph node coverage during combined modality therapy. Metachronous involvement of inguinal lymph nodes is also a poor prognostic indicator: median survival after discovery metachronous lymph node metastases was approximately 12 months in spite of aggressive therapy (49).

Treatment of Anal Cancer in the HIV-Positive Population

With the significant increase in the risk of developing anal cancer in the HIV population, significant attention has been paid to possible modes of treatment in this immune suppressed group, which is known to respond poorly to chemotherapeutic regimens for other tumors. Nonetheless, recent papers have demonstrated reasonable tolerance of combined modality therapy in patients who are HIV positive, but not suffering any AIDS defining illnesses (60,61). However, these same reports demonstrated less successful treatment in patients with AIDS. In spite of initial complete response, most AIDS patients die within months of treatment. Therefore, in HIV-positive patients without ongoing opportunistic infections or evidence of AIDS defining illnesses, use of a modified Nigro protocol for the treatment of anal cancer is appropriate. In patients with AIDS, there is no clear evidence at this time of the benefit of combined modality therapy. However, with the dramatic results that recently have been seen in viral suppression and prolonged life using medication cocktails in patients with AIDS, future experience may show that patients with good viral load control may tolerate chemoradiation therapy with results similar to patients who are HIV positive.

ADENOCARCINOMA OF THE ANAL CANAL

Adenocarcinoma of the anus is rare, accounting for only 5% to 10% of all anal canal cancers in large series. The histological origin is thought to be malignant degeneration of the glandular epithelium lining the anal ducts located at the level of the dentate line. While careful anatomical investigation might show that many anal adenocarcinomas are in fact very low rectal cancers spreading distally, this distinction is probably unimportant, since the treatment is not significantly different.

In a recent report of a survey of the American Society of Colon and Rectal Surgery conducted by Abel et al. (62) information was gathered about the treatment of 52 cases of adenocarcinoma of the anus by the members of the society. The most common presenting complaints included pain, bleeding and the presence of a mass. An associated fistula-in-ano was reported in 54% of the patients, and metastases at presentation was found in 13% of patients. 77% of patients ultimately underwent abdominoperineal resection, while 9% underwent wide local excision. Although the majority of patients underwent some form of adjuvant therapy (53%), no clearly defined role for adjuvant therapy could be determined. Of patients who underwent attempted curative resection, those followed for 3 years (17 patients) had a survival without evidence of disease of 74%; of those followed for 5 years (15 patients), survival was 93%. Overall survival for the group was 62% (follow-up ranged from 6 months to 17 years).

These results were somewhat better than those of Basik et al. (63) who reported a 30% crude 5-year survival rate (five patients died of disease) and 70% recurrence or metastasis in his series of 10 patients. They are significantly better than the series of 21 patients reported by Jensen et al. (64), which demonstrated a 4.8% 5-year crude survival rate. However, 13/21 of Jensen's patients had metastatic disease at presentation. While sampling error may account for the comparatively excellent survival rates in Abel's survey (62), three conclusions can be drawn from the published reports: (a) survival with metastatic disease in dismal, (b) lack of recurrence after 3 years suggests a cure, and (c) aggressive surgery is warranted if appropriate margins can be obtained.

NEOPLASMS OF THE ANAL MARGIN

Squamous Cell Carcinoma

Squamous cell carcinoma of the anal margin occurs at a frequency of about one-fifth that of anal canal squamous cell carcinoma. Average age at presentation is in the sixth to seventh decade, and, in contradistinction to squamous cell cancer of the anal canal, occurs with a significant male predominance of about 4:1. Reports in the literature vary as to the anatomic boundaries for the anal margin, with some describing the proximal limit at the level of the dentate line, at the intersphincteric groove, or at the anal verge. As described earlier, since anatomic considerations are of first importance in the treatment of anal cancer, the most useful proximal border of the anal margin would seem to be the intersphincteric groove, which corresponds closely with the anal verge. In this way tumors of the anal canal, and therefore intimately associated with the anal sphincter, are considered separately from tumors of the anal margin, which are often not intimately associated with the anal sphincter muscle. However, that this is a relatively arbitrary classification, useful mainly to allow comparison between treatment methods, must be kept in mind. Ultimately, with the only exception perhaps being melanoma, decisions regarding treatment of anal tumors are based on the relationship of the tumor to the anal sphincter and whether its size and proximity to the sphincter muscle allow a safe, curative excision. The distal limit is generally defined as 5 cm from the anal verge in all directions.

Presenting symptoms and findings include presence of a palpable mass (Fig. 18-9), bleeding, and pain in a majority of patients (27), and are present for a median duration of 6 months prior to evaluation. Initial misdiagnosis is common, though not as frequent as in cancer of the anal canal (27). Synchronous inguinal lymph node involvement is observed in 15% to 30%, the incidence of which increases with increase in the size of the primary tumor (65,66). Risk factors for squamous cell cancer of the anal margin are similar to those for the anal canal, and include Crohn's disease, smoking, anal receptive intercourse, infection with human papilloma virus (HPV), and immune compromise.

Initial evaluation should include a careful examination under anesthesia and biopsy. Relationship to the sphincter muscles should be documented, the inguinal regions should be carefully inspected for lymphadenopathy, and any enlarged lymph nodes evaluated by FNA. While no randomized

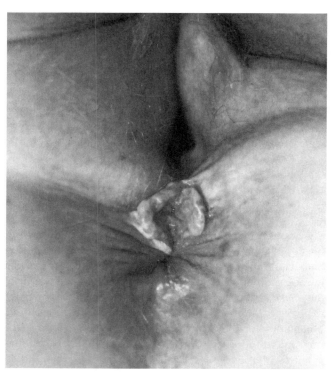

FIG. 18-9. Squamous cell carcinoma of the anal margin.

trials regarding therapeutic options have been (or will most likely be) completed secondary to the small number of cases, several large series have provided data to assist in guiding therapy. Small tumors (less than 2 cm) that do not directly involve the sphincter muscle are excellent candidates for radiation or wide local excision, with or without skin graft. Stage T2 lesions (2 to 5 cm) are at significant risk of inguinal nodal metastasis, and are therefore best treated with radiation, possibly with chemotherapy. Therapy of larger lesions (more than 5 cm, T3 and T4) can be completed along the same guidelines used for anal canal squamous cell cancer, using external beam radiation and 5-FU and mitomycin C for chemotherapeutic potentiation (65,67).

The disease-specific 5-year survival rate following local excision was 88% in one series of 31 patients at Memorial Sloan-Kettering; however, locoregional recurrence was 42%, though response was good following reexcision in seven of nine local recurrences (68). A total of 54 patients treated with radiation with or without local excision demonstrated an 80% disease-specific 5-year survival rate in Papillon's series (65), and in a review of 10 reports in the literature involving 214 total patients, cause-specific 5-year survival rates between 64% and 100% following local excision with or without radiotherapy were reported (69). Recurrence is frequently seen, however, appearing up to many years following apparent curative therapy (64,68). For this reason, postoperative surveillance is critical for at least 10 years posttreatment.

A special consideration is the discovery of invasive squamous cell carcinoma in a hemorrhoidectomy specimen. Generally, cancer found in a hemorrhoidectomy specimen will have been confined to the anal margin. If the excised columns were labeled, reexcision can be done to achieve wide negative margins. If the origin of the specimen is not clear, and margins were negative, the patient can be offered postoperative radiation therapy. Interestingly, a significant number of patients presenting with anal margin cancer have a history of benign anal pathology, and this has been used to support the routine analysis of hemorrhoidectomy specimens. However, in their review of 21,257 hemorrhoidectomy specimens, Cataldo et al. (70) found only one case of unsuspected anal cancer, and it was concluded that hemorrhoidectomy specimens not be routinely analyzed, but that only suspicious lesions be sent to the pathology department.

Basal Cell Carcinoma

Basal cell carcinoma of the anus is an extremely rare tumor, accounting for only 0.2% of anal cancer cases. Present with slight male predominance, they tend to occur in the seventh decade. The appearance is often that of an ulcerated lesion at the anal verge, though extension into the anal canal is also seen. A palpable mass, bleeding and pain are other common complaints. Delay in diagnosis is frequent: in one series, average duration of symptoms prior to treatment was 6 months, and in 10 patients, an erroneous initial diagnosis led to a median delay of treatment of 8 months (71). Identification is made on microscopic analysis, with the most important differential diagnosis being basaloid squamous cell carcinoma. The presence of squamous differentiation in basaloid squamous cell cancer usually permits appropriate classification.

Nielsen and Jensen (71) reported their experience with 34 patients and found that more than 50% had tumors less than 3 cm in diameter, while almost all had tumors with diameters less than 5 cm. Twenty-seven patients underwent wide local excision, while four underwent radical surgery secondary to extension of the tumor into the anal canal. Metastasis was rare, and disease-specific survival was 100% at 5 years. Nonetheless, local recurrence was frequent (27%), and emphasizes the importance of adequate margins and close follow-up. However, with adequate reexcision, excellent long-term survival rates can be expected.

Melanoma

Anal melanoma is a very rare anal tumor, accounting for only 0.5% of anal cancer cases. It is often discovered late and is generally fatal. Its etiology is unknown, and population databases are uncommon. While several hundred cases have been reported in the literature, most series are small or are compilations of case reports (72–75).

Presenting symptoms are nonspecific, including pain, bleeding, change in bowel habits, or a mass (74,75). Average age at presentation is in the sixth to seventh decade, and most series show a slight female majority. Up to one-third of anal melanomas are unpigmented, and 30% to 60% have regional or distant spread at initial diagnosis. Median survival with distant metastasis at presentation was 5 months in one series; median survival if no metastasis was identified at presentation was only moderately better, at 12 months (72). Five-year survival following therapy is uniformly poor regardless of approach (abdominoperineal resection or wide local excision) and generally ranges from 2% to 15%. Recurrence is the rule, and survival following recurrence is very poor. No effective chemotherapeutic regimens have been reported for this aggressive tumor. General recommendations are for palliative care only.

In spite of a dismal prognosis, a recent report offer hope for a subgroup of patients with anorectal melanoma. In their report of 85 patients from Memorial Sloan-Kettering, Brady et al. (74) found that in the nine long-term survivors following abdominoperineal resection, eight had no nodal metastasis, the average tumor size was 2.5 cm (as compared to 4.0 cm for nonsurvivors), and all were women. They concluded that abdominoperineal resection should be considered for patients with small tumors without demonstrable metastasis. While other reports have not shown a survival advantage based on choice of surgical therapy, they have been limited by small numbers of survivors or the lack of adequate subset analysis (72,73).

Paget's Disease

Perianal Paget's disease is an extremely rare intraepithelial adenocarcinoma, with approximately 125 cases having been discussed in the literature (38). Named for Sir James Paget following his description of the classic breast lesion in 1874 (76), the disease most likely originates in apocrine glandular tissue. The average age at presentation is in the seventh decade, and the gender distribution is equal. Patients classically complain of pruritis and bleeding, and on examination, a typical eczematoid, erythematous and scaling perianal rash is observed. The differential diagnosis includes Bowen's disease, leukoplakia, condyloma acuminata, eczema, squamous cell carcinoma, and prolapsed hemorrhoids. Initial diagnosis can be made with a punch biopsy of the lesion in the office, which will show cells with abundant, pale cytoplasm and eccentric nuclei localized in the epithelium (Fig. 18-10). Once the diagnosis has been made, two steps must be taken: a search for any underlying carcinoma, and mapping of the perianal tissue to determine the extent of the disease.

While Paget's disease of the breast is classically associated with an underlying malignancy, perianal Paget's disease is associated with underlying cancer in 50% to 86% of cases, depending on the series (77,78). Therefore, following establishment of the diagnosis, a careful search for associated anal or rectal malignancies must be made. In the absence of an invasive neoplasm, perianal Paget's disease should be treated as a premalignant lesion, since progression to invasive carcinoma has been reported to be as high as 40% in untreated lesions (64). In the presence of a malignancy, treatment is dictated by the appropriate principles regarding the invasive cancer: e.g., for rectal cancer, an abdominoperineal resection is completed, with special attention to the anal area to provide adequate excision of the Paget's disease.

In the absence of a malignancy, Beck and Fazio (77) have described a useful method of mapping which accounts for possible occult spread into normal appearing skin (Fig. 18-3). Under anesthesia, the lesion is identified and biopsies are taken from normal appearing tissue one centimeter from the edge of the lesion. Random frozen section biopsies are then taken in a proscribed fashion from the four quadrants of the anus, at three levels: at the dentate line, at the anal verge, and 3 cm from the anal verge. With the extent of the lesion so defined, a wide local excision with one centimeter margins in all directions is then accomplished. Frozen section biopsies are then again taken from the edge of the resection to rule out residual disease. The defect is then closed primarily or covered with a skin graft if necessary. Given the risk of recurrence of Paget's disease or invasive cancer, long-term

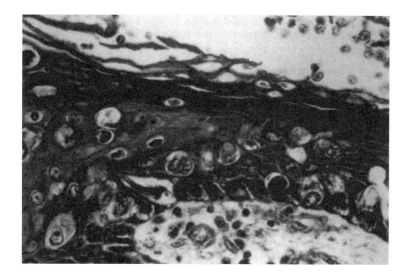

FIG. 18-10. Perianal Paget's disease. (From Beck DE, Wexner SD, eds. *Fundamentals of anorectal surgery*. St. Louis: McGraw-Hill, 1992:233.)

follow-up, including surveillance for adenocarcinoma of the anus and rectum, and biopsies of any suspicious perianal lesions, is necessary.

In the absence of invasive cancer, perianal Paget's disease has an excellent prognosis. As with any rare perianal lesion, however, a high index of suspicion and readiness to biopsy must be maintained regarding any lesion which does not respond to appropriate therapy in a reasonable time course.

REFERENCES

1. Morson BC. The pathology and results of treatment of squamous cell carcinoma of the anal canal and anal margin. *J R Soc Med* 1960;503:416.
2. Beck DE, Wexner SD. Anal neoplasms. In: Beck DE, Wexner SD, eds. *Fundamentals of anorectal surgery*. New York: McGraw-Hill, 1992:222.
3. American Joint Committee on Cancer. *AJCC cancer staging manual*. 5th ed. Philadelphia: JB Lippincott Co, 1997:91.
4. Beck DE, Fazio VW. Perianal Paget's disease. *Dis Colon Rectum* 1986; 30:263.
5. Cintron J. Buschke-Lowenstein tumor of the perianal and anorectal region. *Semin Colon Rectal Surg* 1995;6:135.
6. Beckmann AM, Daling JR, Sherman KJ, et al. Human papilloma virus infection and anal cancer. *Int J Cancer* 1989;43:1042.
7. Pfister H. Relationship of papillomaviruses to anogenital cancer [Review]. *Obstet Gynecol Clin North Am* 1987;14:349.
8. Palefsky JM, Holly EA, Gonzales J, Berline J, Ahn DK, Greenspan JS. Detection of human papillomavirus DNA in anal intraepithelial neoplasia and anal cancer. *Cancer Res* 1991;51:1014.
9. Scholefield JH. The technique of anal colposcopy and the diagnosis of anal intraepithelial neoplasia. *Semin Colon Rectal Surg* 1995;6:150.
10. Daling JR, Sherman KJ, Hislop TG, et al. Cigarette smoking and the risk of anogenital cancer. *Am J Epidemiol* 1992;135:180.
11. Holly EA, Whittemore AS, Aston DA, Ahn DK, Nickoloff BJ, Kristiansen JJ. Anal cancer incidence: genital warts, anal fissure or fistula, hemorrhoids, and smoking. *J Natl Cancer Inst* 1989;81:1726.
12. Holmes F, Borek D, Owen-Kummer M, et al. Anal cancer in women. *Gastroenterology* 1988;95:107.
13. Lin AY, Gridley G, Tucker M. Benign anal lesions and anal cancer [Letter]. *N Engl J Med* 1995;332:190.
14. Frisch M, Glimelius B, van den Brule AJ, et al. Sexually transmitted infection as a cause of anal cancer. *N Engl J Med* 1997;337:1350.
15. Nelson RL, Abecarian H. Do hemorrhoids cause cancer? *Semin Colon Rectal Surg* 1995;6:178.
16. Daling JR, Weiss NS, Hislop TG, et al. Sexual practices, sexually transmitted disease, and the incidence of anal cancer. *N Engl J Med* 1987;317:973.
17. Heino P, Goldman S, Lagerstedt U, Dillner J. Molecular and seriological studies of human papilloma virus among patients with anal epidermoid carcinoma. *Int J Cancer* 1993;53:377.
18. Palmer JG, Scholefield JH, Coates PJ, et al. Anal cancer and human papillomaviruses. *Dis Colon Rectum* 1989;32:1016.
19. Melbye M, Cote TR, Kessler L, Gail M, Biggar R. High incidence of anal cancer among AIDS patients. The Aids/Cancer Working Group. *Lancet* 1994;343:636.
20. Wexner SD, Milsom JW, Daily TH. The demographics of anal cancer are changing. Identification of a high risk population. *Dis Colon Rectum* 1987;30:942.
21. Volm MD, von Roenn JH. Non–AIDS-defining malignancies in patients with HIV infection [Review]. *Curr Opin Oncol* 1996;8:386.
22. Penn I. Cancers of the anogenital region in renal transplant recipients. Analysis of 65 cases. *Cancer* 1986;58:611.
23. Lumley JW, Stitz RW. Crohn's disease and anal carcinoma: an association? A case report and review of the literature [Review]. *Aust N Z J Surg* 1991;61:76.
24. Melbye M, Rabkin C, Frisch M, Biggar RJ. Changing patterns of anal cancer incidence in the United States, 1940–1989. *Am J Epidemiol* 1989;139:772.
25. Goldman S, Glimelius B, Nilsson B, Pahlman L. Incidence of anal epidermoid carcinoma in Sweden 1970–1984. *Acta Chir Scand* 1989; 155:191.
26. Frisch M, Melbye M, Moller H. Trends in incidence of anal cancer in Denmark. *BMJ* 1993;306:419.
27. Jensen SL, Hagen K, Shokouh-Amiri MH, Nielsen OV. Does an erroneous diagnosis of squamous cell carcinoma of the anal canal and anal margin at first physician visit influence prognosis? *Dis Colon Rectum* 1987;30:345.
28. Pintor MP, Northover JM, Nicholls RJ. Squamous cell carcinoma of the anus at one hospital from 1948 to 1984. *Br J Surg* 1989;76:806.
29. Brown DK, Oglesby AB, Scott DH, Dayton MT. Squamous cell carcinoma of the anus: a 25-year retrospective. *Am Surg* 1988;54:337.
30. Beahrs OH, Wilson SM. Carcinoma of the anus. *Ann Surg* 1976;184:422.
31. Boman BM, Moertel CG, O'Connell MJ, et al. Carcinoma of the anal canal. A clinical and pathologic study of 188 cases. *Cancer* 1984; 54:114.
32. Myerson RJ, Shapiro SJ, Lacey D, et al. Carcinoma of the anal canal. *Am J Clin Oncol* 1995;18:32.
33. Goldman S, Glimelius B, Norming U, Pahlman L, Seligson U. Transanal rectal ultrasonography and anal carcinoma. A perspective study of 21 patients. *Acta Radiol* 1988;29:337.
34. Roseau G, Palazzo L, Colardelle P, et al. Endoscopic ultrasonography and staging and follow-up of epidermoid carcinoma of the anal canal. *Gastrointest Endosc* 1994;40:447.
35. American Joint Committee on Cancer. *AJCC cancer staging manual*. 5th ed. Philadelphia: JB Lippincott Co, 1997:91.
36. Finne CO. The role of endorectal sonography and the follow-up of malignant disease of the anorectum. *Semin Colon Rectal Surg* 1995;6:86.
37. Clark J, Petrelli N, Herrera L, Mittelman A. Epidermoid carcinoma of the anal canal. *Cancer* 1986;57:400.
38. Northover J. Malignant tumors. In: Nicholls RJ, Dozois RR, eds. *Surgery of the colon and rectum*. New York: Churchill Livingstone, 1997:309.
39. Glimelius B, Pahlman L. Radiation therapy of anal epidermoid carcinoma. *Int J Radiat Oncol Biol Phys* 1987;13:305.
40. Papillon J, Montbarbon JF. Epidermoid carcinoma of the anal canal. A series of 276 cases. *Dis Colon Rectum* 1987;30:324.
41. Papillon J, Mayer M, Montbarbon JF, Gerard JP, Chassard JL, Bailly C. A new approach to the management of epidermoid carcinoma of the anal canal. *Cancer* 1983;51:1830.
42. Merlini M, Eckert P. Malignant tumors of the anus. A study of 106 cases. *Am J Surg* 1985;150:370.
43. Nigro ND, Vaitkevicius VK, Considine B Jr. Combined therapy for cancer of the anal canal: a preliminary report 1974. *Dis Colon Rectum* 1974;36:709.
44. Nigro, ND. An evaluation of combined therapy for squamous cell cancer of the anal canal. *Dis Colon Rectum* 1984;27:763.
45. Flam MS, John MJ, Mowry PA, Lovalvo LJ, Ramalho LD, Wade J. Definitive combined modality therapy of carcinoma of the anus. A report of 30 cases including results of salvage therapy in patients with residual disease. *Dis Colon Rectum* 1987;30:495.
46. Sischy B, Doggett RL, Krall JM, et al. Definitive irradiation and chemotherapy for radiosensitization in management of anal carcinoma: interim report on Radiation Therapy Oncology Group study No. 8314. *J Natl Cancer Inst* 1989;81:850.
47. Cummings B, Keane T, Thomas G, Harwood A, Rider W. Results and toxicity of the treatment of anal canal carcinoma by radiation therapy or radiation therapy and chemotherapy. *Cancer* 1984;54:2062.
48. Grabenbauer GG, Schneider IH, Gall FP, Sauer R. Epidermoid carcinoma of the anal canal: treatment by combined radiation and chemotherapy. *Radiother Oncol* 1993;27:59.
49. Tanum G, Tveit K, Karlsen KO, Hauer-Jensen M. Chemotherapy and radiation therapy for anal carcinoma. Survival and late morbidity. *Cancer* 1991;67:2462.
50. Cummings BJ, Keane TJ, O'Sullivan B, Wong CS, Catton CN. Epidermoid anal cancer: treatment by radiation alone or by radiation and 5-fluorouracil with and without mitomycin C. *Int J Radiat Oncol Biol Phys* 1991;21:1115.
51. Beck DE, Karulf RE. Combination therapy for epidermoid carcinoma of the anal canal [Review]. *Dis Colon Rectum* 1994;37:1118.
52. Martenson JA, Lipsitz SR, Lefkopoulou M, et al. Results of combined modality therapy for patients with anal cancer (E7283). An Eastern Cooperative Oncology Group study. *Cancer* 1991;76:1731.
53. Flam M, John M, Pajak TF, et al. Role of mitomycin in combination with fluorouracil and radiotherapy, and of salvage chemoradiation in the definitive nonsurgical treatment of epidermoid carcinoma of the anal

canal: results of a phase III randomized intergroup study. *J Clin Oncol* 1996;14:2527.

54. Bartelink H, Roelofsen F, Eschwege F, et al. Concomitant radiotherapy and chemotherapy is superior to radiotherapy alone in the treatment of locally advanced anal cancer: results of a phase III randomized trial of the European Organization for Research and Treatment of Cancer, Radiotherapy and Gastrointestinal Cooperative Groups. *J Clin Oncol* 1997;15:2040.

55. UKCCCR Anal Cancer Trial Working Party. Epidermoid anal cancer: results from the UKCCCR randomized trial of radiotherapy alone versus radiotherapy, 5-fluorouracil, and mitomycin. *Lancet* 1996;348:1049.

56. Longo WE, Vernava AM III, Wade TP, Coplin MA, Virgo CS, Johnson FE. Rare anal canal cancers in the U.S. veteran: patterns of disease and results of treatment. *Am Surg* 1991;61:495.

57. Tanum G. Treatment of relapsing anal carcinoma. *Acta Oncol* 1993;32:33.

58. Rich TA, Ajani JA, Morrison WH, Ota D, Levin B. Chemoradiation therapy for anal cancer: radiation plus continuous infusion of 5-fluorouracil with or without cisplatin. *Radiother Oncol* 1993;27:209.

59. Doci R, Zucali R, La Monica G, et al. Primary chemoradiation therapy with fluorouracil and cisplatin for cancer of the anus: results in 35 consecutive patients. *J Clin Oncol* 1996;14:3121.

60. Peddada AV, Smith DE, Rao AR, Frost DB, Kagan AR. Chemotherapy and low-dose radiotherapy in the treatment of HIV-infected patients with carcinoma of the anal canal. *Int J Radiat Oncol Biol Phys* 1997;37:1101.

61. Holland JM, Swift PS. Tolerance of patients with human immunodeficiency virus and anal carcinoma to treatment with combined chemotherapy and radiation therapy. *Radiology* 1993;193:251.

62. Abel ME, Chiu YS, Russell TR, Volpe PA. Adenocarcinoma of the anal glands. Results of a survey. *Dis Colon Rectum* 1993;36:383.

63. Basik M, Rodriguez-Bigas MA, Penetrante R, Petrelli NJ. Prognosis and recurrence patterns of anal adenocarcinoma. *Am J Surg* 1995;169:233.

64. Jensen SL, Shokouh-Amiri MH, Hagen K, Harling H, Nielsen OV. Adenocarcinoma of the anal ducts. A series of 21 cases. *Dis Colon Rectum* 1988;31:268.

65. Papillon J, Chassard JL. Respective roles of radiotherapy and surgery in the management of epidermoid carcinoma of the anal margin. Series of 57 patients. *Dis Colon Rectum* 1992;35:422.

66. Cummings BJ, Keane TJ, Hawkin NV, et al. Treatment of perianal carcinoma by radiation (RT) or radiation plus chemotherapy (RTCT) [Abstract]. *Int J Radiat Oncol Biol Phys* 1986;12:170.

67. Touboul E, Schlienger M, Buffat L, et al. Epidermoid carcinoma of the anal margin: 17 cases treated with curative intent radiation therapy. *Radiother Oncol* 1995;34:195.

68. Greenall MJ, Quan SH, Stearns MW, Urmacher C, De Cosse JJ. Epidermoid cancer of the anal margin. *Am J Surg* 1985;149:95.

69. Mendenhall WM, Zlotecki RA, Vauthey JN, Copeland EN III. Squamous cell carcinoma of the anal margin [Review]. *Oncology* 1996; 10:1843.

70. Cataldo PA, MacKeigan JM. The necessity of routine pathologic evaluation of hemorrhoid specimens. *Surg Gynecol Obstet* 1992;174:302.

71. Nielsen OV, Jensen SL. Basal cell carcinoma of the anus—a clinical study of 34 cases. *Br J Surg* 1981;68:856.

72. Goldman S, Glimelius B, Pahlman L. Anorectal malignant melanoma in Sweden. Report of 49 patients. *Dis Colon Rectum* 1990;33:874.

73. Cooper PH, Mills SE, Allen MS Jr. Malignant melanoma of the anus: report of 12 patients and analysis of 255 additional cases. *Dis Colon Rectum* 1982;25:693.

74. Brady MS, Kavolius JP, Quan SH. Anorectal melanoma. A 64-year experience at Memorial Sloan-Kettering Cancer Center [Review]. *Dis Colon Rectum* 1995;38:146.

75. Weinstock MA. Epidemiology and prognosis of anorectal melanoma. *Gastroenterology* 1993;104:174.

76. Paget J. On disease of the mammary areola preceding cancer of the mammary gland. *St. Bartholemew Hosp Res Lond* 1874;10:87.

77. Beck DE, Fazio VW. Perianal Paget's disease. *Dis Colon Rectum* 1986;30:263.

78. Tjandra J. Perianal Paget's disease. Report of three cases. *Dis Colon Rectum* 1988;31:462.

CHAPTER 19

Neoplasms of the Appendix

William E. Burak, Jr., and William B. Farrar

Neoplasms of the appendix are relatively rare, accounting for less than 1% of all intestinal malignancies (1). Because the veriform appendix is derived embryologically from the large intestines, similar tumor types are found in the appendix and large intestines, with the exception of carcinoid tumors, which are found with much greater frequency in the appendix (2). Most commonly, appendiceal neoplasms are identified at the time of appendectomy performed for the diagnosis of acute appendicitis; occasionally, they are diagnosed at a much later stage, and the patient will present with an abdominal mass or intestinal obstruction. Appendiceal tumors are classified as benign or malignant, and will be discussed separately. Carcinoid tumors, although occasionally thought to be benign, will be considered malignant, as the majority have metastatic potential.

BENIGN APPENDICEAL NEOPLASMS

Benign lesions of the appendix are seen in Table 19-1. Appendiceal polyps are similar to those found in the remaining large intestines and are classified as hamartomatous, adenomatous, or hyperplastic in nature (3–5). Appendiceal adenomas are distinguished from hyperplastic polyps in that hyperplastic polyps appear to be a response to inflammation as a result of local mucosal injury (4). Adenomas appear more diffuse and villous when compared to colonic adenomas (6,7). A cystadenoma is an adenomatous polyp that produces excessive amounts of mucus and can lead to the formation of a mucocele. The term "mucocele" has been traditionally applied to a group of lesions characterized by one or more of the following features: (a) dilatation of the lumen; (b) alterations of the mucosal lining; (c) hypersecretion of mucus; and (d) occasional extension outside the appendix, either as peritoneal implants (pseudomyxoma peritonei), or, exceptionally, as distant metastatic spread (8). More recently, these lesions have been described more appropriately to include the following: (a) focal or diffuse mucosal hyperplasia (no epithelial atypia, but mild distention of the lumen); (b) mucinous cystadenoma (some degree of atypia and marked luminal distention); and (c) mucinous cystadenocarcinoma (stromal invasion by glands

or epithelial cells in peritoneal implants, pseudomyxoma peritonei) (9). The differentiation between the latter two conditions is often subtle, as cystadenoma often distend with mucous and rupture, leading to a localized collection of mucus surrounding the appendix (9–11). The presence of invasive epithelial cells is required for a lesion to be classified as a cystadenocarcinoma.

Diagnosis

By and large, the majority of benign appendiceal lesions are asymptomatic and are incidentally found on routine examination of an appendectomy specimen (12). Occasionally, a cystadenoma with associated mucocele will present as acute appendicitis, a palpable mass, or intussusception (13,14). Various reports describe mucoceles presenting in more unusual fashions, including ureteral obstruction, hematuria, or as an adnexal mass on pelvic ultrasound (15–17).

Because these neoplasms usually present as incidental findings, preoperative imaging studies are not routinely performed. Occasionally, patients with right lower quadrant masses undergo plain abdominal radiographs, which may reveal dystrophic calcification with upward and medial placement of the appendix. A fluid-filled, variable shaped, thin-walled structure containing low-density material is highly suggestive of a cystadenoma with mucocele when seen on abdominal CT scan (18). With the increased utility of sonography, it is important that this disease process be in the differential diagnosis when similar findings are seen on pelvic ultrasound.

Treatment

Because most benign tumors of the appendix are found incidentally in the appendectomy specimen, no further treatment is required. Appendectomy is curative if the margins of resection are uninvolved. Complete colonoscopy should be performed in patients with adenomatous polyps due to the high frequency of associated colonic polyps (6,7). Patients with cystadenomas associated with mucoceles show resolu-

TABLE 19–1. *Benign tumors of the appendix: benign appendiceal neoplasms*

Hamartomatous polyps
Adenomatous polyps-cystadenoma with mucocele
Hyperplastic polyps
Ganglioneuroma

tion of the mucinous process following appendectomy with excision of the localized mucous deposit (9).

MALIGNANT APPENDICEAL NEOPLASMS

There are four types of malignant neoplasms of the appendix (Table 19-2). These are as follows: (a) carcinoid tumors; (b) mucinous cystadenocarcinoma; (c) adenocarcinoma; and (d) adenocarcinoid tumors (1). All of these malignancies are rare, compromising less than 0.4% of all intestinal neoplasms (19). The reported incidence of malignancy in appendectomy specimens range from 1.08% to 1.35% (20,21). Although the four types of neoplasms can behave quite differently with regard to clinical characteristics and outcome, they are similar in that they all share a 15% to 20% chance of having a metachronous or synchronous malignancy, which is usually also in the gastrointestinal tract (22).

Carcinoid Tumors

Carcinoid tumors of the appendix constitute approximately 85% of all appendiceal neoplasms and at least 50% of all carcinoid tumors originate in the appendix (22). It has been reported that carcinoid tumors of the appendix occur more commonly in females. However, this is due to the fact that more women undergo incidental appendectomy; the actual percentage of carcinoids related to the total number of appendectomies is almost identical (2).

Presentation and Diagnosis

The majority of patients with appendiceal carcinoids will present with symptoms indistinguishable from those of acute appendicitis; however it probably contributes to the disease in less than 25% of cases (11,23). The incidental finding of an appendiceal mass during a laparotomy for another disease process will lead to the diagnosis in some patients. Occasionally, the surgeon will incidentally encounter intraabdominal

metastatic carcinoid tumor during surgery for an acute abdomen or when operating for an unrelated condition. Symptoms of carcinoid syndrome are rare and indicate liver metastases (24,25). Increased urinary 5-hydroxy-indoleacetic acid (5-HIAA) and serotonin levels are often diagnostic and can be used to monitor disease progression. Both CT scanning and somatostatin analogue–based nuclear imaging can be used to diagnose and monitor metastatic disease (26,27).

Pathology

Two populations of neuroendocrine cells are present in the mucosa of the veriform appendix (28–32). Intraepithelial enterochromaffin cells are found within the crypt epithelium and are believed to arise from undifferentiated stem cells rather than from migration of neural crest derived cells. The second group of neuroendocrine cells are found in the lamina propria, lie in close association with Schwann cells, and are thought to be derived from neural crest cells. These subepithelial cells are believed responsible for the formation of carcinoid tumors.

Grossly, most carcinoid tumors appear yellow-white, elliptic, circumscribed, but unencapsulated, and involve the appendiceal tip (22). Occasionally, they will diffusely involve the appendiceal wall and are only recognizable on microscopic examination. Only 7% will involve the base of the appendix, explaining the relative uncommon occurrence of obstructive symptoms. Intraoperatively, the tumor will usually appear as a bulbous enlargement of the tip of the appendix (Table 19-3). Approximately 75% of carcinoids are less than 1.0 cm in diameter, and only 10% are greater than 2.0 cm.

Microscopically, carcinoids are composed of nests of small, uniform argyrophilic cells with occasional acinar formation. Microscopic invasion of the subserosal lymphatics is common, but spread to regional lymph nodes is seen infrequently. Multicentricity is observed in approximately 4% of patients, in contrast to small bowel carcinoids, which show a 29% incidence of multicentricity (2).

Treatment

When considering the potential for metastatic spread from an appendiceal carcinoid, size appears to be the best indicator (2,22). Because most carcinoids of the veriform appendix are under 1 cm in greatest diameter, appendectomy is considered

TABLE 19–2. *Malignant tumors of the appendix: malignant appendiceal neoplasms*

Tumor	Frequency
Carcinoid tumor	85%
Mucinous cystadenocarcinoma	8%
Adenocarcinoma	4%
Adenocarcinoid tumor	2%

Data from ref. 22.

TABLE 19–3. *Site of appendiceal carcinoids: location of carcinoid tumors of the appendix*

Site	Percentage of patients
Distal	62
Midportion	15
Proximal	7
Totality	5
Not reported	10

Data from ref. 2.

curative. If the base of the appendix is involved, excision of the appendix with a normal rim of cecum is considered adequate if final margins are negative. Because of the propensity for lymph node metastasis, right hemicolectomy is recommended in the 10% of patients with tumors larger than 2 cm. There is debate regarding the role of right hemicolectomy in patients with 1- to 2-cm carcinoids: some advocate appendectomy alone (2), whereas others recommend secondary right hemicolectomy if lymphatic permeation, mesenteric invasion, or mucin-producing cells are seen on pathologic examination (33–35). A summary regarding the management of incidental appendiceal carcinoids is seen in Table 19-4.

When an unsuspected carcinoid tumor is found during appendectomy or during another abdominal procedure, the appendix should be removed and a frozen section obtained. If the tumor is larger than 2.0 cm, a right hemicolectomy should be undertaken if the situation permits a primary anastomosis to be performed. Otherwise, interval right hemicolectomy should be performed when the patient is bowel prepped and recovered from the initial surgery. No further treatment is required for tumors less than 2.0 cm (with negative margins) that have no lymphatic permeation or excess mucin production. If any enlarged mesenteric lymph nodes are identified, these should be biopsied and if metastatic cells are present, right hemicolectomy should be undertaken. Treatment should be individualized for patients with 1.0- to 2.0-cm carcinoids with unfavorable characteristics (i.e., lymphatic invasion, mucin production), with right hemicolectomy being offered to younger patients.

When metastatic carcinoid is found in the peritoneal cavity during surgery, a biopsy should be obtained to confirm the diagnosis. If the primary is identified, resection for palliation should be considered to decrease the chance of a future bowel obstruction (especially with primary small bowel carcinoids). It is very uncommon for an appendiceal carcinoid to present in this fashion. Although systemic treatment of metastatic carcinoid is disappointing, most of these tumors are indolent, and long-term survival is possible with no treatment. Aggressive curative surgery has no role in this situation.

TABLE 19–4. *Treatment of carcinoid tumors of the appendix*[a]

Tumor size (before fixation)	Treatment
<1.0 cm	Appendectomy
1.0–2.0 cm	Appendectomy or right hemicolectomy[b]
>2.0 cm	Right hemicolectomy

[a] The recommended surgical management of carcinoid tumors of the appendix varies by the size of the lesion. Small tumors (<1 cm) are treated with simple appendectomy, whereas tumors greater than 2 cm require right hemicolectomy, either at the same setting or as a secondary procedure.

[b] Intermediate size (1–2 cm) lesions can be treated with simple appendectomy if there is no lymphatic or mesenteric invasion and the number of mucin-producing cells is small. Otherwise, interval right hemicolectomy should be performed.

Patients with carcinoid syndrome secondary to an appendiceal primary will invariably have liver metastases; palliative procedures include hepatic resection (for isolated lesions) or hepatic arterial chemoembolization (36), which can be effective in controlling symptoms in up to 80% of patients (Table 19-5). Somatostatin analogues (i.e., octreotide) have been shown to reduce the symptoms (flushing, diarrhea) in 85% of patients and should be considered in all symptomatic patients (37). Fifty percent of patients will have disease stabilization; however, this may be short lived as most patients will eventually progress. Interferon alpha is sometimes effective in patients who progress or do not respond to octreotide (38).

Mucinous Cystadenocarcinoma

Mucinous cystadenocarcinomas are the second most common appendiceal malignancy and often are grouped with primary adenocarcinomas as mucinous adenocarcinomas (which probably constitute the same disease), with a majority of lesions showing cystic changes, hence the term "mucinous cystadenocarcinoma" (39). A mucinous cystadenocarcinoma differs from a cystadenoma in that the former shows invasion of the appendiceal wall by atypical glands and the presence of epithelial cells in the intraperitoneal mucinous collections (22).

Presentation and Diagnosis

Right lower quadrant pain associated with a palpable mass is the most common presentation of this disease (22). Approximately 50% of patients with mucinous cystadenocarcinoma will present with intraabdominal metastases, referred to as "pseudomyxoma peritonei." Preoperative diagnosis of pseudomyxoma peritonei is often possible, although it can be mistaken for carcinomatosis, lymphoma, pyogenic peritoni-

TABLE 19–5. *Treatment of carcinoid syndrome*[a]

Symptoms	Treatment
None or minimal	None recommended
Substantial, secondary to syndrome	Somatostatin analogues (i.e., octreotide) α-Interferon Intrahepatic chemoembolization
Substantial, secondary to tumor compression	Hepatic resection (if surgically feasible) Intrahepatic chemoembolization

[a] The recommended treatment of carcinoid syndrome is based upon the presence or absence of symptoms. Somatostatin analogues are useful in patients with minimal symptoms; however, symptoms will eventually reappear. Hepatic artery chemoembolization with doxorubicin is effective in these patients if the extent of disease does not permit surgical debulking.

tis, or loculated ascites (40). The CT scan findings are very characteristic; ascites with attenuation greater than water, low attenuation soft tissue masses with internal mottles densities, distinctive rim-like calcifications, and compression of abdominal viscera without direct invasion. An additional specific finding is scalloping of the hepatic margin from extrinsic compression by fluid-filled ascitic spaces (Fig. 19-1) (40,41). Ultrasonography shows multiple intraperitoneal multilocular cysts; ascitic septations are considered specific for this disease (42).

Pathology

Histologically, mucinous cystadenocarcinoma shows invasion of the appendiceal wall with malignant glandular elements. Pseudomyxoma peritonei is characterized by a benign appearance, with simple columnar epithelium containing small uniform nuclei and mucin-containing vacuoles (43). The diagnosis of this process requires the presence of epithelial cells in the intraperitoneal collections of mucinous material.

Treatment

The primary treatment of mucinous cystadenocarcinoma is surgery. If the disease is isolated to the appendix, or appendix and cecum, right hemicolectomy is required (22). Pseudomyxoma peritonei is treated with surgical debulking; the primary lesion is resected with the right colon in most cases. Intraabdominal metastases are treated with debulking, as it is impossible to obtain negative surgical margins due to the diffuseness of the process. All gelatinous implants should be attempted to be removed in attempt to reduce the patient to the lowest tumor burden. Very rarely is it necessary to resect

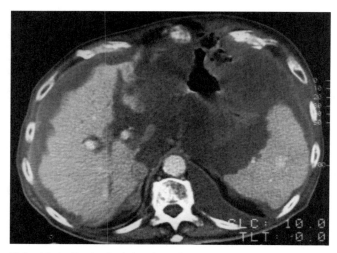

FIG. 19-1. Typical abdominal CT finding of a patient with pseodomyxoma peritonei secondary to a mucinous cystadenocarcinoma. Note the scalloped edges of the hepatic parenchyma and the large amount of gelatinous material surrounding the stomach.

involved visceral organs as the gelatinous implants do not invade the wall of the organ. Omentectomy should be performed as it is often involved in the disease process. Furthermore, repeat operations are often necessary, which may be facilitated by removing the omentum. Recurrent disease should be treated with further cytoreductive surgery, particularly if the patient is symptomatic due to distention, pain, or obstruction. When surgery is no longer feasible, 5-flourouracil (5-FU) chemotherapy results in a small percentage of responses; it may be useful in symptomatic patients however the majority of patients will not benefit.

The 5-year survival of patients with mucinous cystadenocarcinoma is approximately 70%; patients with intraabdominal metastasis in the form of pseudomyxoma peritonei have 50% 5-year survival with aggressive surgical therapy (22). This should be kept in mind when treating the patient who presents with this indolent disease.

Adenocarcinoma

Adenocarcinoma of the appendix is responsible for 4% to 6% of primary malignant appendiceal neoplasms (22,44). Biologically and histologically, these tumors are similar to colonic adenocarcinoma. The peak incidence of adenocarcinoma of the appendix is in the fifth, sixth, and seventh decades of life (45,46), and it is rarely seen in patients under the age of 40.

Presentation and Diagnosis

This disease process, like other appendiceal neoplasms, is very difficult to diagnose preoperatively. This is largely due to the lack of specific historical, physical, clinical, and radiographic findings. The most common initial presentation is right lower quadrant pain, mimicking appendicitis (70%), and less often, an abdominal mass. Quite frequently, the diagnosis is made on histologic examination of the appendix, when it is removed during surgery for presumed appendicitis or because of an unsuspected appendiceal mass found at laparotomy performed for another disease process. The barium enema finding of nonfilling of the appendix and a submucosal mass in a rigid cecal tip has been reported as a characteristic radiographic finding, however this study is rarely obtained preoperatively (22).

Pathology

Adenocarcinoma is identified histologically by invasion of the appendiceal wall by neoplastic cells. Because the muscular wall of the appendix is deficient, any cells that invade the submucosa are subserosal; mesenteric and lymphatic involvement is common. Otherwise, the malignant epithelial cells are identical to those seen in other colonic adenocarcinomas, demonstrating a villous or papillary configuration. Grossly, it may be difficult to determine the origin as to whether it arises from the base of the appendix or the adjacent cecum. An appendiceal primary is present when the majority of the tumor is in the appendix and when adenomatous changes are seen in the remaining appendiceal mucosa (6,7).

Treatment

The treatment of an appendiceal adenocarcinoma is similar to that of a similar tumor in the cecum or right colon, namely right hemicolectomy. If the tumor is found during surgery for an unrelated cause (i.e., appendectomy or unrelated laparotomy) and the operative conditions are not desirable (i.e., peritonitis), an interval right hemicolectomy should be performed once the patient recovers (2 to 6 weeks). Adjuvant chemotherapy should be offered to node positive patients, as it is in patients with adenocarcinoma of the colon (5-FU/levamisole or leucovorin). When similar stages are compared, prognosis is similar to that of colonic adenocarcinoma. Surveillance for secondary colonic neoplasms is recommended due to the high incidence of synchronous or metachronous lesions (Fig. 19-2).

Adenocarcinoid Tumors

Despite the relative rarity of this appendiceal neoplasm, an abundance of literature is available describing this interesting malignancy (47,48). A variety of names have been proposed for this neoplasm: composite tumor, mucinous carcinoid, goblet cell carcinoid, crypt cell carcinoma, and microglandular carcinoma. Adenocarcinoid is a tumor that shares the histologic features of both carcinoids and adenocarcinomas. Biologically, they are more aggressive than carcinoids and less than adenocarcinomas. An interesting feature of these tumors is their propensity for ovarian metastases (Krukenberg tumor) which may lead to misdiagnosis.

Presentation and Diagnosis

Patients with adenocarcinoids are nearly always symptomatic with the most common symptom that of acute appendicitis. Occasionally, the malignancy will present as an abdominal or pelvic (ovarian) mass, or bowel obstruction, or it will be an incidental finding at the time of laparotomy (47). Although symptoms are present, it is difficult to make the diagnosis preoperatively and it is usually a pathological finding.

Pathology

Adenocarcinoids are a combination of tubuloglandular structures and goblet cells (which stain for acid mucin and argyrophilic granules) that arise from the base of the gland, sparing the luminal mucosa (22). Two subgroups have been described: (a) the goblet cell type, which is composed of smooth-bordered nests of cells, the nuclei of which are compressed to the periphery of the cells by abundant intracytoplasmic mucin, and (b) the tubular type, which is composed of small, discrete tubules lined by a single layer of cuboidal or columnar cells (47). Abundant mucin production, areas of concentration of neoplastic elements about the crypts of Lieberkühn, and the absence of any malignant cells in the mucosa are the common characteristics to adenocarcinoids.

Most adenocarcinoid tumors have no characteristic gross appearance. Most are smaller than 2.0 cm in diameter, involve all regions of the appendix, and are often diffusely infiltrative (22). Unlike simple carcinoids, size does not seem to correlate with clinical behavior.

Treatment

The treatment of choice for adenocarcinoid tumors of the appendix is right hemicolectomy, which is usually performed as a secondary procedure after the diagnosis is established. Bilateral oophorectomy should also be undertaken due to the high incidence of ovarian metastases. Patients presenting with Kruckenberg tumors with no identifiable gastrointestinal primary should have an appendectomy performed to avoid missing a small adenocarcinoid of the appendix.

ALGORITHM FOR MANAGEMENT
OF
APPENDICEAL NEOPLASMS

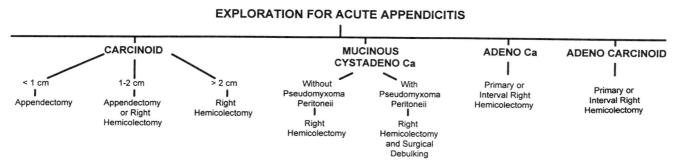

FIG. 19-2. Algorithm for management of appendiceal neoplasms.

The long-term outcome of patients with adenocarcinoid tumors is somewhat variable and falls between that seen with appendiceal carcinoid and adenocarcinoma. The tubular pattern appears to have a more favorable prognosis, with an overall 5-year survival rate of 80%.

Miscellaneous Tumors

A variety of miscellaneous neoplasms of the appendix have been described including metastatic adenocarcinoma, leiomyosarcoma, Kaposi's sarcoma, and lymphoma (49–52). Metastatic carcinoma of the appendix usually results from a primary intraabdominal gastrointestinal adenocarcinoma, although other tumors such as lung and breast have been observed.

CONCLUSION

Benign appendiceal neoplasms are usually incidental operative findings that require no further treatment. Malignant neoplasms are rare tumors that are very difficult to diagnose preoperatively. Their behavior is quite variable, with carcinoids being the most indolent. The mainstay of treatment is surgery; right hemicolectomy is favored for all malignant tumors, with the exception of selected small (less than 2.0 cm) carcinoid tumors. Mucinous cystadenocarcinoma can lead to pseudomyxoma peritonei, in which patients may require multiple operations during the course of this indolent disease.

Although these tumors are quite rare, appendiceal masses identified during laparotomy require appendectomy in order to make an accurate diagnosis and institute proper treatment.

REFERENCES

1. Lyss AP. Appendiceal malignancies [Review]. *Semin Oncol* 1988; 15:129.
2. Moertel CG, Dockerty MD, Judd ES. Carcinoid tumors of the veriform appendix. *Cancer* 1968;21:270.
3. Kitchin AP. Polyps of small intestine with pigmentation of oral mucosa. Report of two cases. *BMJ J* 1953;I:658.
4. Qizilbash AG. Hyperplastic (metaplastic) polyps of the appendix: report of 19 cases. *Arch Pathol* 1974;97:385.
5. Shnitka TK, Sherbaniuk RW. Adenomatous polyps of the appendix in children. *Gastroenterology* 1957;32:462.
6. Wolff M, Ahmed N. Epithelial neoplasms of the veriform appendix (exclusive of carcinoid). I. Adenocarcinoma of the appendix. *Cancer* 1976;37:2493.
7. Wolff M, Ahmed N. Epithelial neoplasms of the veriform appendix (exclusive of carcinoid). II. Cystadenomas, papillary adenomas, and adenomatous polyps of appendix. *Cancer* 1976;37:2511.
8. Bernhardt H, Young JM. Mucocele and pseudomyxoma peritonei of appendiceal origin—clinicopathologic aspects. *Am J Surg* 1965;109:235.
9. Higa E, Rosai J, Pizzimbono CA, Wise L. Mucosal hyperplasia, mucinous cystadenoma, and mucinous cystadenocarcinoma of the appendix. A re-evaluation of appendiceal "mucocele." *Cancer* 1973;32:1525.
10. Gibbs NM. Mucinous cystadenoma and cystadenocarcinoma of the veriform appendix with particular reference to mucocele and pseudomyxoma peritonei. *J Clin Pathol* 1973;26:413.
11. Qizilbash AG. Mucoceles of the appendix. Their relationship to hyperplastic polyps, mucinous cystadenomas and cystadenocarcinomas. *Arch Pathol* 1975;99:548.
12. Deans GT, Spence RA. Neoplastic lesions of the appendix [Review]. *Br J Surg* 1995;82:299.
13. Langsam LB, Raj PK, Galang CF. Intussusception of the appendix. *Dis Colon Rectum* 1985;27:387.
14. Holck S, Wolff M. Intussusception with incarceration of a cystadenoma of the appendix: case report and review of the complications of appendiceal adenomas. *Dis Colon Rectum* 1979;22:133.
15. Risher WH, Ray JE, Hicks TC. Calcified mucocele of the appendix presenting as ureteral obstruction. *J La State Med Soc* 1991;143:29.
16. Vale J, Kirby RS. Haematuria due to mucocele of the appendix. *Br J Urol* 1989;63:218.
17. Landen S, Bertrand C, Maddern GJ, et al. Appendiceal mucoceles and pseudomyxoma peritonei. *Surg Gynecol Obstet* 1992;175:401.
18. Balthazar EJ, Megibow AJ, Gordon RB, Whelan CA, Hulnick D. Computed tomography of the abnormal appendix. *J Comput Assist Tomogr* 1988;12:595.
19. Hesketh K. The management of primary adenocarcinoma of the veriform appendix. *Gut* 1963;4:158.
20. Collins D. 71,000 human appendix specimens. A final report summarizing 40 years study. *Am J Proctol* 1963;14:265.
21. Schmutzer K, Bayar M, Zaki M, Regan JF, Poletti JB. Tumors of the appendix. *Dis Colon Rectum* 1975;18:324.
22. Rutledge RH, Alexander JW. Primary appendiceal malignancies: rare but important [Review]. *Surgery* 1992;111:244.
23. Nwiloh JO, Pillarisetty S, Moscovic EA, Freeman HP. Carcinoid tumors. *J Surg Oncol* 1990;45:261.
24. Markgraf WH, Dunn TM. Appendiceal carcinoid with carcinoid syndrome. *Am J Surg* 1964;107:730.
25. Johnston WH, Waisman J. Carcinoid tumor of the vermiform appendix with Cushing's syndrome. Ultrastructural study of a case. *Cancer* 1971; 27:681.
26. Bomanji J, Mather S, Moyes J, et al. A scintigraphic comparison of iodine-123-metaiodobenzylguanidine and an iodine-labeled somatostatin analog (Tyr-3-octreotide) in metastatic carcinoid tumors. *J Nucl Med* 1992;33:1121.
27. Kvols LK, Brown ML, O'Connor MK, et al. Evaluation of a radiolabelled somatostatin analog (I-123 octreotide) in the detection and localization of carcinoid and islet cell tumors. *Radiology* 1993;187:129.
28. Goddard MJ, Lonsdale RN. The histogenesis of appendiceal carcinoid tumors. *Histopathology* 1992;20:345.
29. Cheng H. Leblond CP. Origin, differentiation and renewal of the four main epithelial cell types in the mouse small intestine. III. Enteroendocrine cells. *Am J Anat* 1974;141:503.
30. Cheng H, Leblond CP. Origin, differentiation and renewal of the four main epithelial cell types in the mouse small intestine. V. Unitarian Theory of the origin of four epithelial cell types. *Am J Anat* 1974;141:537.
31. Rode J, Dhillon A, Papadki L. Serotinin-immunoreactive cells in the lamina propria of the appendix. *Hum Pathol* 1983;14:464.
32. LeDouarin NM, Teillet M. The migration of neural crest cells to the wall of digestive tract in avian embryo. *J Embryo Exp Morphol* 1973;30:31.
33. Syracuse DC, Perzin KH, Price JB, Wiedel PD, Mesa-Tejada R. Carcinoid tumors of the appendix. *Ann Surg* 1979;190:58.
34. Bowman GA, Rosenthal D. Carcinoid tumors of the appendix. *Am J Surg* 1983;176:700.
35. Gouzi JL, Laigneau P, Delalande JP, et al. Indications for right hemicolectomy in carcinoid tumors of the appendix. The French Association for Surgical Research. *Surg Gynecol Obstet* 1993;176:543.
36. Ruszniewski P, Rougier P, Roche A, et al. Hepatic arterial chemoembolization in patients with liver metastases of endocrine tumors. A prospective phase II study in 24 patients. *Cancer* 1993;71:2624.
37. Moertel CG, Johnson CM, McKusick MA, et al. The management of patients with advanced carcinoid tumors and islet cell carcinomas. *Ann Intern Med* 1994;120:302.
38. Janson ET, Ronnblom L, Ahlstrom H, et al. Treatment with alpha-interferon versus alpha-interferon in combination with streptozocin and doxorubicin in patients with malignant carcinoid tumors: a randomized trial. *Ann Oncol* 1992;3:635.
39. Carr, NJ, McCarthy WF, Sobin LH. Epithelial noncarcinoid tumors and tumor-like lesions of the appendix. *Cancer* 1995;75:757.
40. Lee HH, Agha FP, Weatherbee L, Boland CR. Pseudomyxoma peritonei. Radiologic features. *J Clin Gastroenterol* 1986;8(3 Pt 1):312.
41. Yeh HC, Shafir MK, Slater G, Meyer RJ, Cohen BA, Geller SA. Ultrasonography and computed tomography in pseudomyxoma peritonei. *Radiology* 1984;153:507.
42. Hopper KD. Ultrasonic findings in pseudomyxoma peritonei. *South Med J* 1983;76:1051.

43. Ghosh BC, Huvos AG, Whiteley HW. Pseudomyxoma peritonei. *Dis Colon Rectum* 1972;15:420.
44. Gamble HA II. Adenocarcinoma of the appendix: an unusual case and review. *Dis Colon Rectum* 1976;19:621.
45. Didolkar MS, Fanous N. Adenocarcinoma of the appendix: a clinicopathologic study. *Dis Colon Rectum* 1977;20:130.
46. Steinberg M, Cohn I Jr. Primary adenocarcinoma of the appendix. *Surgery* 1967;61:644.
47. Warkel RL, Cooper PH, Helwig EB. Adenocarcinoid, a mucin-producing carcinoid tumor of the appendix, a study of 39 cases. *Cancer* 1978; 42:2781.

48. Isaacson P. Crypt cell carcinoma of the appendix (so-called adenocarcinoid tumor). *Am J Surg Pathol* 1981;5:213.
49. Jones PA. Leiomyosarcoma of the appendix: report of two cases. *Dis Colon Rectum* 1979;22:175.
50. Deziel DJ, Saclarides TJ, Marshall JS, Yaremko LM. Appendiceal Kaposi's sarcoma: a cause of right lower quadrant pain in the acquired immune deficiency syndrome. *Am J Gastroenterol* 1991;86:901.
51. Dieter RA Jr. Carcinoma metastatic to the vermiform appendix: a report of three cases. *Dis Colon Rectum* 1970;13:336.
52. Carpenter BW. Lymphoma of the appendix. *Gastrointest Radiol* 1991; 16:256.

CHAPTER 20

Carcinoid and Other Neuroendocrine Tumors Arising in the Abdomen

Stephen F. Sener and Nancy Schindler

The neuroendocrine system represents a collection of heterogenous cells found in many organs. These enterochromaffin cells secrete amines and peptides, which regulate carbohydrate metabolism and digestion of proteins and fat (1). They exert physiologic control by three mechanisms: (a) humoral endocrine function; (b) neurocrine function, secreting aminergic and peptidergic neuotransmitters; and (c) paracrine function relating to neighboring cells. Tumors that arise from these cells comprise what have been designated as "carcinoid and neuroendocrine tumors," as well as APUDomas and argentaffin tumors.

Lubarsch (2) is credited with the first desciption of a carcinoid tumor in 1888. Oberndorfer (3) coined the term "karzinoide" (carcinoma-like) in 1906 to imply a more benign clinical course for gastrointestinal (GI) carcinoid tumors, and Cassidy (4) first described malignant carcinoid syndrome in 1934. Feyrter (5) in 1938 described a diffuse group of enterochromaffin cells distributed along the entire GI tract, more heavily concentrated in the appendix, ileum, and duodenum, which represented an endocrine epithelial system with paracrine function. In 1968, Pearse (6) discovered amines stored in cytoplasmic secretory granules, with a decarboxylating enzyme that converted precursors to amines or peptides. This finding led to the designation "APUDoma" (amine precursor uptake and decarboxylation). And in 1987, it was determined that gastroenteropancreatic neuroendocrine cells are derived from endoderm instead of neural crest (7). Although the term "APUDoma" may not currently be representative of the common origin of all APUD cells, the concept has been the basis for understanding multiple endocrine neoplasia (MEN) syndromes and the potential for these tumors to be composed of heterogeneous cell types. Most neuroendocrine tumors are designated by the predominant humoral product secreted by the tumor.

These tumors are entopic (produce increased amounts of the native hormone derived from that tissue), ectopic (produce hormones not expected from that tissue), or nonfunctioning (no recognizable hormone secretion despite having neuroendocrine cells on histologic examination). In general, tumors producing entopic hormones are less malignant than those producing ectopic hormones, suggesting that those that produce ectopic hormones are more poorly differentiated (1). Approximately 19 cell types, producing some 40 pharmacologically active substances, have been described.

CARCINOID TUMORS

Pathobiology

Carcinoid tumors account for over 50% of tumors of the neuroendocrine system. About 85% of carcinoids occur in the GI tract, 10% in the bronchi of the lungs, and the remainder in numerous other organs, including esophagus, gall bladder, liver, ampulla of Vater, sacrum, ovary, prostate, kidney, thymus, larynx, and skin (8–17). Table 20-1 describes the embryologic site of origin, involved organs, and types of hormone secretion for abdominal carcinoid tumors.

Although generally uncommon tumors, carcinoids are the most common tumors of the appendix and small bowel. The majority of carcinoids are of midgut origin, with the most frequent location in appendix (46%), followed by small bowel (28%) and rectum (16%) (18,19). Carcinoid tumors are found in one of 300 appendectomies (8). Eighty percent of small bowel carcinoids occur in the distal 2 feet of ileum (20).

Carcinoid tumors are usually firm, with a charactersitic tan to yellow color, located within the wall of the organ of origin, and covered by intact intestinal mucosa. The tumors are composed of solid nests of small cells, arranged in insular, trabecular, or glandular growth patterns.

The malignant potential of carcinoid tumors cannot be determined solely by the histology, but is dependent on several other clinical factors, including site of origin, size of primary tumors, depth of penetration, multicentricity, nuclear DNA content, and growth pattern (21–24) (Table 20-2). Carcinoids of the appendix and rectum are uncommonly multicentric, but 30% of small bowel tumors are multiple.

TABLE 20–1. *Carcinoid tumors: site of embryologic origin, organs, and types of hormone secretion*

Site of origin	Organs	Hormone secretion
Foregut	Bronchus, pancreas, stomach, duodenum	Multiple
Midgut	Jejunum through right colon, ovary	Single
Hindgut	Left colon, rectum	Multiple

Clinical Presentation and Surgical Management of Primary Tumor

Although carcinoid tumors are indeed uncommon, the constellation of symptoms, including a long history of abdominal pain, cramping, intermittent intestinal obstruction, and diarrhea, should pique the physician's attention to the possibility of carcinoid tumor. Patients with carcinoid tumors have urinary 5-hydroxyindolacetic acid (5-HIAA) levels (normal, less than 6 mg/day) that are typically elevated in the range of 50 to 150 mg/day in those without carcinoid syndrome and 100 to 2,500 mg/day in those with carcinoid syndrome (25).

One might expect early detection of gastroduodenal and colorectal carcinoid tumors by endoscopic screening techniques, but other areas in the abdominal cavity are not amenable to early detection of these tumors. Capitalizing on the fact that most neuroendocrine tumors have somatostatin cell surface receptors, somatostatin-receptor scintigraphy using 111-Indium–labeled pentetreotide has been used successfully as a diagnostic tool for determining extent of disease in patients with newly diagnosed carcinoid tumors prior to laparotomy (26). However, somatostatin receptors are also expressed in other conditions, such as inflammatory bowel and granulomatous diseases (27).

Carcinoid tumors are usually found incidentally during exploration for another indication, unless associated with the syndrome or obstructive symptoms. Obstruction may be a manifestation of intussusception, but more likely results from an intense desmoplastic reaction around either primary tumor, or retroperitoneal or mesenteric node metastases. Based on the factors associated with malignant potential, ex-

TABLE 20–2. *Carcinoid tumors: risk of metastatic disease based of location, size, and depth of tumor penetration*

Factor	Risk of metastasis (%)
Location	
Appendix (rarely multiple)	2
Ileum (30% multiple)	35
Colon (<5% multiple)	60
Size	
T < 1 cm (75% of tumors)	2
T 1–2 cm (20% of tumors)	50
T > 2 cm (5% of tumors)	85
Depth of penetration	
Submucosa	Near 0
Muscularis propria	10
Beyond serosa	70

ploration of the abdomen should be performed, searching for multicentricity and metastatic disease in mesentery and liver.

The design of the operative procedure for a carcinoid is based on the malignant potential of the tumor, regardless of whether the tumor is found incidentally. Thus, the goals of surgical therapy are to determine the extent of disease, to resect tumor with curative intent when possible, to palliate symptoms when tumor is unresectable, and to extend survival time.

Small gastroduodenal tumors that have not invaded the muscularis are treated by local excision, but larger, more invasive tumors may require subtotal gastrectomy or pancreatoduodenectomy with appropriate lymph node dissection. In addition, of patients with the most common gastric carcinoid tumors that arise in the fundus, about 10% develop metastases when they are hypergastrinemic, whereas in those whose tumors arise in eugastrinemic states, about 50% have metastases (28).

Small bowel carcinoids found incidentally are important because multiple tumors will be found in about 30% of patients, and other primary GI malignancies will be present in 30% (29). These tumors are treated by intestinal excision with mesenteric node dissection, because 20% of patients with ileal carcinoid tumors of less than 1 cm have nodal metastases at the time of presentation. Thus, an ileal carcinoid should be treated by right hemicolectomy, even in the presence of hepatic metastases. An incidentally discovered Meckel's diverticulum should also be explored to exclude the possibility of harboring a carcinoid tumor (30).

Appendiceal carcinoids greater than 2 cm or those between 1 and 2 cm and associated with local invasion should also be removed by right hemicolectomy. Appendiceal carcinoids of less than 1 cm without metastases or local invasion may be treated by appendectomy (31,32).

Rectal carcinoids of less than 1 cm may be locally excised, but larger or invasive tumors may require low anterior or abdominoperineal resection. However, one report has questioned the value of aggressive surgical treatment for advanced rectal tumors (33).

Carcinoid Syndrome

Serotonin was first extracted from a carcinoid tumor at autopsy in 1953 and was thus identified as the cause of the syndrome (34). A thorough description of the vasomotor changes, bronchospasm, and valvular heart disease was provided in 1954 by Thorson et al. (35).

Serotonin is formed by hydroxylation and decarboxylation of dietary tryptophan, and is metabolized in the liver to

5-HIAA. The syndrome occurs in less than 10% of patients with carcinoid tumors, when serotonin escapes metabolism by the liver and is secreted into the systemic circulation. This happens most frequently in patients with liver metastases or those with metastases drained by the systemic circulation, such as retroperitoneal, ovarian, or bronchial tumors.

The syndrome is typically caused by mid-gut carcinoids, and consists of vasomotor, cardiopulmonary, and GI symptoms. Cutaneous flushing occurs in 95% of patients, diarrhea (not coincident with flushing) in 85%, abdominal cramping in 50%, heart valve lesions in 50%, and wheezing in 6%. Many substances have been identified that contribute to the syndrome, including amines (histamine, dopamine, 5-HIAA), kinins (kallikrein), peptides (pancreatic polypeptide, chromogranins, neurotensin, motilin), and prostaglandins.

Surgical Treatment of Advanced Abdominal Carcinoid Tumors

In patients with carcinoid syndrome resulting from hepatic metastases, several surgical strategies have been used to palliate clinical symptoms. Hepatic resection for curative intent or palliative debulking, as well as hepatic artery ligation or embolization, cryosurgical ablation for unresectable tumor, and orthotopic liver transplantation for massive but resectable liver disease have been used with mixed results (36–39). Somatostatin analogues, antidiarrheal agents, and bronchodilators have been used to ameliorate the symptoms of the syndrome. Interferon with hepatic artery embolization has also shown efficacy in the control of cutaneous flushing (40).

Carcinoid crisis, manifested by severe cutaneous flushing, hypotension and vascular collapse, can occur in patients with carcinoid syndrome during the induction of anesthesia and the surgical or radiologic manipulation of bulky tumors (41). Intravenous somatostatin analogue, in doses of 50 to 100 μg, has successfully been used to reverse hypotension associated with the crisis. Induction of anesthesia is safely accomplished using fentanyl, diazepam, and vecuronium with adequate intravascular volume repletion (42). Thiopentone, histamine-releasing muscle relaxants (atracurium and d-tubocurarine), adrenergic agonists (epinephrine, norepinephrine, and dopamine), and succinylcholine may foster release of vasoactive substances and should therefore be avoided.

Selected patients with advanced extrahepatic disease may also benefit from debulking procedures (43). Soreide et al. (44) reported that in a series of 65 patients, there was 50% 5-year survival rate in unresectable patients and 70% in those having debulking procedures. McEntee et al. (45) reported a 62% survival rate at 2 years in 23 patients having debulking, even in the face of hepatic metastases. Though patients with advanced abdominal disease may live for years without resection, there appears to be a role for debulking of advanced extrahepatic disease. Unfortunately, many of these patients are unresectable because of complex obstructions, fistulas and bowel infarction resulting from the dense mesenteric and retroperitoneal desmoplastic reaction seen in carcinoid tumors.

Nonsurgical Treatment of Advanced Abdominal Carcinoid Tumors

Cytotoxic chemotherapeutic agents have been used, with limited success in reducing bulky disease burden. Combination chemotherapy with 5-fluorouracil and streptozotocin resulted in a 32% response rate with a mean duration of three months (46). However, more recently, somatostatin receptor scintigraphy has been used to predict the efficacy of octreotide in the inhibition of hormone release and tumor regression. It has been suggested that patients with a positive scan respond to octreotide, whereas those with negative scans do not respond. Patients with the anaplastic variant of carcinoid tumor would be expected to have negative scans and do pursue a more malignant disease course. However, Moertel et al. (47) demonstrated that 67% of patients with the anaplastic variant had objective tumor regression using intravenous etoposide and cisplatin. Thus, somatostatin receptor scintigraphy may aid not only to localize tumors, but also to focus selection of therapy between octreotide and combination chemotherapy for patients with advanced disease (48,49).

Prognosis

The prognosis in patients with carcinoid tumors depends on the factors present at the time of presentation (50). Those with noninvasive, small tumors of the appendix and rectum have 5-year survival rates near 100%. Patients with tumors greater than 2 cm have 5-year survival rates less than 50%, and those with hepatic metastases have 5-year survival rates of 20 to 40%.

PERIPANCREATIC NEUROENDOCRINE TUMORS

Pathobiology

Insulinoma

Insulinomas arise from beta cells of the pancreatic islets and account for nearly half of all noncarcinoid neuroendocrine tumors found in the abdominal cavity (1). Ninety percent of these tumors are single, benign adenomas, equally distributed throughout the pancreas, but on rare occasions can be found in the duodenal wall, splenic hilum, or gastrocolic ligament. They are small, encapsulated, and brownish in color, with nearly half being less than 1 cm in diameter. About 10% are malignant, and those are usually larger tumors (more than 5 cm) with liver metastases (51). Multiple tumors occur in about 10% of cases and are typically associated with MEN-1 (Table 20-3).

The diagnosis of insulinoma is suggested by the classic Whipple's triad: (a) hypoglycemic symptoms precipitated by fasting or exercise, (b) fasting blood glucose of less than 50 mg/dL, and (c) relief of symptoms by administration of oral or intravenous glucose. However, the symptoms may be protean and are related to the rapidity of the drop in blood glucose levels. In addition, the triad of symptoms is not

TABLE 20–3. *Peripancreatic nueroendocrine tumors*

Tumor	Islet cell of origin	Location	Associated with MEN	Percentage malignant
Insulinoma	Beta	Equal distribution through pancreas	Most with multiple tumors	10%
Gastrinoma	Nonbeta	"Gastrinoma triangle"	25% of multiple tumors	>90%
Glucagonoma	Alpha	Body/tail pancreas	No	>90%
VIPoma	Neural	Body/tail pancreas	5%	50%
Nonfunctioning	Islet	Head of pancreas	No	>90%

specific to insulinoma, and the differential diagnosis includes the other causes of hypoglycemia-functional (ethanol overdose), organic (pancreatic and nonpancreatic tumors, nesidioblastosis), hepatogenic (liver enzyme defects), factitious, and iatrogenic (sulfonylureas) (1).

Because nearly one-third of patients with insulinoma will have insulin concentrations within the normal range, a 72-h fasting test is generally used, during which excessively high levels of insulin and low levels of glucose are identified. An insulin (microunit/mL)-to-glucose (mg/dL) ratio of more than 0.3 is diagnostic of organic hyperinsulinemia (52). Because insulinoma cells also secrete C-peptide fragment, increased concentrations of this peptide may be diagnostic when attempting to differentiate exogenous use of insulin from tumor as the source of hyperinsulinemia.

Gastrinoma

In 1955, Zollinger and Ellison (53) characterized a syndrome consisting of ulcer diathesis, abdominal pain, and diarrhea, and postulated that a substance secreted by a pancreatic tumor resulted in hyperacidity and GI trophic effects. In 1960, gastrin was isolated from tumor extracts, confirming the hypothesis (54).

Gastrinomas are usually malignant and originate from gastrin-secreting, non–beta islet cells in pancreatic and extrapancreatic sites. As many as two-thirds of gastrinomas may occur outside the pancreas, most commonly in the duodenal wall but also in lymph nodes, stomach, jejunum, mesentery, liver, ovary, and kidneys (1). Sporadic gastrinomas in the intestinal wall are solitary, small (most less than 1 cm), and submucosal, and they frequently metastasize to regional nodes. Those arising in the pancreas frequently also metastasize to the liver. About half of patients with MEN-1 have multiple tumors, and about 25% of patients with multiple tumors have MEN-1 (55). Ninety percent of tumors are found in the gastrinoma triangle with corners at the junction of cystic and common bile duct, the junction of the second and third portion of the duodenum, and the junction of the neck and body of the pancreas.

The diagnosis is made with the combination of an elevated fasting serum gastrin level (more than 100 picograms/mL) and an elevated basal gastric acid output (more than 15 meq/h). The differential diagnosis of hypergastrinemia also includes a(hypo)chlorhydria, gastric outlet obstruction, antral G-cell hyperplasia, retained gastric antrum post antrectomy, postvagotomy state, renal failure, and small bowel resection. A secretin stimulation test may be necessary for those patients who present with a normal serum gastrin level (56).

Glucagonoma

Glucagonomas are uncommon neuroendocrine tumors that originate in alpha cells of the pancreas. Most tumors are solitary, large (more than 5 cm), occur in the body and tail of the pancreas, and are almost never extrapancreatic. Most are malignant, metastasize to regional nodes and liver, and about 70% are associated with the glucagonoma syndrome. These tumors are usually not associated with MEN-1 syndrome.

The glucagonoma syndrome is characterized by mild diabetes, normocytic normochromic anemia, and migratory necrolytic erythema, which is a pathognomonic dermatitis. The rash typically has exacerbations and remissions with a one to two week cycle, begins as scaly papules on face abdomen, perineum, and extremities, then becomes blistered and confluent. Healing of the rash is accompanied by hyperpigmentation in the scar (57). The rash responds to the parenteral administration of amino acids.

Glucagonomas are usually associated with fasting serum glucagon levels of more than 1,000 picograms/mL, and may have concomitant elevations of carcinoembryonic antigen (CEA) and carbohydrate antigen (CA 19-9).

Nonfunctioning Islet Cell Tumor

Nonfunctioning tumors arise from pancreatic islet cells but are not associated with a recognized clinical syndrome. They are usually large (more than 10 cm), solitary, and occur predominantly in the head of the pancreas, thus presenting more like the usual pancreatic neoplasm with pain, weight loss, and jaundice. Most of these tumors are malignant, metastasizing primarily to regional nodes and liver.

VIPoma

VIPomas probably arise from neural cells which produce the neurotransmitter vasoactive intestinal peptide (VIP). Of the approximately 200 patients reported in the literature, 90% had solitary, large tumors in the pancreatic body and tail, with the remaining instances being in the pancreatic head and in extrapancreatic locations such as retroperitoneum, lung, esophagus, and jejunum (1). About 5% of patients with VIPoma have associated MEN-1.

The result of excessive secretion of VIP is the syndrome of watery diarrhea, hypokalemia, hypochlorhydria, and acidosis (WDHHA). Patients have a profuse, secretory diarrhea with hypovolemia, which responds well to somatostatin analogue (59). About 50% of patients also have hypophosphatemia, hypercalcemia, and glucose intolerance, leading to speculation that there may be multiple peptide hormones secreted. Fasting plasma levels of VIP of more than 200 picograms/mL are suggestive of the diagnosis, and elevated levels of pancreatic polypeptide, prostaglandin PGE_2, and calcitonin are confirmatory. About 50% of VIPomas have been malignant to date.

Principles of Surgical Management

Preoperative Evaluation

Because many patients with syndromes related to excess autonomous hormone secretion present with primary tumors of less than 1 cm in diameter and may not have established metastatic disease, localization and operative management of these tumors can be vexing for the surgeon. Once serum hormone levels have adequately explained the clinical syndrome, preoperative radiologic imaging is done to locate the primary tumor and to stage the disease, identifying those patients whose metastatic disease precludes surgical exploration.

Whether one uses conventional computed tomography (CT), spiral CT, or gadolinium enhanced magnetic resonance imaging (MRI) depends on available equipment and expertise of individual radiologists. Invasive testing may also include celiac-superior mesenteric artery angiography with CT portography, since most neuroendocrine tumors are hypervascular and demonstrate a blush following contrast injection of surrounding arteries. Angiography may also be combined with provocative stimulation tests to provide localization information on gastrinoma and insulinoma, employing selective injection of secretogogue into the arteries supplying the pancreas and simultaneous collection of blood from hepatic veins for hormone assay (58).

Somatostatin receptor scintigraphy (SRS) has been used to localize peripancreatic neuroendocrine tumors, as well as carcinoids. In a prospective study of 55 patients, Kisker et al. (26) reported that SRS was not effective imaging insulinomas and nonfunctioning islet cell tumors. Of newly diagnosed gastrinomas evaluated by a combination of CT, transabdominal ultrasound, and SRS, 10 of 17 primary tumors and metastases in 9 of 9 patients were detected.

Endoscopic ultrasound (EUS) has been reported to be more sensitive than transabdominal ultrasound for localization of neuroendocrine tumors, but few studies have compared EUS to intraoperative ultrasound.

Medical control of the symptoms related to hormone secretion from peripancreatic neuroendocrine tumors is an important part of the preoperative management. For patients with gastrinoma, continuous infusion of intravenous H2-antagonists at doses titrated to control basal acid output are begun prior to operation and maintained through the immediate postopertive period, since even after tumor excision the hypertrophied gastric parietal cell mass may continue to hypersecrete acid. For those with insulinoma, continuous infusion of intravenous D10W solution will generally maintain serum glucose concentrations in a normal range through the period when operative manipulation of tumor may cause exaggerated hyperinsulinemia. For those with VIPomas, control of hypovolemia and electrolyte imbalance is facilitated by somatostatin analogue to control the diarrhea (59).

Operative Management

For all peripancreatic neuroendocrine tumors, the only available curative treatment is surgical excision. Given the propensity for extrapancreatic tumors, the abdominal examination must be thorough and include liver, small and large intestine, pelvic structures, omentum, and retroperitoneum. Careful examinatiion of the pancreas through the lesser sac requires an extensive Kocher maneuver and mobilization along the inferior rim of the pancreas to dissect the plane between the posterior pancreas and the retroperitoneal fat.

Intraoperative B-mode ultrasonography (IOUS) using a 10 MHz transducer within a sterile sheath has become an important adjunct to physical examination of the liver and pancreas. With increasing experience, IOUS provides additional information useful in planning tumor excision, even when the tumor is palpable. Tumors are generally hypoechoic, and knowledge of the relationship of tumor to bile duct, pancreatic duct, and vascular structures aids in the decision of whether to enucleate a tumor or perform a formal pancreatectomy. For occult gastrinomas the search is initially focused within the gastrinoma triangle, whereas for occult insulinomas the entire gland is at risk to harbor the tumor.

Further evaluation for occult tumor may be performed using intraoperative endoscopy with transillumination of the intestinal wall. The endoscopist may insufflate and distend the lumen of the bowel to aid in locating the occult tumor. For patients in whom tumor remains occult after these maneuvers, a longitudinal duodenotomy in the anterior wall of the second portion of the duodenum may be done, which facilitates evaluation of the difficult medial wall of the duodenum from the pylorus to the ligament of Treitz. At times, the relationship between tumor and the ampulla is unclear. In this circumstance, cholecystectomy and passage of a balloon-tipped biliary catheter through the cystic and common bile ducts through the ampulla not only identifies the ampulla but demonstrates the path of the intrapancreatic bile duct, facilitating excision of tumor in the medial duodenal wall (60) (Table 20-4).

In recent years, the success of H2-antagonists has resulted in fewer instances when total gastrectomy is required for Zollinger-Ellison syndrome. With earlier diagnosis and much better medical control of ulcer disease, fewer patients succumb to complications of severe peptic ulcer disease and more are thus exposed to the mortality risk from metastatic tumor.

TABLE 20-4. *Operative Management of Gastrinoma*

Exploration, including operative ultrasound	
Aids: intraoperative endoscopy, longitudinal duodenotomy, cholecystectomy, common duct exploration	
If	*Then*
Small noninvasive tumor of duodenal wall/pancreas	Enucleation with regional node dissection
Small invasive tumor, multiple nodes, multiple tumors	Pancreatoduodenectomy
Occult primary tumor	Regional node dissection, consider total gastrectomy, avoid blind pancreatoduodenectomy
Advanced disease	Debulk, total gastrectomy

This change in the natural history of the disease has fostered newer concepts in the resection of gastrinomas. Small, noninvasive gastrinomas of the duodenal wall or pancreas in the absence of node metastases, may be locally excised or enucleated. Regional lymph nodes, whether suspicious or not, and resectable liver metastases should be removed. Pancreatoduodenectomy may be necessary for small but invasive tumors with multiple node metastases or for multiple tumors. For those patients in whom primary tumor remains occult, regional lymphadenectomy is appropriate because in up to 40% of these cases node removal results in long-term biochemical cure. For those with advanced disease, surgical debulking and total gastrectomy may still be necessary to prolong survival and control peptic ulcer disease.

The situation may arise in which the tumor remains occult despite localization attempts, prompting the protracted discussion in the operating room regarding blind pancreatic resection. For patients with insulinoma, the entire gland is at risk to harbor the tumor, the risk of malignancy is low, and localization techniques continue to evolve with time. For these reasons it may be preferable to avoid blind resection in favor of follow-up localization procedures. For those with Zollinger-Ellison syndrome, blind resection of the gastrinoma triangle is probably not indicated. But total gastrectomy to eliminate the complications of ulcer diathesis is an option that must be considered, because the procedure provides the only reliable method of avoiding the long-term effects of acid hypersecretion (61).

MEN-1 and Zollinger-Ellison Syndrome

The surgical approach to MEN-1 patients with Zollinger-Ellison syndrome is predicated upon the preoperative localization of gastrin secretion from discrete tumors rather than islet cell hyperplasia or nesidioblastosis. Based on extensive experience, Thompson et al. reported that all MEN-1 patients with Zollinger-Ellison syndrome and localized gastrin secretion should be explored, in the absence of liver metastases demonstrated by a CT scan (62). A 6-cm longitudinal duodenotomy with complete exploration of the duodenal wall from the pylorus to the ligament of Treitz revealed that most MEN-1

patients had multiple, functional gastrinomas within the gastrinoma triangle. Peripancreatic and periduodenal nodes were aggressively removed, and 60% had occult node metastases. Although IOUS was helpful, most pancreatic tumors were palpable and were enucleated. In addition, almost all patients had tumors in the pancreatic body or tail which required distal pancreatectomy. Most patients were rendered eugastrinemic during early follow-up, with the long-term results of this strategy still pending.

REFERENCES

1. Delcore R, Friesen SR. Gastrointestinal neuroendocrine tumors [Review]. *J Am Coll Surg* 1994;178:187.
2. Lubarsch O. [Uber den primaren Krebs des Ileums. Bemerkungen uber das gleichzeitige Vorkommen von Krebs und Tuberculose] [German]. *Arch Pathol Anat* 1888;111:280.
3. Oberndorfer S. [Ueber die kleinen Dunndarmcarcinome] [German]. *Verh Dtsch Ges Pathol* 1907;11:1213.
4. Cassidy M. Abdominal carcinomatosis associated with vasomotor distubances. *Proc R Soc Med* 1934;27:220.
5. Feyrter F. [Ueber diffuse endokrine epitheliale Organe] [German]. *Zbl Inn Med* 1938;59:545.
6. Pearse AG. Common cytochemical and ultrastructural characteristics of cells producing polypeptide hormones (the APUD series) and their relevance to thyroid and ultimobranchial C cells and calcitonin. *Proc R Soc Lond B Biol Sci* 1968;170:71.
7. Pearse AG. Genesis of the neuroendocrine system. In: Friesen SR, Thompson NW, eds. *Surgical endocrinology*. Philadelphia: JB Lippincott, 1990:15.
8. Moertel CG. Karnofsky memorial lecture. An odyssey in the land of small tumors. *J Clin Oncol* 1987;5:1502.
9. Partensky C, Chayvialle JA, Berger F, Souquet JC, Moulinier B. Five-year survival after transhiatal resection of esophageal carcinoid tumor with a lymph node metastasis. *Cancer* 1993;72:2320.
10. Khetan N, Bose NC, Arya SV, Gupta HO. Carcinoid tumor of the gallbladder: report of a case [Review]. *Surg Today* 1995;25:1047.
11. Krishnamurthy SC, Dutta V, Pai SA, et al. Primary carcinoid tumor of the liver: report of four resected cases including one with gastrin production [Review]. *J Surg Oncol* 1996;62:218.
12. Feurle GE. Argyrophil cell hyperplasia and a carcinoid tumour in the stomach of a patient with sporadic Zollinger-Ellison syndrome. *Gut* 1994;35:275.
13. Modlin IM, Gilligan CJ, Lawton GP, Tang LH, West AB, Darr U. Gastric carcinoids. The Yale experience. *Arch Surg* 1995;130:250.
14. Thomas RM, Baybick JH, Elsayed AM, Sobin LH. Gastric carcinoids. An immunohistochemical and clinicopathologic study of 104 patients. *Cancer* 1994;73:2053.
15. Emory RE Jr, Emory TS, Goellner JR, Grant CS, Nagorney DM. Neuroendocrine ampullary tumors: spectrum of disease including the first

report of a neuroendocrine carcinoma of non–small cell type. *Surgery* 1994;115:762.

16. Wilkowske MA, Hartmann LC, Mullany CJ, Behrenbeck T, Kvols LK. Progressive carcinoid heart disease after resection of primary ovarian carcinoid. *Cancer* 1994;73:1889.
17. Schnee CL, Hurst RW, Curtis MT, Friedman ED. Carcinoid tumor of the sacrum: case report [Review]. *Neurosurgery* 1994;35:1163.
18. Godwin JD II. Carcinoid tumors. An analysis of 2,837 cases. *Cancer* 1975;36:560.
19. Moertel CG, Dockerty MB, Judd ES. Carcinoid tumors of the vermiform appendix. *Cancer* 1968;21:270.
20. Cheek RC, Wilson H. Carcinoid tumors. *Curr Probl Surg* 1970;7:34.
21. Zeitels J, Naunheim K, Kaplan EL, Strauss F II. Carcinoid tumors: a 37-year experience. *Arch Surg* 1982;117:732.
22. Moertel CG, Sauer WG, Dockerty MB, Bogenstoss AH. Life history of the carcinoid tumor of the small intestine. *Cancer* 1961;14:901.
23. Falkmer S, Erhardt K, Auer G, Martensson H, Nobin A. Patterns of DNA distribution and neurohormone immunoreactivity in tumour cells: tools for the histopathological assessment of gastrointestinal carcinoids. *Digestion* 1986;35[Suppl 1]:144.
24. Johnson LA, Lavin PT, Moertel CG, et al. Carcinoids: the association of histologic growth patterns and survival. *Cancer* 1983;51:882.
25. Sjoblom SM. Clinical presentation and prognosis of gastrointestinal carcinoid tumours. *Scand J Gastroenterol* 1988;23:779.
26. Kisker O, Bartsch D, Weinel RJ, et al. The value of somatostatin-receptor scintigraphy in newly diagnosed endocrine gastroenteropancreatic tumors. *J Am Coll Surg* 1997;184:487.
27. Reubi JC, Mazzucchelli L, Laissue JA. Intestinal vessels express a high density of somatostatin receptors in human inflammatory bowel disease. *Gastroenterology* 1994;106:951.
28. Solcia E, Capella C, Fiocca R, Cornaggia M, Bosi F. The gastroenteropancreatic endocrine system and related tumors [Review]. *Gastroenterol Clin North Am* 1989;18:671.
29. Thompson GB, van Heerden JA, Martin JK Jr, et al. Carcinoid tumors of the gastrointestinal tract: presentation, management, and prognosis. *Surgery* 1985;98:1054.
30. Ohmori T, Okada K, Arita N, Tabei R. Multiple ileal carcinoid and appendiceal endocrine carcinoma in association with Meckel's diverticulum. A histochemical and immunohistochemical study. *Arch Pathol Lab Med* 1994;118:283.
31. Moertel CG, Weiland LH, Nagorney DM, Dockerty MB. Carcinoid tumor of the appendix: treatment and prognosis. *N Engl J Med* 1987;317:1699.
32. Roggo A, Wood WC, Ottinger LW. Carcinoid tumors of the appendix [Review]. *Ann Surg* 1993;217:385.
33. Sauven P, Ridge JA, Quan SH, Sigurdson ER. Anorectal carcinoid tumors. Is aggressive surgery warranted? *Ann Surg* 1990;211:67.
34. Lembeck F. 5-Hydroxytryptamine in a carcinoid tumor. *Nature* 1953;172:910.
35. Thorson A, Biorck G, Bjorkman G, et al. Malignant carcinoid of the small intestine with metastases to the liver, valvular disease of the right side of the heart (pulmonary stenosis and tricuspid regurgitation without septal defects), peripheral vasomotor symptoms, bronchoconstriction, and an unusual type of cyanosis. *Am Heart J* 1954;47:795.
36. Creutzfeldt W, Stockmann F. Carcinoids and carcinoid syndrome [Review]. *Am J Med* 1987;82:4.
37. Therasse E, Breittmayer F, Roche A. Transcatheter chemoembolization of progressive carcinoid liver metastasis. *Radiology* 1993;189:541.
38. Johnson LB, Krebs T, Wong-You-Cheong J, et al. Cryosurgical debulking of unresectable liver metastases for palliation of carcinoid syndrome. *Surgery* 1997;121:468.
39. Schweizer RT, Alsina AE, Rosson R, Bartus SA. Liver transplantation for metastatic neuroendocrine tumors. *Transplant Proc* 1993;25:1973.
40. Nobin A, Lindblom A, Mansson B, Sundberg M. Interferon treatment in patients with malignant carcinoids. *Acta Oncol* 1989;28:445.

41. Kvols LK, Martin JK, Marsh HM, Moertel CG. Rapid reversal of carcinoid crises with a somatostatin analogue. *N Engl J Med* 1985;313:1229.
42. Parris WC, Oates JA, Kambam J, Shmerling R, Sawyers JF. Pretreatment with somatostatin in the anesthetic management of a patient with carcinoid syndrome. *Can J Anaesth* 1988;35:413.
43. Norton JA. Surgical management of carcinoid tumors: role of debulking and surgery for patients with advanced disease [Review]. *Digestion* 1994;55[Suppl 3]:98.
44. Soreide O, Berstad T, Bakka A, et al. Surgical treatment as a principle in patients with advanced abdominal carcinoid tumors. *Surgery* 1992;111:48.
45. McEntee GP, Nagorney DM, Kvols LK, Moertel CG, Grant CS. Cytoreductive hepatic surgery for neuroendocrine tumors. *Surgery* 1990;108:1091.
46. Moertel CG, Hanley JA. Combination chemotherapy trials in metastatic carcinoid tumor and the malignant carcinoid syndrome. *Cancer Clin Trials* 1979;2:327.
47. Moertel CG, Kvols LK, O'Connell MJ, Rubin J. Treatment of neuroendocrine carcinomas with combined etoposide and cisplatin. Evidence of major therapeutic activity in anaplastic variants of these neoplasms. *Cancer* 1991;68:227.
48. Reubi JC. Clinical relevance of somatostatin receptor imaging. *Eur J Endocrinol* 1994;131:575.
49. Janson ET, Westlin JE, Eriksson B, Ahlstrom H, Nilsson S, Oberg K. [111-In-DTPA-D-Phe1] octreotide scintigraphy in patients with carcinoid tumours: the predictive value for somatostatin analogue treatment. *Eur J Endocrinol* 1994;131:577.
50. Agranovich AL, Anderson GH, Manji M, Acker BD, Macdonald WC. Carcinoid tumour of the gastrointestinal tract: prognostic factors and disease outcome. *J Surg Oncol* 1991;47:45.
51. Thompson NW, Eckhauser FE. Malignant islet cell tumors of the pancreas. *World J Surg* 1984;8:940.
52. Vinik AI, Pavlic-Renar I. Insulin-producing tumors. In: Mazzaferri EL, Bar RS, Kreisberg RA, eds. *Advances in endocrinology and metabolism.* Vol. 4. St. Louis: Mosby–Year Book, 1993:1.
53. Zollinger RM, Ellison EH. Primary peptic ulcerations of the jejunum associated with islet cell tumors of the pancreas. *Ann Surg* 1955;14:709.
54. Gregory RA, Tracy HJ, French JM, et al. Extraction of a gastrin-like substance from a pancreatic tumor in a case of Zollinger-Ellison syndrome. *Lancet* 1960;1:1045.
55. Pipeleers-Marichal M, Somers G, Willems G, et al. Gastrinomas in the duodenums of patients with multiple endocrine neoplasia type 1 and the Zollinger-Ellison syndrome. *N Engl J Med* 1990;322:723.
56. Townsend CM Jr, Thompson JC. Up-to-date treatment of the patient with hypergastrinemia [Review]. *Adv Surg* 1987;20:155.
57. Bloom SR, Polak JM. Glucagonoma syndrome [Review]. *Am J Med* 1987;82:25.
58. Thom AK, Norton JA, Doppman JL, et al. A prospective study of the use of intrarterial secretin injection and portal venous sampling to localize duodenal gastrinomas. *Surgery* 1992;112:1002.
59. Vinik AI, Tsai ST, Moattari AR, et al. Somatostatin analogue (SMS 201-995) in the management of gastroenteropancreatic tumors and diarrhea syndromes. *Am J Med* 1986;81:23.
60. Fraker DL, Alexander HR. The surgical approach to endocrine tumors of the pancreas [Review]. *Semin Gastrointest Dis* 1995;6:102.
61. Tasiopoulos JN, Meiselman M, Chiao G, Levy R, Sener SF, Townsend CM. Zollinger-Ellison syndrome. In: Winchester DP, Brennan MF, Dodd GD, et al., eds. *Tumor board: case management.* Philadelphia: Lippincott–Raven Publishers, 1997:128.
62. Thompson NW, Pasieka J, Fukuuchi A. Duodenal gastrinomas, duodenotomy, and duodenal exploration in the surgical management of Zollinger-Ellison syndrome. *World J Surg* 1993;17:455.

CHAPTER 21

Image-Directed Breast Biopsy Techniques

David S. Robinson and Magesh Sundaram

The diagnosis of nonpalpable breast cancer through image guidance has become important for many general surgeons. The reasons for this growing interest, the techniques themselves, and the decision about how to approach an imaged lesion comprise the substance of this chapter.

Just over half a century following Roentgen's discovery of x-rays, mammography found its earliest beginnings in the 1950s, and during the next one and one half decades it proved its efficacy through prospective trials (1). As a result, women engaged in ongoing screening mammography have realized a 30% decrease in mortality (2). Despite that observation, mammography remained underutilized. In 1985, the number of women eligible under the American Cancer Society's guidelines who chose to undergo screening mammography was barely 15%; with an increased awareness that early detection may both save lives and often improve cosmetic outcome, the compliance rate is now approaching 70% (3). Of all imaging studies, mammography is now the second most common behind the chest x-ray. In absolute numbers, increased by "baby-boomers" who have come of age, it is anticipated that 47.5 million women will undergo mammography in the United States in the year 2000. With this increase comes a proportionate number of image-directed biopsies. Currently, 2% to 3% of patients undergoing screening or diagnostic mammography receive a recommendation to undergo a subsequent biopsy. If that level remains consistent, by the end of this century 1.25 million women will undergo a breast biopsy annually. By current estimates, based on the projected number of stereotactic tables that will be in use, 75% of those biopsies will be performed stereotactically (3).

Several factors drive this trend to a less invasive approach. The cost of a stereotactic procedure is significantly less than that of an open biopsy performed in an operating room. In addition, the use of this technology has expanded beyond the radiology suite and into the surgical corridors, creating a competitive market. Clearly, both disciplines will continue to participate with expertise using these tissue-sampling techniques. Along with the "gold standard" of needle localization and open breast biopsy, these new techniques are important

in the armamentarium of any general surgeon who deals with breast disease.

When it was realized three decades ago that mammography could find a breast cancer before it became palpable, a collegial relationship between the radiologist and the surgeon developed. To sample a mammographically suspicious lesion, the radiologist placed a hypodermic needle (and later a guide wire) using mammographic imaging, which would then direct the surgeon to the nonpalpable lesion to be biopsied. Now, with the advent of newer technology, the technical need for both specialists to perform an image-guided breast biopsy may be less pressing. This has created a turf war, the fires of which are fanned by economic issues. While the costs of sampling are lowered, the doctor who collects both imaging and biopsy fees has enhanced profits, and with increased recognition as an expert, that doctor is better perceived in his or her community.

A radiologist who can take the image and then the biopsy may eliminate participation by the surgeon. This is important to the economics of general surgery because the diagnosis and treatment of breast disease ranks fourth in the generation of income for the general surgeon, as a close runner-up to (a) office visits, (b) laproscopic cholecystectomy, and (c) hernia repair. Therefore, the general surgeon must be assertive in maintaining a presence in breast cancer diagnosis, not for financial reasons, but because the diagnosis and treatment of breast disease is a significant part of general surgery. The American College of Surgeons (ACoS) is taking an affirmative stand in developing criteria for the eligibility to perform stereotactic and ultrasound-directed biopsies with the American Academy of Radiologists (4). The ACoS has also proactively developed a program to provide training to surgeons in both the cognitive and technical aspects of stereotactic and ultrasound-guided biopsies. Those engaged in this process clearly recognize that general surgeons are and will continue to be involved in image-directed biopsies.

BASIC CONCEPTS AND RULES OF THE ROAD

Regardless of the approach, the basic concept for all image-guided techniques remains to translate a suspicious two-dimensional image into a three-dimensional location in the breast to obtain tissue for diagnosis. Although some images are suspicious enough to be considered diagnostic, a true diagnosis of primary breast cancer can only be made by a histologic assessment of cells or tissues. This does not in any way diminish the importance of imaging; it simply puts the technique in perspective.

Recently, the American College of Radiology has proposed a system called the "Breast Imaging Reporting and Data System" (BI-RADs) to standardize the approach to mammographic reporting of densities and microcalcifications (4). Although there are no fixed criteria, the system evaluates shapes and sizes of masses and numbers, shapes, sizes, and distribution of microcalcifications to develop a scale leading to one of five categories from "completely normal" through "highly suspicious of malignancy." The BI-RADs concept on clinical prospective evaluation appears a reliable approach for the development of an acuity scale based on images for uniform reporting (5). For lesions that appear to be suspicious of demonstrating malignancy, the use of images to obtain tissue is important. Placement of a needle localization to a mammographically suspicious lesion requires that the lesion be seen in two films from different views to gain a three-dimensional sense of its location; depth cannot be obtained from a lesion recognized on only one mammographic view. Using ultrasound for needle localization, the viewer gains depth perception because the mobility of the imaging probe through a narrow field of view can quickly (in real time) provide a sense of the lesion's location. Using either approach, a needle and guide wire can be placed for an open biopsy very close to or through the lesion to be biopsied. Core sampling employs the same principles of depth, but when using stereotactic mammography the core needle is passed using two images taken from different angles in the same arc to triangulate the depth.

Once a sample has been obtained either by needle localization with open biopsy or by core sampling, image validation that the appropriate tissue has been removed is an important part of the biopsy process. Because the reason for the biopsy is to determine whether a nonpalpable x-ray–discovered change in the tissue is cancer, it is important to prove that the tissue giving rise to this x-ray abnormality has been removed. A specimen mammogram of an open biopsy is the time-honored approach. Validation is straightforward using ultrasonography because the core-sampling needles or localizing needle/guide wire enter under direct observation. The non-calcified mass that is a stereotactically biopsied can be validated by observing the pre- and postfire positions of the core-sampling device, and after the samples have been removed a mid-axial film is taken to compare with the prebiopsy scout film. For microcalcifications, stereotactic cores should be imaged to confirm that microcalcifications are in the specimen. This can be taken stereotactically or by analog mammography; the cores in a petri dish are either taped to the stereotactic imaging plate or placed on the mammography stage. In addition, validation should extend to the pathology report.

When core samples containing microcalcifications are sent, the request sheet must ask pathologist to specifically state that there are or are not microcalcifications seen in the histologic specimen.

Finally, biopsy-directed images cannot be transposed from one medium to another. For example, an ultrasonographic density cannot be stereotactically biopsied. What is seen by one imaging method may very well produce a different image by another approach. Moreover, a specimen that has been removed using one imaging approach cannot be confirmed with another; for example, a lesion that has been ultrasonographically localized cannot be validated with specimen mammography.

These are some of the general principles that apply to all imaged biopsies. We will now examine the techniques in more detail.

NEEDLE LOCALIZATION AND OPEN BIOPSY

The initial and still the most frequent approach to a nonpalpable image lesion is mammographic needle localization by a radiologist prior to surgical incision. When taking the patient's history, the surgeon should ask if she is taking an anticoagulant such as Coumadin or aspirin. These medications should be discontinued well in advance of the operative procedure. If anticoagulation must be maintained, then the patient may be placed on short-acting heparin injections, not requiring monitoring and administered twice daily; this should be discontinued 12 h before the image-directed biopsy.

In the mammography suite prior to needle placement, the patient's mammograms will be reviewed by the radiologist, who may want additional confirmatory x-rays or ultrasound prior to placement of the alpha-numeric grid. The schedule should anticipate enough time for the radiologist to place the needle prior to the biopsy.

When the patient presents with a mammographic change that appears to correspond with a palpable mass, the surgeon should communicate with the radiologist to be certain that the visualized and palpable lesions are the same. If there is any question, the mammography technician can demonstrate a correlation by placing a radiopaque skin marker over the palpable mass prior to taking mammograms. Even with that, if there is any question it is often safer to perform an image-directed biopsy with needle/wire localization prior to an open biopsy; if the palpable and mammographic lesions are not the same, both should be removed. For the prominently palpable lesion that correlates with the skin marker, image-directed guidance is not necessary, but if there is even a scintilla of doubt, a specimen radiogram should be taken to confirm that the visualized and palpable lesions are the same and that the imaged lesion has been removed.

If the preneedle localization mammograms show the density or microcalcifications on only one view, needle localization is impossible. At that juncture, either a stereotactic needle localization or core sampling can be performed, or the patient should return for repeat films to reevaluate the lesion.

Local anesthesia for needle placement is usually not needed. Mammograms after placement confirm the needle's tip to be near the lesion. Orthogonal views complete the localization, and a guide wire is passed through the needle and deployed. Once in place, the needle and guide wire are secured, and the area is dressed in such a way so as not to move the position of the needle.

The patient with her mammograms is taken into the operating room. The surgeon evaluating the films determines the relative position of the needle to the lesion and gauges the position of the incision and depth required to reach that area.

With regard to planning the incision, in the operating suite the surgeon should carefully evaluate the needle's entry and its position deep within the breast tissue. If the needle enters through a cosmetically acceptable site (one that would not be seen in most circumstances), the surgeon may chose to make his or her incision around the needle and follow its track, creating a tissue core around the needle itself down to the level at which he or she wishes to take the specimen. If the needle enters through a cosmetically sensitive area (for example, the upper inner quadrant of the breast) and the needle's tip is found to lie centrally within the breast, then the incision should be placed in a more central location, with subsequent dissection toward the tip without following it. In addition, the surgeon should have a relatively good idea of what therapeutic procedure the patient might wish to pursue should the biopsy demonstrate malignancy. If a modified radical mastectomy is anticipated, the surgeon may wish to place an incision within the skin island that will be resected; if a lumpectomy and axillary dissection are anticipated, then the incision may be placed in an entirely different location. In general terms, biopsy and lumpectomy incisions placed in the lower quadrants are generally radial or "spoke-like," whereas those placed in the upper quadrants are curvilinear, paralleling the areolar margin and following Langer's lines.

After antiseptic preparation and draping, local anesthesia is usually sufficient for many straightforward needle localization biopsies. The analgesic agent will vary with the surgeon's preference; ours is a 1% solution of lidocaine with 1:100,000 epinephrine to which sodium bicarbonate is added. By itself, lidocaine with epinephrine is painful upon injection because of the acidity to extend shelf-life. This pain can be abrogated with an addition of 7.5% sodium bicarbonate to the lidocaine by the scrub nurse; we prefer seven parts of the analgesic to three parts of sodium bicarbonate.

After the anesthetic is injected, creating a skin weal, deeper infiltration is carried out using a generous amount of the analgesic in the corridor of the proposed dissection and around the site to be excised. This is important because every patient waits anxiously for pain to occur. Like all of us, she will remain calm as long as no pain is encountered, but once pain occurs the anxiety associated with it will make the remaining time spent in performance of the biopsy far more unpleasant for both the surgeon and the patient. Through a 25-gauge or smaller needle at a relatively low pressure, the injection is painless.

To quell anxiety, some patients may require preincisional sedation; here our preference is the intravenous administration of 1 to 4 mg of Versed and 25 mg of Demerol. Oxygen saturation and ECG monitoring are observed by an operating room nurse. Very rarely is general anesthesia needed for a breast biopsy. After the procedure has been completed and the sedated patient has recovered, she must be accompanied home.

The electrocautery is often used deep to the skin incision to effectively divide the tissue while providing hemostasis down to the level of tissue to be removed; dissection near the specimen should avoid the electrocautery because electrical damage and polarization of the nuclei (often into a picket fence alignment) may render a histologic analysis difficult.

In performing the operative procedure, if the needle track is to be followed, an incision is carried out and a core of tissue is left around the needle itself. Often with an Allis clamp in place around the needle, this core can be extended to the depth of the sample. As the area of the lesion is reached, the diameter of tissue taken should be widened to insure removing the target. Careful assessment of the guide wire's position in relation to the lesion is important because it is often difficult to return to the cavity to take more tissue when the lesion is missed. We advise expanding the area to be biopsied to increase the certainty of the removal of the imaged lesion.

After removal, while waiting for confirmation by the specimen mammogram, a sterile field should be maintained, but the surgeon, if confident that the lesion has been accurately removed, may begin closure so that the operation is completed as the confirmatory report is received.

In closure, we rarely recommend drainage. The internal seroma created will often cosmetically fill the space, leaving the contour appearing much as it did preoperatively. The skin overlying the breast is a forgiving envelope. If the patient has no history of hypertrophic scarring, interrupted dermal sutures of 4-0 monoglycolic or polyglycolic acid followed by a running subcuticular suture will provide a tensionless skin reapproximation. For the patient with tendency to keloid formation, very few absorbable sutures should be placed because the biochemical process of suture disintegration causes a local inflammatory response that can increase hypertrophic scarring. Nylon suture or staples should be used in this circumstance.

While there is disagreement about whether a diagnostic biopsy can serve as a therapeutic lumpectomy, because cancer has been found in 50% to 75% of the reexcised tissue following a diagnostic biopsy, we believe that most image-guided procedures should be only diagnostic. The exception to this would be removal of a cancer less than 1 cm in diameter with a cuff of normal tissue of 1 or more cm around the lesion seen in two orthogonal mammograms. In every event specimens should be sent to pathology with a copy of the specimen mammogram to orient the pathologist to the location of lesion and the specimen should be marked with colored ink, sutures or staples or at least two sutures to assist the pathology. In the event that the cancer is near to one surface, that facet of the cavity can be removed rather than undertaking a reexcision of the entire cavity.

Both verbal and written instructions should be given to the patient prior to leaving the recovery area. A cold pack (often a rubber glove containing ice) can be placed on the wound for approximately 2 h following the operative procedure to decrease nerve conduction and with it the level of pain. The incidence of postoperative infection following breast biopsy is low, and the use of prophylactic antibiotics is at the discretion of the surgeon. Analgesic control is important, and the level of postbiopsy pain is highly variable. For that reason, we send patients home with a prescription for a limited number of oral narcotic analgesics as well as for a moderate number of nonnarcotic analgesics. Patients should be asked to return in 1 week for wound evaluation. Finally, we suggest to each patient that she may take a light shower 24 h after a biopsy, but should avoid exercise, baths, and swimming for 1 week.

STEREOTACTIC BREAST BIOPSY

The stereotactic breast biopsy is a mammographic method of obtaining core samples of nonpalpable suspicious lesions. Through advances in digital mammography, computer science, and minimal invasive surgical techniques, stereotactic mammographic instruments have come into widespread use. First reported for fine-needle aspiration in the 1977, this technique is now a widely accepted approach to core sampling of mammographically discovered lesions (6).

Stereotactic Biopsy Technique

In the same way that a child's three-dimensional slide viewer looks at two images in the same plane from slightly two different perspectives, the stereotactic approach uses a computer to evaluate two mammographic images 30 degrees apart to triangulate the area to be biopsied within the patient's breast. Lying prone, the patient's breast is passed through a port in the stereotactic table to be compressed against the charge coupled device (CCD) or a Bucky grid by a compression plate with a 5 × 5 cm window. A "scout" image assures that the tissue to be sampled is within the working window, and each of the offset images, 15 degrees from this central axis, provide localization. The operator then selects the site for biopsy on each of these pictures through an electronic cursor and the computer determines the three-dimensonal position of the lesion within the breast. The computer instructs small motors attached to the stage to align the vertical and horizontal positions of the needle for biopsy, and the surgeon then selects the depth or Z axis and places a 2- to 3-mm incision under local anesthesia for passage of the stereotactic needle. Once the needle is in place, offset images are obtained to ensure that the needle has been correctly positioned at the target. In the event that spring-loaded 14-gauge device core samples are to be taken, pre- and postfire images should show that the needle was placed superficial to the lesion and then through it. If the align-

ment is not correct, then the needle can be repositioned at that point. With more recently available instruments, such as Biopsys' Mammotome or the Abbi core system, the sampling device (Biopsys) or guide wire (Abbi) is placed to the center of the lesion itself, and the sample is taken after this single passage. After the samples have been obtained, either a single mid-axial view should be taken for comparison with the scout film or stereotactic views should be taken to compare with the prebiopsy offset images demonstrating that the target has been appropriately sampled.

Once the sampling instrument has been withdrawn and the postbiopsy films taken, the patient may then be released from the table. A small stab wound (up to 11 gauge) is steri-stripped. If a 20-mm core is taken, the cavity is made hemostatic through loop cauterization and the skin incision is sutured. Before being discharged, the patient should be given written and verbal instructions to return within 1 week for a wound evaluation and discussion of the histology.

Indications for Stereotactic Biopsy

Just as they are for needle localization and open biopsy, the indications for stereotactic biopsy are the establishment of a tissue diagnosis for a nonpalpable density or a suspicious focus of microcalcifications. Because of its minimally invasive approach, stereotactic biopsy has a distinct advantage in two circumstances. First, when a mammogram shows a suspicious lesion on only one film, but it cannot be found on its orthogonal counterpart, the lesion can still be stereotactically biopsied because the two observational points are in the same plane. Second, a stereotactic biopsy is especially helpful in sampling a lesion immediately adjacent to a breast prosthesis. The stereotactic approach carries a lower risk than free hand needle placement because the computerized positioning of the stereotactic needle can be imaged to within 1 mm of the intended target (Table 21-1).

The stereotactic technique is also ideally suited for tissue sampling of several foci of microcalcifications in different quadrants of the breast thus eliminating multiple large incisions.

Some authors have suggested that the stereotactic biopsy be reserved for less suspicious mammographic findings. The indication should not be so narrow. On review, the stereotactic technique can be used for lesions of the same degree of suspicion as for needle localization and open biopsy. When a solid density is discovered that may be core sampled either stereotactically or by ultrasound, the latter is preferred by many because it is less cumbersome to arrange and less expensive.

Contraindications and Warnings

Some of the features of the stereotactic biopsy that make it attractive also may make it difficult for some patients. Because the patient is required to lie absolutely still in a prone position for 20 to 45 min, anxious patients, those with a cough, or patients with shoulder or cervical arthritis who sim-

TABLE 21–1. *Indications for image-directed biopsies*

	Needle localization and open biopsy	Stereotactic mammographic biopsy	Ultrasound biopsy
Microcalcifications	Yes	Yes	No
Mammographic density	Yes	Yes	No
Architectural distortion	Yes	Yes	Yes
Large *en bloc* field required (e.g., microcalcifications)	Yes	No	No
Multiple small foci of microcalcifications	No	Yes	No
A lesion on one mammographic view	No	Yes	No
Density close to the chest wall	Yes	No	Yes
Lateral lesion in the tail of Spence	Yes	No	Yes

ply cannot lie still for that length of time should be treated with a needle localization and open biopsy. It is recommended by the producers of stereotactic tables that morbidly obese patients, who weigh more than 300 lb, are poor candidates; the tables are not licensed to hold patients of that weight. Technically, lesions very close to the chest wall can pose a difficulty in bringing the tissue into the working field. Neither a stereotactic nor a mammographic approach is easy in this situation, but when a lesion cannot be stereotactically brought into view, a needle localization and open biopsy must be considered (Table 21-2).

ULTRASOUND-GUIDED BIOPSY

In the main, ultrasonography is better suited for the small dense breast, and the stereotactic approach is preferable for the larger fat-replaced breasts. Most dense solid lesions can be biopsied under ultrasound guidance, but microcalcifications are reserved for stereotactic or needle localization biopsy. Asymmetric changes, radial scars, and architectural distortion that require *en bloc* observation of architectural features should be reserved for needle localization and open biopsy (7).

Most ultrasound biopsies are currently taken by a spring-loaded 14-gauge Trucut needle. Under local anesthesia and following a 2- to 3-mm stab wound, the needle is placed under ultrasonic guidance so that the point is at or near the edge of the lesion, the needle is then fired under direct observation, and it can be seen after firing that the lesion itself will move with the needle in the postfired position. The needle is then removed, the sample is taken out, and the process is repeated. Up to five cores may be required if the observer is not entirely certain that the lesion has been adequately sampled. All of this is usually performed with the patient lying supine on an examining table and under sterile technique through a fenes-

trated drape. Validation of the needle's position must be made at the time of sampling. Ultrasonic images taken following the sample may or may not demonstrate that the needle passed through the area of concern. In the event that the patient has a histologically benign diagnosis, she should present in 4 to 6 months for an ultrasonic image to evaluate the size, shape, and nature of the lesion to discern if there has been any change.

GENERAL ISSUES OF CONCERN

A core diagnosis of atypical ductile hyperplasia (ADH) or ductal carcinoma *in situ* (DCIS) usually obtained stereotactically from microcalcifications with 14-gauge biopsies are of concern because they may underdiagnose the lesion. In one study, up to 44% of patients who had a diagnosis of ADH were found to have breast cancer at the time of a definitive therapeutic surgical incision (8). For that reason, if a 14-gauge Trucut sampling is used by a spring-activated gun system and a diagnosis of atypical ductile hyperplasia is made, then that patient should undergo a needle localization and open biopsy to confirm the diagnosis. The same issue holds true for ductal carcinoma *in situ,* which later may be found to contain an invasive component. Obviously, both of the these findings would change the course of treatment. A true, focal DCIS would be treated by a lumpectomy and, perhaps radiation therapy, and an invasive cancer should be considered for a sentinel axillary node biopsy or a lymphadenectomy with a lumpectomy followed by radiation therapy. The use of an 11-gauge vacuum-assisted core biopsy or a single 20-mm core may decrease the instance of histologic underdiagnosis. Recent reports suggest an advantage to these newer sampling techniques (9); clinical studies will be needed to confirm their efficacy.

In the main, accuracy of core biopsy is dependent on the number of cores taken. For 14-gauge Trucut cores, six appear

TABLE 21–2. *Contraindications to stereotactic biopsy*

Inability to lie prone and still for 20–45 min (arthritis, anxiety, cough)
Weight of greater than 300 lb
Lesion that cannot be brought into field (too close to the chest wall, or in the tail of Spence)
Architectural distortion or radial scar

to be an optimal number (10); for the vacuum-assisted biopsy of 14- or 11-gauge cores, the needle is placed one time, and because it is fairly straightforward to take 15 to 25 samples quickly, the minimal number to ensure accuracy has not been an issue. No reports regarding a minimal number have been described for this approach. With the 20-mm single core, one sample is taken, and no additional samples are submitted. The accuracy is dependent in the initial placement of the guide wire. Again, there has been limited reporting of this new technique.

DOCUMENTATION AND FOLLOW-UP

There is disagreement about the importance and the interval of follow-up. Several radiologists, when queried about a 6-month follow-up, have stated that this was arbitrarily chosen some time ago and that there has been no clinical validation of this interval. While the interval is not clear, we may presume that in the event that the finding might be due to cancer, a 1-year exposure to a possible cancer may be putting the patient at an unknown, but undue risk. Follow-up films may not be necessary if the biopsied lesion is both discrete and benign (e.g., fibroadenoma). If the lesion is an area of asymmetry or a focus of microcalcifications of moderate to high suspicion that, on subsequent biopsy, was found to be benign, it is important to restudy that patient before 1 year passes to be certain that there has not been a sampling error. The simplest way to confirm that the proper site had been biopsied would be to take another mammogram to demonstrate that the lesion is mammographically absent after the biopsy.

CREDENTIALING AND TRAINING

The affirmative position taken by the American College of Surgeons that general surgeons should be trained and able to perform both stereotactic and ultrasound core biopsies has led to the issues of training and credentialing. The American College of Surgeons itself has taken an unprecedented step in offering postgraduate training to general surgeons in these techniques. These and other image-guided biopsy courses should permit the general surgeon to have both a cognitive and "hands-on" experience in this technology.

The issue of credentialing is currently being analyzed by a panel of interested participants, both from the American College of Surgeons and from the American Academy of Radiology. While early recommendations are being formulated, more definitive guidelines will be forthcoming. Yet to be addressed is the incorporation of this technology into surgical training progress.

CONCLUSION

We have discussed the general principles of image-directed biopsy and have given a focused approach to the technique to needle localization, stereotactic biopsy, and ultrasonically directed biopsy. In addition, the indications, contraindications, and areas of concern in image-directed biopsy have been presented as well as a discussion of credentialing. Image-directed biopsies of breast disease are important now and will become increasingly important. With regard to credentialing of surgeons and radiologists in the performance of stereotactic biopsies, the major issue is patient safety, but it is clear that both groups share an economic interest in this domain. General surgeons interested in the diagnosis and treatment of early breast cancer should take an active role in shaping the destiny of image-directed biopsy technology and it use.

REFERENCES

1. Shapiro S, Strax P, Venet L. Periodic breast cancer screening in reducing mortality from breast cancer. *JAMA* 1971;215:1777.
2. Cady B, Stone MD, Schuler JG, Thakur R, Wanner MA, Lavin PT. The new era in breast cancer. *Arch Surg* 1996;131:301.
3. Nields M. Cost-effectiveness of image-guided core needle biopsy versus surgery in diagnosing breast cancer. Personal communication, 1997.
4. Suggestions for accreditation of surgeons who perform image-directed breast biopsies [Editorial]. *Bull Am Coll Surg* 1996;181:37.
5. Baker JA, Kornguth PJ, Floyd CE. Breast imaging reporting and data system: standardized mammography lexicon. *AJR* 1996; 166:773.
6. Sickles EA. Management of probably benign breast lesions. *Radiol Clin North Am* 1995;33:1123.
7. Stavros AT, Thickman D, Rapp CL, Dennis MA, Parker SH, Sisney GA. Solid nodules: use of sonography to distinguish between benign and malignant nodules. *Radiology* 1995;196:123.
8. Liberman L, Cohen MA, Dershaw DD, Abramson AF, Hann LE, Rosen PP. Atypical ductal hyperplasia diagnosed at stereotactic core biopsy of breast lesions: an indication for surgical biopsy. *AJR Am J Radiol* 1995;164:1111.
9. Burbank F. Stereotactic breast biopsy of atypical ductal hyperplasia and ductal carcinoma *in situ* lesions: improved accuracy with directional vacuum-assisted biopsy. *Radiology* 1997;202:843.
10. Liberman L, Dershaw DD, Rosen PP, Abramson AF, Deutch BM, Hann LE. Stereotactic 14-gauge breast biopsy: how many core specimens are needed? *Radiology* 1994;192:793.

CHAPTER 22

Early Stage Breast Cancer

David J. Winchester and S. Eva Singletary

During the past two decades, there has been a stage migration to increase the proportion of early breast cancer in relationship to advanced stage disease (1). This shift reflects an increased public awareness and, most importantly, the implementation of screening mammography (2). Early detection of breast cancer has been responsible for the reduction in the mortality of this disease (3,4).

Guidelines for screening mammography have been scrutinized, with consensus conferences reaching differing conclusions (5–7). Although survival data have not been as compelling for women under the age of 50, as it is for those older than 50, recent data from Sweden have established an important benefit for yearly mammography for women between ages 40 and 49 (8,9). Recently, this approach has been uniformly advocated by the American Cancer Society and the National Institutes of Health (6). As an important adjunct, a thorough breast examination should be performed on an annual basis and ideally, occurring at the time of mammography to facilitate a correlation between findings. Monthly breast self-examination should also be encouraged.

DETECTION AND DIAGNOSIS

With the method of detection, the diagnostic evaluation varies considerably. The identification of a palpable breast lesion suspicious for carcinoma should be approached in the least invasive fashion to establish a diagnosis (Fig. 22-1). In most settings, this should consist of a fine-needle aspiration (FNA) cytology. This can be accomplished with a 22-gauge needle, without anesthesia, and provide a diagnosis within an hour in an organized breast center. Equivocal readings or suspicious findings should be followed up with additional diagnostic studies depending upon the index of suspicion. This may consist of either a repeat aspiration cytology, a core needle biopsy, or an open incisional or excisional biopsy depending upon the size of the lesion. Prior to any therapeutic procedure, it is imperative to evaluate both breasts with screening mammography to identify occult multicentric or bilateral disease that may affect therapeutic choices.

In the setting of a mammographically detected, nonpalpable abnormality, several methods of diagnosis may be selected depending upon the location of the abnormality and its imaging characteristics. If a lesion is imaged sonographically, ultrasound-guided FNA or core biopsy may prove to be the easiest and least invasive approach. Microcalcifications are typically difficult to image sonographically and may be analyzed best with a stereotactic core biopsy providing technical criteria are met including a cooperative patient capable of lying prone for 45 min and the abnormality located away from the skin or chest wall so that the breast parenchyma may be adequately compressed during the localization and insertion of the needle. If the cluster of microcalcifications is small, core biopsy sampling may create difficulties with future localizations for definitive treatment procedures. In this setting, a metallic marker should be placed within the lesion at the time of the biopsy or alternatively, an open image-directed biopsy should be performed. With lesions located laterally, along the chest wall, or close to the skin, a guidewire directed open biopsy may be preferable. Guide wire placement can be performed under ultrasound or mammographic guidance and the guidewire position can be confirmed after placement. In any of these approaches for nonpalpable lesions, it is critical to examine the specimen radiographically to confirm that the lesion of interest is included within the specimen.

Most cases of ductal carcinoma *in situ* (DCIS) are diagnosed with screening mammography through the identification of microcalcifications. Although corresponding masses are occasionally appreciated on physical examination, most cases of DCIS are nonpalpable, requiring image-directed biopsy. Stereotactic core needle biopsy is a reliable means of addressing the histologic features of a mammographic finding (10). Identification of atypical ductal hyperplasia with this technique is associated with an increased risk of a false-negative study and should be followed by an open excisional biopsy (11). Establishing a diagnosis of cancer with stereotactic core biopsy can be followed by a therapeutic procedure and has the benefit of allowing the surgeon to approach the disease with a one-step operation with the initial intention of achieving an adequate margin of resection and staging the

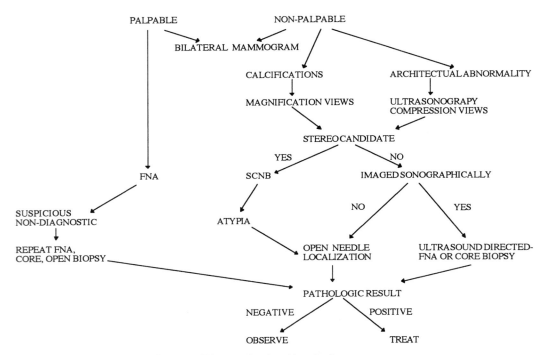

FIG. 22-1. Diagnostic algorithm for breast cancer.

nodal basins with sentinel node biopsy with or without a standard axillary dissection if an invasive tumor is identified in the diagnostic biopsy.

In the event of performing an open procedure, it is desirable to place a curvilinear incision directly over the mammographic abnormality. Frequently, this may be a considerable distance from the guidewire or blue dye injection site. If a guidewire is used, palpation of the breast and movement of the external portion of the wire may help to identify proximity within the breast. This in combination with the review of the localization films and communication with the radiologist should help in determining the placement of the incision. Once the incision is made and the guidewire is identified, it can be drawn through the guidewire insertion site and into the biopsy cavity without difficulty. Peripheral incisions or incisions placed away from the lesion should be avoided. If a mastectomy becomes necessary, peripheral incisions may be difficult to include within the specimen. Tunneling should also be avoided as this will create more difficulty in reexcising involved margins. Meticulous hemostasis should be achieved with electrocautery. Postoperative hematomas will complicate follow-up mammography and physical examinations and lead to more difficult reexcisions if necessary.

Once a cancer diagnosis is established, a concerted effort can be made to perform a one stage therapeutic operation. The most important preoperative evaluation after establishing a diagnosis consists of a careful history and physical examination. Routine chest radiographs, serum chemistry analysis, and bone scans rarely identify metastatic disease in early breast cancer patients and should not be included for staging purposes in the absence of complaints or physical findings that support their utility.

THERAPY

The treatment of breast cancer, for all stages, has increasingly utilized a multimodality approach. The stage of disease is important in defining the selection and order of surgery, chemotherapy, hormonal therapy, and radiotherapy (Fig. 22-2). The TNM staging system defines survival according to the size of the primary tumor, the presence of nodal metastases, and the presence of distant metastases (12) (Tables 22-1, 22-2). Adjuvant systemic therapy and radiotherapy are given selectively based upon empirical decisions that compare the risks and benefits of treatment. Surgery represents the initial treatment in most stage 0, I, and II disease. The presence and extent of *in situ* disease and the patient's risk factors for breast cancer also become important in defining the locoregional treatment approach.

In Situ Carcinoma

Lobular carcinoma *in situ* has no unique features of identification. It is not palpable and has no characteristic mammographic findings. It is most commonly detected serendipitously during the evaluation of other findings. Its significance relates to addressing the risk of breast cancer in both breasts. It does not require treatment and can correctly be perceived as a marker of risk and not as a cancerous or precancerous lesion that requires therapy. The management of this lesion consists of two approaches; close observation for early detection or

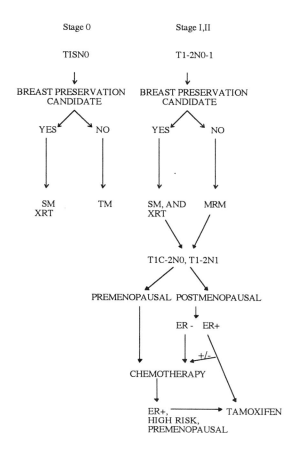

SM = SEGMENTAL MASTECTOMY
TM = TOTAL MASTECTOMY
MRM = MODIFIED RADICAL MASTECTOMY
AND = AXILLARY NODE DISSECTION
ER = ESTROGEN RECEPTOR

FIG. 22-2. Treatment algorithm for early breast cancer.

surgical intervention for cancer prevention. If surveillance is deemed appropriate, monitoring should include yearly bilateral mammography and biannual physical examination, augmented by additional magnification views, sonography, or biopsy when necessary. Because the risk of subsequent cancer is equivalent for both breasts, the surgical management should consist of a bilateral total mastectomy. The choice between these two options is dependent upon other risk factors for breast cancer including a personal history of breast cancer, a family history of premenopausal breast cancer in one or more first degree relatives, or the identification of a breast cancer susceptibility gene mutation through genetic testing. Other factors influencing this decision include the patient's perception of her risk and risk reduction with surveillance and the degree of difficulty of evaluating the breast by physical examination and mammography.

The incidence, presentation, and treatment of ductal carcinoma *in situ* continues to change (13). With the introduction of screening mammography, ductal carcinoma *in situ* has evolved from a palpable lesion to a nonpalpable mammo-

graphic finding leading to fewer instances of coexistent invasive disease. During the past decade, the proportion of DCIS cases has progressively increased on an annual basis (13). Along with other stages of breast cancer, there has been a significant shift to tissue preservation with the majority of cases of DCIS managed with a segmental mastectomy (13).

Several treatment options are available for patients with ductal carcinoma *in situ.* These include a total mastectomy with or without reconstruction, and a segmental mastectomy with or without radiotherapy. None of these options should include an axillary dissection with the exception of a diffuse presentation, where the exclusion of an invasive component becomes difficult with the limitations of an extensive histologic evaluation. The choice between these modalities can be controversial, with little information based upon randomized clinical trials (14). Retrospective studies have confirmed that recurrence rates following total mastectomy are low, ranging from 1% to 2% (15–17). Recurrence rates determined in retrospective analyses following segmental mastectomy vary according to the use of radiotherapy, analysis of surgical margins, extent of resection, histologic category, and method of detection. In most series, the risk of recurrence more than doubles when comparing 5 and 10 years of follow-up (18,19), indicating the necessity of long term evaluation to determine the efficacy of treatment approaches.

There are several important considerations in choosing local therapy for DCIS. Magnification views of the involved breast best define the extent of disease (20). The mammographic extent of disease usually correlates but frequently underestimates the pathologic extent of disease (21). By all criteria, extensive, multiquadrant DCIS is best managed with a total mastectomy. The decision to perform a total mastectomy should also be accompanied by a discussion of immediate and delayed reconstructive options.

Selection criteria for breast preserving therapy relate to the extent of disease and the expected cosmetic deformity and risk of recurrence. Involvement of microscopic margins leads to a two- to threefold increase in risk of local recurrence (22) and if identified, should be followed by either reexcision or total mastectomy.

Postoperative radiotherapy following breast preserving surgery lowers the risk of local recurrence for ductal carcinoma *in situ* (14,23). Although intended for the study of invasive breast cancers, the National Surgical Adjuvant Breast Project (NSABP) B-06 compared these two therapeutic modalities directly in 78 patients with DCIS, suggesting a benefit from irradiation after a short follow-up (23). All local recurrences involved the same quadrant as the primary and 50% were of invasive histology. More importantly, NSABP B-17 compared segmental mastectomy with and without postoperative radiation. In this prospective randomized study with a mean follow-up of 43 months, there was a statistically significant local disease-free survival advantage for those women receiving postoperative radiotherapy (14). A subsequent but limited subset analysis identified comedo necrosis as an independent risk factor for local recurrence (22). Other risk factors

TABLE 22–1. *Tumor-node-metastasis (TNM) classification system for breast cancer*

Primary tumor (T)
TX Primary tumor cannot be assessed
T0 No evidence of primary tumor
Tis Carcinoma *in situ* or Paget's disease of the nipple with no associated tumor
T1 Tumor ≤2 cm in greatest dimension
     T1a ≤0.5 cm
     T1b >0.5 and ≤1.0 cm
     T1c >1.0 and ≤2.0 cm
T2 Tumor >2 and ≤5 cm in greatest dimension
T3 Tumor >5 cm in greatest dimension
T4 Tumor of any size with direct extension to chest wall or skin
     T4a Extension to chest wall
     T4b Edema, ulceration, or satellite nodules
     T4c Both T4a and T4b
     T4d Inflammatory carcinoma
Regional lymph nodes (N)
NX Regional lymph nodes cannot be assessed
N0 No regional lymph node metastasis
N1 Metastasis to ipsilateral axillary lymph node(s)
N2 Metastasis to ipsilateral axillary node(s) fixed to one another or to other structures
N3 Metastasis to ipsilateral internal mammary lymph node(s)
Distant metastasis (M)
MX Presence of distant metastasis cannot be assessed
M0 No distant metastasis
M1 Distant metastasis, includes metastases to supraclavicular lymph node(s)

for recurrence include the size of the lesion, the grade of the tumor, and the involvement of microscopic margins. In an attempt to define therapy according to these variables, Silverstein et al. (24) have advocated a scoring system based upon these identified risk factors for recurrence. Most patients who develop a local recurrence after segmental mastectomy and radiation can be rendered disease-free by total mastectomy.

No systemic therapy is indicated for DCIS. If breast preserving surgery is performed, a postoperative mammogram should be obtained to confirm removal of the microcalcifications. Ideally, this should be performed when the patient can tolerate compression of her breast, prior to the initiation of radiotherapy. Follow-up should consist of annual mammography and physical examination at 6-month intervals.

Invasive Breast Cancer

The treatment of invasive breast cancer has also evolved to a multimodality approach. Clinical trial data have confirmed the equivalency in survival between breast preserving treatment and mastectomy (25,26). Treatment selection between these two options is dependent upon the size of the tumor, the expected cosmetic deformity and the presence of coexistent *in situ* or multiquadrant disease.

After establishing a diagnosis, it is best to address the overall treatment plan before initiating therapy. With this approach, staging and management strategies of the axilla can be addressed preoperatively. For T2 tumors, neoadjuvant chemotherapy may be preferable in order to facilitate a breast preserving operation. This approach has not been shown to influence survival but it may lead to a lesser surgical procedure.

A modified radical mastectomy becomes preferable over a breast preserving operation in situations where radiotherapy cannot be delivered due to coexistent medical conditions including connective tissue disorders or because of patient preference. In patients with small invasive tumors accompanied by diffuse ductal carcinoma *in situ,* the treatment of the non-invasive component becomes equally important, necessitating a modified radical mastectomy. Premenopausal patients presenting with a significant family history of breast or ovarian carcinoma also raise the issue of addressing prophylaxis and treatment. The first priority is to treat the cancer that has been identified but in situations where an early, favorable lesion has been detected, both prophylaxis and treatment may

TABLE 22–2. *Current stage grouping of breast carcinoma*

Stage	T	N	M
0	Tis	N0	M0
I	T1	N0	M0
IIA	T0	N1	M0
	T1	N1	M0
	T2	N0	M0
IIB	T2	N1	M0
	T3	N0	M0
IIIA	T0	N2	M0
	T1	N2	M0
	T2	N2	M0
	T3	N1 or N2	M0
IIIB	T4	Any N	M0
	Any T	N3	M0
IV	Any T	Any N	M1

be addressed simultaneously with a bilateral mastectomy. Such an aggressive management strategy should only be selected after a thoughtful discussion with the patient and preferably following consultation with a genetic counselor. In any situation where either a unilateral or bilateral mastectomy is being contemplated, it is useful to have a plastic surgeon involved in the decision process in order to limit surgical procedures and allow for optimal cosmetic results. In patients with clinically evident nodal disease or a large tumor, systemic chemotherapy has a greater likelihood of having a survival impact. Under such circumstances, simultaneous breast reconstruction carries a more significant consequence if an operative complication delays chemotherapy. A strategy implementing neoadjuvant chemotherapy or delayed reconstruction may avoid treatment conflicts for patients with more advanced disease.

For most cases of stage I or II breast cancer, a breast preserving operation should be the first step in treatment (Fig. 22-2). Adjuvant systemic therapy follows the surgical treatment for most patients providing their primary tumor is greater than 1 cm in diameter or if there is involvement of the axillary lymph nodes. For most patients, radiotherapy to the breast is indicated after breast preserving surgery to minimize risk of local recurrence (25). Although not supported by randomized clinical trial data, exceptions would include elderly patients with significant comorbidity or patients with small tumors with favorable histologic findings. Current clinical trials are comparing disease-free and overall survival in elderly patients randomized to receive tamoxifen with or without radiotherapy to the breast.

Segmental Mastectomy

Although the histologic features differ between an invasive breast cancer and ductal carcinoma *in situ,* the operative approach to these two subtypes are similar. A breast preserving operation should be defined by preoperative mammography and physical findings with an intention to achieve a margin-free resection, encompassing a margin of normal breast tissue around the malignancy. For invasive cancer, the most important variables to predict recurrence are the age of the patient, margin involvement, the extent of resection, and the use of radiotherapy (22,27–29). Three of these four variables are under the control of the patient and surgeon. Although the risk is much lower for patients with clear surgical margins as compared to involved margins, local recurrences still occur, indicating the imprecise nature of margin assessment. To limit this shortcoming, a more generous extent of resection beyond the identifiable tumor translates into a lower risk of recurrence (27). Supporting this concept, analysis of mastectomy specimens by serial subsections indicates that the frequency of occult microscopic disease decreases as a function of the distance from the macroscopic tumor (28). If close or involved microscopic margins are identified, reexcision of the respective margin should be performed. After two attempts at reexcision, the cosmetic value of a breast preserving approach should be assessed. If extensive margin involvement is identified following the initial procedure, it may be preferable to proceed with total mastectomy. Radiotherapy may sterilize residual disease but a critical threshold of tumor burden and radiosensitivity most likely define the risk of a local recurrence.

Axillary Lymphadenectomy

The most sensitive indicator of breast cancer recurrence and survival is the presence of axillary lymph node metastases (30). Entry criteria for current clinical trials comparing chemotherapy regimens are strongly tied into the presence and extent of lymph node metastases. Aside from clinical trial participation, there are situations in which the staging information from an axillary dissection does not alter the patient's treatment plan. In the absence of clinically involved lymph nodes, elderly patients with a T1c or greater tumor will most likely receive tamoxifen if hormone receptors are expressed in the primary tumor. Thus, the identification of axillary disease will not change the decision to add tamoxifen to the patient's treatment regimen. With clinically involved axillary lymph nodes, an axillary node dissection should be performed, if technically feasible, for regional control.

In a similar fashion, if a T1c tumor or greater is diagnosed in a premenopausal patient, the perceived benefit of adjuvant chemotherapy would be defined without axillary staging information. Based upon the National Surgical Adjuvant Breast protocol B-04 (31), many believe that in the absence of clinically evident axillary disease, there is no survival benefit in performing an axillary dissection. Others, however, would argue that the conclusions from this and other trials were not valid because of study size limitations and by the limited extent of the lymphadenectomy performed in a major portion of the study patients. In addition, the local recurrence risk in an untreated axilla is clearly higher than in one treated with either radiotherapy or surgery (31). Although the risk of regional recurrence is affected by treating the axilla with either radiotherapy or surgery, overall survival was equivalent in this study and in a recent metaanalysis (31,32).

Alternative strategies of assessing axillary lymph node involvement consist of evaluating features of the primary tumor, radiographic imaging studies of the axilla, and sentinel lymph node biopsy. To date, there are no reliable features of the primary tumor to define axillary lymph node involvement but a combination of the tumor size, grade, and the age of the patient can define a low risk category patient (33). Computed axial tomography (CAT), magnetic resonance imaging (MRI), and ultrasonography are neither sensitive nor specific in identifying axillary disease. Positron emission tomography (PET) scanning has been reported as a specific indicator of axillary disease but not adequate in excluding regional disease (34). With advances in imaging technology and refined molecular diagnostics, histologic evaluation of the axilla may eventually become unnecessary for staging purposes.

Sentinal Lymph Node Biopsy

Sentinel node biopsy appears to have the most promise in immediately altering the surgical management of breast cancer. If confirmed to be accurate, it offers the benefits of leaving the axilla essentially undisturbed, thus avoiding the long term complications of lymphedema and intercostal brachial cutaneous nerve paresthesias. It also may allow a more accurate means of staging the axilla by virtue of identifying a more limited specimen to examine for micrometastases. In addition, it has the potential to selectively remove internal mammary chain lymph nodes that may be involved in the absence of axillary lymph node metastases.

The optimization of the technique, the selection criteria for its use, and its sensitivity have yet to be defined in large scale clinical trials. However, preliminary information supports the technique as being highly predictive and sensitive in small series of patients (35,36). Critical issues left to be addressed include the size limitations of the primary tumor, applicability for patients treated with neoadjuvant chemotherapy, the approach of nonpalpable lesions, and technical issues regarding the use of either a vital blue dye (isosulphan blue) or a radio-labelled protein ([99]technitium sulfur colloid) or a combination of both. If it proves to be a sensitive indicator, it may potentially replace the standard axillary dissections for T1N0 and T2N0 lesions. The identification of micrometastases may also be sufficient in certain settings without having to complete a full axillary lymph node dissection.

Although no study has directly compared isosulphan blue to sulfur colloid in breast cancer patients, there are theoretical benefits of both techniques. Isosulphan blue migrates more rapidly and works well in situations where the primary tumor is in close proximity to the draining nodal basin. Its disadvantage is that it requires a greater experience and also involves lymphatic mapping or defining the draining lymphatics to the sentinel lymph node. In the axilla, where the lymphatic plexus is three-dimensional, it may be difficult to identify multiple draining lymphatics and sentinel nodes. In contrast, the use of technetium sulfur colloid allows *ex vivo* confirmation of radionucleotide concentration within specific lymph nodes and a subsequent diminution of radioactivity in the draining nodal basin. In addition, radioactivity can be identified within the internal mammary chain with little difficulty. If the primary tumor is in close proximity to the draining internal mammary chain or axillary nodal basin, it may be difficult to distinguish the primary injection site from the sentinel lymph node. A combination of both the vital blue dye and technetium techniques offers the combined advantages of both but requires separate injections because of the more rapid transit time of isosulphan blue.

If patients have nonpalpable lesions, the first step in their surgical procedure is placement of a guidewire. One microcurie of [99]technitium in a total volume of 8 mL is injected in four quadrants around the palpable tumor or the preoperatively placed guidewire. Lymphoscintigraphy is optional but accomplishes two objectives: it indicates when the radionu-

cleotide has migrated from the injection sites to the sentinel lymph node(s) and it helps to identify multiple draining nodal basins. A hand-held gamma probe may also accomplish these same objectives.

If isosulphan blue is used in addition or in place of sulfur colloid, injection around the primary tumor is done in the operating room using a 3- to 5-mL volume in a similar fashion. The breast may be massaged and after a 10-min interval an axillary incision is made. Lymphatic channels containing the vital dye are then identified and followed to sentinel nodes that concentrate the substance.

Intraoperatively, it is best to use two set-ups in breast preserving operations in order to address the tumor first. When using technetium, this allows for a reduction in the background radioactivity and facilitates the identification of sentinel lymph nodes. The breast, internal mammary chain, and axillary nodal basins should be scanned in a systematic fashion to identify areas of increased uptake. Once identified, incisions are made accordingly and the gamma probe is used to identify radioactive lymph nodes. *Ex vivo* measurement of lymph node radioactivity and reexamination of the nodal basin are important to confirm that all sentinel nodes are identified.

Lymph node specimens are processed by permanent section and are serially sectioned and analyzed by hematoxylin and eosin staining at 5- to 10-μm intervals. Ongoing clinical trials are analyzing molecular staging of homogenized lymphatic tissue with polymerase chain reactions however, the clinical significance of submicroscopic metastases remains unclear. If all sentinel lymph nodes are negative, no additional lymphadenectomy is necessary. If there are involved sentinel nodes, a level I to II lymph node dissection may be performed depending upon the impact of identifying additional micrometastases. In most situations a segmental mastectomy and sentinel node biopsy can be performed under local anesthesia, as an outpatient procedure and without the use of an axillary drain.

Until the technical details, indications, and accuracy of sentinel lymph node biopsy are defined by those performing the technique, a level I to II axillary lymph node dissection should be performed to provide reliable staging information for the patient.

Adjuvant Therapy

After the surgical management is completed, either radiotherapy or systemic therapy is initiated. For small (less than 1 cm), favorable tumors with uninvolved axillary lymph nodes, radiation therapy becomes the next and last step in the treatment. For patients with involved lymph nodes or with larger or less favorable lesions, chemotherapy is started after the surgical incisions are securely closed and all drains have been removed. Typically, this occurs 3 to 4 weeks following the operation.

Standard chemotherapy regimens vary with regional preferences but are usually comprised of one of two combinations containing either cyclophosphamide, doxorubicin, and 5-fluorouracil (5-FU) or cyclophosphamide, methotrexate, and 5-FU. Four to eight cycles are given each over a 2- to 4-week interval. The choice between these two standard regimens is often subjective but evidence supports the use of a doxorubicin based regimen for patients with greater than four involved lymph nodes (37). Prior to initiating doxorubicin chemotherapy a baseline multigated acquisition (MUGA) scan should document a normal cardiac ejection fraction. If given as a continuous infusion and not as a bolus injection, cardiotoxicity of doxorubicin is minimal. The combination of doxorubicin and radiotherapy to the left breast may increase the risk of cardiac dysfunction, although significant improvement in the precision of radiotherapy delivery using tangential fields has lessened this complication. Nonetheless, in patients with a poor or borderline cardiac function, a non-doxorubicin regimen may represent a safer approach, providing cytotoxic chemotherapy is advised.

The simultaneous combination of chemotherapy and radiation therapy is accompanied by significant toxicity, necessitating sequential treatment. Delay in the delivery of either modality is associated with an increased risk of failure but the most significant risk of failure is the development of systemic metastases. For this reason, chemotherapy is given prior to radiotherapy. In addition, chemotherapy may help to reduce the risk of a regional recurrence but radiotherapy does not affect distant disease-free survival.

If the patient's local therapy was a total mastectomy, the risk of a locoregional recurrence varies between 2% and 20% depending upon the stage of disease, extent of lymph node involvement, and adjuvant therapy (38). Patients with limited nodal involvement do not achieve a significant improvement in local disease-free survival with the addition of radiation therapy (38). For patients with four or more involved axillary lymph nodes, radiation therapy following a total mastectomy may decrease the risk of locoregional recurrence (38). Recently, two reports have suggested a significant overall survival advantage for women treated with mastectomy and postoperative radiotherapy (39,40). In patients treated with breast preservation, the use of postoperative radiotherapy will lead to a threefold reduction in risk of local recurrence (32). An overall survival advantage has not been demonstrated in patients treated with breast preservation (32,38).

Because hormonal therapy is currently given over a 5-year period, it either succeeds radiotherapy or is delivered simultaneously. Receptor data can be reliably obtained with immunohistochemical techniques, utilizing a minimal amount of tissue preserved in formalin. For patients expressing estrogen or progesterone receptors, the standard dose is 10 mg given twice daily for 5 years. Alternatively, it may also be delivered as a 20-mg tablet with a delayed delivery, providing equivalent pharmacokinetics. Because tamoxifen is teratogenic, it should not be given in premenopausal patients without birth control. Although tamoxifen provides an equivalent reduction in breast cancer mortality as seen with cytotoxic chemotherapy, it may also provide an additive reduction in mortality when combined with chemotherapy (41). Because there are known complications including thromboembolic disorders, an increase risk of uterine cancer, and retinopathy, tamoxifen should be used judiciously, taking into account the perceived risks and benefits of its use.

POSTOPERATIVE EVALUATION AND FOLLOW-UP

For those patients undergoing an axillary lymph node dissection, it is important to examine the patient during the first 6 weeks following surgery to insure that a full range of motion of the affected limb is reestablished. It may become necessary to involve a physical therapist to achieve this goal. In most situations, thorough preoperative instruction and daily exercises will be sufficient.

Breast cancer recurrences are most common during the first 3 years following therapy. Accordingly, follow-up should be most intensive during this time period, consisting of history and physical examination at a 3-month interval. A bilateral mammogram should be obtained yearly. After a 2-year interval, physical examinations may be extended to a 6-month period. Beyond 5 years, a yearly interval becomes appropriate. In addition to evaluating the patient on a periodic basis for recurrent disease, it is equally important to monitor the contralateral breast and the remaining ipsilateral breast tissue for the development of a new primary breast cancer.

When a local or regional recurrence is detected, the patient should be restaged for evidence of metastatic disease. A local recurrence is the harbinger of metastatic disease in 50% of patients. With risk of systemic failure, most local recurrences are treated in a multimodality fashion. For patients initially treated with breast preservation and radiotherapy, a completion mastectomy is the safest approach to reestablish local control. This may then be followed by either hormonal or cytotoxic therapy. Patients with a chest wall or axillary recurrence should undergo wide excision with a goal of achieving clear histologic margins. If followed carefully for recurrences, a formal chest wall resection is seldom necessary. In such situations, closure of the chest wall defect may involve the use of a myocutaneous flap, particularly if radiation therapy was a component of the initial treatment regimen.

Screening for metastatic disease with the periodic use of bone scanning, serum chemistry analysis, and radiographs of the chest and abdomen are not sensitive for micrometastases and have not been shown to impact on altering the survival of a patient with metastatic disease. These tests should be reserved for those patients presenting with a history or physical findings suggestive of distant failure and not as routine screening tests. Unlike locoregional recurrences where intervention may lead to a cure, the identification of distant metastases signifies an incurable patient and treatment efforts are directed towards palliation.

REFERENCES

1. Winchester DP, Osteen RT, Menck HR. The National Cancer Data Base report on breast carcinoma characteristics and outcome in relation to age. *Cancer* 1996;78:1838.
2. Busch E, Kemeny M, Fremgen A, Osteen RT, Winchester DP, Clive RE. Patterns of breast cancer care in the elderly. *Cancer* 1996;78:101.
3. Cody HS III. The impact of mammography in 1096 consecutive patients with breast cancer, 1979–1993: equal value for patients younger and older than age 50 years. *Cancer* 1995;76:1579.
4. De Koning HJ, Fracheboud J, Boer R, et al. Nation-wide breast cancer screening in The Netherlands: support for breast-cancer mortality reduction. National Evaluation Team for Breast Cancer Screening (NETB). *Int J Cancer* 1995;60:777.
5. National Institutes of Health Consensus Development Conference Statement. Breast Cancer Screening for Women Ages 40–49, January 21–23, 1997. National Institutes of Health Consensus Development Panel [Review]. *J Natl Cancer Inst* 1997;89:1015.
6. Marwick C. NIH consensus panel spurs discontent [News]. *JAMA* 1997;277:519.
7. Leitch AM, Dodd GD, Costanza M, et al. American Cancer Society guidelines for the early detection of breast cancer: update 1997. *CA Cancer J Clin* 1997;47:150.
8. Bjurstam N, Bjorneld L, Duffy SW. The Gothenburg breast cancer screening trial: results from 11 years follow-up [Abstract]. Presented at the NIH Consensus Development Conference: Breast Cancer Screening for Women, Ages 40–49. Bethesda, MD, Jan. 21–23, 1997.
9. Andersson I. Results from the Malmo breast screening trial. Presented at the NIH Consensus Development Conference: Breast Cancer Screening for Women, Ages 40–49 [Abstract]. Bethesda, MD, Jan. 21–23, 1997.
10. Israel PZ, Fine RE. Stereotactic needle biopsy for occult breast lesions: a minimally invasive alternative. *Am Surg* 1995;61:87.
11. Liberman L, Dershaw DD, Glassman JR, et al. Analysis of cancers not diagnosed at stereotactic core breast biopsy. *Radiology* 1997;203:151.
12. American Joint Committee on Cancer. In: Beahrs OH, Henson DE, Hutter RVP, Kennedy BJ, eds. *Manual for staging of cancer.* 4th ed. Philadelphia: JB Lippincott Co, 1992:149.
13. Winchester DJ, Menck HR, Winchester DP. National treatment trends for ductal carcinoma *in situ* of the breast. *Arch Surg* 1997;132:660.
14. Fisher B, Constantino J, Redmond C, et al. Lumpectomy compared with lumpectomy and radiation therapy for the treatment of intraductal breast cancer. *N Engl J Med* 1993;328:1581.
15. Kinne DW, Petrek JA, Osborne MP, Fracchia AA, DePalo AA, Rosen PP. Breast carcinoma *in situ. Arch Surg* 1989;124:33.
16. Rosen PP, Senie R, Schottenfeld D, Ahikari R. Noninvasive breast carcinoma: frequency of unsuspected invasion and implications for treatment. *Ann Surg* 1979;189:377.
17. Silverstein MJ, Cohlan BF, Gierson ED, et al. Duct carcinoma *in situ:* 227 cases without microinvasion. *Eur J Cancer* 1992;28:630.
18. Silverstein MJ, Barth A, Poller DN, et al. Ten-year results comparing mastectomy to excision and radiation therapy for ductal carcinoma *in situ* of the breast. *Eur J Cancer* 1995;31:1425.
19. Solin LJ, Kurtz J, Fourquet A, et al. Fifteen-year results of breast-conserving surgery and definitive breast irradiation for the treatment of ductal carcinoma *in situ* of the breast. *J Clin Oncol* 1996;14:754.
20. Morrow M, Schmidt R, Hassett C. Patient selection for breast conservation therapy with magnification mammography. *Surgery* 1995;118:621.
21. Holland R, Hendriks JH, Vebeek AL, Mravunac M, Schuurmans Stekhoven JH. Extent, distribution, and mammographic/histological correlations of breast ductal carcinoma *in situ. Lancet* 1990;335:519.
22. Fisher ER, Costantino J, Fisher F, Palekar AS, Redmond C, Mamounas E. Pathologic findings from the National Surgical Adjuvant Breast Project (NSABP) protocol B-17. Intraductal carcinoma (ductal carcinoma *in situ*). *Cancer* 1995;75:1310.
23. Fisher ER, Sass R, Fisher B, Wicherham L, Paik SM. Pathologic findings from the National Surgical Adjuvant Breast Project (protocol 6). I. Intraductal carcinoma (DCIS). *Cancer* 1986;57:197.
24. Silverstein MJ, Lagios MD, Craig PH, et al. A prognostic index for ductal carcinoma *in situ* of the breast. *Cancer* 1996;77:2267.
25. Fisher B, Anderson S, Redmond CK, Wolmark N, Wickerham L, Croin WM. Reanalysis and results after 12 years of follow-up in a randomized clinical trial comparing total mastectomy with lumpectomy with or without irradiation in the treatment of breast cancer. *N Engl J Med* 1995;333:1456.
26. Veronesi U, Banfi A, Del Vecchio M, et al. Comparison of Halsted mastectomy with quadrantectomy, axillary dissection, and radiotherapy in early breast cancer: long-term results. *Eur J Cancer Clin Oncol* 1986; 22:1085.
27. Ghossein NA, Alpert S, Barba J, et al. Breast cancer: importance of adequate surgical excision prior to radiotherapy in the local control of breast cancer in patients treated conservatively. *Arch Surg* 1992;127:411.
28. Holland R, Veling SH, Mravunac M, Hendriks JH. Histologic multifocality of Tis, T1-2 breast carcinomas. Implications for clinical trials of breast-conserving surgery. *Cancer* 1985;56:979.
29. Fisher ER, Anderson S, Redmond C, Fisher B. Ipsilateral breast tumor recurrence and survival following lumpectomy and irradiation: pathological findings from NSABP protocol B-06. *Semin Surg Oncol* 1992; 8:161.
30. Ciatto S, Cecchini S, Iossa A, Grazzini G. "T" category and operable breast cancer prognosis. *Tumori* 1989;75:18.
31. Fisher B, Montague E, Redmond C, et al. Comparison of radical mastectomy with alternative treatments for primary breast cancer. A first report of results from a prospective randomized clinical trial. *Cancer* 1977;39[Suppl]:2827.
32. Early Breast Cancer Trialists Collaborative Group. Effects of radiotherapy and surgery in early breast cancer. An overview of the randomized trials. *N Engl J Med* 1995;333:1444. [For erratum, see *N Engl J Med* 1996;334:1003.]
33. Mustafa IA, Cole B, Wanebo HJ, Bland KI, Chang HR. The impact of histopathology on nodal metastases in minimal breast cancer [Review]. *Arch Surg* 1997;132:384.
34. Utech CI, Young CS, Winter PF. Prospective evaluation of fluorine-18 fluorodeoxyclucose positron emission tomography in breast cancer for staging of the axilla related to surgery and immunocytochemistry. *Eur J Nucl Med* 1996;23:1588.
35. Giuliano AE, Dale PS, Turner RR, Morton DL, Evans SW, Krasne DL. Improved axillary staging of breast cancer with sentinel lymphadenectomy [Review]. *Ann Surg* 1995;222:394.
36. Giuliano AE. Lymphatic mapping and sentinel node biopsy in breast cancer. *JAMA* 1997;277:791.
37. Buzzoni R, Bonadonna G, Valagussa P, Zambetti M. Adjuvant chemotherapy with doxorubicin plus cyclophosphamide, methotrexate, and fluorouracil in the treatment of resectable breast cancer with more than three positive axillary nodes. *J Clin Oncol* 1991;9:2134.
38. Griem KL, Henderson IC, Gelman R, et al. The 5-year results of a randomized trial of adjuvant radiation therapy after chemotherapy in breast cancer patients treated with mastectomy. *J Clin Oncol* 1987;5:1546.
39. Overgaard M, Hansen PS, Overgaard J, et al. Postoperative radiotherapy in high-risk premenopausal women with breast cancer who receive adjuvant chemotherapy. *N Engl J Med* 1997;337:949.
40. Ragaz J, Jackson SM, Le N, et al. Adjuvant radiotherapy and chemotherapy in node-positive premenopausal women with breast cancer. *N Engl J Med* 1997;337:956.
41. Fisher B, Redmond C, Legault-Poisson S, et al. Postoperative chemotherapy and tamoxifen compared with tamoxifen alone in the treatment of positive-node breast cancer patients aged 50 years and older with tumors responsive to tamoxifen: results from the National Surgical Adjuvant Breast and Bowel Project B-16. *J Clin Oncol* 1990;8:1005.

CHAPTER 23

Locally Advanced Breast Cancer

S. Eva Singletary and David J. Winchester

Although locally advanced breast cancer now accounts for less than 5% to 10% of breast cancers detected in mammographically screened populations, the surgeon should be aware of the appropriate management of this disease entity (1). In medically underserved areas of the United States and in many other countries, locally advanced breast cancer still represents 30% to 50% of newly diagnosed breast cancer cases.

Historically, patients with locally advanced breast cancer were felt to have a predestined poor survival outcome. In 1943, Haagensen and Stout (2) reported the clinical features of locally advanced breast cancer treated with radical mastectomy alone that predicted a 50% or greater chance of local recurrence and a 0% 5-year survival rate: extensive edema involving more than two-thirds of the breast, satellite skin nodules, "inflammatory" carcinoma, or edema of the arm. A local recurrence rate of 13% to 32% and a 5-year survival rate of 5% to 36% were possible with radical mastectomy in patients with less extensive skin edema (one-third of the breast), skin ulcerations, tumor fixation to the chest wall, or fixed axillary lymph nodes. However, if two or more of these features were present, the local recurrence rate increased to 40% and the long-term survival rate decreased to less than 5%. Because of the poor results seen with surgery alone, high-dose radiotherapy replaced surgery as the local therapy of choice in the 1950s and 1960s. Although a 5-year overall survival rate of 21% was achieved with radiotherapy in combined series (3,4), high-dose radiotherapy was often associated with severe side effects, such as chest wall fibrosis and skin ulceration, brachial plexopathy, and lymphedema of the arm. In the 1970s, the integration of systemic chemotherapy into a combined modality approach with local therapy led to local control rates of greater than 80% and 5-year survival rates of 35% to 70%.

Today, because therapeutic options in the management of locally advanced breast cancer are so diverse, the clinical decision-making process requires the interaction of a team of multidisciplinary specialists. To communicate effectively and to participate fully in the treatment plan, the surgeon must understand the concepts of locally advanced breast cancer and the staging system and current therapeutic strategies for this disease. The goal is to attempt to cure the patient's disease while maintaining optimal quality of life for the patient. This chapter addresses the initial evaluation of the disease, induction (preoperative) chemotherapy, the surgical approaches used in combination with chemotherapy and irradiation, and the cost-effective pathways of follow-up care.

INITIAL EVALUATION

The first step in the evaluation of a patient with locally advanced breast cancer is to clinically stage the cancer using the tumor-node-metastasis system (see Table 22-1 in Chapter 22) of the American Joint Committee on Cancer. Major changes in this staging system were made in 1988 (5,6): T3N0 disease was classified as stage IIB rather than stage IIIA, and metastases to the supraclavicular nodes were classified as distant (stage IV) rather than regional disease (see Table 22-1 in Chapter 22).

Locally advanced breast cancer is defined as primary breast tumors larger than 5 cm in diameter (T3, stage IIB), with skin or chest wall involvement (T4, stage IIIB), or with matted or fixed axillary lymph nodes (N2, stage IIIA). Although patients with supraclavicular lymph node metastases are now classified as having stage IV disease (M1) according to the revised American Joint Committee on Cancer staging system (5,6), these patients are often included in the treatment protocols for locally advanced breast cancer as both local and distant control is achievable in approximately 30% of such patients. A special type of locally advanced breast cancer is inflammatory breast cancer (T4d stage IIIB), which is defined by a rapid onset (empirically defined as within 3 months) of the clinical triad of erythema, "peau d'orange" or dermal lymphatic involvement, and ridging of the skin overlying the breast mound (Fig. 23-1).

Tissue for histologic diagnosis and determination of hormone receptor status and proliferative markers (S-phase fraction determined by flow cytometry or measurement of Ki67 expression) is usually obtained by fine-needle aspiration or a core-needle biopsy. If there is no clinical evidence of invasion, such as skin involvement or proven nodal metastases, a core-needle biopsy is required to confirm actual invasion rather than the presence of a large palpable mass of in situ

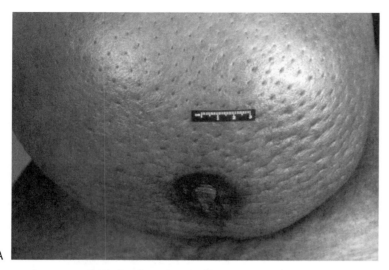

A

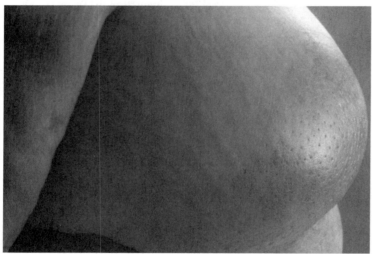

B

FIG. 23-1. Inflammatory breast cancer with clinical presentation of erythema, skin edema, and skin ridging of rapid onset.

(noninvasive) disease. A punch biopsy of the skin may be performed if dermal lymphatic involvement is suspected. However, the results of the skin biopsy are helpful only if they are positive. A negative finding on skin biopsy does not reliably rule out a dermal lymphatic tumor process if the clinical features are consistent with this finding.

A careful review of bilateral mammograms is performed, with particular attention given to identifying possible synchronous bilateral disease or ipsilateral multicentricity. Skin edema is often reflected on the mammograms as a thickening of the skin contour of the central breast. A baseline ultrasound examination of the breast and nodal basins is useful to delineate tumor size and the presence of nonpalpable nodal disease. If the patient may be a candidate for breast conservation surgery after tumor downstaging with chemotherapy, radiopaque clips may be inserted percutaneously in the epicenter of the primary tumor under ultrasound guidance. These clips can serve as markers for subsequent surgical excision of the tumor region if an excellent clinical response is achieved with chemotherapy. The staging work-up for possi-

ble distant metastases includes a chest x-ray, bone scan, and ultrasound or computed tomographic scan of the abdomen. A complete blood count, serum liver function tests, serum calcium level, and platelet count are routinely obtained. Some oncologists also order tests for the tumor markers carcinoembryonic antigen and CA 15-3. Levels of these tumor markers are often initially elevated; decreasing levels may reflect response to therapy.

INDUCTION CHEMOTHERAPY

The standard of care for most patients with locally advanced breast cancer is the combined-modality approach, which includes induction chemotherapy, surgery, radiation therapy, and postoperative chemotherapy (Fig. 23-2). Initially, the use of chemotherapy prior to surgery for patients with resectable disease was controversial. This controversy was based on concerns that (a) the surgeon might miss a "window of opportunity" to resect operable disease if tumor progression occurred during induction chemotherapy, (b) the histologic stag-

Locally Advanced Breast Cancer

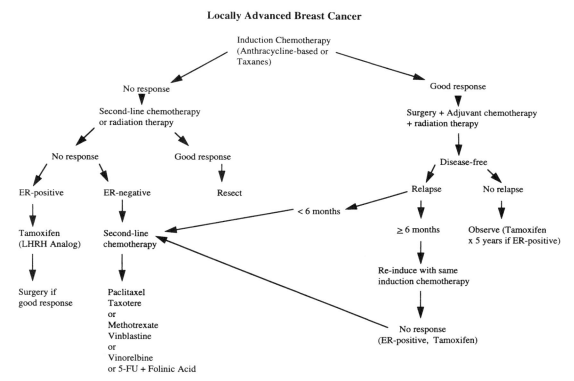

FIG. 23-2. Algorithm for choice of local and systemic therapy for locally advanced breast cancer.

ing information from surgery after chemotherapy might not be a prognostic indicator, and (c) the incidence of surgical complications would be higher. All three concerns have now been allayed with the long-term experience with induction preoperative chemotherapy.

Most patients (80%) have significant tumor shrinkage after three or four cycles of chemotherapy, especially if the drug regimen is based on doxorubicin or paclitaxel. Approximately 15% to 20% of patients will have a complete clinical remission. Tumor progression rarely occurs (less than 2% of patients) during induction chemotherapy. Patients who do experience disease progression while receiving chemotherapy usually have a poor prognosis and early onset of distant metastases.

Induction chemotherapy has been shown not to interfere with prognostic staging information gained from surgical treatment. In The University of Texas M. D. Anderson Cancer Center series of patients with locally advanced noninflammatory breast cancer treated with doxorubicin-based induction chemotherapy (7), the actuarial 5-year survival rate after surgery was 70% for patients with histologically negative nodes, 62% for patients with one to three positive nodes, 47% for patients with four to 10 positive nodes, and 21% for patients with more than 10 positive nodes. For patients treated at M. D. Anderson Cancer Center with inflammatory breast cancer protocols, the amount of residual tumor on histologic examination was also highly predictive of disease-specific and disease-free survival. For patients with microscopic or no

residual disease in the mastectomy specimen who had negative or only one to three positive axillary nodes on histologic examination, the 5-year disease-specific and disease-free survival rates were 71% and 59%, respectively, compared to 31% and 26% in patients with gross macroscopic residual disease or four or more positive nodes (8).

Although studies such as the National Surgical Adjuvant Breast and Bowel Project protocol B-18 have not yet confirmed a survival advantage for patients who receive induction chemotherapy, the use of chemotherapy in patients with intact tumors prior to surgical intervention may identify patients with chemoresistant disease and an associated worse prognosis who could then qualify for investigational studies. Conversely, if the tumor is chemosensitive, tumor downstaging may allow breast conservation surgery.

Induction chemotherapy is usually well tolerated. If the tumor is resectable, surgery is performed at the time of hematologic recovery (granulocyte count of at least 1,000 cells/μL). In patients receiving high-dose chemotherapy, the surgeon needs to be aware that only neutropenia and not anemia or thrombocytopenia is corrected by granulocyte colony-stimulating factor. If necessary, erythropoietin (Epogen) can be used to correct the chemotherapy-induced anemia prior to surgery. Blood transfusions are rarely indicated. The surgical procedures can usually be completed without an increased risk of infection or delayed wound healing (9). However, if the tumor just barely meets the criteria for resectability, consideration should be given to a cross-over chemotherapy regimen or preoperative irradiation. Tight or very thin mastectomy skin flaps should be avoided.

Elderly patients with cardiac disease and other significant comorbidity may not be candidates for induction chemotherapy, limiting their treatment options for locally advanced disease. Patients with resectable T3N0 or T3N1 tumors may be treated surgically as the first step in their management. In most cases, a modified radical mastectomy would be required but a breast preserving approach remains an option providing the patient is capable and willing to be treated with postoperative radiotherapy. Surgical resection may not be possible as the initial step in patients with more progressive disease involving larger T3 tumors, disease involving the skin (T4), or matted axillary nodes (N2). Providing hormone receptors are present, a 3- to 6-month trial of tamoxifen or other estrogen analogues may lead to a resectable tumor as might be observed with induction chemotherapy. Patients with unresectable tumors lacking receptors will usually not benefit from this approach and are best managed with an initial course of external beam radiation, followed by reassessment for resectability. Patients who have a reasonable life expectancy should be referred to a radiotherapist following their surgical treatment for consideration of postoperative radiotherapy. Those patients with tumors expressing hormone receptors should receive tamoxifen for the ensuing five years.

All patients with locally advanced breast cancer should be considered for radiotherapy at some point during their course of treatment. In most cases, this will occur as one of the final steps, following chemotherapy and surgery regardless of the decision to preserve the breast. Following mastectomy, radiotherapy lowers the risk of locoregional recurrence and should be directed to the chest wall using tangential fields. Internal mammary chain (IMC) recurrences seldom develop (10), regardless of inclusion of the IMC in the radiation port and should only be considered in patients with extensive axillary adenopathy or with locally advanced inner quadrant tumors. After completing the induction chemotherapy and locoregional treatment, additional systemic chemotherapy may be given according to the discretion of the patient's physicians. The identification of extensive axillary disease following the surgical management raises the risk of distant failure and represents a common indication for additional therapy.

Tamoxifen alone or in combination with retinoids or other estrogen analogues should be considered for all patients with locally advanced breast cancer. For elderly postmenopausal patients, it represents the first line therapy. In those patients treated with induction cytotoxic chemotherapy, there may be an additive benefit of tamoxifen, providing that hormone receptors are present on the tumor. For each of these scenarios, a five year course of therapy is appropriate.

BREAST CONSERVATION SURGERY AFTER TUMOR DOWNSTAGING

The question as to whether breast conservation surgery should be performed for locally advanced disease was prompted by patients who had no or minimal evidence of residual tumor in their mastectomy specimens after induction chemotherapy. Patients with substantial tumor reduction had difficulty understanding why the entire breast had to be sacrificed. The present concern with preserving the breast for locally advanced disease is whether occult tumor is in other quadrants of the breast. In a retrospective review at M. D. Anderson (11) of 143 patients with stage IIB through selected stage IV (positive supraclavicular nodes) breast cancer who responded with at least 50% tumor shrinkage to induction combination chemotherapy—5-fluouracil (5-FU), doxorubicin, and cyclophosphamide—and then underwent mastectomy, the factors most often associated with tumor involvement in multiple quadrants of the breast were persistent skin edema of the breast (65% of such patients had multiple-quadrant involvement), residual tumor size larger than 4 cm (56% of patients), extensive intramammary lymphatic invasion (20% of patients), and known mammographic evidence of multicentric disease (16% of patients). According to the eligibility criteria for breast conservation surgery used in this study (Table 23-1), 33 (23%) of the 143 patients could have had a segmental mastectomy (wide local excision) and axillary node dissection rather than a modified radical mastectomy. None of these 33 patients were found to have tumor in other quadrants of the breast in the mastectomy specimen, and at a median follow-up of 34 months, none had experienced a chest wall recurrence. In contrast, of 110 patients who were considered poor candidates for breast conservation surgery, 55 (50%) had tumor in other quadrants: 22 involving two quadrants, nine involving three quadrants, and 24 involving the entire breast.

Using the same criteria (Table 23-1) for determining if a patient was a candidate for breast conservation surgery, a subsequent M. D. Anderson clinical trial was initiated in 1989. Among 203 evaluable patients with node-positive stage IIA (primary tumors larger than 2 cm but not exceeding 5 cm), stage IIB, stage IIIA-B, or selected stage IV (positive supraclavicular lymph nodes) noninflammatory breast cancers who completed four cycles of induction chemotherapy, breast conservation surgery was elected and performed in 51 patients (25%). Because of persistent central skin edema, the rate of breast conservation surgery in patients with dermal lymphatic involvement (stage IIIB) was only 6%. With a median follow-up of greater than 60 months, only five patients had relapses in the breast, and three of these patients remained disease free after mastectomy. For patients with inflammatory breast

TABLE 23-1. *Criteria for breast conservation surgery after induction chemotherapy for locally advanced breast cancer*

Resolution of skin edema (peau d'orange)
Residual tumor size of less than 5 cm
Absence of extensive intramammary lymphatic invasion
Absence of extensive suspicious microcalcifications
No known evidence of multicentricity
Patient's desire for breast preservation

cancer, breast conservation surgery is not recommended even in patients who have a complete response to the induction chemotherapy. In the M. D. Anderson experience of patients treated on inflammatory breast cancer protocols, the clinical response correlated poorly with the extent of residual tumor. Of patients who had a clinical complete response and underwent mastectomy, 38% had gross macroscopic disease within the mastectomy specimen, 33% had one to three positive axillary nodes, and 56% had four or more positive nodes (8).

If a patient is considered to be a candidate for breast conservation surgery, a referral to the radiotherapist prior to surgery is important to ensure that the radiotherapist agrees with the treatment plan and that the patient understands the potential short-term and long-term effects and complications of irradiation. A mammogram should also be obtained after the induction chemotherapy and prior to surgery to determine the radiographic extent of the residual tumor. Occasionally, in tumors that respond to chemotherapy, extensive microcalcifications develop within the previous tumor field during chemotherapy; this precludes a conservative surgical approach. If the tumor is not palpable, needle localization should be performed with either mammography or ultrasound. If metal clips have previously been inserted to mark the tumor location, intraoperative ultrasound is a useful approach.

Before surgery, the surgeon and the patient should discuss whether the patient desires to proceed with a complete mastectomy if negative margins cannot be obtained at the time of surgery. This decision should not be placed on the family members in the waiting room during the operation. If the patient desires immediate reconstruction, it is usually more practical to defer the mastectomy and perform it as a second-stage procedure, especially when an autogenous-tissue-flap reconstruction is likely. If a free-flap reconstruction with a microvascular anastomosis to the thoracodorsal vessels is considered a possibility, it is best to defer the axillary node dissection until the time of the completion mastectomy.

The surgical procedure for breast conservation should be similar to that used for early-stage breast cancer. The skin incision should be placed directly over the residual breast mass. An ellipse of skin should be included if the lesion is superficial or has previously been biopsied. Usually a curvilinear transverse incision that conforms to the contour of the breast achieves the best cosmetic result (10) (Fig. 23-3). However, if the patient is a borderline candidate for breast preservation, the skin incision should be oriented so that it can be easily included in a mastectomy specimen, especially if there is a high probability of performing a skin-sparing mastectomy with immediate reconstruction. For larger lesions or if considerable skin sacrifice is required, particularly for tumors in the lower aspect of the breast, it is helpful to consult a plastic surgeon before attempting a wide local excision. Potential strategies for avoiding a poor cosmetic result, such as a Z-plasty closure or local flap rotation, can be discussed before surgery. However, if the anticipated defect is large enough to require a large tissue flap, the preferred option is to proceed with a total mastectomy with standard reconstruction techniques.

A separate skin incision from the segmental mastectomy site should be used for the axillary node dissection. Separate incisions diminish retraction of the breast toward the axilla after irradiation and allow the radiotherapist the option of delivering a radiation boost to the tumor bed if needed.

An *en bloc* excision around the tumor or biopsy cavity should be performed with a margin of normal breast tissue of approximately 1 cm or larger obtained in all three dimensions. The skin flaps should be relatively thick unless the tumor is superficial. For lesions deep in the breast, the pectoralis fascia may be included. If the tumor is invading the pectoralis major muscle, a wide local excision of the involved muscle should be performed.

The surgeon should orient the specimen for the pathologist with at least two of the margins identified by either hemoclips or sutures, and should request that any close margins be checked with frozen section examination. If the residual tumor was nonpalpable and needle localization under mammographic guidance was performed or if metal markers were previously inserted at the tumor site, a specimen radiograph should be obtained before the specimen is sectioned to document that the lesion has indeed been removed. The specimen should be inked and serially sectioned to include all margins within each section. A second specimen radiograph of the sections is often helpful for locating a nonpapable lesion or microcalcifications and provides a relative guide to the adequacy of the margins. A portion of the tumor should be sent for hormone receptor assays and flow cytometric analysis if these were not performed on initial evaluation. For very small residual disease, receptor status may be determined by immunostaining of slides from either the frozen section or the paraffin block.

Radiopaque hemoclips are used to mark the tumor resection bed for the planning of the radiotherapy fields. These clips should be placed at the periphery and the base of the surgical defect. The defect inside the breast should not be closed with sutures, and drains are not necessary. The skin should be closed with absorbable interrupted inverted sutures of the deep dermis followed by a running subcuticular 4-0 or 5-0 absorbable suture. Steristrips should be used to approximate the skin edges. Bulky pressure dressings and heavy tape are not necessary and are uncomfortable to the patient. A lightweight stretch bra supports the breast and may decrease tension on the incision from the weight of the breast itself.

AXILLARY NODE DISSECTION

The current standard of care for operable invasive breast cancer is to perform a level I and II axillary node dissection (lymph nodes lateral and posterior to the pectoralis minor muscle). In patients with limited life expectancy or severe comorbid conditions, the value of the surgical procedure must be weighed against the possible complications or side effects. The extent of the axillary node dissection should be the same regardless of whether breast conservation surgery or modified radical mastectomy is performed.

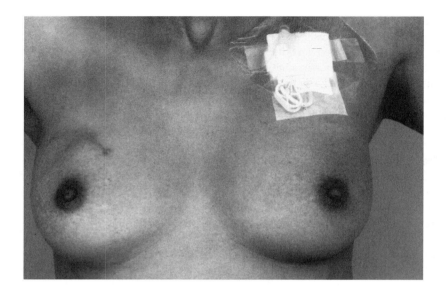

FIG. 23-3. A 40-year-old woman with T2 N2 M0 carcinoma of the left breast who underwent segmental mastectomy and axillary node dissection after four cycles of induction chemotherapy with 5-FU, doxorubicin, and cyclophosphamide (FAC). No residual tumor was found in the breast or axillary nodes. Postoperatively, she received 4 cycles of FAC followed by radiation to the breast and peripheral lymph nodes. She was free of disease at the 38-month follow-up. (Reprinted with permission from Singletary SE. Surgical management of locally advanced breast cancer. *Semin Radiat Oncol* 1994;4:254.)

A subject of controversy today is whether an axillary node dissection can be omitted if patients are receiving systemic therapy on the basis of the initial size of the tumor. The staging information from an axillary node dissection still has prognostic value in this situation and may be helpful in selecting patients to participate in dose-intensive chemotherapy trials or other investigational studies. However, there is still no conclusive evidence that high-dose chemotherapy significantly prolongs survival in the subset of patients with tumors that are resistant to standard chemotherapy.

Another controversy surrounding axillary node dissection is whether if is necessary to achieve local control of disease in the axilla. In the National Surgical Adjuvant Breast and Bowel Project B-04 trial, which compared radical mastectomy and total mastectomy with or without irradiation for patients with invasive tumors up to 4 cm in size with a clinically negative axilla (12), 20% of patients who were treated with total mastectomy alone required a delayed axillary node dissection; fewer than 2% presented with an inoperable axilla. Even in recent studies with stage I breast cancer, axillary relapse rate of 15% to 20% have been reported for the nondissected axilla (12–15).

Whether modern-day chemotherapy can substitute for surgical control of the axilla is not yet known. A lower rate of locoregional recurrences (the majority of which occurred on the chest wall) has been demonstrated with the use of adjuvant chemotherapy as compared with mastectomy or radiotherapy alone (16). The lowest regional recurrence rate is achieved by using both systemic therapy and irradiation. The addition of irradiation has been shown to decrease the rate of recurrence in the nondissected clinically negative axilla to less than 3% (17). The ability to control the axilla nonsurgically for more advanced primary disease is unknown. The current protocol at M. D. Anderson for patients with T2-3, N0-1 breast cancers initially randomizes patients to receive either four cycles of paclitaxel (Taxol) or four cycles of 5-FU, doxorubicin, and cyclophosphamide before surgery. If the patient's tumor is downstaged enough that breast preservation can be considered and if the axilla becomes clinically negative, patients are offered a second randomization to receive either irradiation of the axilla or a standard level I and II axillary node dissection. After surgery, four cycles of 5-FU, doxorubicin, and cyclophosphamide are administered. The breast and nodal basin are treated with irradiation, which includes the axilla if it was not dissected and, in selected patients, the supraclavicular fossa.

The recently described technology of lymphatic mapping and sentinel lymph node biopsy raises the possibility that a proportion of patients could be spared a complete axillary dissection. However, the role of sentinel node biopsy for locally advanced breast cancer has not been fully explored. The lymphatic drainage of the breast is ambiguous, and tumors may drain directly to level I, II, or III axillary lymph nodes, internal mammary nodes, or a combination of these. The major advantage of sentinel node biopsy is that it allows for a selective approach to the axilla (18,19). If the sentinel node is negative for metastatic disease, then a formal axillary node dissection can be avoided. If the sentinel node is positive, the patient can have a complete node dissection for local control and additional staging information. Another advantage is that the pathologist can perform a more in-depth examination of the sentinel node than is possible with the entire axillary contents. This sentinel node can be probed for evidence of metastatic tumor cells using molecular and immunohistological markers.

The major disadvantage of sentinel lymph node biopsy is that it yields reproducible and accurate results only in the hands of a surgeon experienced in this technique. Another obstacle is the use of lymphatic mapping in patients who have had excisional biopsy with removal of the primary tumor, which may disrupt the lymphatic draining channels. At present, lymphatic mapping is an investigational tool and should be done in conjunction with an axillary node dissection unless the patient is enrolled in a formal protocol.

Thus, since axillary node dissection is still a major component of breast cancer surgery, the surgeon must be familiar with the anatomy of the axilla and the appropriate surgical technique. The technique is as follows: A single dose of a preoperative antibiotic at the time of surgery may decrease the likelihood of wound infection (20). The patient is placed in the supine position with the ipsilateral arm extended. A small roll is placed beneath the patient's back longitudinally to elevate the axilla from the operating table. Folded sheets should be used to raise the extended arm to the same height as the axilla to avoid possible brachial plexus injury from excessive traction. The arm must not be hyperextended. The entire breast and ipsilateral arm are prepared. The opposite breast should be included within the prepared field if immediate reconstruction is planned so that the plastic surgeon can compare symmetry between the opposite breast and the reconstructed breast mound. The ipsilateral arm is draped separately from the field so that, if necessary, the surgeon can lift the arm to gain exposure of the high axilla either for removal of nodal disease or for control of any unexpected hemorrhage.

A separate skin incision is made for the axillary node dissection if the patient is undergoing breast conservation surgery. A transverse S-shaped incision made approximately 2 to 3 cm beneath the axillary skin fold allows better exposure of the axillary contents with retractors. The anterior cephalad extension of the S-shaped incision is the lateral border of the pectoralis major muscle, while the posterior caudad extension is the anterior border of the latissimus dorsi muscle. It is preferable that the incision be placed below the hair follicles to facilitate the patient's shaving of the axilla in the future.

The superior skin flap is raised within a plane of dissection of approximately 5 mm beneath the skin to ensure adequate cutaneous blood supply. Identification of the cephalad portion of the pectoralis major muscle serves as a guide to the anticipated location of the axillary vein. The inferior skin flap is then elevated to at least the level of the fifth intercostal space to ensure that the lowest axillary lymph nodes are included with the specimen and the lateral border of the pectoralis major muscle is exposed. After the anterior border of the latissimus dorsi muscle is identified, the dissection traces the tendinous insertion of this muscle until the axillary vein is located. Incising the axillary fascia immediately medial to the anterior border of the latissimus muscle exposes the thoracodorsal vessels. The fascia on the anterior surface of the thoracodorsal vascular pedicle is then dissected free to allow the vessels and the thoracodorsal nerve to fall laterally as the specimen is retracted medially. A landmark for the long thoracic nerve is a perpendicular branch from the medial side of the thoracodorsal vessels. By incising the fascia anterior to the long thoracic nerve, the specimen is moved more medially. It is important to identify the thoracodorsal trunk and long thoracic nerve throughout their course up to the axillary vein so that these structures are carefully preserved throughout the course of the axillary node dissection.

The nodal tissue is dissected from the axillary vein either from a lateral to a medial direction or vice versa depending on the surgeon's preference. The fascia covering the pectoralis major muscle is incised, exposing the underlying pectoralis minor muscle. It is preferable to preserve the pectoralis minor neurovascular bundle because often a nerve branch to the lateral third of the pectoral major muscle courses through this bundle. To avoid traction injury to this neurovascular bundle, a small perpendicular branching vessel arising from the curve of this vascular trunk should be carefully divided. The pectoralis minor muscle may be retracted medially to gain exposure to the level II lymph nodes. Division of the pectoralis minor muscle is rarely necessary. If obvious nodal disease is detected medial to the pectoralis minor muscle, inclusion of level III axillary lymph nodes with the dissection should be considered. If an attempt is made to preserve any of the intercostal brachial cutaneous nerves, the specimen may need to be bivalved where the cutaneous nerves enter the chest wall. As the specimen is dissected from the chest wall, the fascia of the serratus anterior muscle can be left intact.

After meticulous hemostasis is achieved, a 0.25-inch closed-suction drainage catheter is inserted through the inferior skin flap. The catheter is placed into the axilla so that it is not in direct contact with the axillary vein. The most distal perforations of the catheter should be positioned far enough from the exit site to avoid an air leak. A single 3-0 nylon suture is used to secure the catheter to the skin. The suture should not loop the skin so tightly that later removal of the suture is difficult, but the loop also should not be so large that the catheter can slide in and out of the axilla, risking contamination. The skin flaps are reapproximated with 3-0 or 4-0 synthetic absorbable sutures on the deep dermis and a running subcuticular 4-0 or 5-0 synthetic absorbable suture on the skin. Steristrips are applied along the length of the wound for coverage. A small (4 × 4 inch) gauze dressing with a small amount of antibacterial ointment can be placed over the drain site. Bulky pressure dressings are unnecessary and are uncomfortable to the patient.

TIMING OF BREAST RECONSTRUCTION

Although immediate breast reconstruction is considered acceptable for early-stage breast cancer, controversy exists about whether breast reconstruction should be delayed until completion of both adjuvant chemotherapy and irradiation in patients with locally advanced breast cancer. The M. D. Anderson experience suggests that immediate reconstruction does not interfere with the resumption of chemotherapy (21) as the risk of complications is very low, especially with the use of autogenous tissue for the reconstruction. Irradiation of a breast mound reconstructed from autogenous tissue has not been shown to impair the flap's blood supply or affect the cosmetic result if there is no pre-existing significant fat necrosis. If fat necrosis is present, irradiation tends to increase the fibrosis and volume loss of the reconstructed breast mound. In the series of 19 patients from M. D. Anderson (22) who received postoperative radiotherapy after reconstruction with a transrectus rectus abdominous myocutaneous flap either for known local recurrence (4 patients) or as adjuvant therapy for high risk of recurrence (15 patients), the cosmetic result was dependent on the initial outcome of the reconstruction.

However, the use of tissue expansion for implant reconstruction with anticipated irradiation has usually had poor results. In the M. D. Anderson series of patients who received submuscular implants, the rates of capsular contracture (Baker III or greater), pain, implant exposure, and implant removal were significantly higher in 13 patients with implants within an irradiated field than in 230 patients with implants that were not irradiated (23). Although results are slightly improved with the use of implants placed beneath autogenous tissue, the optimal result is obtained by avoiding implants and using only autogenous tissue for reconstruction in patients who will receive radiotherapy.

Prior to a final decision regarding the immediate reconstruction, the radiotherapist should be consulted to ensure that no special radiotherapy planning is required. For selected patients, such as those with internal mammary node involvement or dermal lymphatic tumor, the radiotherapist usually prefers to delay the reconstruction. Certainly, if the patient is unsure whether she desires reconstruction, the best course of action is to reassure the patient that delaying the reconstruction will not adversely affect her well-being or later cosmetic result. The first priority of treatment should be to control the tumor.

POSTOPERATIVE CARE AND FOLLOW-UP

With thorough instruction in wound care for the patient and her personal caregiver, most patients can be discharged from the hospital as soon as they recover from the general anesthesia—usually within 24 h. It is critical that the patient and her family be educated before surgery on the treatment plan and the home management of the suction catheters. This involvement of the patient and family members in discussions about the diagnosis, treatment options, side effects, and postoperative care enhances their ability to adjust to the disease and its treatment. Patients are instructed to call if their temperature exceeds 101°F, if they have excessive bloody drainage (200 mL or more over an 8-h period), or if any signs of infection or difficulty with the drainage system are present (24). Suction catheters are removed when the drainage is less than 30 mL over a 24-h period. Although movement of the ipsilateral arm is not restricted, range-of-motion exercises are deferred until the day following catheter removal. Patients are then seen the week after drain removal to check for seroma formation in the axilla and to ensure that the range of motion of the affected arm is improving. Most seromas can be managed by needle aspiration; however, if a seroma reaccumulates rapidly or after several aspirations, it is usually more convenient to the patient to reinsert a catheter.

If a patient has had a mastectomy with immediate breast reconstruction, the hospital stay averages 5 days. In addition, range-of-motion exercises are delayed for 2 weeks if a microvascular procedure is done.

Every patient, regardless of the type of surgical procedure, should be offered support services, such as the American Cancer Society's program "Reach to Recovery." As patients are now discharged home soon after surgery, the best time for this psychosocial interaction is prior to surgery.

Routine long-term follow-up includes a thorough history and physical examination every 3 to 4 months for the first 2 years, every 6 months during years 3 through 5, and yearly thereafter for the patient's lifetime (25). Annual diagnostic mammograms of the contralateral breast and, if intact, the treated breast are required. For patients who underwent breast conservation surgery, a mammogram 6 months after completion of radiotherapy is useful as a baseline for future comparisons. Routine mammograms of the reconstructed breast mound are not helpful as most local recurrences will be detected in the skin and subcutaneous tissue of the mastectomy flaps by physical examination. Extensive laboratory or radiologic studies obtained on routine patient follow-up have not been shown to affect survival or quality of life in the absence of symptoms and are not cost-effective (26–28).

REFERENCES

1. Leitch AM, Garvey RF. Breast cancer in a county hospital population: impact of breast screening on stage of presentation. *Ann Surg Oncol* 1994;1:516.
2. Haagensen CD, Stout AP. Carcinoma of the breast. II. Criteria of operability. *Ann Surg* 1943;118:859.
3. Baclesse F. Roentgen therapy as the method of treatment of cancer of the breast. *Am J Roentgenol* 1949;62:311.
4. Fletcher GH, Montague ED. Radical irradiation of advanced breast cancer. *Am J Roentgenol* 1965;93:573.
5. American Joint Committee on Cancer. *Manual for staging of cancer.* 3rd ed. Philadelphia: JB Lippincott Co, 1988:145.
6. American Joint Committee on Cancer. Beahrs OH, Henson DE, Hutter RV, Kennedy BJ, eds. *Manual for staging of cancer.* 4th ed. Philadelphia: JB Lippincott Co., 1992:164.
7. McCready DR, Hortobagyi GN, Kau SW, Smith TL, Buzdar AU, Balch CM. The prognostic significance of lymph node metastases after preoperative chemotherapy for locally advanced breast cancer. *Arch Surg* 1989;189:21.
8. Fleming RY, Asman L, Buzdar AU, et al. Effect of mastectomy by response to induction chemotherapy for control of inflammatory breast carcinoma. *Ann Surg Oncol* 1997;4:452.
9. Broadwater JR, Edwards MJ, Kuglen C, Hortobagyi GN, Ames FC, Balch CM. Mastectomy following preoperative chemotherapy. *Ann Surg* 1991;213:1265.
10. Singletary SE. Surgical management of locally advanced breast cancer. *Semin Radiat Oncol* 1994;4:254.
11. Singletary SE, McNeese MD, Hortobagyi GN. Feasibility of breast conservation surgery after induction chemotherapy for locally advanced carcinoma. *Cancer* 1992;69:2849.
12. Fisher B, Redmond C, Fisher ER, et al. Ten-year results of a randomized clinical trial comparing radical mastectomy and total mastectomy with or without radiation. *N Engl J Med* 1985;312:674.
13. Baxter N, McCready D, Chapman J, et al. The clinical behavior of untreated axillary nodes following local treatment for primary breast cancer. *Ann Surg Oncol* 1996;3:235.
14. Martelli G, DePalo G, Rossi N, et al. Long-term follow-up of elderly patients with operable breast cancer treated with surgery without axillary dissection plus adjuvant tamoxifen. *Br J Cancer* 1995;72:1251.
15. Haffty BG, McKhann C, Beinfield M, Fischer D, Fischer JJ. Breast conservation therapy without axillary dissection. *Arch Surg* 1993;128:1315.
16. Buzdar AU, McNeese MD, Hortobagyi GN, et al. Is chemotherapy effective in reducing the local failure rate in patients with operable breast cancer? *Cancer* 1990;65:394.

17. Recht A, Pierce SM, Abner A, et al. Regional nodal failure after conservative surgery and radiotherapy for early-stage breast carcinoma. *J Clin Oncol* 1991;9:988.
18. Guiliano AE, Dale PS, Roderick R, Morton DL, Evans SW, Krasne DL. Improved axillary staging of breast cancer with sentinel lymphadenectomy. *Ann Surg* 1995;222:394.
19. Albertini JJ, Lyman GH, Cox, et al. Lymphatic mapping and sentinel node biopsy in the patient with breast cancer. *JAMA* 1996;276:1818.
20. Mansfield PM, Berger DH, Hohn DC, et al. A prospective randomized double-blinded trial of cefonicid for prophylaxis during axillary node dissection [Abstract]. Presented at the 49th Annual Cancer Symposium Society Surgical Oncology, 1996.
21. Schusterman MA, Kroll SS, Miller MJ, et al. The free TRAM flap for breast reconstruction: one center's experience with 211 consecutive cases. *Ann Plast Surg* 1994;32:234.
22. Hunt KK, Baldwin BJ, Strom EA, et al. Feasibility of postmastectomy radiation therapy after TRAM flap breast reconstruction. *Ann Surg Oncol* 1997;4:377.
23. Evans GR, Schusterman MA, Kroll SS, et al. Reconstruction and the radiated breast: is there a role for implants? *Plast Reconstr Surg* 1995;96:1111.
24. Burke CC, Zabka CL, McCarver KJ, Singletary SE. Patient satisfaction with 23-hour short stay observation following breast cancer surgery. *Oncol Nurs Forum* 1997;24:645.
25. Judkins AF, Peterson SK, Singletary SE. Satisfaction of breast cancer patients with a nonphysician-provider model of long-term follow-up care. *Breast Dis* 1996;9:1339.
26. Yeh KA, Fortunato L, Ridge JA, Hoffman JP, Eisenberg BL, Sigurdson ER. Routine bone scanning in patients with T1 and T2 breast cancer: a waste of money. *Ann Surg Oncol* 1995;2:319.
27. Del Turco MR, Palli D, Cariddi A, Ciatto S, Pacini P, Distante V. Intensive diagnostic follow-up after treatment of primary breast cancer. A randomized trial. *JAMA* 1994;271:1593.
28. GIVIO Investigators. Impact of follow-up testing on survival and health-related quality of life in breast cancer patients. A multicenter randomized controlled trial. *JAMA* 1994;271:1587.

CHAPTER 24

Ovarian Cancer: Considerations for the General Surgeon

Edward E. Partridge

In the United States, ovarian cancer is the leading cause of death from gynecologic malignances. There are an estimated 26,800 new cases and 14,200 deaths associated with the epithelial form of this malignancy annually (1). Surgical confirmation of the suspected diagnosis, surgical staging, and aggressive surgical removal of disease are all essential elements in the care of women with this disease. Approximately one in five women with ovarian cancer will have a general surgeon as their primary surgeon because either a gynecologic oncologist is not available or, more commonly, the cancer is encountered unexpectedly (2). It is therefore incumbent upon all surgeons who operate in the abdomen and pelvis to understand this disease, with special emphasis on prevention, screening and diagnosis, and surgical management.

RISK FACTORS

Advancing age is probably the most significant risk factor for developing ovarian cancer. This risk increases from 17.5 to 54 per 100,000 as one ages from 40 to 79 years (3). The strongest risk factor, other than age, for the development of ovarian cancer is a familial history of the disease. It is estimated that at least 5% to 10% of all epithelial ovarian carcinomas result from hereditary predisposition (4,5). This results from the germline inheritance of a mutant gene conferring autosomal dominant susceptibility with high penetrance (4–6). The average age for the development of ovarian cancer cases with genetic predisposition is lower by up to 10 years than that of ovarian cancer cases in general (6,7).

Three specific ovarian cancer hereditary syndromes have been identified and are important to the general surgeon because two of the three involve cancers traditionally managed by the general surgeon. These syndromes include the following: (a) breast and ovarian cancer syndrome, in which both cancers are seen in excess and on occasion in the same individual; (b) ovarian cancers associated with an excess of colorectal and endometrial cancers [hereditary nonpolyposis colon cancer syndrome (HNPCC)]; and (c) site-specific ovarian cancer syndrome. The breast and ovarian cancer syndrome is the most common, accounting for 65% to 75% of all hereditary ovarian cancer cases, with HNPCC and site-specific syndrome probably accounting for only 10% to 15% each (8).

It is now clear that most breast and ovarian cancer families are linked to the *BRCA1* gene (9). The majority of those that are not linked to *BRCA1* are linked to the *BRCA2* gene (10,11). The penetrance of the *BRCA1* mutation is estimated to be about 95%, providing a cumulative risk of about 63% for the development of ovarian cancer by age 70 (7).

Other risk factors for this disease include nulliparity, early menarche, and late menopause. It is of considerable importance to know that women who use oral contraceptives *reduce* their risk for the development of this disease by 30% to 60% (12). Pregnancy and lactation also reduce the risk. One hypothesis to explain the above observations is that greater numbers of ovulations lead to a greater number of repairs of the ovarian epithelium, leading in turn to a higher risk of inadequate or aberrant repair, which in turn may progress to carcinogenesis. It has also been suggested that both tubal ligation and hysterectomy reduce the risk of ovarian cancer. It is postulated that this reduction is secondary either to an interruption in the ability of cocarcinogens to get to the ovary via the genital tract or a change in the hormonal milieu of the ovary secondary to the surgery (13).

PREVENTION

The major risk factor for the development of ovarian cancer, advancing age, is unalterable. Since oral contraceptives are known to decrease risk for the development of this disease, they should be strongly considered as a method of birth control, particularly in women with a suggestion of a hereditary predisposition. As previously noted, both hysterectomy and tubal ligation may afford some protection, and this should be taken into account when permanent sterilization is contemplated.

Prophylactic oophorectomy should be strongly considered in women with a hereditary predisposition to ovarian cancer.

Although an earlier study suggested that the risk of development of intraperitoneal carcinomatosis following oophorectomy in these women was substantial (as high as 10%) (14), a more recent publication of a larger group of women suggested a rate closer to 1.8% (15). Since the risk of development of ovarian cancer in a *BRCA1* mutation carrier exceeds 60%, it would seem clear that ovarian cancer can be prevented in a number of these women by prophylactic oophorectomy. The issues related to genetic testing—technical, ethical, legal, and psychosocial—are formidable and beyond the scope of this text.

It has been suggested that families with a total of five or more breast or ovarian cancers in first or second degree relatives qualify as having the breast and ovarian cancer syndrome (16), as do families with at least three cases of early onset (before age 60) breast or ovarian cancer (9). Genetic testing should be considered in these families; however, it should be performed in conjunction with established research programs that have a certified laboratory, pre- and posttest counseling, and continued emphasis of the ethical, legal, and psychosocial aspects of genetic testing.

Recommendations by the American College of Obstetricians and Gynecologists, published in 1994 prior to our current knowledge of genetic testing, include the consideration of bilateral oophorectomy based on documentation of (a) two or more first degree relatives with epithelial ovarian cancer, suggesting either maternal or paternal transmission; (b) a pedigree of multiple occurrences of nonpolyposis colorectal cancer, endometrial cancer, and ovarian cancer; and (c) a pedigree of multiple cases of breast or ovarian cancer (17).

SCREENING

An optimal screening test is distinguished by high sensitivity, specificity, patient acceptance, and ease of performance. Unfortunately, the three screening tests available at this time (pelvic exam, CA-125, and vaginal ultrasound) do not actually diagnose ovarian cancer; each requires a laparotomy for definitive diagnosis. Based upon the prevalence of ovarian cancer in the population, the positive predictive value of a screening test for ovarian cancer with a 99% specificity in women 45 to 75 years of age is estimated to be approximately 4%. This would lead to 24 negative laparotomies for each case of ovarian cancer detected. None of the single tests noted above reaches this level of specificity.

The pelvic examination, which is the current standard for screening women with ovarian cancer, is of limited value since its sensitivity for detecting a 4 × 6 cm mass is only 67%. A 15-year study evaluating pelvic examinations found six ovarian cancers in 1,319 women who underwent 18,753 pelvic examinations, further demonstrating the inadequacy of this method of screening (18).

The CA-125 is the most extensively studied tumor marker used in screening for ovarian cancer. CA-125 is a high molecular weight glycoprotein that is recognized by the murine OC-125 monoclonal antibody as an immunogen. The normal value has been established as 35 U/mL.

CA-125 levels are elevated (more than 35 U/mL) in 85% of epithelial ovarian cancers, but in only 50% of patients with stage I disease—the stage at which mortality is most likely to be affected. It should also be noted that the CA-125 can be elevated in a number of other disease processes, including endometriosis, pelvic inflammatory disease, adenomyosis, liver disease, pancreatitis, peritonitis, and many other benign processes. It also may be elevated in a number of other malignant processes, including endometrial adenocarcinoma, biliary tract tumors, hepatic, pancreatic, breast, and colon carcinomas. A recent review of several large studies using CA-125 and other markers concluded that the CA-125 does not have adequate specificity to warrant its use in mass screening (19).

Although transabdominal and transvaginal ultrasound have both been investigated as noninvasive screening modalities, the transvaginal ultrasound is the preferred method at present because of its superior ability to image the ovary. Again, the major problem with transvaginal ultrasound is lack of sufficient specificity. Morphologic scoring systems have been proposed to increase specificity. Criteria being studied include size/volume, papillary projections from the cyst wall, and cyst complexity. A large study of 3,220 women utilizing transvaginal ultrasound and morphologic index provided a specificity of 98.7% and a positive predictive value of 6.8%. Forty-four laparotomies were required to find three cancers, two of which were stage I (20).

Color Doppler imaging coupled with transvaginal ultrasound to detect specific flow patterns related to malignant disease has been proposed. This is of course a more expensive screening methodology. A study of 1,601 women with a family history of ovarian cancer ended with 61 patients having surgery. Six ovarian cancers were found (five stage I and one stage III), and three were low malignant potential (21).

A summary of five studies using transabdominal ultrasound, transvaginal ultrasound, morphologic index and color Doppler indices in various combinations screened 11,283 women. Four hundred eighty-six of these women required laparotomy for definitive diagnosis. Twenty-two cases of cancer were found, 13 of which were stage I, five of which were invasive. This provides a specificity for ovarian cancer of 95.8% and a positive predictive value of 3.1 (22).

In 1994, the NIH held a Consensus conference on ovarian cancer. After careful deliberation including review of all available data, it was concluded that there is no evidence that screening with CA-125 and/or transvaginal ultrasound can be used effectively to reduce ovarian cancer mortality or decrease morbidity (23). These tests are not recommended for routine screening at this time. The PLCO (prostate, lung, colon, and ovary) cancer screening trial sponsored by the NCI is currently testing the efficacy of pelvic examination, transvaginal ultrasound, and CA-125 in detecting ovarian cancer in women between the ages of 60 and 74; future recommendations await the completion of this prospective randomized trial (24).

However, the appropriateness of screening women who are high risk based on genetic studies or family history continues to be debated. Beyond the recommended routine gynecologic examination, measurement of serum CA-125 levels and transvaginal sonography have not been systematically studied in this group of women. Screening procedures may well prove more effective in the early detection of ovarian cancer in women with genetic predisposition; however, clinical trials are needed to test this hypothesis. For now, the American College of Obstetricians and Gynecologists recommends an annual rectovaginal examination, CA-125, and transvaginal ultrasound in women at high risk until childbearing is complete or to age 35, at which point prophylactic oophorectomy should be considered (23).

The general surgeon who sees high-risk members of HNPCC families has an even more formidable challenge because of the numerous cancers seen in these patients. The consensus recommendations of the International Collaborative Group on HNPCC include the option of prophylactic total abdominal hysterectomy and bilateral salpingooophorectomy in women who are undergoing subtotal colectomy following the diagnosis of colon cancer or in asymptomatic high-risk members of HNPCC families with severe cancer phobias. Otherwise, surveillance guidelines for high-risk individuals include, in addition to colonoscopy procedures, endometrial curettage, transvaginal ultrasound, possibly Doppler color blood flow imaging of the ovaries, and serum CA-125 measurement annually after the age of 30 (25).

The most recent recommendations for follow-up care in individuals with an inherited predisposition to cancer come from a task force convened by the Cancer Genetics Studies Consortium, organized by the National Human Genome Research Institute (26,27). For patients with HNPCC-associated mutations, colonoscopy every 1 to 3 years starting at age 25 is recommended. Endometrial cancer screening is recommended as well. The task force felt that there was insufficient evidence to recommend surveillance for ovarian cancer, but noted that some experts have recommended this. No recommendation is made for or against prophylactic surgery (i.e., colectomy, hysterectomy), but these surgeries are an option for mutation carriers.

Early breast cancer and ovarian cancer screening is recommended for individuals with *BRCA1* mutations and early breast cancer screening for women with *BRCA2* mutations. Again, no recommendation is made for or against prophylactic surgery (i.e., mastectomy, oophorectomy), but these surgeries are an option for mutation carriers.

SIGNS AND SYMPTOMS

Ovarian cancer has traditionally been called the "silent killer" by both the medical and lay community. This is based upon the belief that early-stage disease is usually asymptomatic and that symptoms become recognized by the patient only after the disease becomes more advanced. However, several studies have suggested that women with localized disease in fact have symptoms that are quite similar to and occur as often as women with non-localized disease (28,29). The most common symptoms include abdominal swelling, abdominal

pain, intestinal symptoms, and vaginal bleeding or discharge. Many of these symptoms are fairly nonspecific; therefore, it is important that physicians consider the possibility of ovarian neoplasm when these symptoms persist. Diagnostic tests to be considered in these cases include a pelvic exam and perhaps a CA-125 and pelvic ultrasound, particularly in a patient with persistent symptoms and a normal pelvic examination.

DIAGNOSTIC TESTS

The evaluation of a suspected pelvic mass is basically designed to determine whether or not the mass is likely to be malignant and who should therefore be the appropriate surgeon to perform the laparotomy when indicated (Fig. 24-1).

Basically all masses, whether solid or cystic, found in premenarchal children and adolescents and in all postmenopausal women should be considered abnormal and potentially malignant. Surgery is indicated in all of these patients. The only exception is when an ultrasound in a postmenopausal woman reveals a completely cystic mass, less than 5 cm in diameter with no septations, and the CA-125 is normal. When these criteria are met, the patient may be followed conservatively without laparotomy as the likelihood of malignancy is quite low. The tests should be repeated in 3 months to confirm that there is no change (30).

In the premenarchal female, all solid masses have the potential to be neoplastic. Germ cell tumors should be strongly considered in this age group. Tumor markers, including alpha-fetoprotein (aFP), human chronic gonadotropin (HCG), CA-125, and LDH, can help guide the surgeon to the most likely diagnosis. Alpha-fetoprotein is elevated in endodermal sinus tumors, HCG is elevated in choriocarcinoma and both are elevated in embryonal cell tumors. LDH and low levels of HCG are present in dysgerminomas. Children and young women with solid masses and elevated tumor markers should have their surgical procedures performed by a gynecologic oncologist or pediatric surgeon.

Pelvic masses found in women of reproductive and postmenopausal age must be evaluated preoperatively to determine the probability of malignancy. This is important to assure that the surgeon(s) who is to perform the laparotomy has the appropriate skills and training to complete the necessary procedures.

A pelvic mass in a woman of reproductive age may be a functional cyst, particularly if the mass is cystic, less than 6 to 8 cm in diameter, unilateral, and mobile. If all of these criteria are present, it is appropriate to re-examine the patient in 4 to 6 weeks. If the mass persists or has enlarged, then exploratory laparotomy is indicated.

A pelvic mass in the presence of ascites or with a markedly elevated CA-125 is likely to be cancer regardless of the age of the patient. Certainly a solid or partially cystic mass in a postmenopausal woman should be considered malignant until proven otherwise. Women who have a solid or partially cystic mass, ascites, and/or elevated CA-125 should be operated upon by a gynecologic oncologist or by surgical teams that

MANAGEMENT OF WOMEN WITH PELVIC MASS

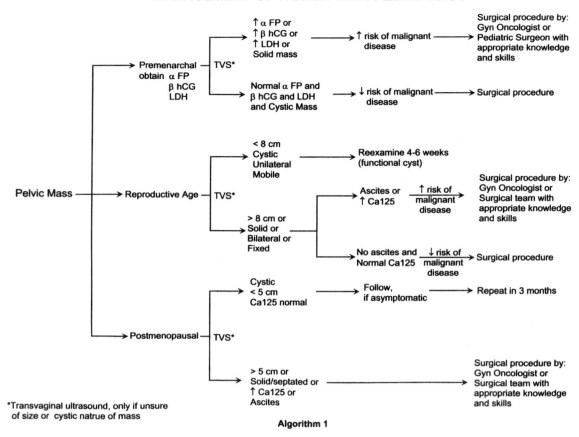

Algorithm 1

FIG. 24-1. Management of women with pelvic mass.

possess the necessary skills to appropriately surgically stage or debulk the disease and have a knowledge of the natural history of the disease and the appropriate surgical approach to be taken in each case.

It is important to note that in a 1988 patient care evaluation study from the Commission on Cancer, surgical procedures on 45% and 18.8% of ovarian cancer cases were performed by general obstetrician gynecologists and general surgeons respectively. In comparison with gynecologic oncologists, general surgeons and general obstetrician gynecologists do fewer biopsies of the peritoneum, diaphragm, bowel and lymphatic structures, all areas in which the same study revealed a high positivity rate (2). It has also been demonstrated that optimal debulking rates for gynecologic oncologists and gynecologists were 40–45% compared to 25% for general surgeons. This difference in optimal debulking rates also translated into a significantly reduced survival for those women operated upon by the general surgeons (31). It is therefore incumbent upon all general surgeons and general obstetrician gynecologists to understand the need for appropriate surgical staging and debulking surgery when caring for women with ovarian cancer. The appropriate operative procedures for

early and advanced stage ovarian cancer will be discussed in the next sections.

STAGING

Ovarian cancer is a surgically staged disease. Almost all ovarian cancers are approached operatively unless there is a significant medical contraindication to the procedure. The staging schema is shown in Table 24-1. It should be noted that since 1988, stage III disease has been subdivided into three substages based upon the greatest dimension of upper abdominal disease prior to cytoreductive surgery. This information should be recorded in the operative report. It is essential that the appropriate staging procedures be performed, particularly in those women with early-stage disease.

SURGICAL TREATMENT

The initial approach to the treatment of ovarian cancer is almost always surgical. The purpose of surgery is to establish or confirm the suspected diagnosis; to surgically stage the patient in apparent early stage disease; and in the event of advanced

TABLE 24–1. *International Federation of Gynecology and Obstetrics (FIGO) American Joint Committee on Cancer (AJCC) staging for ovarian carcinoma[a]*

TNM	FIGO	
T1	**Stage I**	Tumor limited to the ovaries (one or both)
T1a	Stage IA	Tumor limited to one ovary; capsule intact, no tumor on ovarian surface. No malignant cells in ascites or peritoneal washings[b]
T1b	Stage IB	Tumor limited to both ovaries; capsules intact, no tumor on the ovarian surface. No malignant cells in ascites or peritoneal washings[b]
T1c	Stage IC	Tumor limited to one or both ovaries with any of the following: capsule ruptured, tumor on ovarian surface, malignant cells in ascites or peritoneal washings
T2	**Stage II**	Tumor involves one or both ovaries with pelvic extension.
T2a	Stage IIA	Extension and/or implants on uterus and/or tube(s). No malignant cells in ascites or peritoneal washings
T2b	Stage IIB	Extension to other pelvic tissues. No malignant cells in ascites or peritoneal washings
T2c	Stage IIC	Pelvic extension (2a or 2b) with malignant cells in ascites or peritoneal washings
T3 and/or N1	**Stage III**	Tumor involves one or both ovaries with microscopically confirmed peritoneal metastasis outside the pelvis and/or regional lymph node metastasis
T3a	Stage IIIA	Microscopic peritoneal metastasis beyond pelvis
T3b	Stage IIIB	Macroscopic peritoneal metastasis beyond pelvis 2 cm or less in greatest dimension
T3c and/or N1	Stage IIIC	Peritoneal metastasis beyond pelvis more than 2 cm in greatest dimension and/or regional lymph node metastasis
M1	**Stage IV**	Distant metastasis (excludes peritoneal metastasis)

[a] Staging of ovarian carcinoma is based on findings at clinical examination and by surgical exploration. The histologic findings are to be considered in the staging, as are the cytologic findings as far as effusions are concerned. It is desirable that a biopsy be taken from suspicious areas outside of the pelvis.

[b] The presence of nonmalignant ascites is not classified. The presence of ascites does not affect staging unless malignant cells are present. Note: Liver capsule metastases are T3/Stage III; liver perenchymal metastasis, M1/Stage IV. Pleural effusion must have positive cytology for M1/Stage IV.

stage disease, to remove as much disease as possible—i.e., debulk or cytoreduce the tumor.

Early-Stage Disease

It is of paramount importance to properly stage women who are found to have malignant ovarian neoplasms visibly confined to one or both ovaries or to the pelvis only. Prognosis is established and therapeutic decisions, to be discussed later, are made on the basis of the information obtained by this procedure. A thorough inspection and surgical evaluation of the upper abdomen and pelvis is necessary. An organized approach to the laparotomy is shown in Table 24-2 and discussed below.

Any ascitic fluid should be removed and sent for cytology. In the absence of obvious ascites, peritoneal washings should be obtained from the right and left paracolic gutters, the pelvis and the subdiaphragmatic areas.

The primary mass should be removed and sent for frozen section, if necessary, to establish the diagnosis. If fertility is not an issue, total abdominal hysterectomy and bilateral salpingoooophorectomy should be performed. Any masses or implants in the pelvis should be removed. In the absence of any mass in this area, biopsies of the right and left pelvic peritoneum, cul-de-sac, and bladder peritoneum should be obtained. When disease is confined to the ovary(ies) or the pelvis, it is necessary to biopsy pelvic and para-aortic nodes in order to complete the surgical staging and to guide post surgical treatment recommendations. The procedure for removal of pelvic and para-aortic nodes adopted by the Gynecologic Oncology Group (GOG) is as follows:

A. Pelvic Node Sampling
  1. Identify the bifurcation of the common iliac, external iliac, hypogastric arteries and veins and the ureter.
  2. Any enlarged or suspicious nodes are excised or biopsied if unresectable.
  3. Nodal tissue from the distal one-half of each common iliac artery should be removed.
  4. The nodal tissue from the anterior and medial aspect of the proximal one-half of the external iliac artery and vein is excised.
  5. The distal one-half of the obturator fat pad anterior to the obturator nerve is excised.
  6. Ligation of the proximal and distal attachments of the nodal tissue is recommended.
B. Aortic Node Sampling
  1. The bifurcation of the aorta, the inferior vena cava, the ovarian vessels, the inferior mesenteric artery, the ureters and duodenum should be identified.
  2. Any enlarged or suspicious nodes are excised or biopsied if unresectable.
  3. The nodal tissue over the distal vena cava from the level of the inferior mesenteric artery to the mid right common iliac artery is removed.
  4. The nodal tissue between the aorta and the left ureter from the inferior mesenteric artery to the left mid common iliac artery is removed.

TABLE 24–2. *Surgical staging procedure for apparent early stage disease*

Remove primary tumor intact, send for frozen section if necessary. If apparently confined to ovaries or pelvis:
1. Thoroughly inspect pelvis and upper abdomen.
2. Submit any free fluid for cytology.
3. If no free fluid, peritoneal washings should be obtained.
4. Biopsy any adhesions or suspicious areas. If none, biopsy multiple areas of the peritoneum.
5. Sample right diaphragm by biopsy or scraping sent for cytology.
6. Infracolic omentectomy.
7. Biopsy/remove pelvic and periaortic lymph nodes.

5. Ligation of the proximal and distal nodal tissue is recommended.
6. Dissection cephalad to the inferior mesenteric artery is restricted to those cases with palpably suspicious nodes above that level.

Any disease noted in the omentum should be removed and in the absence of gross disease an infracolic omentectomy should be performed. The right hemidiaphragm should be biopsied or a scraping made with a sterile tongue blade, fixed to a glass slide and sent to cytology.

Removal of a unilateral adnexa with preservation of the contralateral adnexa and uterus is appropriate in patients with apparent stage IA disease who desire maintenance of fertility. This conservative approach can be considered in women with epithelial cancers, borderline tumors, stromal tumors, and malignant germ cell tumors confined to one ovary (Fig. 24-2).

Surgical staging that includes all of the above steps is absolutely essential in the care of women with early-stage disease. Otherwise, consideration will have to be given to re-exploration with the appropriate evaluation before definitive adjunctive therapy or no treatment decisions can be safely made (Fig. 24-3).

Laparoscopy has been proposed and utilized as an alternative to open laparotomy even in the management of masses suspicious for malignancy. Childers and coworkers performed laparoscopy on 138 patients with suspicious adnexal masses based upon a combination of elevated CA-125, abnormal ultrasound and/or mass greater than 10 cm in size. Malignancies were found in 19 patients and 14 (74%) were able to have surgery completed via the laparoscope (32). The laparoscopic approach does increase the chance of rupture of

SURGICAL PROCEDURE FOR OVARIAN CANCER

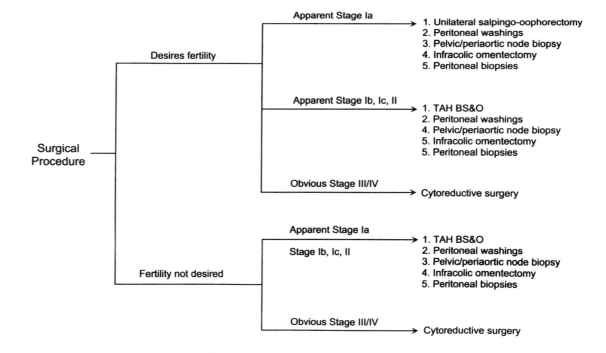

Algorithm 2

FIG. 24-2. Surgical procedure for ovarian cancer.

APPROACH TO DISEASE WHEN DIAGNOSED BY PREVIOUS SURGERY

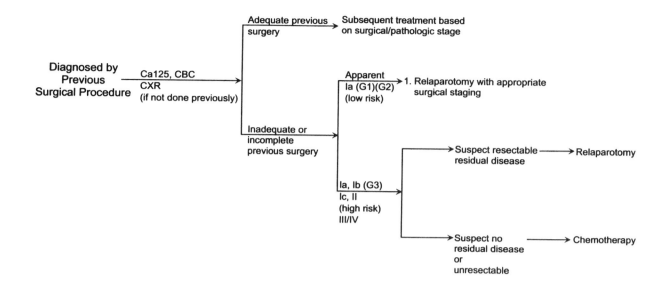

Algorithm 3

FIG. 24-3. Approach to disease when diagnosed for previous surgery.

the primary disease and should be performed only by those surgeons who are skilled in and knowledgeable about the open approach. More data is needed regarding the efficacy and safety of this approach before it is widely adopted.

Advanced Stage Disease

In contrast to early-stage disease, the goal of surgery in obviously advanced disease is primary cytoreduction. Because of the tendency of ovarian cancer to remain confined to the peritoneal cavity and not invade deeply or into the hollow organs, it is often amenable to surgical resection. The superficial nature of the disease allows itself to the removal of disease in many cases without resection of major organs.

There is little debate that patients whose largest residual disease is less than 2 to 3 cm in diameter have survival rates superior to those with larger volume disease. Multiple retrospective studies have demonstrated this difference. A summary of these studies demonstrated a median survival of 36.7 months in 388 patients who were optimally cytoreduced versus 16.6 months in 537 patients with large volume residual disease (33). Unfortunately, these studies do not prove beyond question that cytoreductive surgery that leads to small volume disease is the key element in improved survival. It may well be that the ability to adequately debulk, and subsequent survival, is more reflective of the biology of the disease. How-

ever, given the preponderance of retrospective evidence that cytoreductive surgery is beneficial, most gynecologic oncologists and others who treat this disease regularly believe in its value. Although a randomized, prospective clinical trial is the only way to definitively answer the question, this is unlikely to ever happen. Practical and ethical problems in the design and physician participation would likely be problematic.

Optimal cytoreduction has been defined variously and arbitrarily at 5 mm to 3 cm. It has been demonstrated by the GOG that survival for patients with advanced ovarian cancer progressively decreases as the maximum residual disease increases from microscopic to 2 cm (34) (Fig. 24-4). The GOG also found that the upper threshold at which no survival improvement takes place is 2 cm (34) (Fig. 24-5). Thus, less than or equal to 2 cm is accepted by most as the goal of cytoreduction. The removal of all tumor should, of course, be the surgeon's initial goal; however, if this is not technically feasible, then an attempt should be made to reduce residual disease to 2 cm or less. Bowel resections or other aggressive surgical procedures should not be attempted if the maximum residual of less than or equal to 2 cm is not possible with the resection.

The aggressiveness, patience and training of the surgeon determines the percentage of patients with advanced ovarian cancer who are optimally debulked. A summary of nine retrospective studies reveals that 42% of 925 patients were

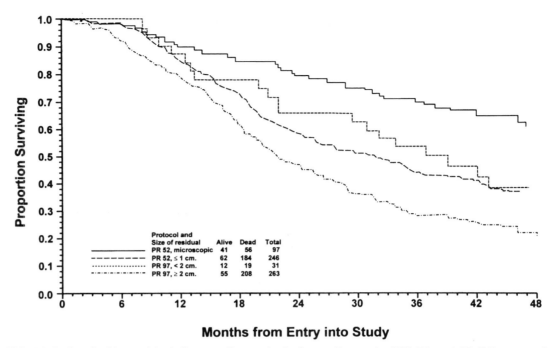

FIG. 24-4. Survival by residual disease, Gynecologic Group Protocols (PR) 52 and 97. PR, protocol. (Reprinted with permission from Hoskins WJ, McGuire WP, Brady MF, et al. The effect of diameter of largest residual disease on survival after primary cytoreductive surgery in patients with suboptimal residual epithelial ovarian carcinoma. *Am J Obstet Gynecol* 1994;170:974.)

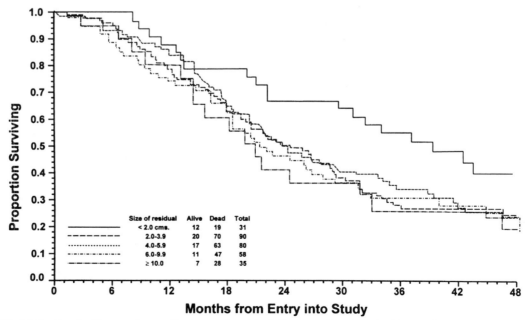

FIG. 24-5. Survival by maximum diameter of residual disease. (Reprinted with permission from Hoskins WJ, McGuire WP, Brady MF, et al. The effect of diameter of largest residual disease on survival after primary cytoreductive surgery in patients with suboptimal residual epithelial ovarina carcinoma. *Am J Obstet Gynecol* 1994;170:974.)

optimally cytoreduced (33); however, in the most contemporary of these series 87% of the patients were optimally cytoreduced (35).

Disease located in the pelvis can almost always be optimally resected. Many patients will require only a total abdominal hysterectomy and bilateral salpingooophorectomy to accomplish this goal. Others however, particularly those patients with a so-called socked in pelvis, will require radical pelvic surgery. This type of surgery includes a retroperitoneal approach and requires resection of pelvic peritoneum, cardinal ligaments, uterosacral ligaments, a portion of the sigmoid colon or rectum, and possibly partial resection of the lower urinary tract. This type of surgery has been described previously and has been called radical oophorectomy, modified posterior exenteration, and reverse hysterocolpsigmoidectomy (36,37).

Resection of a portion of sigmoid colon and/or rectum is the most frequent ancillary component to the total abdominal hysterectomy and bilateral salpingooophorectomy when resecting pelvic disease. With modern surgical stapling devices, most of these patients do not require a colostomy, and every consideration should be given to reanastomosis of the resected area (36,37). Pre-operative mechanical and antibiotic bowel preparation should be completed.

The value of cytoreduction of the pelvic and para-aortic nodes in ovarian cancer is not completely clear. At least two studies have demonstrated a survival advantage in those patients with advanced stage disease undergoing a lymphadenectomy (38,39). Another report, however, demonstrated no difference in survival in patients with stages III and IV disease with negative, microscopically positive, or macroscopically positive nodes (40).

Although a randomized clinical trial would be required to prove the benefit of nodal resection in advanced ovarian cancer, it is probably reasonable to perform a pelvic and para-aortic lymphadenectomy in patients in whom optimal intraperitoneal resection has been accomplished.

Areas that cannot be entirely cytoreduced from a technical standpoint include agglutination of the liver and diaphragm with disease, extensive liver parenchymal disease, positive nodes above the level of the renal vessels with involvement of the superior mesenteric artery, extensive disease in the lesser sac of the omentum, and involvement of the mesentery of the small bowel causing agglutination of the mesentery in the central abdomen.

It is important that the general surgeon understand the concept of debulking when it is technically feasible. As noted earlier, a patient care evaluation study from the Commission on Cancer suggests that general surgeons are less aggressive in this disease than they should be (31).

Secondary Cytoreductive Surgery

The value of secondary cytoreductive surgery—i.e., surgery following a course of chemotherapy—continues to be controversial, and a discussion of the pros and cons of this procedure is beyond the scope of this text. The GOG is currently conducting a randomized trial of interval secondary cytoreductive surgery following three courses of cisplatin and paclitaxel in patients with stage IIIC suboptimally resected disease. The results of this study should answer the question regarding the appropriateness of this surgical procedure.

Patients who are under consideration for secondary cytoreduction have a confirmed diagnosis of ovarian cancer and should therefore be referred to a gynecologic oncologist for any discussion regarding the appropriateness of this procedure and performance of the secondary cytoreductive surgery if indicated.

Second Look Surgery

The true second look operation is defined as a systematic surgical exploration in an asymptomatic patient who has completed a course of chemotherapy, has no clinical evidence of disease by physical examination and/or radiographic studies, and has a negative CA-125. The rationale for this surgical procedure is to accurately determine the disease status in order to select appropriate subsequent therapy or safely terminate first-line chemotherapy.

There is no evidence, however, that second look laparotomy is a therapeutic procedure. Retrospective studies comparing survival in patients who underwent a second look laparotomy compared to those who did not have the procedure failed to show a difference in survival (41).

Many gynecologic oncologists no longer consider a second look laparotomy part of the routine care of women with ovarian cancer. This is strengthened by the realization that current standard second-line therapies are largely ineffective. Thus, second look laparotomies are now confined to clinical trials evaluating innovative therapies and are not justified if only current standard salvage clinical management is anticipated.

POSTSURGICAL CHEMOTHERAPY

Early-Stage Disease

Patients with early-stage disease who have been appropriately surgically staged can be separated into two categories—favorable and unfavorable based on prognostic factors (Table 24-3). The GOG performed two randomized trials in these groups. The first group consisted of patients with surgical stage IA, IB, G1, G2 tumors—i.e., favorable prognosis. These patients were randomized to Melphalan versus no further treatment. Survival was excellent with no difference between the two groups (42). Thus, there is general agreement that observation is appropriate in the group of patients in whom comprehensive surgical evaluation detects no high-risk factors.

In the less favorable group, patients were randomized to either intraperitoneal radioactive phosphorous (p32) or Melphalan. Again, no difference in survival was demonstrated, but both arms had a survival rate 20% less than the favorable group (42). p32 was chosen as the superior arm and was subsequently compared to cisplatin and cyclophosphamide in patients with

TABLE 24–3. *Early stage ovarian cancer prognostic factors*

Favorable prognosis (low risk)
    Stage Ia and Ib
        Well differentiated (GI)
        Moderately well differentiated (GII)
Unfavorable prognosis (high risk)
    Stage II
    Stage I with any of the following characteristics
        Poorly differentiated (GIII)
        Malignant ascites
        Ruptured capsule
        Excrescences on surface of ovary

early-stage high-risk disease. Although this study has been closed, it is too early to make any conclusions. The GOG is currently evaluating three versus six courses of combination chemotherapy with paclitaxel and cisplatin in this group. Thus, the optimum therapy for this group of patients is still unclear (Fig. 24-6).

Chemotherapy for Germ Cell Tumors

It is also important for the general surgeon to know that all stage I germ cell tumors, with the exception of immature teratomas grade 1 and dysgerminomas require adjunctive chemotherapy with bleomycin, etoposide and platinol (43). The general surgeon must recognize that patients with stage I choriocarcinoma, endodermal sinus tumor, and embryonal cell carcinoma and mixed germ cell tumors all require adjunctive chemotherapy and must be referred to the appropriate specialist or subspecialist for this treatment. It is inappropriate for these patients to undergo observation only, even when surgically proven to be stage I.

Advanced Stage Disease

All patients with advanced stage ovarian cancer should receive postoperative chemotherapy irrespective of whether or not all disease is resected at surgery (Fig. 24-6). Paclitaxel and cisplatin were recently compared to cyclophosphamide and cisplatin in a randomized, prospective trial in patients with advanced stage, suboptimally resected disease. This trial showed a median survival advantage of 12 months for the paclitaxel and cisplatin group and this combination is now accepted as standard therapy (44). Carboplatin has been substituted for cisplatin based on two trials showing no difference in survival between patients receiving cisplatin and cyclophosphamide versus carboplatin and cyclophosphamide but less neurotoxicity, ototoxicity, nephrotoxicity, nausea and vomiting in the carboplatin arm (45,46). Thus, the standard regimen for first-line chemotherapy in advanced stage disease is currently carboplatin and paclitaxel.

FOLLOW-UP

Following completion of definitive treatment with either surgery alone or surgery and chemotherapy or radiation, the

POST-SURGICAL TREATMENT

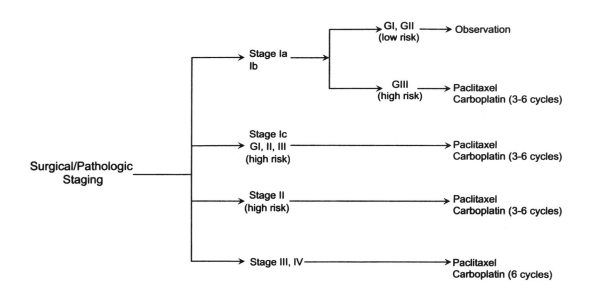

Algorithm 4

FIG. 24-6. Postsurgical treatment.

patient with no clinical evidence of disease should be followed with pelvic and abdominal examinations at 3- to 4-month intervals for the first few years and at 6-month intervals until 5 years from original diagnosis.

The value of expensive studies, such as MRI, CT scan, and ultrasound, in the asymptomatic patient is unclear and should not be advocated at this point. A CA-125 can be considered at each examination although there is considerable controversy regarding the appropriateness of second-line therapy for increasing CA-125s in the absence of clinical disease. A doubling of the CA-125 from the upper limits of normal confirmed by a further elevated sample, however, has been shown to be very specific in predicting ultimate clinical recurrence (47).

TREATMENT FOR RECURRENT DISEASE

Salvage or second-line chemotherapy for recurrent ovarian cancer is essentially palliative in nature as cures are rarely, if ever, obtained. It is therefore reasonable to withhold treatment until symptoms occur. Another alternative for the patient who has documented and measurable recurrent disease is investigational therapy. These patients should preferentially be placed on clinical trials when available.

The likelihood of response to second-line chemotherapy is heavily influenced by the patient's response to first-line therapy. Those patients with a complete clinical response to first-line chemotherapy and a long treatment-free interval are more likely to respond to second-line therapy.

A number of agents have demonstrated activity as secondary or salvage chemotherapy, including paclitaxel, carboplatin, cisplatin, ifosfamide, hexamethylmelamine, etoposide, tamoxifen, and topotecan (48).

Patients with recurrent or progressive carcinoma of the ovary will often develop signs and symptoms of intestinal obstruction, which may be relieved by major surgical intervention. The decision to surgically intervene is dependent upon a number of factors, including risk assessment and life expectancy. If the patient has begun to lose weight and has a poor performance status—i.e., a life expectancy of 2 months or less—a less invasive approach might be nasogastric suction or placement of a percutaneously introduced gastrostomy tube.

The surgeon should also be aware that abdominal carcinomatosis often present in ovarian cancer can lead to a paralytic ileus that can mimic an obstruction. Operative intervention in these cases is futile. If doubt exists regarding the presence of small bowel obstruction versus an ileus from carcinomatosis, a small bowel series to rule out obstruction is appropriate. It should be understood that surgery for intestinal obstruction in the face of recurrent or progressive ovarian carcinoma improves survival by only a few months, but does allow about 50% of patients to at least avoid prolonged hospitalization (49).

CONCLUSION

The general surgeon will be called upon to manage women with ovarian cancer. Although screening of the general population is not advocated at this time, women with a hereditary predisposition to development of the disease should be screened with pelvic examination, transvaginal ultrasound, and CA-125. The surgeon should be aware of those syndromes that increase the risk of ovarian cancer and other cancers traditionally cared for by the general surgeon. Prophylactic oophorectomy should also be considered in these women at completion of childbearing or after age 35.

At surgery for a suspected ovarian cancer or when an ovarian cancer is encountered unexpectedly, the general surgeon must be prepared to perform the appropriate surgical procedures. In apparent early-stage disease, thorough surgical staging is mandatory for subsequent treatment decisions. In advanced stage disease, an attempt should be made to surgically cytoreduce the tumor to a residual of less than 2 cm.

Most women with ovarian cancer will require postoperative chemotherapy and should be referred to the appropriate specialist or subspecialist for their care.

REFERENCES

1. American Cancer Society. *Cancer facts and figures 1997*. Atlanta: American Cancer Society, 1997.
2. Averette HE, Hoskins W, Nguyen HN, et al. National survey of ovarian carcinoma. I. A patient care evaluation study of the American College of Surgeons. *Cancer* 1993;71[Suppl]:1629.
3. Fiorica JV, Roberts WS. Screening for ovarian cancer. *Cancer Cont* 1996;3:120.
4. Greggi S, Genuardi M, Benedetti-Panici P, et al. Analysis of 138 consecutive ovarian cancer patients: incidence and characteristics of familial cases. *Gynecol Oncol* 1990;39:300.
5. Houlston RS, Collins A, Slack J, et al. Genetic epidemiology of ovarian cancer: segregation anaylsis. *Ann Hum Genet* 1991;55:291.
6. Piver MS, Baker TR, Jishi MF, et al. Familial ovarian cancer. A report of 658 families from the Gilda Radner Familial Ovarian Cancer Registry 1981–1991. *Cancer* 1993;71[Suppl]:582.
7. Lynch HT, Watson P, Bewtra C, et al. Hereditary ovarian cancer. Heterogeneity in age at diagnosis. *Cancer* 1991;67:1460.
8. Bewtra C, Watson P, Conway T, Read-Hippee C, Lynch HT. Hereditary ovarian cancer: a clinicopathological study. *Int J Gynecol Pathol* 1992;11:180.
9. Narod SA, Ford D, Devilee P, et al. An evaluation of genetic heterogeneity in 145 breast-ovarian cancer families. Breast Cancer Linkage Consortium. *Am J Hum Genet* 1995;56:254.
10. Wooster R, Neuhausen S, Mangion J, et al. Localization of a breast cancer susceptibility gene, *BRCA2*, to chromosome 13q12-13. *Science* 1994;265:2088.
11. Narod S, Ford D, Devilee P, et al. Genetic heterogeneity of breast-ovarian cancer revisited. Breast Cancer Linkage Consortium [Letter]. *Am J Hum Genet* 1995;57:957.
12. Anonymous. Epithelial ovarian cancer and combined oral contraceptives. The WHO collaborative study of neoplasia and steroid contraceptives. *Int J Epidemiol* 1989;18:538.
13. Hankinson SE, Hunter DJ, Colditz GA, et al. Tubal ligation, hysterectomy, and risk of ovarian cancer. *JAMA* 1993;270:2813.
14. Tobacman JK, Tucker MA, Kase R, Greene MH, Costa J, Fraumeni JF Jr. Intra-abdominal carcinomatosis after prophylactic oophorectomy in ovarian-cancer prone families. *Lancet* 1982;2:795.
15. Piver MS, Jishi MF, Tsukada Y, Nava G. Primary peritoneal carcinoma after prophylactic oophorectomy in women with a family history of ovarian cancer. A report of the Gilda Radner Familial Ovarian Cancer Registry. *Cancer* 1993;71:2751.
16. Easton DF, Bishop DT, Ford D, Crockford GP. Genetic linkage analysis in familial breast and ovarian cancer: results from 214 families. The Breast Cancer Linkage Consortium. *Am J Hum Genet* 1993;52:678.
17. American College of Obstetricians and Gynecologists. *Prophylactic bilateral oophorectomy to prevent epithelial ovarian cancer*. ACOG criteria set 2. Washington DC: ACOG, 1994.

18. MacFarlane C, Sturgis MC, Fetterman FC. Results of an experience in the control of cancer of the female pelvic organs: a report of a 15-year research. *Am J Obstet Gynecol* 1956;69:294.
19. Squatrito RC, Buller RE. Use of serum CA-125 for monitoring and prognosticating outcome in patients with epithelial ovarian cancer. *Fem Pat* 1994;19:14.
20. DePriest PD, van Nagell JR Jr, Gallion HH, et al. Ovarian cancer screening in symptomatic postmenopausal women. *Gynecol Oncol* 1993; 51:205.
21. Bourne TH, Campbell S, Reynolds KM, et al. Screening for early familial ovarian cancer with transvaginal ultrasonography and colour flow imaging. *BMJ* 1993;306:1025.
22. Karlan BY, Platt LD. The current status of ultrasound and color Doppler imaging in screening for ovarian cancer [Review]. *Gynecol Oncol* 1994;55:S28.
23. NIH Consensus conference. Ovarian cancer: screening, treatment, and follow-up. NIH Consensus Development Panel on Ovarian Cancer [Review]. *JAMA* 1995;273:491.
24. Kramer BS, Gohagan J, Prorok P, Smart C. A National Cancer Institute sponsored screening trial for prostatic, lung, colorectal, and ovarian cancers. *Cancer* 1993;71[Suppl]:589.
25. Menko FH, Wijnen JT, Khan PM, Vasen HF, Oosterwijk MH. Genetic counseling in hereditary nonpolyposis colorectal cancer. *Oncology* 1996;10:71.
26. Burke W, Petersen G, Lynch P, et al. Recommendations for follow-up care of individuals with an inherited predisposition to cancer. I. Hereditary nonpolyposis colon cancer. Cancer Genetics Studies Consortium [Review]. *JAMA* 1997;277:915.
27. Burke W, Daly M, Garber J, et al. Recommendations for follow-up care of individuals with an inherited predisposition to cancer. II. *BRCA1* and *BRCA2*. Cancer Genetics Studies Consortium [Review]. *JAMA* 1997; 277:997.
28. Flam F, Einhorn N, Sjovall K. Symptomatology of ovarian cancer. *Eur J Obstet Gynecol Reprod Biol* 1988;27:53.
29. Finn CB, Luesley DM, Buxton EJ, et al. Is stage I epithelial ovarian cancer overtreated both surgically and systemically? Results of a five-year cancer registry review. *Br J Obstet Gynecol* 1992;99:54.
30. Goldstein SR. Postmenopausal adnexal cysts: how clinical management has evolved [Review]. *Am J Obstet Gynecol* 1996;175:1498.
31. Nguyen HN, Averette HE, Hoskins W, Penalver M, Sevin B, Steren A. National survey of ovarian carcinoma. Part V. The impact of physician's specialty on patients survival. *Cancer* 1993;72:3663.
32. Childers JM, Nasseri A, Surwit EA. Laparoscopic management of suspicious adnexal masses. *Am J Obstet Gynecol* 1996;175:1451.
33. Hoskins WJ. Epithelial ovarian carcinoma: principles of primary surgery [Review]. *Gynecol Oncol* 1994;55:S91.
34. Hoskins WJ, McGuire WP, Brady MF, et al. The effect of diameter of largest residual disease on survival after primary cytoreductive surgery in patients with suboptimal residual epithelial ovarian carcinoma. *Am J Obstet Gynecol* 1994;170:974.
35. Piver MS, Lele SB, Marchetti DL, Baker TR, Tsukada Y, Emrich LJ. The impact of aggressive debulking surgery and cisplatin-based chemotherapy on progression-free survival in stage III and IV ovarian carcinoma. *J Clin Oncol* 1988;6:983.
36. Eisenkop SM, Nalick RH, Teng NN. Modified posterior exenteration for ovarian cancer. *Obstet Gynecol* 1991;78:879.
37. Barnes W, Johnson J, Waggoner S, Barter J, Potkul R, Delgado G. Reverse hysterocolposigmoidectomy (RHCS) for resection of panpelvic tumors. *Gynecol Oncol* 1991;42:151.
38. Burghardt E, Pickel H, Lahousen M, Stettner H. Pelvic lymphadenectomy in operative treatment of ovarian cancer. *Am J Obstet Gynecol* 1986;155:315.
39. Kigawa J, Minagawa Y, Ishihara H, Kanamori Y, Itamochi H, Terakawa N. Evaluation of cytoreductive surgery with lymphadenectomy including para-aortic nodes for advanced ovarian cancer. *Eur J Surg Oncol* 1993;19:273.
40. Spirtos NM, Gross GM, Freddo JL, Ballon SC. Cytoreductive surgery in advanced epithelial cancer of the ovary: the impact of aortic and pelvic lymphadenectomy. *Obstet Gynecol* 1995;56:345.
41. Ozols RF, Rubin SC, Dembo AJ, et al. Epithelial ovarian cancer. In: Hoskins WJ, Perez CA, Young RC, eds. *Principles and practice of gynecologic oncology.* 3rd ed. Philadelphia: JB Lippincott Co, 1992:731.
42. Young RC, Walton LA, Ellenberg SS, et al. Adjuvant therapy in stage I and stage II epithelial ovarian cancer. *N Engl J Med* 1990;322:1021.
43. Young RC, Perez CA, Hoskins WJ. Cancer of the ovary. In: DeVita VT Jr, Hellman S, Rosenberg SA, eds. *Cancer: principles & practice of oncology.* 4th ed. Philadelphia: JB Lippincott Co, 1993:1226.
44. McGuire WP, Hoskins WJ, Brady MF, et al. Cyclophosphamide and cisplatin compared with paclitaxel and cisplatin in patients with stage III and stage IV ovarian cancer. *N Engl J Med* 1996;334:1.
45. Alberts DS, Green S, Hannigan EV, et al. Improved therapeutic index of carboplatin plus cyclophosphamide versus cisplatin plus cyclophosphamide: final report by the Southwest Oncology Group of a phase III randomized trial in stages III and IV ovarian cancer. *J Clin Oncol* 1992;10:706. [For erratum, see *J Clin Oncol* 1992;10:1505.]
46. Swenerton K, Jeffrey J, Stuart G, et al. Cisplatin-cyclophosphamide versus carboplatin-cyclophosphamide in advanced ovarian cancer: a randomized phase III study of the National Cancer Institute of Canada Clinical Trials Group. *J Clin Oncol* 1992;10:718.
47. Rustin GJ, Nelstrop AE, Tuxen MK, Lambert HE. Defining progression of ovarian carcinoma during follow-up according to CA-125; a North Thames group study. *Ann Oncol* 1996;7:361.
48. Thigpen JT, Vance RB, Khansur T. Second-line chemotherapy for recurrent carcinoma of the ovary [Review]. *Cancer* 1993;71[Suppl]:1559.
49. Robin SC, Hoskins WJ, Benjamin I, Lewis JL Jr. Palliative surgery for intestinal obstruction in advanced ovarian cancer. *Gynecol Oncol* 1989; 34:16.

CHAPTER 25

Soft Tissue Sarcomas

Peter W. T. Pisters and Raphael E. Pollock

Soft tissue sarcomas are a group of relatively rare, anatomically and histologically diverse malignant neoplasms. The majority of these tumors share a common embryologic origin, arising primarily from mesodermal tissues. Given that the skeleton and somatic soft tissues account for as much as 75% of total body mass, neoplasms of the soft tissues are remarkably rare, accounting for only 1% of adult malignancies and 15% of pediatric malignancies (1). In the United States, approximately 7,000 new cases of soft tissue sarcoma are diagnosed annually, and about 4,300 patients per year die of soft tissue sarcoma (1). Although the mortality rate approaches 50%, a substantial proportion of patients can be cured with careful selection of unimodality or multimodality treatment strategies.

This chapter focuses on the diagnosis and multimodality treatment of patients with primary sarcoma of the extremities. The management of locally recurrent and metastatic sarcoma is also briefly addressed. The anatomic and histologic diversity of these lesions precludes detailed discussion of all forms of soft tissue sarcoma. For further information, the reader is referred to existing detailed reviews of this disease (2,3).

ETIOLOGY AND EPIDEMIOLOGY

No specific etiologic agent is identified in the majority of patients with soft tissue sarcoma. There are, however, a number of recognized associations between environmental factors and the subsequent development of sarcoma. These include therapy with ionizing radiation (4,5); exposure to alkylating chemotherapeutic agents; occupational exposure to phenoxy acetic acids, chlorophenols, vinyl chloride, or arsenic; or exposure to the previously employed intravenous contrast agent Thorotrast. In addition, chronic lymphedema of congenital origin, infectious etiology (filariasis), or postsurgical or post-irradiation etiology has been implicated in the development of lymphangiosarcoma.

In clinical practice, the most commonly observed nongenetic predisposing factors are previous radiation and chronic lymphedema. By definition, radiation-induced sarcomas arise no sooner than 3 years after completion of therapeutic radiation and often decades later (4). The vast majority of these sarcomas are high grade (87%), and the predominant histology of radiation-induced sarcomas is osteosarcoma (4), possibly due to the greater absorption of radiation by bone than by soft tissue. Chronic lymphedema is seen as a contributing factor in the development in lymphangiosarcoma arising in the chronically lymphedematous arms of women treated for breast cancer with radical mastectomy (Stewart-Treves syndrome).

A number of genetic conditions are also associated with increased risk for development of soft tissue sarcoma. These conditions include neurofibromatosis, Li-Fraumeni syndrome, familial retinoblastoma, and Gardner's syndrome. Genetically related soft tissue sarcomas occur most commonly in patients with neurofibromatosis or Gardner's syndrome. Patients with neurofibromatosis have a 7% to 10% lifetime risk of developing a malignant neurofibrosarcoma or fibrosarcoma (6,7). Gardner's syndrome is characterized by colonic polyposis associated to a variable extent with extracolonic benign and malignant manifestations. Desmoid tumors occur in 8% to 12% of patients with the Gardner's variant of familial polyposis (8). The precise etiology of an individual sarcoma is of little clinical significance because it does not effect therapeutic decision-making beyond the obvious fact that patients who have sarcomas arising in a previously irradiated field usually cannot receive further external-beam radiotherapy.

PATHOLOGY OF SOFT TISSUE SARCOMAS

Anatomic Distribution

Soft tissue sarcomas have been found in virtually all anatomic sites. Approximately half of all soft tissue sarcomas occur in the extremities (lower, 38%; upper, 15%), where the most common histopathologies are liposarcoma (30%) and malignant fibrous histiocytoma (22%) (2). Retroperitoneal and intraabdominal sarcomas constitute 14% of all soft tissue sarcomas, with liposarcoma being the predominant histologic subtype (41%). Visceral sarcomas account for 13% and head and neck sarcomas for approximately 5% of all soft tissue sarcomas (2).

Classification

The most common classification scheme for soft tissue sarcoma is based on histogenesis. This classification system is reproducible for the better differentiated tumors. However, as the degree of histologic differentiation declines, the determination of cellular origin becomes increasingly difficult. In particular, despite advanced immunohistochemical techniques and electron microscopy, determining the cellular origin for many spindle cell and round cell soft tissue tumors is difficult and sometimes impossible. This leads to significant disparities in findings among pathologists. A discrepancy between the original histologic diagnosis and that of a subsequent expert reviewer has been noted in up to 25% of cases (9). However, in general, the specific histologic diagnosis is usually of secondary importance because, with the possible exceptions of leiomyosarcoma, fibrosarcoma, and malignant peripheral nerve tumors, histologic subtype is not directly related to biologic behavior.

One of the pathologic hallmarks of soft tissue sarcoma distinguishing it from carcinoma is sarcoma's tendency to spread by hematogenous means. Lymph node metastases are uncommon in sarcoma (10). Indeed, in one comprehensive study, nodal metastasis was noted at presentation in only 2.7% of more than 1,700 adult soft tissue sarcoma patients (10). The histologic types with the highest incidence of lymph node metastasis were epithelioid sarcoma (16.7%), embryonal rhabdomyosarcoma (13.6%), and angiosarcoma (13.5%) (10).

Histologic Grading

Biologic aggressiveness can be best predicted based on histologic grade. The spectrum of grades varies among specific histologic subtypes (Fig. 25-1). In careful comparative multivariate analyses, histologic grade is the most important prognostic factor in assessing the risk for distant metastasis and tumor-related mortality (11,12). Several grading systems have been proposed, but there is no consensus regarding the specific morphologic criteria that should be employed in the grading of soft tissue sarcomas.

Two of the most commonly employed grading systems are the U.S. National Cancer Institute (NCI) system developed by Costa et al. (13) and the FNCLCC system (*Federation Nationale des Centres de Lutte Contre le Cancer*) developed by the French Federation of Cancer Centers Sarcoma Group (14). The NCI system is based on the tumor's histologic type or subtype, location, and amount of tumor necrosis, but cellularity, nuclear pleomorphism and mitosis count are also to be considered in certain situations. The FNCLCC system employs a score generated by evaluation of three parameters: tumor differentiation, mitotic rate, and amount of tumor necrosis. The prognostic values of these two grading systems were retrospectively compared in a population of 410 adult patients with nonmetastatic soft tissue sarcoma (15). Univariate and multivariate analyses suggested that the FNCLCC system has a slightly better ability to predict distant metastasis development and tumor-related mortality. Significant discrepancies were observed in one third of cases. An increased number of grade

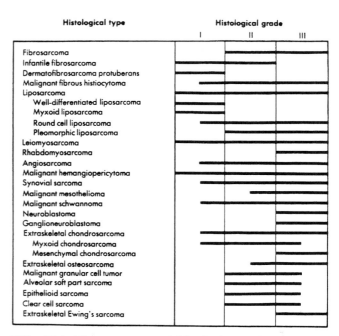

FIG. 25-1. The spectrum of histologic grades observed among histologic subtypes of soft tissue sarcoma. (Reprinted with permission from Enzinger FN, Weiss SW, eds. *Soft tissue tumors.* 3rd ed. St. Louis: Mosby, 1995.)

III tumors, reduced number of grade II tumors, and better correlation with overall and metastasis-free survival within subpopulations with discordant grades were observed in favor of the FNCLCC system (15).

CLINICAL PRESENTATION

The clinical presentation of patients with soft tissue sarcoma is highly variable. This reflects the anatomic heterogeneity of these lesions. The majority of patients with extremity sarcomas present with a painless soft tissue mass. Delay in diagnosis is common, with the most common misdiagnoses, including intramuscular hematoma ("pulled muscle"), sebaceous cyst, and benign lipoma. Symptoms are often not experienced until these tumors grow large enough to press directly on nearby neurovascular structures, causing pain, numbness, or swelling.

Patients with intraabdominal or retroperitoneal sarcomas commonly present with vague, nonspecific abdominal pain or a palpable abdominal mass. Retroperitoneal and intraabdominal tumors can also produce symptoms of nausea, vomiting, abdominal distention, or early satiety. Sarcomas arising from specific viscera may produce symptoms or signs related to the organ involved. For example, patients with a gastrointestinal or uterine leiomyosarcoma may present with symptoms related to gastrointestinal or uterine bleeding.

DIAGNOSTIC EVALUATION

Physical examination should include an assessment of the size and mobility of the mass. The relationship of the mass to the muscular fascia (superficial versus deep) and nearby neuro-vascular and bony structures should be noted. A site-specific neurovascular examination and assessment of regional lymph nodes should also be performed.

The diagnostic evaluation of patients with suspected soft tissue sarcoma involves appropriate biopsy and imaging of the primary tumor together with complete staging evaluation. The following comments focus primarily on patients with extremity sarcomas since the extremities are the site of the majority of soft tissue sarcomas. Important considerations in the evaluation and staging of retroperitoneal sarcomas are noted separately.

Biopsy of the primary tumor is essential for most patients presenting with primary soft tissue masses. In general, any soft tissue mass in an adult that is asymptomatic or enlarging, is larger than 5 cm, or persists beyond 4 to 6 weeks should be biopsied. The preferred biopsy approach is generally the least invasive technique required to allow a definitive histologic diagnosis and assessment of grade. In most centers, core-needle biopsy provides satisfactory tissue diagnosis (16). Superficial lesions can commonly be biopsied using direct palpation, but less accessible sarcomas often require an image-guided biopsy to safely sample the most heterogeneous component of the mass. In some centers, fine-needle aspiration (FNA) may be an acceptable biopsy technique provided that an experienced sarcoma cytopathologist is available. However, because of the frequent difficulty in accurately diagnosing these lesions even when adequate tissue is available, the major utility of FNA in most centers is in the diagnosis of suspected recurrent sarcoma.

Incisional or excisional biopsy is rarely required but may be performed when a definitive diagnosis cannot be achieved by less invasive means. Several technical points merit comment. Relatively small, superficial masses that can easily be removed should be biopsied by complete excision with microscopic assessment of surgical margins. Incisional and excisional biopsies should be performed with the incision oriented longitudinally (for extremity lesions) to facilitate subsequent wide local excision. The incision should be centered over the mass at its most superficial point. Care should be taken not to raise tissue flaps. Meticulous hemostasis should be ensured to prevent dissemination of tumor cells into adjacent tissue planes by hematoma. All excisional biopsy specimens should be sent fresh, sterile, and anatomically oriented for pathologic analysis. At definitive resection of a previously biopsied sarcoma, the previous surgical biopsy scar should be excised *en bloc* with the tumor.

Biopsy of radiographically resectable, presumed primary retroperitoneal (extravisceral) masses by either FNA or core-needle biopsy is not indicated. This is because the overall therapeutic plan is rarely altered by preoperative histologic diagnosis and the histologically heterogeneous nature of individual lesions precludes a plan of observation for biopsies that are read as benign or indeterminant. Preoperative image-directed biopsy is invasive, expensive, and rarely modifies treatment for patients in whom surgical exploration is planned. However, there are specific circumstances in which biopsy of primary retroperitoneal masses should be performed. These include

(a) clinical suspicion of lymphoma or germ cell tumor, (b) tissue diagnosis for preoperative treatment, (c) tissue diagnosis of radiographically unresectable disease, and (d) suspected retroperitoneal or intraabdominal metastasis from another primary tumor. In the main, however, for patients for whom exploratory laparotomy is planned, surgical resection is the best means of establishing a tissue diagnosis of a resectable retroperitoneal mass; intraoperative incisional biopsy is appropriate if the lesion proves to be unresectable.

Optimal imaging of the primary tumor is dependent on anatomic site. For extremity sarcomas, magnetic resonance imaging (MRI) has been regarded as the imaging modality of choice for soft tissue masses. This is because MRI enhances the contrast between tumor and muscle and between tumor and adjacent blood vessel (17), and provides multiplanar definition of the lesion. However, a recent study by the Radiation Diagnostic Oncology Group that compared MRI and computed tomography (CT) showed no specific advantage of MRI over CT (18). For pelvic lesions, the multiplanar capability of MRI may provide superior single-modality imaging. In the retroperitoneum and abdomen, CT usually provides satisfactory anatomic definition of the lesion. Occasionally, MRI with gradient sequence imaging can delineate the relationship of the tumor to midline vascular structures, particularly the inferior vena cava and aorta (Fig. 25-2). More invasive studies such as angiography or cavography are almost never required for evaluation of soft tissue sarcomas.

Cost-effective imaging to exclude the possibility of distant metastatic disease is dependent on the size, grade, and anatomic location of the primary tumor. In general, patients with low-grade and intermediate grade tumors or high-grade tumors smaller than 5 cm require only a chest x-ray for satisfactory evaluation for thoracic disease. This directly reflects the comparatively low risk for pulmonary metastases at presentation in these patients. In contrast, patients with high-grade tumors larger than 5 cm should undergo more thorough staging by chest CT. Patients with retroperitoneal and intraabdominal visceral sarcomas should undergo MRI or CT of the liver to exclude the possibility of synchronous hepatic metastases since the liver is a more common site of first metastasis for these lesions.

STAGING

The relative rarity of soft tissue sarcomas, the anatomic heterogeneity of these lesions, and the presence of more than 30 recognized histologic subtypes of variable grade have made it difficult to establish a functional system that can accurately stage all forms of this disease. Staging systems employed for soft tissue tumors include the International Union Against Cancer (UICC) system (19), the Musculoskeletal Tumor Society system (20), and the Memorial Sloan-Kettering Cancer Center (MSKCC) system (21). Of these, the recently revised UICC staging system is the most widely employed. This staging system is a modification of the American Joint Committee on Cancer (AJCC) system, which was first published in 1977, that incorporates histologic grade into the conventional TNM sys-

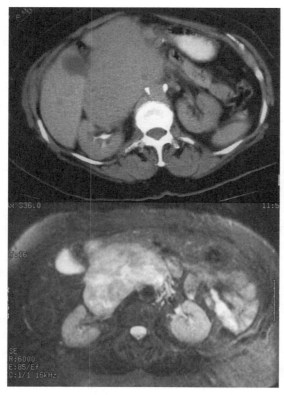

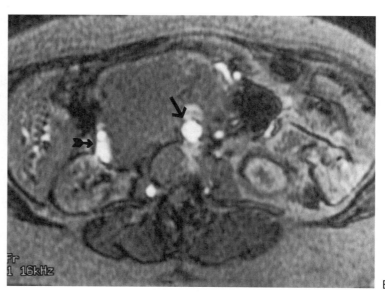

FIG. 25-2. A: A large midline right retroperitoneal sarcoma imaged by CT *(top panel)* and contrast-enhanced T2 MRI with fat suppression *(bottom panel)*. Note the improved contrast resolution of MRI. **B:** Gradient sequence MRI of a large retroperitoneal sarcoma occupying the interaortocaval groove. This technique enhances signal intensity from vascular structures and allows optimal imaging of the relationship between midline lesions and the large midline vessels. Note the almost angiographic appearance of the inferior vena cava *(left arrow)* and aorta *(right arrow)*.

tem (Table 25-1). Four distinct histopathologic grades are recognized, ranging from well-differentiated to undifferentiated. Histologic grade and tumor size are the primary determinants of clinical stage (Table 25-1). Tumor size is further substaged as a (superficial tumor arising outside the investing fascia) or b (a deep tumor that arises beneath the fascia or extends through the fascia). At this time, data validating this revised staging system have not been published. The original data used to validate the initial version of this staging system in 1977 are plotted by stage in Fig. 25-3.

A major limitation of the present staging systems is that they do not take into account the anatomic heterogeneity of these lesions. The present staging systems are optimally designed to stage patients with extremity tumors. Anatomic site, however, is an important determinant of outcome. Patients with retroperitoneal and visceral sarcomas have a worse overall prognosis than do patients with extremity tumors. Although site is not incorporated as a specific component of any present staging system, outcome data should be reported on a site-specific basis.

PROGNOSTIC FACTORS

The majority of published multivariate analyses of prognostic factors in extremity sarcoma have been small single-institution

reports with fewer than 300 patients per report. Three recently reported detailed analyses of prognostic factors in soft tissue sarcoma merit comment (11,12,22). The initial study of prognostic factors in extremity sarcoma from the MSKCC evaluated clinicopathologic prognostic factors in a series of 423 patients with extremity soft tissue sarcoma seen from 1968 to

TABLE 25–1. *UICC/AJCC staging system for extremity soft tissue sarcomas*

Stage	G	T	N	M
Stage IA	G1, 2	T1a, b	N0	M0
Stage IB	G1, 2	T2a	N0	M0
Stage IIA	G1, 2	T2b	N0	M0
Stage IIB	G3, 4	T1a, b	N0	M0
Stage IIC	G3, 4	T2a	N0	M0
Stage III	G3, 4	T2b	N0	M0
Stage IV	Any G	Any T	N1	M0
	Any G	Any T	Any N	M1

T1, ≤5cm; T1a, superficial to muscular fascia; T1b, deep to muscular fascia; T2, >5 cm; T2a, superficial to muscular fascia; T2b, deep to muscular fascia.

N1, regional nodal involvement.

G1, well differentiated; G2, moderately differentiated; G3, poorly differentiated; G4, undifferentiated.

Adapted from AJCC Cancer Staging Manual (19).

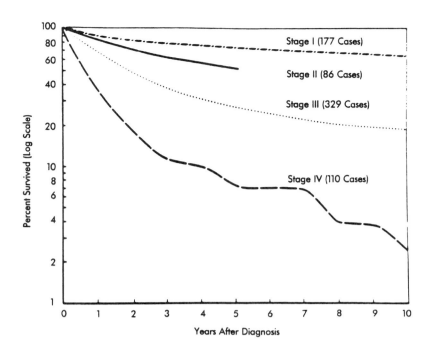

FIG. 25-3. Overall survival by AJCC stage. (Reprinted with permission from Russell O, et al. *Cancer* 1977;40:1562.)

1978 (22). This analysis, among the first to discriminate between among specific clinical end points, clearly established the clinical profile of what is now accepted as the high-risk patient with extremity soft tissue sarcoma: the patient with a large (more than 5 cm), high-grade, deep lesion. The adverse prognostic significance of a high tumor grade, deep tumor location, and tumor size of less than 5 cm were also noted in the recent report of the French Federation of Cancer Centers study of 546 patients with sarcomas of the extremities, head and neck, trunk wall, retroperitoneum, and pelvis (12).

A follow-up report from MSKCC evaluated clinicopathologic prognostic factors that had been documented prospectively in a population of 1,041 patients with extremity soft tissue sarcoma (11). The end points for the multivariate analyses were local recurrence, distant recurrence (metastasis), and disease-specific survival. Results of the regression analyses for each of these end points are summarized in Table 25-2. These results, using prospectively acquired data, confirm the observations made initially by Gaynor et al. (22). In addition, the previously unappreciated prognostic significance of specific histopathologic subtypes and the increased risk for adverse outcome associated with either a microscopically positive surgical margin or locally recurrent disease were noted.

TABLE 25–2. *Multivariate analysis of prognostic factors in patients with extremity soft tissue sarcoma*

Endpoint	Adverse prognostic factor	Relative risk
Local recurrence	Age >50 years	1.6
	Local recurrence at presentation	2.0
	Microscopically positive margin	1.8
	Fibrosarcoma	2.5
	Malignant peripheral nerve tumor	1.8
Distant recurrence	Size 5.0–9.9 cm	1.9
	Size ≥10.0 cm	1.5
	High grade	4.3
	Deep location	2.5
	Local recurrence at presentation	1.5
	Leiomyosarcoma	1.7
	Nonliposarcoma histology	1.6
Disease-specific survival	Size ≥10.0 cm	2.1
	Deep location	2.8
	Local recurrence at presentation	1.5
	Leiomyosarcoma	1.9
	Malignant peripheral nerve tumor	1.9
	Microscopically positive margin	1.7
	Lower extremity site	1.6

Adapted from Pisters et al. (11).

The adverse prognostic factors for local recurrence are different from those that predict distant metastasis and tumor-related mortality. Therefore, staging systems that are designed to stratify patients for risk of distant metastasis and tumor-related mortality using these prognostic factors will not stratify patients for risk of local recurrence. Conversely, patients with a constellation of adverse prognostic factors for local recurrence are not necessarily at increased risk for distant metastasis or tumor-related death. The results of these analyses should be incorporated in the design of new staging systems and clinical trials for soft tissue sarcoma, and the identification of individual patients at high risk for distant recurrence and death.

TREATMENT OF LOCALIZED PRIMARY SOFT TISSUE SARCOMA

A general stage-specific treatment algorithm for patients with primary sarcomas of the extremity and superficial trunk is outlined in Fig. 25-4. The data substantiating these treatment approaches are summarized below with specific emphasis on the findings from randomized prospective trials. The treatment of patients with retroperitoneal sarcomas is presented at the end of this chapter.

Surgery

Surgical resection remains the cornerstone of therapy for localized disease. Over the past 20 years, there has been a marked decline in the rate of amputation as the primary therapy for extremity soft tissue sarcoma. With application of multimodality treatment strategies, less than 10% of patients presently undergo amputation (23). The current use of limb-sparing multimodality treatment approaches for patients with extremity sarcoma is largely based on a remarkable randomized prospective study from the NCI in which patients with extremity sarcomas amenable to limb-sparing surgery were randomized to receive amputation or limb-sparing surgery with postoperative radiotherapy (24). Both arms of this trial included postoperative

chemotherapy with doxorubicin, cyclophosphamide, and methotrexate. With greater than 9 years of follow-up evaluation, five of 27 patients randomized to receive limb-sparing surgery and postoperative radiation with chemotherapy had local recurrences as compared to one of 17 patients in the amputation plus chemotherapy arm ($p = 0.22$) (25). The disease-free survival rate was 63% for limb-sparing surgery versus 71% for amputation ($p = 0.52$), and the overall survival rate was 70% for limb-sparing surgery versus 71% for amputation ($p = 0.97$). This study established that for patients for whom limb-sparing surgery is an option, a multimodality approach employing limb-sparing surgery combined with postoperative radiotherapy yields disease-related survival rates comparable to those for amputation while simultaneously preserving a functional extremity.

Currently, at least 85% of patients with localized extremity sarcomas can undergo limb-sparing procedures (26). Most surgeons consider definite major vascular, bony, or nerve involvement as relative indications for amputation. Complex *en bloc* bone, vascular, and nerve resections with interposition grafting can be undertaken, but the associated morbidity is high. Therefore, for a few patients with critical involvement of major bony or neurovascular structures, amputation remains the only surgical option but offers the prospect of prompt rehabilitation with excellent local control and survival comparable to limb-sparing approaches (26).

Satisfactory local resection involves resection of the primary tumor with a margin of normal tissue around the lesion. It is clear that dissection along the tumor pseudocapsule (enucleation) is associated with local recurrence rates ranging between 33% and 63% (27). Wide local excision with a margin of normal tissue around the lesion is associated with local recurrence rates in the range of 12% to 31% as noted in the control arms (surgery alone) of the randomized trials evaluating adjuvant radiotherapy (28,29). Unlike for malignant melanoma, a disease for which there are randomized data to address the size of an adequate margin, there are no comparable data available to define what constitutes a satisfactory gross resectional margin for a sarcoma.

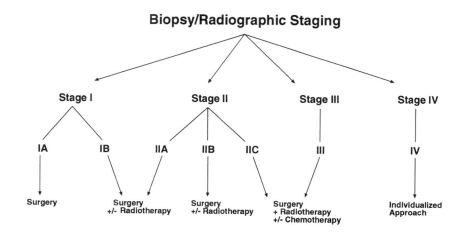

FIG. 25-4. Treatment algorithm for patients with extremity or superficial trunk sarcomas based on UICC clinical stage. For UICC/AJCC Stage System, see Table 25-1. Surgery, wide local resection with assessment of microscopic surgical margins; radiotherapy, pre- or postoperative (50 or 65 Gy, respectively) external-beam radiotherapy or brachytherapy (42 to 50 Gy) for suitable patients with G3/4 sarcomas; chemotherapy, doxorubicin and/or ifosfamide-based pre- or postoperative chemotherapy, optimally as part of the clinical trial. (Reprinted with permission from Pisters PW. Combined modality treatment of extremity soft tissue sarcomas. *Ann Surg Oncol* 1998;5:464–472.

Although the majority of patients with extremity soft tissue sarcoma should be treated with pre- or postoperative radiotherapy, recent reports suggest that concomitant radiotherapy may not be required for selected patients with completely resected, small soft tissue sarcomas (Table 25-3). Rydholm et al. (30) have reported their experience with 70 patients with subcutaneous or intramuscular extremity sarcomas. These patients were treated with wide surgical resection and microscopic assessment of surgical margins. Negative histologic margins were obtained for 32 of 40 subcutaneous and 24 of 30 intramuscular tumors. The 56 patients with microscopically negative margins received no postoperative radiotherapy, yet only four (7%) developed local recurrence. These favorable local recurrence rates in this select population are comparable to local recurrence rates observed with conventional multi-modality therapy incorporating pre- or postoperative radiotherapy (28,29,31). Similar findings have been reported from the Brigham and Women's Hospital in a series of 54 patients with small (less than 5 cm) soft tissue sarcomas (AJCC stage IA, IIA, or IIIA) treated with surgical resection without radiotherapy (32). Resection margins were microscopically clear for all but one patient. Only four (7%) of 54 patients developed subsequent local recurrence, and distant metastases were observed in four patients (7%) with intermediate grade or high-grade lesions. These data support the hypothesis that selected patients with small, primary soft tissue sarcomas can be treated with surgical resection alone without pre- or postoperative radiotherapy.

It is difficult to provide a precise estimation of what, if any, size restriction should be used to identify patients who can safely undergo surgery without radiotherapy. In the study by Rydholm and colleagues, the median tumor size of the deep lesions treated with wide surgical resection was 7 cm. Other studies, however, utilized a smaller tumor size as a criterion for surgery without radiotherapy (Table 25-3). The most conservative recommendation that can be made at this time would be to use 5 cm as an approximate size cutoff. Treatment of patients with large (more than 5 cm) primary lesions by surgery alone should not be done outside the confines of a clinical trial.

Pre- or Postoperative Radiotherapy

Radiotherapy has been combined with conservative (limb-sparing) surgery to optimize local control for patients with localized soft tissue sarcoma. Concomitant radiotherapy can be administered preoperatively, postoperatively, or by interstitial techniques (brachytherapy). The randomized data supporting combined-modality treatment are outlined below.

Data from two randomized prospective trials (28,29) have confirmed several retrospective reports suggesting that surgery combined with radiotherapy results in superior local control compared to surgery alone (31,33,34). Yang et al. (29) from the NCI recently reported a randomized prospective trial of postoperative external-beam radiotherapy. A total of 141 patients with localized extremity soft tissue sarcomas amenable to limb-sparing resection were randomized to receive adjuvant postoperative external-beam radiotherapy or no radiotherapy. All patients with high-grade lesions received postoperative chemotherapy. In the subset of 91 patients with high-grade lesions, there have been no local recurrences noted in the 44 patients who received postoperative radiotherapy (with chemotherapy) versus nine local recurrences in the 47 patients who received postoperative chemotherapy alone ($p = 0.0003$). In the 50 patients with low-grade sarcomas, one of 26 patients who received adjuvant radiotherapy has had a local recurrence versus eight of 24 patients treated by surgical resection alone ($p = 0.016$). However, there was no improvement in survival noted with adjuvant radiotherapy in the entire cohort of patients or in any subgroups.

The second randomized trial of postoperative radiotherapy was conducted at MSKCC, where investigators studied adjuvant brachytherapy for patients with extremity and superficial trunk soft tissue sarcomas (28). A total of 164 patients with extremity or superficial trunk soft tissue sarcomas were randomized following complete resection of their sarcomas to receive adjuvant brachytherapy (42 to 45 Gy with an iridium-192 implant) or no postoperative radiotherapy. Sixty-eight of 119 patients with high-grade tumors also received chemotherapy. With a median follow-up of 76 months, 5-year actuarial local control rates were significantly better in the group treated with adjuvant brachytherapy (82%) than in those who received surgery alone (69%). Subset analysis demonstrated that the local control advantage of brachytherapy was confined to patients with high-grade lesions, for whom the 5-year local control rate was 89% (versus 66% in the surgery-only group) (Fig. 25-5). Patients with low-grade soft tissue sarcomas did not appear to experience the same local control benefit with adjuvant brachytherapy (28). As noted in the NCI randomized trial, the improvement in local control did not translate into any detectable survival difference between the brachytherapy and control arms of the trial.

TABLE 25–3. *Results of surgery alone for selected patients with soft tissue sarcoma*

First author	Institution	No.	Selection criteria	No. adjuvant RT	Local recurrence (%)	Distant recurrence (%)
Geer	MSKCC	174	T1 size, primary tumor	117	10	5
Rydolm	Lund, Sweden	56	G/M margin negative	0	7	NR
Healey	BWH	54	T1 size, G/M margin negative	0	4	4

MSKCC, Memorial Sloan-Kettering Cancer Center; G/M, gross/microscopic; NR, not reported; BWH, Brigham and Women's Hospital. (Reprinted with permission from Pisters PW. Combined modality treatment of extremity soft tissue sarcomas. *Ann Surg Oncol* 1998;5:464–472.)

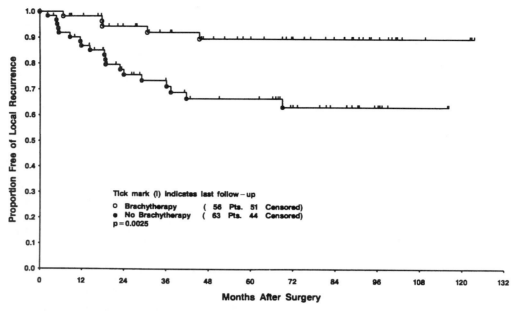

FIG. 25-5. Local recurrence-free survival in patients with high-grade sarcoma treated in the Memorial Sloan-Kettering Cancer Center randomized trial of postoperative brachytherapy versus surgery alone. There is a statistically significant improvement in local recurrence-free survival with brachytherapy (*p* = 0.0025.) (Reprinted with permission from Pisters PW, Harrison LB, Leung DH, Woodruff JM, Casper ES, Brennan MF. Long-term results of a prospective randomized trial of adjuvant brachytherapy in soft tissue sarcoma. *J Clin Oncol* 1996;14:859–868.)

Local failure rates with combined-modality regimens incorporating surgery and radiotherapy are generally less than 15% (Table 25-4). Despite theoretical advantages that may favor preoperative radiation, brachytherapy, or postoperative radiation, there does not appear to be a major difference in local control rates among these radiation techniques, although no presently available data directly compare the techniques. However, a phase III trial of preoperative external-beam radiotherapy compared to postoperative external-beam radiotherapy for patients with localized extremity soft tissue sarcoma is presently nearing completion under the direction of the National Cancer Institute of Canada Clinical Trials Group/Canadian Sarcoma Group (CSG). The results of this important study may provide insight into the comparative efficacy and

complication rates of these two options for external-beam radiotherapy.

In the absence of a clear local control advantage to any specific radiation technique, clinicians have considered other factors in formulating standards of care. Such factors have included wound complication rates, financial costs, and patient convenience. It is clear that while field size and radiation dose may be minimized with preoperative radiotherapy, major wound complications following preoperative radiotherapy and surgery have been reported to be in the 20% to 30% range (35,36). This fact alone has caused some groups to favor postoperative radiotherapy. On the other hand, with brachytherapy, the patient's entire local treatment (surgery plus radiation) can be completed within 10 to 14 days. This has significant cost ad-

TABLE 25–4. *Local control with surgery and radiotherapy for localized soft tissue sarcoma*

Radiotherapy approach	First author	Radiation dose (Gy)	Study design	*n*	Local failure (%)
Preoperative EBRT	Suit	50–56	Retrospective	89	17
	Barkley	50	Retrospective	110	10
	Brant	50.4	Retrospective	58	9
Brachytherapy	Pisters	42–45	Prospective (RCT)	119	9 (high grade)
				45	23 (low grade)
Postoperative EBRT	Lindberg	60–75	Retrospective	300	22
	Karakousis	45–60	Retrospective	53	14
	Suit	60–68	Retrospective	131	12
	Yang	45+18	Prospective (RCT)	91	0 (high grade)
				50	5 (low grade)

EBRT, external beam radiotherapy; RCT, randomized control trial. (Reprinted with permission from Pisters PW. Combined modality treatment of extremity soft tissue sarcomas. *Ann Surg Oncol* 1998;5:464–472.)

vantages (37) and also has significant implications in terms of overall patient convenience. In the absence of comparative data addressing the efficacy of these techniques in achieving local control, these additional considerations assume increased importance. Until data from the CSG phase III comparative study are available, it appears reasonable to treat most patients with postoperative external-beam radiotherapy since local control rates are comparable to preoperative techniques but major wound complication rates are significantly lower. Where the necessary expertise is available for brachytherapy, this technique provides an excellent, cost-effective alternative for patients with high-grade lesions. Brachytherapy should not be used for patients with low-grade sarcomas (28,38).

Postoperative Chemotherapy

The role of postoperative chemotherapy in the management of patients with localized soft tissue sarcoma remains controversial. Table 25-5 outlines 10 published randomized trials evaluating adjuvant chemotherapy in patients with extremity soft tissue sarcoma. Each of these trials had a control arm that received no adjuvant therapy and a treatment group that received postoperative systemic therapy with doxorubicin alone or doxorubicin-based combination therapy. Four of the trials reported significantly improved relapse-free survival, but only one of 10 trials found a statistically significant improvement in overall survival (Table 25-5).

All of the randomized trials of adjuvant chemotherapy published thus far contain recognized deficiencies in design and conduct. The most commonly cited deficiencies of these trials as a group relate to the relatively small sample size and to the fact that small differences in survival require relatively large numbers of patients to detect with sufficient statistical

power. The statistical tool of meta-analysis is designed to address these deficiencies by examining a group of similarly designed clinical trials. Recently, the Sarcoma Meta-Analysis Collaboration (SMAC) group reported on a comprehensive meta-analysis of the published randomized trials evaluating local therapy plus adjuvant doxorubicin-based chemotherapy versus local therapy alone (39). This meta-analysis demonstrated statistically significant improved local recurrence-free survival and disease-free survival rates in patients who received doxorubicin-containing postoperative chemotherapy (Table 25-6). However, there was no statistically significant improvement in overall survival rates in this meta-analysis of individual patient data. Since a significant improvement in survival with postoperative chemotherapy has not been detected with these advanced statistical techniques, it appears reasonable to conclude that if such a benefit exists, it must be quite small. Indeed, the meta-analysis suggests that if a survival benefit exists, it may be 5% or less (Table 25-6).

Recent investigations have focused on the possible benefits of newer agents in the postoperative treatment of localized soft tissue sarcomas. A recently reported randomized trial of five cycles of epirubicin (120 mg/m^2) and ifosfamide (9 g/m^2) following definitive local therapy versus local therapy alone showed a significant survival advantage in favor of the group receiving postoperative chemotherapy (40). This study was reported with a relatively short 21-month median follow-up and has been criticized for the unexplained comparatively poor outcome in the group treated with local therapy alone (median survival, 13 months). Indeed, comparison of the outcome of the control group in this study with the aggregate control group in the SMAC meta-analysis or the treatment groups in the existing randomized trials of adjuvant radiotherapy (i.e., other groups treated with local therapy alone) reveals significantly

TABLE 25–5. *Randomized trials of adjuvant doxorubicin-based chemotherapy versus observation in extremity soft tissue sarcoma*

Group	Regimen	Total no. patients	Median follow-up (months)	Disease-free survival (%) CTx	Disease-free survival (%) Obs	p	Overall survival (%) CTx	Overall survival (%) Obs	p
EORTC	ACVD	317	80	56	43	0.007	63	56	NS
MDACC	ACVAd	43	120	60	35	0.05	75	61	NS
NCI	ACM	67	85	75	54	0.037	83	60	NS
Mayo	AVDAd	48	64	88	67	NS	83	63	NS
UCLA	A	119	28	58	54	NS	84	80	NS
Scand	A	154	40	62	56	NS	75	70	NS
Rizzoli	A	76	120	56	27	<0.02	NR	NR	0.04
MGH/DFCI	A	26	46	90	71	NS	89	81	NS
ISTSS	A	41	20	77	50	NS	72	62	NS
ECOG	A	18	59	70	63	NS	61	63	NS

Studies of extremity lesions only and subset analyses of studies that included extremity lesions.
Ctx, chemotherapy; Obs, observation; NS, not significant; NR, not reported; EORTC, European Organization for Research and Treatment of Cancer; MDACC, M. D. Anderson Cancer Center; NCI, U.S. National Cancer Institute; Mayo, Mayo Clinic; UCLA, University of California at Los Angeles; Scand, Scandinavian Sarcoma Group; Rizzoli, Istituto Ortopedico Rizzoli; MGH/DFCI, Massachusetts General Hospital/Dana Farber Cancer Institute; ISTSS, Intergroup Sarcoma Study Group; ECOG, Eastern Cooperative Oncology Group; A, doxorubicin (Adriamycin); C, cyclophosphamide; V, vincristine, D, dacarbazine; Ad, dactinomycin; M, methotrexate.

TABLE 25–6. *Sarcoma metaanalysis collaboration group's metaanalysis of randomized doxorubicin-based postoperative chemotherapy in soft tissue sarcoma*

Endpoint	Hazard ratio	Absolute benefit	p
Local recurrence-free interval	0.74	6% (75% → 81%)	0.024
Distant recurrence-free interval	0.69	10% (60% → 70%)	0.0003
Overall recurrence-free interval	0.69	13% (45% → 58%)	0.000008
Overall recurrence-free survival	0.74	11% (40% → 51%)	0.00008
Overall survival	0.87	5% (50% → 55%)	0.087

Adapted from (39).

worse outcome for the patients treated with local therapy alone in this recent randomized trial. These preliminary observations are noteworthy, but longer follow-up and additional studies are needed. At this time, given the overall results of the SMAC meta-analysis and the preliminary nature of this recent positive trial of adjuvant epirubicin and ifosfamide, postoperative chemotherapy cannot be considered standard therapy for patients with localized soft tissue sarcoma. Potentially toxic postoperative chemotherapy should be optimally provided within the context of a clinical trial and should be reserved for selected patients who present with adverse prognostic factors for overall survival. These factors include large tumor size, deep tumor location, and high histologic grade (11,12,22).

Preoperative Chemotherapy

The theoretical advantages of preoperative chemotherapy in the treatment of soft tissue sarcomas are reviewed elsewhere (41). Investigators from the University of Texas M. D. Anderson Cancer Center (MDACC) have reported long-term results with doxorubicin-based preoperative chemotherapy for AJCC Stage IIIB extremity soft tissue sarcomas (41). In a series of 76 patients treated with doxorubicin-based preoperative chemotherapy, radiographic response rates were complete response (CR), 9%; partial response (PR), 19%; minor response, 13%; stable disease, 30%; and progression of disease, 30%. The overall objective major response rate (CR-PR) was 27%. At a median follow-up of 85 months, 5-year actuarial rates of local recurrence-free survival, distant metastasis-free survival, disease-free survival, and overall survival were 83%, 52%, 46%, and 59%, respectively. Comparison of responding patients (CR-PR) and nonresponding patients did not reveal any significant differences in event-free outcome (41).

In a prospective study from MSKCC, 29 patients with AJCC stage IIIB soft tissue sarcomas larger than 10 cm were treated with two cycles of a similar regimen prior to local therapy (42). Subjective changes in the degree of primary tumor firmness and in imaging characteristics of the tumor (intratumoral necrosis and hemorrhage) were observed in many patients but were not quantifiable. Only one patient met standard criteria for a partial response. Survival results in this population of high-risk patients were similar to those in historical controls treated with postoperative doxorubicin or patients treated with local therapy alone. The reasons for the apparent discrepancy in response rates between the reports from

MDACC and MSKCC are unknown but may include differences in patient populations, differences in chemotherapeutic drug dosing and number of cycles, and differences in the definition of major response.

Recently, ifosfamide-containing combinations have been used in the preoperative setting. Selected patients treated with aggressive doxorubicin- and ifosfamide-based regimens have had major responses, and preliminary results suggest that response rates may be higher than in historical controls treated with non–ifosfamide-containing regimens (43). A randomized trial of preoperative chemotherapy (50 mg/m² doxorubicin; 5 g/m² ifosfamide) versus local therapy alone has recently been completed by the European Organization for the Research and Treatment of Cancer Bone and Soft Tissue Sarcoma Group (EORTC protocol 62874). Toxicity results of this trial have been presented (44), but event-free outcome has not yet been formally reported.

Combined Preoperative Chemotherapy and Radiotherapy

With the advances made with combined-modality treatment of other solid tumors, there has been interest in combined-modality preoperative treatment (concurrent or sequential chemotherapy and radiation) for patients with localized soft tissue sarcomas. Concurrent doxorubicin-based chemoradiation has been employed extensively by investigators at the University of California, Los Angeles. This treatment protocol involved intraarterial doxorubicin with 35 Gy of external-beam radiotherapy delivered over 10 days or 17.5 Gy delivered over 5 days (45,46). A subsequent prospective randomized trial compared preoperative intraarterial doxorubicin to intravenous doxorubicin, both followed by 28 Gy of radiation delivered over 8 days followed by surgical resection (45). No differences in local recurrence or survival were noted.

Investigators from the Massachusetts General Hospital employed sequential chemoradiation in the treatment of patients with localized, high-grade, large (more than 8 cm) extremity soft tissue sarcomas. This treatment protocol involved alternating courses of chemotherapy and radiotherapy: three courses of doxorubicin, ifosfamide, mesna, and dacarbazine, and two 22-Gy courses of radiation (11 fractions each) for a total preoperative radiation dose of 44 Gy. This was followed by surgical resection with careful microscopic assessment of surgical margins. An additional 16-Gy (eight fractions) boost was delivered for microscopically positive surgical margins. The outcome of 26 patients treated with this regimen has been compared to that of matched historical controls, with a 13-month (range, 3 to 76 months) median follow-up (47). Five-year actuarial local control, disease-free survival, and overall survival rates for the sequential chemoradiation group are 100%, 84%, and 93%, respectively. For the matched historical controls, these rates are 97%, 45%, and 60%, respectively. These encouraging preliminary results will require longer follow-up and additional studies for confirmation. An ongoing Radiation Therapy Oncology Group protocol (RTOG-95-14) is further investigating this treatment approach.

Hyperthermic Isolated Limb Perfusion and Whole-Body Hyperthermia With Chemotherapy

Hyperthermic isolated limb perfusion (HILP) and whole-body hyperthermia with chemotherapy are two investigational techniques that have received considerable recent attention in the treatment of soft tissue sarcomas. HILP is an experimental technique that has been evaluated for treatment of extremity sarcomas in the setting of (a) locally advanced extremity soft tissue sarcomas amenable only to amputation and (b) locally advanced extremity lesions with synchronous pulmonary metastases where HILP is employed in an effort to preserve a functional extremity for the short survival anticipated in the setting of stage IV disease. A multicenter phase II trial has evaluated a series of 55 patients with radiographically unresectable extremity soft tissue sarcomas treated with HILP using high-dose tumor necrosis factor-a, interferon-g, and melphalan (48). A major tumor response was seen in 87% of patients: complete responses in 20 (36%) and partial responses in 28 (51%). Limb salvage was achieved in 84% of patients. Regional toxicity was limited, and systemic toxicity was minimal to moderate. There were no treatment-related deaths. This approach is presently being further evaluated in the United States in a multicenter study conducted through the NCI.

Whole-body hyperthermia combined with ifosfamide and carboplatin has also been evaluated for treatment-refractory small cell sarcomas (49). Hyperthermia is achieved with extracorporeal heating of blood. Other investigators have employed regional hyperthermia (accomplished with an external electromagnetic field, phased-array system) combined with ifosfamide and etoposide in the treatment of patients with locally advanced soft tissue sarcomas (50).

TREATMENT OF SARCOMA PATIENTS AT SPECIALTY CENTERS

Recent data on other tumor types have demonstrated improved outcome for patients requiring complex treatment who are treated at specialty centers (51). The most comprehensive data addressing this issue in soft tissue sarcoma come from Sweden, where Gustafson and colleagues analyzed the quality of treatment in a population-based series of 375 patients with primary soft tissue sarcomas arising in the ex-

tremities (n = 329) or the trunk (n = 46) (52). Comparison was made between patients referred to a specialty soft tissue tumor center prior to surgery (n = 195), those referred after surgery (n = 102), and those not referred for treatment of the primary tumor (n = 78). The total number of operations for the primary tumor was 1.4 times higher in patients not referred, and 1.7 times higher in patients referred after surgery than in patients referred prior to surgery. Of greatest significance, however, was the finding that the local recurrence rate was 2.4 times higher in patients not referred and 1.3 times higher in patients referred after surgery than in patients referred to a specialty soft tissue tumor center prior to any manipulation of their tumor. These findings support the principle of centralizing treatment of these rare tumors, which frequently require complex multimodality therapy.

TREATMENT OF LOCALLY RECURRENT SOFT TISSUE SARCOMA

Despite optimal multimodality therapy, local recurrence develops in a substantial number of patients. Not surprisingly, local recurrence rates are a function of the primary site and are highest for retroperitoneal and head and neck sarcomas. This is due to the fact that adequate surgical margins are technically more difficult to attain in these locations. In addition, employment of high dose pre- or postoperative radiotherapy is often limited in these sites by the relative radiosensitivity of surrounding structures. These factors result in local recurrence rates of 38% to 50% for retroperitoneal sarcomas (53), and 48% for head and neck sarcomas (54) as compared to less than 15% for extremity soft tissue sarcomas (28,29).

Treatment approaches for patients with locally recurrent soft tissue sarcoma need to be individualized based on local anatomic constraints and the limitations on present treatment options imposed by prior therapies. In general, all such patients should be evaluated for reresection of their local recurrence. The results of such salvage surgery are good, with two-thirds of patients experiencing long-term survival (55). For patients who have not had prior radiotherapy to the area of recurrence, optimal treatment of the local recurrence includes surgery and pre- or postoperative radiotherapy. In addition, it may be reasonable to consider pre- or postoperative chemotherapy for patients with locally recurrent high-grade tumors because of the adverse prognostic significance of local recurrence (11,12) and the fact that the SMAC meta-analysis of randomized postoperative chemotherapy trials (Table 25-6) suggests a specific local control advantage for patients receiving doxorubicin-based postoperative chemotherapy (39).

Few data have been published on the use of additional radiotherapy in patients who develop local recurrence in or at the margin of a previous external-beam radiation field. Nori and colleagues at MSKCC have pioneered the use of brachytherapy for treatment of patients with locally recurrent disease arising in a previously irradiated field (56). These authors have reported a very acceptable 69% local control and minimal toxicity in 40 patients treated with surgery and adjuvant brachytherapy in a previously irradiated field. An important limitation of reirradiation by brachytherapy, however, is its apparent ineffectiveness against low-grade sarcomas (28,38).

TREATMENT OF METASTATIC SOFT TISSUE SARCOMA

The most common site of metastasis from soft tissue sarcoma is the lung. Indeed, the lung is the only site of recurrence in approximately 20% of patients with extremity and trunk soft tissue sarcomas (57). Primary visceral and gastrointestinal sarcomas also commonly metastasize to the liver. Extrapulmonary metastases are uncommon forms of first metastasis and usually occur as a late manifestation of widely disseminated disease (58). Median survival from the time of development of metastatic disease is 8 to 12 months. Optimal treatment of patients with metastatic soft tissue sarcoma requires an understanding of the natural history of the disease and individualized selection of treatment options based on specific patient factors, disease factors, and limitations imposed by prior treatment.

Surgical Resection of Metastatic Disease

Carefully selected patients may benefit from surgical resection of metastatic sarcoma. Unfortunately, this treatment approach benefits only a small fraction of patients who develop pulmonary metastases. This is best illustrated by data from MSKCC, where a population of 716 patients with primary extremity sarcoma were followed for the subsequent development and treatment of pulmonary metastases (Fig. 25-6). Of the initial cohort of 716 patients, 148 patients (21%) developed subsequent pulmonary metastases. Isolated pulmonary metastases occurred in 135 (91%) of these 148 patients. Of the 135 patients with pulmonary-only metastases, 78 (58%) were considered to have operable disease and 65 (83%) of

those taken to thoracotomy were able to undergo complete resection of all their pulmonary metastatic disease. Median survival from the time of complete resection was 19 months, and the 3-year survival rate was 23%. All patients who did not undergo thoracotomy died within 3 years. For the entire cohort of 135 patients developing pulmonary-only metastases, the 3-year survival rate was only 11% (Fig. 25-6).

The rather disappointing overall treatment results for patients with metastatic disease underscore the importance of careful patient selection for resection of pulmonary metastases. The following criteria are generally agreed upon: (a) the primary tumor is controlled or is controllable; (b) there is no extrathoracic disease; (c) the patient is a medical candidate for thoracotomy and pulmonary resection; and (d) complete resection of all disease appears possible (59). With careful patient selection, the morbidity of thoracotomy can be limited to the subset of patients who are most likely to benefit from this aggressive treatment approach. Three-year survival rates following thoracotomy for pulmonary metastases range from 23% to 42% as outlined in Table 25-7.

Chemotherapy for Metastatic Soft Tissue Sarcoma

Systemic treatment of metastatic disease remains the only therapeutic option for the majority of patients with metastatic soft tissue sarcoma. Detailed review of the single-agent and combination chemotherapeutic approaches for advanced sarcoma is beyond the scope of this text but has been reviewed elsewhere (2,3).

The combination of cyclophosphamide, vincristine, doxorubicin, and dacarbazine (CyVADIC) has been considered the standard of care for well over a decade. Response rates in excess of 40% have been observed with this regimen. However, a randomized trial comparing CyVADIC to doxorubicin alone revealed no significant difference in response rates or survival (60). On the basis of these data, many investigators now consider single-agent doxorubicin to be the

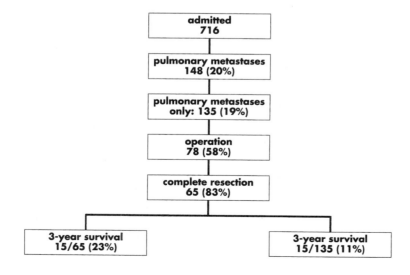

FIG. 25-6. Risk for and subsequent management of pulmonary metastases in 716 patients with primary or locally recurrent extremity soft tissue sarcoma. (Reprinted with permission from Brennan MF. The surgeon as a leader in cancer care: lessons learned from the study of soft tissue sarcoma. *J Am Coll Surg* 1996;182:520.)

TABLE 25–7. *Survival following complete resection of pulmonary metastases from soft tissue sarcoma in adults*

First author(s)/ institution (year)	Total	No. of patients Pulmonary metastases	Surgical treatment	Complete resection (%)	Median survival (months)	Three-year survival (%)
Creagan/Mayo (1979)	112	112	112	64 (57%)	18	29
Putnam/Roth/NCI (1984, 1985)	487	93	68	51 (75%)	23	32
Jablons/NCI (1989)	74	57	57	49 (86%)	27	35
Casson/MDACC (1992)	68	68	68	58 (85%)	25	42
Verazin/Roswell (1992)	78	78	78	61 (78%)	21	21.5 (5-year)
Gadd/MSKCC (1993)	716	135	78	65 (83%)	19	23
van Geel/EORTC (1996)	255	255	255	255 (100%)	NR	54

Mayo, Mayo Clinic; Roswell, Roswell Park Cancer Institute; NCI, U.S. National Cancer Institute; MDACC, M. D. Anderson Cancer Center; MSKCC, Memorial Sloan-Kettering Cancer Center; EORTC, European Organization for Research and Treatment of Cancer; NR, not reported.

present standard of care against which new combinations should be evaluated.

Ifosfamide, an analogue of cyclophosphamide, has been reported to produce significant response rates in the range of 30% to 40% in patients with advanced soft tissue sarcoma. Higher response rates have been reported with small cell sarcomas such as rhabdomyosarcoma and synovial sarcoma. The evaluable phase III trials with ifosfamide-containing treatment arms are summarized in Table 25-8. The most comprehensive comparative study performed to date was reported by the EORTC (60). In that study, 663 eligible patients were randomly assigned to receive doxorubicin (75 mg/m²) (arm A); CyVADIC (arm B); or ifosfamide (5 mg/m²) plus doxorubicin (50 mg/m²) (arm C). There was no statistically significant difference detected among the three study arms in terms of response rate (arm A, 23.3%; arm B, 24.4%; and arm C, 28.1%), remission duration, or overall survival (median 52 weeks for arm A, 51 weeks for arm B, and 55 weeks for arm C). The degree of myelosuppression was significantly greater for the combination of ifosfamide and doxorubicin than for the other two regimens. Cardiotoxicity was also more frequent in arm C. This study and others suggest that single-agent doxorubicin is still the standard against which more intensive or new drug treatment should be compared.

TREATMENT OF RETROPERITONEAL SARCOMAS

Surgical resection with negative margins remains the ideal standard primary treatment for patients with retroperitoneal sarcoma. Because *en bloc* multiorgan resection may be necessary to achieve negative margins, all patients should have preoperative bowel preparation and assessment of bilateral renal function by CT. Overall resectability rates in recent series combining patients with primary and recurrent retroperitoneal sarcomas range from 53% to 59%. For patients with primary retroperitoneal soft tissue sarcomas, grossly complete resection may be possible in 80% to 90% of patients. The most common reasons for unresectability are the presence of major vascular involvement (aorta or vena cava), peritoneal implants, or distant metastases (53). In many cases, resection of adjacent retroperitoneal or intraabdominal organs may be necessary to facilitate complete resection. Partial resections or debulking procedures have been performed, but there is no evidence that partial resection improves survival (53,61). In general, deliberate partial resection of retroperitoneal sarcomas should be reserved for relief of bowel obstruction or palliation of other critical manifestations of advanced disease. Results from recent series demonstrate 5-year

TABLE 25–8. *Randomized phase III trials with ifosfamide-containing treatment arms in advanced soft tissue sarcoma*

Group	Treatment arm (dose in mg/m²)	No. patients	Response rate (%)	Median survival (months)
SWOG/CALGB	A (60), D (1000)	170	17	12
	A (60), D (1000), I (7.5)	170	32[a]	13[a]
ECOG	A (80)	90	20	9
	A (60), I (7.5)	88	34[a]	12
	M (8), A (40), P(60)	84	32	10
EORTC[60]	A (75)	263	23	13
	A (50), I (5)	258	28	12.8
	Cy (500), V (1.5), A (50), D (750)	142	28	13.8

[a] p < 0.05.

SWOG, Southwest Oncology Group; CALGB, Cancer and Leukemia Study Group B; ECOG, Eastern Cooperative Oncology Group; EORTC, European Organization for Research and Treatment of Cancer; A, doxorubicin (Adriamycin); D, dacarbazine; I, ifosfamide; M, mitomycin C; P, cisplatin; Cy, cyclophosphamide; V, vincristine; response rate, complete response + partial response.

actuarial survival rates in the range of 54% to 64% for patients with completely resected retroperitoneal sarcomas. Recurrent disease remains a significant problem, with local and/or distant recurrences developing in the majority of patients (53% to 68%) (53,62).

Although postoperative radiotherapy has been shown to reduce local recurrence rates for extremity and superficial trunk sarcomas, gastrointestinal and neurological toxicities frequently limit the delivery of sufficient radiation doses to the retroperitoneum. Several retrospective reports have suggested that postoperative external-beam radiotherapy improves local control after surgical resection but there are no randomized trials addressing this question. A randomized trial from the NCI demonstrated that surgical resection with intraoperative (IORT) and subsequent postoperative external-beam radiotherapy resulted in improved local control versus treatment with resection and postoperative high dose external-beam radiotherapy (63). However, IORT was associated with significant neurotoxicity (47%). This technique remains investigational at this time and is generally limited to specialty centers because of the need for a dedicated operating room.

Retrospective studies have not demonstrated any benefit to preoperative or postoperative doxorubicin-based chemotherapy for retroperitoneal sarcomas. A small (15 patients) randomized trial from the NCI comparing postoperative doxorubicin, cyclophosphamide, and methotrexate to surgery alone revealed no advantage for the group receiving postoperative chemotherapy. Thus, at present, there are no data from randomized trials supporting pre- or postoperative chemotherapy as a standard treatment for retroperitoneal sarcomas. These patients should be encouraged to enter clinical trials investigating novel multimodality treatment strategies.

REFERENCES

1. Landis SH, Murray T, Bolden S, Wingo PA. Cancer statistics, 1998. *CA Cancer J Clin* 1998;48:6–29.
2. Pisters PWT, Brennan MF. Sarcomas of soft tissue. In: Abeloff M, Armitage J, Lichter A, Niederhuber J, edis. *Clinical oncology.* New York: Churchill Livingstone, 1995:1799.
3. Brennan MF, Casper ES, Harrison LB. Soft tissue sarcoma. In: DeVita VT Jr, Hellman S, Rosenberg SA, eds. *Cancer: principles and practice of oncology.* 5th ed. Philadelphia: JB Lippincott Co, 1996:1738.
4. Feigen M. Should cancer survivors fear radiation-induced sarcomas? *Sarcoma* 1997;1:5.
5. Brady MS, Gaynor JJ, Brennan MF. Radiation-associated sacoma of bone and soft tissue. *Arch Surg* 1992;127:1379.
6. Sorensen SA, Mulvihill JJ, Nielsen A. Long-term follow-up of von Recklinghausen neurofibromatosis. Survival and malignant neoplasms. *N Engl J Med* 1986;314:1010.
7. Zoller ME, Rembeck B, Oden A, Samuelsson M, Angervall L. Malignant and benign tumors in patients with neurofibromatosis type 1 in a defined Swedish population. *Cancer* 1997;79:2131.
8. Jones IT, Jagelman DG, Fazio VW, Lavery IC, Weakley FL, McGannon E. Desmoid tumors in familial polyposis coli. *Ann Surg* 1986;204:94.
9. Presant CA, Russell WO, Alexander RW, Fu YS. Soft-tissue and bone sarcoma histopathology peer review: the frequency of disagreement in diagnosis and the need for second pathology opinions. The Southeastern Cancer Study Group experience. *J Clin Oncol* 1986;4:1658.
10. Fong Y, Coit DG, Woodruff JM, Brennan MF. Lymph node metastasis from soft tissue sarcoma in adults. Analysis of data from a prospective database of 1772 sarcoma patients. *Ann Surg* 1993;217:72.
11. Pisters PW, Leung DH, Woodruff J, Shi W, Brennan MF. Analysis of prognostic factors in 1041 patients with localized soft tissue sarcomas of the extremities. *J Clin Oncol* 1996;14:1679.
12. Coindre JM, Terrier P, Bui NB, et al. Prognostic factors in adult patients with locally controlled soft tissue sarcoma: a study of 546 patients from the French Federation of Cancer Centers Sarcoma Group. *J Clin Oncol* 1996;14:869.
13. Costa J, Wesley RA, Glatstein E, Rosenberg SA. The grading of soft tissue sarcomas: results of a clinicohistopathologic correlation in a series of 163 cases. *Cancer* 1984;53:530.
14. Trojani M, Contesso G, Coindre JMR, et al. Soft-tissue sarcomas of adults: study of pathological prognostic variables and definition of a histopathological grading system. *Int J Cancer* 1984;33:37.
15. Guillou L, Coindre J, Bonichon F, et al. Comparative study of the National Cancer Institute and French Federation of Cancer Centers Sarcoma Group grading systems in a population of 410 adult patients with soft tissue sarcoma. *J Clin Oncol* 1997;15:350.
16. Ball AB, Fisher C, Pittam M, Watkins RM, Westbury G. Diagnosis of soft tissue tumours by Tru-Cut biopsy. *Br J Surg* 1990;77:756.
17. Chang AE, Matory YL, Dwyer AJ, et al. Magnetic resonance imaging versus computed tomography in the evaluation of soft tissue tumors of the extremities. *Ann Surg* 1987;205:340.
18. Panicek DM, Gatsonis C, Rosenthal DI, et al. CT and MR imaging in the local staging of primary malignant musculoskeletal neoplasms: report of the Radiology Diagnostic Oncology Group. *Radiology* 1997;202:237.
19. Soft tissue carcinoma. In: *American Joint Committee on Cancer*, 5th ed. Philadelphia: Lippincott-Raven, 1997:149.
20. Enneking WF. A system of staging musculoskeletal neoplasms. *Clin Orthop* 1986;9–24.
21. Hajdu SI. History and classification of soft tissue tumors. In: *Pathology of soft tissue tumors.* Philadelphia: Lea & Febiger, 1979:1.
22. Gaynor JJ, Tan CC, Casper ES, et al. Refinement of clinicopathologic staging for localized soft tissue sarcoma of the extremity: study of 423 adults. *J Clin Oncol* 1992;10:1317.
23. Brennan MF, Casper ES, Harrison LB, Shiu MH, Gaynor J, Hajdu SI. The role of multimodality therapy in soft-tissue sarcoma. *Ann Surg* 1991;214:328.
24. Rosenberg SA, Tepper J, Glatstein E, et al. The treatment of soft-tissue sarcomas of the extremities: prospective randomized evaluations of (1) limb-sparing surgery plus radiation therapy compared with amputation and (2) the role of adjuvant chemotherapy. *Ann Surg* 1982;196:305.
25. Yang JC, Rosenberg SA. Surgery for adult patients with soft tissue sarcomas. *Semin Oncol* 1989;16:289.
26. Williard WC, Collin C, Casper ES, Hajdu SI, Brennan MF. The changing role of amputation for soft tissue sarcoma of the extremity in adults. *Surg Gynecol Obstet* 1992;175:389.
27. Cantin J, McNeer GP, Chu FC, Booher RJ. The problem of local recurrence after treatment of soft tissue sarcoma. *Ann Surg* 1968;168:47.
28. Pisters PW, Harrison LB, Leung DH, Woodruff JM, Casper ES, Brennan MF. Long-term results of a prospective randomized trial of adjuvant brachytherapy in soft tissue sarcoma. *J Clin Oncol* 1996;14:859.
29. Yang JC, Chang AE, Baker AR, et al. A randomized prospective study of the benefit of adjuvant radiation therapy in the treatment of soft tissue sarcomas of the extremity. *J Clin Oncol* 1997;16:197.
30. Rydholm A, Gustafson P, Rooser B, et al. Limb-sparing surgery without radiotherapy based on anatomic location of soft tissue sarcoma. *J Clin Oncol* 1991;9:1757.
31. Suit HD, Mankin HJ, Wood WC, et al. Treatment of the patient with stage M0 soft tissue sarcoma. *J Clin Oncol* 1988;6:854.
32. Healey B, Corson J, Demetri G, Singer S. Surgery alone may be adequate treatment for select stage IA-IIIA soft tissue sarcomas [Abstract]. *Proc Am Soc Clin Oncol* 1995;4:517.
33. Lindberg RD, Martin RG, Romsdahl MM, Barkley HT Jr. Conservative surgery and postoperative radiotherapy in 300 adults with soft-tissue sarcomas. *Cancer* 1981;47:2391.
34. Barkley HT Jr, Martin RG, Romsdahl MM, Lindberg R, Zagars GK. Treatment of soft issue sarcomas by preoperative irradiation and conservative surgical resection. *Int J Radiat Oncol Biol Phys* 1988;14:693.
35. Bujko K, Suit HD, Springfield DS, Convery K. Wound healing after preoperative radiation for sarcoma of soft tissues. *Surg Gynecol Obstet* 1993;176:124.
36. Peat BG, Bell RS, Davis A, et al. Wound-healing complications after soft-tissue sarcoma surgery. *Plast Reconstr Surg* 1994;93:980.
37. Janjan NA, Yasko AW, Reece GP, et al. Comparison of charges related to radiotherapy for soft tissue sarcomas treated by preoperative external

beam irradiation versus interstitial implantation. *Ann Surg Oncol* 1994; 1:415.

38. Pisters PW, Harrison LB, Woodruff JM, Gaynor JJ, Brennan MF. A prospective randomized trial of adjuvant brachytherapy in the management of low-grade soft tissue sarcomas of the extremity and superficial trunk. *J Clin Oncol* 1994;12:1150.

39. Adjuvant chemotherapy for localised resectable soft-tissue sarcoma of adults: metaanalysis of individual data. Sarcoma Meta-analysis Collaboration. *Lancet* 1997;350:1647.

40. Frustaci S, Gherlinzoni F, De Paoli A, et al. Preliminary results of an adjuvant randomized trial on high-risk extremity soft tisssue sarcomas (STS). The interim analysis [Abstract]. *Proc Am Soc Clin Oncol* 1997; 16:1785.

41. Pisters PW, Patel SR, Varma DG, et al. Preoperative chemotherapy for stage IIIB extremity soft tissue sarcoma: long-term results from a single institution. *J Clin Oncol* 1997;15:3481.

42. Casper ES, Gaynor JJ, Harrison LB, Panicek DM, Hajdu SI, Brennan MF. Preoperative and postoperative adjuvant combination chemotherapy for adults with high-grade soft tissue sarcoma. *Cancer* 1994;73:1644.

43. Patel SR, Vadhan-Raj S, Papdopolous N, et al. High-dose ifosfamide in bone and soft tissue sarcomas: results of phase II and pilot studies—dose-response and schedule dependence. *J Clin Oncol* 1997;15:2378.

44. Gortzak E, Rouesse J, Verwey J, et al. Randomised phase II study of neoadjuvant chemotherapy in soft tissue sarcomas in adults. Protocol 62874 [Abstract]. *Eur J Cancer* 1993;29A[Suppl 6]:S183.

45. Eilber F, Giulano A, Huth JH, Mirra J, Rosen G, Morton D. Neoadjuvant chemotherapy, radiation, and limited surgery for high-grade soft tissue sarcoma of the extremity. In: Ryan JR, Baker LO, eds. *Recent concepts in sarcoma treatment*. Boston: Kluwer Academic, 1988:115.

46. Eilber FR, Giulano AE, Huth JF, Morton DL. Postoperative adjuvant chemotherapy (Adriamycin) in high-grade extremity soft tissue sarcoma: a randomized prospective trial. In: Salmon SE, ed. *Adjuvant therapy of cancer V*. 5th ed. Orlando: Grune & Stratton, 1987:719.

47. Spiro IJ, Suit H, Gebhardt M, Springfield D, et al. Neoadjuvant chemotherapy and radiotherapy for large soft tissue sarcomas [abstract]. *Proc Am Soc Clin Oncol* 1996;15:524.

48. Eggermont AM, Shraffordt Koops H, Lienard D, et al. Isolated limb perfusion with high-dose tumor necrosis factor—in combination with interferon-v and melphalan for nonresectable extremity soft tissue sarcomas: a multicenter trial. *J Clin Oncol* 1996;14:2653.

49. Wiedemann GJ, d'Oleire F, Knop E, et al. Ifosfamide and carboplatin combined with 41.8 degrees c whole-body hyperthermia in patients with refractory sarcoma and malignant teratoma. *Cancer Res* 1994; 54:5346.

50. Issels RD, Prenninger SW, Nagele A, et al. Ifosfamide plus etoposide combined with regional hyperthermia in patients with locally advanced sarcomas: a phase II study. *J Clin Oncol* 1990;8:1818.

51. Lieberman MD, Kilburn H, Lindsey M, Brennan MF. Relation of perioperative deaths to hospital volume among patients undergoing pancreatic resection for malignancy. *Ann Surg* 1995;222:638.

52. Gustafson P, Dreinhofer KE, Rydholm A. Soft tissue sarcoma should be treated at a tumor center. A comparison of quality of surgery in 375 patients. *Acta Orthop Scand* 1994;65:47.

53. Jaques DP, Coit DG, Hajdu SI, Brennan MF. Management of primary and recurrent soft-tissue sarcoma of the retroperitoneum. *Ann Surg* 1990;212:51.

54. Kraus DH, Dubner S, Harrison LB, et al. Prognostic factors for recurrence and survival in head and neck soft tissue sarcomas. *Cancer* 1994;74:697.

55. Singer S, Antman K, Corson JM, Eberlein TJ. Long-term salvageability for patients with locally recurrent soft-tissue sarcomas. *Arch Surg* 1992;127:548.

56. Nori D, Schupak K, Shiu MH, Brennan MF, Schupak K. Role of brachytherapy in recurrent extremity sarcoma in patients treated with prior surgery and irradiation. *Int J Radiat Oncol Biol Phys* 1991;20:1229. [For erratum, see *Int J Radiat Oncol Biol Phys* 1991;21:1683.]

57. Brennan MF. The surgeon as a leader in cancer care: lessons learned from the study of soft tissue sarcoma. *J Am Coll Surg* 1996;182:520.

58. Potter DA, Glenn J, Kinsella T, et al. Patterns of recurrence in patients with high-grade soft-tissue sarcomas. *J Clin Oncol* 1985;3:353.

59. McCormack P. Surgical resection of pulmonary metastases. *Semin Surg Oncol* 1990;6:297.

60. Santoro A, Tursz T, Mouridsen H, et al. Doxorubicin versus CYVADIC versus doxorubicin plus ifosfamide in first-line treatment of advanced soft tissue sarcomas: a randomized study of the European Organization for Research and Treatment of Cancer Soft Tissue and Bone Sarcoma Group. *J Clin Oncol* 1995;13:1537.

61. Pisters PW, Brennan MF. Retroperitoneal tumours. In: Taylor I, Cooke TG, Guillou P, eds. *Essential general surgical oncology*. 1st ed. London: Churchill Livingstone, 1996:361.

62. Dalton RR, Donohue JH, Mucha P Jr, van Heerden JA, Reiman HM, Chen SP. Management of retroperitoneal sarcomas. *Surgery* 1989;106:725.

63. Sindelar WF, Kinsella TJ, Chen PW, et al. Intraoperative radiotherapy in retroperitoneal sarcomas. Final results of a prospective, randomized, clinical trial. *Arch Surg* 1993;128:402.

Subject Index

Page numbers followed by *f* indicates figure; page numbers followed by *t* indicates table.

for colon carcinoma, 46, 47t, 51–53, 53t
(*See also under* Colon cancer)
cost in, 44–45
cost-effective analysis in, 44
decision analysis and, 45
decision matrix in, 45–46, 46f
managed care and, 43–44
outcome analysis and, 45
Costoclavicular scissors phenomenon,
60–61, 61f
Cowden's disease genes, 4t, 6
Cryosurgery, for hepatocellular carcinoma,
217
Cuffs, catheter, 55
Cystadenocarcinoma
mucinous, of appendix, 259–260, 260f,
261f
of pancreas, 196, 196f

D

DCC gene, 227–228
DCH (delayed cutaneous hypersensitivity),
34
DCIS (ductal carcinoma *in situ*)
diagnosis of, 279
treatment of, 280–282
DDS (Denys-Drash syndrome), 15
Decision analysis, 45
Decision matrix, 45–46
Delayed cutaneous hypersensitivity
(DCH), 34
Denys-Drash syndrome (DDS), 15
Dermatofibrosarcoma protuberans (DFSP),
131–132
Disease outcome, 45
Distal purse string closure, 76
Ductal carcinoma *in situ* (DCIS)
diagnosis of, 279
treatment of, 280–282
Duodenal tumors, 196–197
Dysplastic nevus syndrome, 13–14

E

Early postoperative bowel obstruction
(EPOBO), 79
Elective lymph node dissection (ELND),
146–148
EMP (extramammary Paget's disease),
125–126, 125f
Endocrine cancers. *See also* Neuroendocrine tumors; specific cancers
genes for, 4t, 9–12
Endoscopic retrograde cholangiopancreatography (ERCP), 199, 199f
Endoscopic ultrasound, 19–23, 20f–22f,
20t, 23t
Enteral feeding. *See also* Nutrition
gastrointestinal complications of, 36, 36t
mechanical complications of, 36, 37t

metabolic complications of, 36, 37t
preoperative, 34–35
Enterochromaffin cells, 265
Epidermoid cancer of the anal canal,
245–251, 245f–248f, 249t. *See
also under* Anal neoplasms
EPOBO (early postoperative bowel obstruction), 79
ERCP (endoscopic retrograde cholangiopancreatography), 199, 199f
Errant-dilator phenomenon, 63–64, 63f
Esophageal cancer, 155–171
cell types in, 156–157
clinical manifestations of, 158–159,
159t
diagnosis of, 159–160, 159f
environmental factors in, 156
genetic and family factors in, 155–156
incidence of, 155
laparoscopy and preoperative staging of,
24–25, 25f
macroscopic appearance of, 157
pathology of, 156–158
preexisting esophageal diseases in, 156
spread of, 157–158, 158f, 158t, 159t
staging of
pathologic, 162, 162t
preoperative, 160–162, 160f, 161f
treatment of, 163–171, 163f
chemoradiotherapy in, 168–169
chemotherapy in, 168
neoadjuvant (induction) therapy in,
169
palliative measures in, 169–171
radiation therapy in, 168
surgical resection in, 163–168
en-bloc esophagectomy in, 165
lymphadenectomy in, 165–166,
166t
operative morbidity and mortality
in, 167–168
reconstruction in, 166–167, 167f
transhiatal esophagectomy in,
164–165
transthoracic esophagectomy in,
163–164
tumor location in, 157
Esophagectomy
en-bloc, 165
transhiatal, 164–165
transthoracic, 163–164
Ethanol injection, for hepatocellular carcinoma, 217
Extramammary Paget's disease (EMP),
125–126, 125f

F

Facial nerve, 90
False-negative (FN) ratio, 45
Familial adenomatous polyposis (FAP)

colon cancer and, 227
genes for, 4t, 6–8
Familial atypical multiple-mole melanoma
(FAMMM) syndrome, 13–14,
138–139, 138f
Familial juvenile polyposis (FJP) syndromes, genes for, 9
Familial polyposis syndromes, genes for,
4t, 6–8
Familial retinoblastoma, soft tissue sarcomas and, 309
FAMMM (familial atypical multiple-mole
melanoma syndrome), 13–14,
138–139, 138f
FAP (familial adenomatous polyposis)
colon cancer and, 227
genes for, 4t, 6–8
Fibroxanthoma, atypical, 132
Fine-needle aspiration (FNA) cytology, in
breast cancer, 279
FJP (familial juvenile polyposis), genes
for, 9
FN (false-negative) ratio, 45
FNA (fine-needle aspiration) cytology, in
breast cancer, 279
Follicular thyroid carcinoma, 100, 100t
staging and treatment of, 103t, 104–105,
106f

G

Gallbladder carcinoma, 221–224
diagnosis of, 221, 222f
epidemiology of, 221
follow-up of, 224
recommendations for, 224
treatment of, 221–224
cholecystectomy and partial hepatectomy in, 221–223, 222t, 223f,
223t
with incidentally/laparoscopically discovered disease, 223–224
Gardner's syndrome, soft tissue sarcomas
and, 309
Gastric cancer, 173–192. *See also* Gastrointestinal malignancies
adjuvant chemotherapy for, 188–189
adjuvant radiotherapy for, 189–190
classification of
Lauren, 175–176, 176f
macroscopic, 177, 177f
Ming, 176–177
WHO, 177
clinical manifestations of, 178
diagnosis of, 178, 179t
environmental influences on, 174, 175f
epidemiology of, 173–174
gastric carcinoids, 192
gastric lymphoma, 192
gastric sarcoma, 192
Helicobacter pylori and, 175

Polyps
colorectal, 227
hyperplastic (gastric), 174
ω-3 Polyunsaturated fatty acids (PUFA),
40–41
Portal vein resection, 205–206
Positional cloning, 2
Predictive value (PV), 46
Preferred provider organizations (PPOs),
43–44
Proband, 1
Prognostic nutritional index (PNI), 34
Protein requirement, 36
Protooncogenes, 1
PTEN gene, 4t, 6
PUFA (ω-3 polyunsaturated fatty acids),
40–41
Purse string closure, distal, 76
PV (predictive value), 46

R

Radioimmunoguided surgery (RIGS), in
colon cancer, 229–230
Radioimmunoscintigraphy (RIT), of gas-
trointestinal/abdominal malignancies, 23–24
Radiolabeled monoclonal antibody imaging, of gastrointestinal/abdomi-
nal malignancies, 23–24
RB gene, 4t, 12
Rectal cancer, 235–242. *See also* Colon
cancer
adjuvant therapies for, 239–241
chemotherapy for, 240–241
evaluation of, 235–236
incidence of, 235
management of, 236
metastatic, 241–242
operative management of, 236–239,
237f, 239t
abdominoperineal resection in, 236
fulguration and local destruction in,
239
functional results of LAR with
coloanal anastomosis in, 238
local excision in, 238–239, 239t
low anterior resection with sphincter
preservation in, 236–238
patient selection in, 238
transendoscopic microsurgery in, 239
postoperative monitoring/surveillance
in, 241, 241t
presentation of, 235
radiation for, 239–240, 240t
recurrent, 241–242
surgery for (*See also* Pelvic surgery)
long-term consequences of, 79–80
Rectum, visceral compartment of, 72, 72f
Red-port reversal phenomenon, 65, 66f

Resting energy expenditure (REE), 31, 32t
measurement of, 35, 35t
Retinoblastoma, familial
genes for, 4t, 12
soft tissue sarcomas and, 309
Retractors, self-retaining, in pelvic
surgery, 73
Rhomboid flap closure, 144, 145f
RIGS (radioimmunoguided surgery), in
colon cancer, 229–230
RIT (radioimmunoscintigraphy), of gas-
trointestinal/abdominal malignancies, 23–24
RNA, as supplement, 40–41

S

Salivary gland, 90
Salivary gland tumors, 89–96
adjuvant treatment for, 96
anatomy and, 89–90, 90f
clinical presentation of, 90–92
diagnostic evaluation of, 93
follow-up with, 96
histology of, 92–93, 92t
lymphatic management with, 95–96
major, 89
pediatric, 92
staging of, 93–94, 94t
surgical management of, 94–95, 94f, 95f
Sarcoma(s)
gastric, 192
genes for, 4t, 12–13
soft tissue, 309–322 (*See also* Soft tissue
sarcomas)
Satellosis, 142, 143f
SBLA (sarcoma, breast cancer, leukemia,
and adrenocortical cancer), 2
genes for, 4t, 5
SCC (squamous cell carcinoma), 117–120,
117f, 118f, 119t. *See also* Squamous cell carcinoma
Schwannomin gene, 13
S-curve phenomenon, 64, 64f
Sebaceous gland carcinoma (SGC),
124–125
Seldinger technique, 61
Self-retaining retractors, 73
Sensitivity, 45
Sentinel lymph node (SLN) biopsy,
148–150, 149f, 150f
in breast cancer management, 284, 292
Sentinel lymph node (SLN) mapping,
148–150, 149f, 150f
in breast cancer management, 292
Serotonin, in carcinoid syndrome, 266–267
Serum tumor markers. *See also* specific
tumor markers and cancers
in breast cancer, 48
Sexual behavior, anal neoplasms and, 247

Sexual dysfunction, after rectal cancer
surgery, 79–80
SGC (sebaceous gland carcinoma),
124–125
Sister Mary Joseph's nodule, 178
Skew-plane phenomenon, 61–62, 62f
Skin cancer
melanoma, 137–153 (*See also*
Melanoma)
nonmelanoma, 111–134
angiosarcoma, 126–127
basal cell carcinoma, 111–117, 112f,
113f, 114t, 115t, 116t (*See also*
Basal cell carcinoma)
environmental and medical conditions
in, 111, 112t
epidemiology of, 111
extramammary Paget's disease,
125–126, 125f
Kaposi's sarcoma, 127–131, 128t,
129f, 130f (*See also* Kaposi's
sarcoma)
keratoacanthoma, 120–122, 120f
Merkel cell carcinoma, 122–123
microcystic adnexal carcinoma,
123–124
risk factors for, 111, 112t
sebaceous gland carcinoma, 124–125
soft tissue sarcomas, 131–134
atypical fibroxanthoma, 132
dermatofibrosarcoma protuberans,
131–132
leiomyosarcoma, 133–134
malignant fibrous histiocytoma,
132–133
squamous cell carcinoma, 117–120,
117f, 118f, 119t (*See also* Squamous cell carcinoma)
SLN (sentinel lymph node) mapping and
biopsy, 148–150, 149f, 150f
in breast cancer management, 284, 292
Smoking
anal neoplasms and, 246
colon cancer and, 227
Soft tissue sarcomas, 131–134, 309–322
anatomic distribution of, 309
atypical fibroxanthoma, 132
classification of, 310
clinical presentation of, 310
dermatofibrosarcoma protuberans,
131–132
diagnostic evaluation of, 310–311, 312f
etiology and epidemiology of, 309
histologic grading of, 310, 310f
incidence of, 309
leiomyosarcoma, 133–134
malignant fibrous histiocytoma,
132–133
pathology of, 309–310
prognostic factors in, 312–314, 313t